CW01289963

OPERATING THEATRE TECHNIQUE

*To My Wife Anne
and Son Nigel*

OPERATING THEATRE TECHNIQUE

A Textbook for Nurses, Technicians, Operating Department Assistants, Medical Students, House Surgeons and others associated with the Operating Theatre

RAYMOND J. BRIGDEN SRN

Nursing Officer,
Department of Health and Social Security,
London

FOURTH EDITION

CHURCHILL LIVINGSTONE
EDINBURGH LONDON AND NEW YORK 1980

CHURCHILL LIVINGSTONE
Medical Division of the Longman Group Limited

Distributed in the United States of America by
Churchill Livingstone Inc., 19 West 44th Street, New York,
N.Y. 10036, and by associated companies,
branches and representatives throughout
the world.

© E. & S. Livingstone 1962, 1969
© Longman Group Limited 1974, 1980

All rights reserved. No part of this publication
may be reproduced, stored in a retrieval system,
or transmitted in any form or by any means,
electronic, mechanical, photocopying, recording
or otherwise, without the prior permission of the
publishers (Churchill Livingstone, Robert Stevenson
House, 1–3 Baxter's Place, Leith Walk,
Edinburgh, EH1 3AF).

First edition 1962
Second edition 1969
Third edition 1974
Fourth edition 1980

ISBN 0 443 01999 1

British Library Cataloguing in Publication Data
Brigden, Raymon John
   Operating theatre technique.—4th ed.
   1. Surgery, Operative
   I. Title
   617′.91   RD32   79-40318

Printed and bound in Great Britain by
William Clowes (Beccles) Limited
Beccles and London

PREFACE TO THE FOURTH EDITION

The basic principles of theatre technique remain essentially unchanged since publication of the third edition. However, following the pattern of previous years, a number of important developments have once again resulted in extensive revision of *Operating Theatre Technique*. Two new Chapters have been added, and the second half of the book has been ammended to include more illustrations of operative procedures.

The first ten Chapters still contain detailed information on theatre technique and have been updated, additional material being included where appropriate. An innovation is the introduction of colour which it is hoped, the reader will consider has enhanced the presentation of appropriate illustrations. Colour has also been used to reproduce photographs taken through endoscopes and the operating microscope. The emphasis is now on metric measurements, although imperial sizes are included in parathesis where appropriate; for the present, it was still considered necessary to include 'BP' sizes for ligatures and sutures, in addition to the metric measurements, which are again given prominence. Fahrenheit has been omitted in preference to Celsius.

The development of microsurgery and the increasing use of the fibrescope has resulted in separate Chapters on those subjects. Operating microscopes are now used in many surgical specialities including ENT, ophthalmic, neuro- and vascular surgery. The facility has enabled the introduction of microsurgical techniques which have revolutionalised operative procedures in these specialties. The Chapter aims to give a broad description of the various microscopes now available. Detailed information on procedures requiring microsurgical techniques are included in the appropriate chapter on specific operations.

In the third edition, fibreoptics were given a cursory mention in the Chapter on urology. The most significant advance in this field has been the development of flexible gastroduodenal endoscopes, although the principles of fibreoptics extend to other instruments, including flexible and rigid bronchoscopes and cysto urethroscopes. Hence, the main portion of the new Chapter is devoted to the field of gastrology.

The Chapters on operative procedures have undergone considerable revision. Where possible, obsolete operations, or those less frequently carried out, have been discarded to make way for new procedures, including renal transplantation; for example, one procedure omitted is that for transfusion, originally included under peripheral vascular operations. It is considered that the reader is able to obtain information on this procedure by referring to other text books. The Chapters on ENT, ophthalmology and cardiovascular surgery are now up-to-date and more detailed.

Following the suggestions of many readers, the appendix of instruments has now been discarded and absorbed into the text where appropriate. Through the generosity of other authors and publishers this edition has been enhanced by the inclusion of more illustrations of operative procedures. The books from which these have been reproduced are excellent sources of reference and are recommended for further reading and study.

As in previous editions, emphasis has been placed on a fully comprehensive index with adequate cross-referencing. The references included in various Chapters have been selected on the basis that they provide detailed information of practical interest or use to the reader.

Once again, I wish to express my sincere and grateful thanks to all those who have helped in some way during the preparation of the new edition. Many individuals have co-operated in providing material for inclusion and this applies particularly to the manufacturers whose instruments and equipment are illustrated throughout the book.

Space does not permit the inclusion by name of everyone who has helped in this work, but nevertheless grateful thanks are due to all. Special mention must be made of colleagues and staff of the Royal Berkshire Hospital, Reading, who provided facilities for preparing illustrations included in the first part of the book and chapter on urology. In particular, the author would like to thank Miss G. E. Griffiths, Nursing Officer, Sister R. G. Clarke and Mr L. F. Williams, medical photographer. Thanks are due also to Mr T. Hayworth, FRCS, who provided a critical appraisal of the ENT Chapter; and Mr A. B. Richardson, FRCS and Sister A. S. Cleveland who were very helpful with the Chapter on ophthalmic surgery. Mr G. Power of Carl Zeiss Ltd. provided the material for the Chapter on operating microscopes.

The work associated with revision has been detailed and prolonged and I am very appreciative of the patience and encouragement of my wife and family at all times. Much of the typing was undertaken, often at short notice, by Mrs P. McGee, and I would like to express gratitude for her help. As usual, the staff of Churchill Livingstone have patiently borne with the idiosyncrasies of the author in a venture which, over the years, has developed into a very satisfactory partnership.

It must be clearly understood that the contents of this book and the opinions expressed are those of the author and do not necessarily reflect the policy of the Department of Health.

London 1980   R.J.B.

PREFACE TO THE FIRST EDITION

For some time now the author has felt there is a need for a comprehensive textbook on theatre technique to which nurses, technicians and medical students can refer and supplement their practical experience.

This book is written primarily for personnel who intend to specialise in theatre duties, but it is hoped that house surgeons and others who may be associated with this work may derive some benefit also.

Theatre technique is now a very complex subject, and it would be impossible to include all the operations and procedures associated with the various specialities without producing a rather unwieldy volume. The author appreciates that techniques vary considerably and wishes to impress upon the reader that this book must be regarded as a basis for practical experience and study in individual units. It is hoped that advantage will be taken of the various references which have been listed if a more detailed study of a particular subject is required.

The Chapters on electricity and static electricity have been included because it is felt that these subjects are of increasing importance to theatre staff. A better understanding of electrical apparatus and lighting will ensure a sensible approach to the use of such equipment in a modern operating theatre.

Emphasis has been placed upon a packet system of sterilisation and the use of heat rather than chemicals whenever possible. Although nylon has been described as a wrapping material, it is accepted that many units are using paper or linen for this purpose. This is, of course, a matter of individual preference.

The Chapter on ligature and suture materials has been made comprehensive in order that it may be used for reference. The sizes and technical data quoted are in accordance with BP standards.

'Assisting the surgeon and draping the operation area' is intended to help the reader to understand how this is done, combined, of course, with practical instruction from the surgeon, theatre superintendent or charge nurse. Again, methods of draping the operation area must be adapted to individual needs, but those described, if carried out correctly, will ensure the drapes remain in position during the course of operation.

The instruments described for various operations are those in common use and are arranged in sets. Substitution of instruments may be necessary according to a surgeon's individual preferences, but those shown should be adequate for the particular procedure. The outline of procedure for each operation is not intended to replace the many excellent textbooks on operative procedure, but it is hoped will act as a general guide and handy source of reference. The reader is referred to the appropriate surgery textbook if further details are required.

The Appendix of instruments is an extraction of those in common use from the multitude illustrated in the surgical instrument catalogues. An opportunity has been taken to list technical data of orthopaedic implants as this information is not easily available from other sources at present.

Coventry 1962   R.J.B.

ACKNOWLEDGEMENTS

Acknowledgement is given to the following authors and publishers who have kindly provided illustrations for this edition:

Adams, J. Crawford (1972) *Standard Orthopaedic Operations*. Edinburgh: Churchill Livingstone.
Ballantyne, J. (1976) *Operative Surgery – The Ear, Nose and Throat*. London: Butterworths.
Bruce, J., Walmsley, R. & Ross, J. A. (1964) *Manual of Surgical Anatomy*. Edinburgh: Churchill Livingstone.
Cleland, W. P. (1968) *Operative Surgery – Thorax*. London: Butterworths.
Farquharson, E. L. & Rintoul, R. F. (1972) *Textbook of Operative Surgery*. Edinburgh: Churchill Livingstone.
Garrey, M. M., Govan, A. D. T., Hodge, C. H. & Callander, R. (1972) *Gynaecology Illustrated*. Edinburgh: Churchill Livingstone.
Gillingham, F. G. (1970) *Operative Surgery – Neurosurgery*. London: Butterworths.
Hall, I. S. & Coleman, B. H. (1976) *Diseases of the Nose, Throat and Ear*. Edinburgh: Churchill Livingstone.
Hall, R. M. (1972) *Air Instrument Surgery*. New York: Springer Verlag.
Howkins, J. & Bourne, G. (1977) *Shaw's Textbook of Operative Gynaecology*. Edinburgh: Churchill Livingstone.
Illingworth, C. (1973) *A Short Textbook of Surgery*. Edinburgh: Churchill Livingstone.
Irvine, W. T. (1971) *Modern Trends in Surgery*. London: Butterworths.
MacFarlane, D. A. & Thomas, L. P. (1972) *Textbook of Surgery*. Edinburgh: Churchill Livingstone.
McGregor, I. A. (1975) *Fundamental Techniques of Plastic Surgery*. Edinburgh: Churchill Livingstone.
MacLeod, D. & Hawkins, J. (1966) *Bonney's Gynaecological Surgery*. London: Baillière, Tindall & Cassell.
Martin, P. (1963) *Indications and Techniques in Arterial Surgery*. Edinburgh: Churchill Livingstone.
Movair, T. J. (1972) *Hamilton Bailey's Emergency Surgery*. Bristol: Wright.
O'Brien, B. McC. (1977) *Microvascular Reconstructive Surgery*. Edinburgh: Churchill Livingstone.
Rank, B., Wakefield, A. R. & Hueston, J. T. (1973) *Surgery of Repair as Applied to Hand Injuries*. Edinburgh: Churchill Livingstone.
Robb, C. (1976) *Operative Surgery – Vascular Surgery*. London: Butterworths.
Robinson, J. O. (1965) *Surgery*. London: Longman.
Stallard, H. B. (1973) *Eye Surgery*. Bristol: Wright.
Stradling, P. (1976) *Diagnostic Bronchoscopy*. Edinburgh: Churchill Livingstone.
Swinney, J. & Hammersley, D. P. (1963) *Handbook of Operative Urology*. Edinburgh: Churchill Livingstone.
Wilson, J. N. (1976) *Watson-Jones Fractures and Joint Injuries*. Edinburgh: Churchill Livingstone.

Acknowledgement to manufacturers who have kindly provided illustrations of supplies or equipment for this edition, is given as appropriate in each chapter.

CONTENTS

1	The Theatre or Operating Department	1
2	Operating Theatre Lighting and Electromedical Equipment	33
3	Static Electricity	66
4	The Operation Table and Positions Used for Surgery	71
5	Preparation of the Operating Theatre and Sterile Supplies	86
6	Sterilisation	126
7	Ligature and Suture Materials	164
8	Storage and Handling of Ligature Materials and Associated Instruments	182
9	Draping Operation Areas and Assisting the Surgeon	194
10	Anaesthetics and the Anaesthetic Room	228
11	Glossary of Technical Terms and Words Commonly Used in the Theatre	286
12	Operating Microscopes	296
13	Fibre Optic Endoscopy	308
14	General Instruments	322
15	General Operations on the Abdomen	327
16	Operations on the Breast	374
17	Dental Operations	379
18	Ear, Nose and Throat Operations	385
19	Operations on the Face	428
20	Gynaecological and Obstetric Operations	429
21	Neurosurgical Operations	452
22	Ophthalmic Operations	488
23	Orthopaedic Operations	511
24	Plastic Operations	617
25	Urological Operations	644
26	Operations on the Thyroid and Neck	681
27	Thoracic Operations	688

28	Cardiovascular Operations	712
29	Abdominal Vascular Operations	737
30	Peripheral Vascular Operations	742
31	Plaster of Paris Technique	755
32	Radioactive Materials in the Theatre	775
	Appendices	778
	Index	791

1
THE THEATRE OR OPERATING DEPARTMENT

When describing the theatre or operating department for the purpose of a textbook it is usual to list those features which are considered to be ideal. Hundreds of new operating departments have been built during the last decade but nevertheless many hospitals have still to utilise facilities which are not ideal, despite extensive upgrading schemes. But even new departments cannot be expected to fulfil all theoretical requirements, as new ideas are constantly being developed, and by the time they are incorporated into buildings, fresh ones take their place on the drawing board. Definitions of the terms operating department, suite and theatre are as follows:

1. *Operating Department.* This is a unit consisting of one or more operating suites together with the ancillary accommodation including such common-use rooms as changing and rest rooms, reception, transfer and recovery areas and circulation space.

2. *Operating Suite.* This comprises the operating theatre or room together with its immediate ancillary areas such as anaesthetic room; sterile lay-up or preparation room; disposal room; a scrub-up and gowning area; and an exit room or area which may be part of the circulating space of the operating department.

3. *Operating Theatre.* This is the room in which surgical operations and certain diagnostic procedures are carried out.

OPERATING DEPARTMENT PERSONNEL

All personnel must aim to reach the highest possible standard, taking into consideration the equipment available, the limits of the operating department facilities and the surgical specialities. Strict asepsis would perhaps not be achieved during tonsillectomy operations as compared with a bone graft, but the same amount of care must be taken during the preparation of each. Speed and accuracy, with absolute efficiency are the goals to which all must aim. The ability of professional nurses to work in an operating team and create a happy professional atmosphere helps toward the attainment and maintenance of the high standard so desired.

The pattern of staffing will depend to some extent on local preferences and circumstances. Due consideration must be given not only to the overall shortage of nurses and, particularly, trained theatre nurses but also to the difficulties of recruiting suitable ancillary staff, often in competition with industry for their services. For many years the operating department was regarded almost exclusively as the domain of nurses; ancillary staff were usually restricted mainly to orderlies, porters and domestics. It is, perhaps, ironical that changes in composition of the theatre team are due both to an increased complexity in the technical aspects of surgery and an increasing shortage of nursing staff. Without entering too deeply into the controversy in some quarters of nurses versus technicians (or operating department assistants), a sensible approach is to acknowledge that each has an important role in the modern theatre team.

Whether or not the nurse will continue to co-ordinate the services of the operating department will depend upon sufficient numbers wishing to pursue a career in operating department management. The nurse's role, however, must be clearly defined and some interchangeability of present duties should enable better deployment of trained nurses in the operating department where it is considered their skills are essential. Trained operating department technicians or assistants can play an increasingly full part as members of the team, including responsibility for acting as the 'scrub or instrument assistant' and assisting the anaesthetist. (Already, highly trained technicians provide special services such as the operation of cardiological equipment including cardio-pulmonary by-pass procedures. These technicians are generally members of departments normally outside the jurisdiction of the operating department manager but providing a service to the theatre team when required. The term 'manager' refers to the person in charge of/accountable for the operating department services. It could apply equally to a nursing officer, superintendent, supervisor or sister.)

In order to ensure a continuing high standard of care for patients undergoing surgery it is essential to set up well-planned induction and training programmes for all grades of operating department staff. Student and pupil nurses should, as part of their training, have adequate experience in the operating department and be taught pre- and post-anaesthetic care of patients and acquire some understanding of surgical procedures. The General Nursing Council 1969 syllabus and practical experiences required for admission to the general part of the Register (77/19/B), indicates that student nurses should have a minimum of two weeks' observation in the anaesthetic room and operating theatre, and one week's experience in the recovery room.

When student nurses are in a department for only three weeks, hospitals should regard them as supernumerary to the establishment and even when they are there for longer it is important to maintain a practical ratio between trained and untrained staff. Although the General Nursing Council for Scotland does not stipulate the period of time pupil nurses should gain experience in the operating department, the GNC for England and Wales suggest that pupil nurses should receive eight weeks practical experience either in the operating department or in the accident/emergency or in the out-patient departments.

An understanding of work carried out in the operating department is important if nurses are to be encouraged to undertake a 'theatre' career when their training is completed.

Ancillary staff

In all operating departments, irrespective of age or size, a critical appraisal should be made of the duties undertaken by skilled staff. Whenever possible, duties not requiring their skills should be delegated to clerical and ancillary staff (Lewin Report, 1970). Some clerical assistance for the operating department manager is essential and where there are four or more operating theatres it may be necessary to employ a full-time receptionist in addition to a clerk/typist (see Appendix for duties).

The development of Central Sterile Supply Departments (CSSD), Theatre Sterile Supply Units (TSSU) adjacent to operating departments, and more recently, Hospital Sterilising and Disinfecting Units (HSDU), enable theatre staff to be relieved of the task of cleaning and processing instruments. Where such facilities exist these duties should be performed by ancillary staff, after appropriate in-service training, their work being supervised by skilled staff. These units should be under the jurisdiction of the CSSD manager, with the closest co-operation with the operating department.

Whilst preparation of the operating theatre between cases and operating sessions will be the responsibility of the team of nurses, technicians/assistants and other immediate ancillary staff, major cleaning including walls, ceilings and 24-hour cleaning in the operating department should be carried out under arrangements made with the domestic manager or supervisor. Domestic staff should be employed to care for staff changing rooms, rest rooms and offices and where necessary for serving refreshments to staff. 'Care' in this context includes duties such as disposal of used items, replenishment of supplies including linen and general tidiness. These are not duties for which skilled operating department staff should be employed.

Tasks undertaken by operating department porters vary considerably from hospital to hospital. In some cases their duties may be restricted to the transfer of patients between wards and theatres, in others their work extends to duties which may normally be carried out by technicians/assistants. Specification of their role is of course a matter for local arrangement, but where there is a strict demarcation between the 'outside' and 'clean' zones a practical solution is to employ 'outside' duty porters from the general portering pool and retain portering or orderly services exclusive to the 'clean' zone.

Operating department manager

The person in charge of an operating department influences to a great extent the degree of co-operation between members of the team (Douglas, 1962; Yeager, 1965). This person essentially should be a good leader with a generally placid nature and qualifications of kindness, tolerance and a sense of responsibility. The capability of planning ahead with good judgment, and the ability to take orders and accept constructive criticism are very important. There should always be a willingness to adapt to developments in surgery and operating theatre technique. Loyalty to the patient, surgeon, co-worker and hospital is vital and obvious. In short, a good 'manager' but essentially a leader of a nursing and technical team.

The visible signs of good leadership can be summed up in seven observable qualities (McKenzie, 1971).

1. A leader should be able and willing to assist his team and individual members of the team to carry out their roles, and in so doing think out clearly what are the roles and functions of all members of the team and then facilitate their carrying out of these functions.

2. He is capable of thinking out and bringing about *desirable* changes, for not all changes result in progress.

3. Since changes may be resisted, the leader will know the most acceptable and effective method of introducing them.

4. He will be seen and known to assist the team and members of the team to overcome difficulties and hardships.

5. The leader will observe and develop initiative and potentialities of members of his team.

6. He will preserve and transmit those appropriate features of the team pattern which are desirable.

7. Finally, the leader will encourage and help the members of his team to express, whether in words or actions, their hopes, desires, apprehensions and wishes.

The manager of an operating department will ensure delegation of tasks which staff are adequately trained to perform. He or she will ensure also that a suitable working environment is established in the operating department so as to secure the safety and welfare of staff and in addition review local rules from time to time to avoid the imposition of unnecessary restrictions upon staff.

An essential quality for an operating department manager, indeed any nurse or technician/assistant working in the operating theatre, is the ability to assimilate practical, mechanical and electronic information related to the correct use and simple maintenance of surgical instruments and equipment. It is probably for this reason that men are particularly attracted towards a career in operating theatre work.

MANAGEMENT

A multiplicity of textbooks devoted to management techniques exist. Many of these are equally as applicable to the operating department as to hospital management in general. A list of suitable books are included in the bibliography on page 31 and readers may seek specialised information from these. However, the organisation and management of operating departments does include aspects which are not readily available from these sources and it is useful to mention some at this stage.

It should be unnecessary to stress that operating departments cannot be organised in isolation from the work of the hospital as a whole. An obvious example is that the provision of surgical facilities must relate to surgical bed turn-over, admission and theatre requirements from diagnostic and other departments of the hospital (Lewin Report, 1970). The organisation of the department must relate to the overall policy decisions of the hospital and for this reason there must be close liaison between the operating department manager and administrative, medical and nursing colleagues responsible for other areas of the hospital. The establishment of a good management structure along the lines of the Salmon and Cogwheel Reports (Salmon, 1966; Cogwheel, 1967, 1974) should contribute towards this liaison. Liaison with administration is probably best established by a member of the hospital's administrative staff having a special interest in the operating department. The formation of an 'Operating Department Committee' will help to preserve liaison with surgeons, anaesthetists and others who are directly concerned with day-to-day matters.

Operating department committee

Although the operating department manager has overall accountability for the service provided, there is a need for a broadly based operating department committee to advise on the overall organisational requirements of the users. Where the hospital is large it will require its own committee but in the case of smaller hospitals it may be more practical to arrange for one committee to serve a number of hospitals in a group.

The function of this committee will vary according to local circumstances. Essentially the committee is advisory to the operating department manager but it may have an executive function also. Examples of executive function include ensuring the most effective use of facilities and staff; to keep under review the incidence of infection; recommending the purchase of new instruments and equipment within financial constraints and a general monitoring of the standards of care and skill in the department. In their advisory role the committee could, for example, make proposals for changes in the organisation of the department which may effect other departments in the hospital or group; advise on staffing patterns and training programmes.

The chairman of this committee should be a surgeon or other suitable person nominated by the Medical Executive Committee. A small committee is more efficient and therefore it is suggested that the remaining members would normally be restricted to the operating department manager, a representative of the anaesthetic staff, a representative of the surgical staff, a member of the junior surgical staff and a senior member of the administrative staff. Other members can be co-opted as required, for example representatives of the general nursing service, CSSD manager, microbiologist, pharmacist, radiologist, domestic supervisor and hospital engineer. It is important that these specialists are invited to attend when matters of particular concern are being discussed and similarly they should also have access to the committee to bring up any matters affecting their own specialty. The committee should meet regularly, at least once a quarter. Minutes should be kept and circulated to interested parties.

Pattern of work

The pattern of work in an operating department should be arranged so as to achieve the most effective utilisation of accommodation, operating time and manpower consistent with the best interests of patients and staff.

Preparation of operation lists by medical staff in collaboration with the operating department manager and ward sisters should ensure that typed copies are available for distribution to all departments concerned not later than the afternoon previous to the operations taking place. The schedule drawn up should be realistic and one which can reasonably be expected to be completed by the surgeons within a defined period. The Lewin Committee (1970) considered that the average length of an elective operating session should be three and a half to four hours, with the afternoon session starting at a time which allows it to finish ideally before 17.00 hours.

Abbreviations should never be used on an operation list which should be typed and include the following information:
1. Surname and first name(s) of patient
2. Age
3. Sex
4. Registered hospital or unit number
5. Nature, site and side of operation
6. Ward or unit
7. Date and time of operation
8. Name of surgeon
9. Name of anaesthetist
10. Special requirements.

Self adhesive labels incorporating identity information, and suitable for attachment to request and other forms, are being used increasingly in hospitals. In the preparation of operation lists these are eminently suitable for indicating the information listed under items 1 to 4. They are an additional safeguard in avoiding errors of transcription.

Last minute changes in operating lists cause concern and possible risk or error. A distinct policy should be laid down by the Operating Department Committee for the procedure to be adopted for any changes to the operation list, in order that all relevant personnel are informed (Medical Defence Union and Royal College of Nursing, 1977). Procedures for checking the identity of patients undergoing surgery are described in Chapter 10.

Records

It is of vital importance that adequate records of operations performed and personnel involved are maintained. The records should be entered and *numbered serially* either in a bound book or filed in a specially designed loose leaf folder. The latter procedure is of particular use where there are a number of theatres in an operating department and a separate page can be used for each. The information should include the following:
1. Surname and first name(s) of the patient
2. Age and sex
3. Registered hospital or unit number
4. Operation serial number
5. Nature of the operation
6. Ward

7. Special remarks (e.g. drug therapy, drainage tubes)
8. Names of surgeon, anaesthetist and assistants
9. A record of staff present during an operation, which can be of value in monitoring sources of cross infection
10. Type of anaesthetic
11. Signatures of two persons checking swabs and instruments.

It is valuable also to keep some record of theatre utilisation and although the day-to-day responsibility for the maintenance of records of this kind rests with the operating department manager, the system employed should be kept under periodic review by the Operating Department Committee. Operation records and swab checking procedures are discussed further in Chapter 5.

DESIGN

Nowadays the need is recognised to group together operating department facilities in a hospital for this provides the maximum economic use of equipment and skilled personnel. Many planners advocate the centralisation of all intensive care facilities, with operating theatres and labour suites immediately adjacent to the intensive therapy unit and near to the accident/emergency and X-ray departments. Planning constraints may preclude this in entirety but the relationship between these departments, surgical wards, Hospital Sterilising and Disinfecting Unit (HSDU) and laboratory facilities are important.

The operating department should be constructed so that it is separate from the independent of general traffic and air movement in the rest of the hospital (Medical Research Council, 1962; DHSS, 1968). In the past the department was often placed on the top floor of a tall building but in order to reduce solar heat-gain, a position at a lower level is now favoured. Noise transmission from ventilation plants sited on the roof is also reduced as they are no longer immediately above the operating department.

Clean and dirty streams of traffic in an operating department should as far as practicable be segregated. Although adequately bagged soiled equipment can be routed via a clean corridor without risk of bacteriological contamination, the provision of a separate disposal corridor has distinct advantages. Such a corridor provides direct access to the point of disposal and reduces traffic congestion in the clean circulation areas.

There should be a transfer or changeover section at the entrance to an operating department providing the first stage entry/exit to the sterile zone. This 'protective' zone includes also the recovery area, plaster room and changing rooms for staff and other personnel; various offices and seminar or teaching facilities may be sited here. The recovery area can be sited just outside the protective zone, although with such a design there are problems of access for the anaesthetist working in the clean zone and some barrier gowning procedure must be devised for him to enter and leave these zones.

Rooms of the department should be so arranged that there is a continued progression from the entrance through zones that increasingly approach sterility to finally the operating theatre and sterile preparation room. The 'clean' zone consists of scrub room and gowning, anaesthetic room, exit lobby, clean movement and rest areas and sterile store. The operating theatre and lay-up or sterile preparation room form the 'sterile' zone. The least clean area of the whole department is the disposal or sluice room and disposal corridor; this is termed the 'disposal' zone.

The clean zone must include adequate storage rooms for equipment or general supplies in addition to sterile packets; an X-ray darkroom may be provided. There is a need for a staff base or floor office in the clean zone of a multisuite operating department.

If possible the processing and sterilisation of drape and instrument packets should be centralised, ideally in the Hospital Sterilising and Disinfecting Unit (HSDU) which

Fig. 1.1 Single theatre suite, type 1. On the left, the surgeon's equipment panel with ventilation controls; in the background anaesthetic and recovery rooms, note the 'through' drug cupboard just above the socket outlets; and the ceiling pendants for oxygen, nitrous oxide, vacuum and compressed air. (Newcastle Regional Health Authority.)

Fig. 1.2 A Medic modular operating theatre showing wall-mounted equipment which allows clear space for the surgical team. (Seacroft Hospital, Leeds – Medical Installations Company Limited.)

Fig. 1.3 Layout and fittings of a single theatre. (Newcastle Regional Health Authority.)

Fig. 1.3 – continued.

Fig. 1.4 Sketch plan of Northwick Park Operating Department. (Llewelyn-Davis, Weeks, Forestier-Walker and Bar.)

operates in association with the main CSSD. Alternatively, this is carried out in the Theatre Sterile Supply Unit where this is built adjacent to the operating department (Buxton Hopkin, 1962; DHSS, 1968).

Personnel working within the department should be able to move from one clean area to another without having to pass through unprotected or traffic areas. Ventilation should be on the principle that the direction of air-flow is from the clean to the less clean areas (Medical Research Council, 1962). Heating and ventilation should also allow comfortable climatic conditions for the patient, surgeons, anaesthetists and other personnel. There should be no movement of air between one theatre suite and another.

The construction must be such that a high standard of cleanliness may be obtained (Houghton and Hudd, 1967). All surfaces should be washable and all joins between walls, ceilings and floors curved to minimise the collection of dust.

Types of operating departments

The general layout is frequently dependent on the total hospital plan. Sometimes the operating department may have been built after the hospital was established, and in this case may probably have been fitted into an existing space. One assumes that active steps have been taken to upgrade these facilities and it is taken for granted that such improvements include the elementary features of an adequate ventilation system.

Fig. 1.5 Picture of interior of theatres depicted in Figure 1.4.
 1. Pipeline suction apparatus.
 2. Stand with unopened packet containing sterile hand lotion bowl.
 3. Diathermy machine.
 4. Mobile supplementary operating light fitting.
 5. Swab count board.
 6. X-ray viewing screen.
 7. Main shadowless operating light fitting.
 8. Swab or sponge checking rack.
 9. Trolley with packet containing sterile instruments and drapes, outer layers only have been opened.
 10. Operation table.
 11. Anaesthetic machine.

Fig. 1.6 Sketch plan of an operating department, type 4, with twin theatre suites. (Prince of Wales General Hospital, Tottenham, London.) (Medical Installations Company Limited.)

The Theatre or Operating Department 13

Fig. 1.7 Standard theatre air flow.

Fig. 1.8 Medic modular operating theatre showing traffic flows. (Medical Installations Company Limited.)

Operating departments constructed in new buildings or extensions to buildings should be of a more satisfactory and compact layout. Readers will find, however, that operating departments may generally be classed in five main categories:

1. The single theatre suite containing operating theatre; scrub-up and gowning area; anaesthetic room; sterile preparation room; exit lobby and disposal area. Ancillary accommodation within and outside the clean areas includes storage space, rest rooms, probably an X-ray darkroom, changing rooms, offices, conference and teaching rooms (Fig. 1.1).

2. The two theatre suite with facilities similar to number 3 but with duplicated ancillary accommodation immediate to each operating theatre; sharing other accommodation such as changing rooms and offices etc.

3. Multiple theatre departments of three or more operating suites with ancillary accommodation similar to numbers 1 and 2 (Fig. 1.4).

4. The now rather outdated single theatre with combined sterilising and utility accommodation. There are the usual ancillary rooms such as anaesthetic accommodation and exit lobby.

5. Similar to the above but arranged as a twin theatre suite with shared ancillary accommodation.

Construction

The operating theatre itself should have walls of an impervious semi-matt surface (Jolly, 1950). The finish can be laminated plastic sheet, vinyl sheet or an epoxy resin type of paint. If the latter is used then the plaster should be a high impact type incorporating fibre glass. Tiles are not ideal due to the crevices formed between each. The most important point is that the surface be easily washable and withstand the repeated application of detergents and disinfectants in general use.

A semi-matt wall surface reflects less light than a highly gloss-finish and is less tiring to the eyes of surgeons and staff. With this in mind the colour is important also, pale blue, grey or green being the most generally suitable colours.

The floor should be impervious also, either of terrazzo, rubber or vinyl. The same considerations should apply regarding the colour, and the floor must be of an anti-static composition, or tiling which is well earthed to minimise the danger of an explosion due to static spark. Measures to reduce risks associated with static electricity are dealt with more fully in Chapter 3.

Well established in Europe is the Medic prefabricated modular operating theatre. This is constructed from factory-made prefabricated sections consisting of a framework of interlocking metal members and wall panels coated with a plastic skin which forms a jointless surface. The unit which is basically hexagonal can be erected relatively quickly either within existing buildings or a simple standard shell.

The unit is designed to take the maximum advantage of the space available. Several variations in layout can be achieved ranging from the single operating theatre to a complete unit of ancillary rooms also. The method provides a speedy means of improving facilities in an existing, outdated operating suite.

Lighting

At one time it was considered important to have windows large enough to admit good diffused daylight into the operating theatre. However, as all operations are performed with the aid of artificial light this is no longer important; although the complete absence of windows is alleged to be psychologically disadvantageous to staff.

If windows are fitted they should be small to reduce the amount of solar gain or loss and facilitate the control of heating and ventilation, and provision must be made to blackout the operating areas if endoscopic operations are to be performed. This is best achieved by dust enclosed blinds, preferably between windows, or alternatively by a power-operated roller blind fitted exteriorly.

An efficient system of artificial lighting which incorporates adequate emergency measures is absolutely essential. If the mains or fuses fail there must be sufficient light to complete the operation, and in emergency commence others. The emergency system must be fully automatic.

Ventilation

An efficient ventilation system should be provided in the operating department to achieve three functions: (1) to supply heated or cooled, humidified, contamination-free air to the operating theatre and adjacent clean areas; (2) to introduce air into these rooms so that it removes the contaminants liberated therein; and (3) prevent the entry of air from adjacent contaminated areas.

The minimum bacteriological requirements are:

1. The air delivered should not contain detectable *Clostridium sp.* or coagulase-positive *Staphylococcus aureus*. Aerobic cultures on non-selective medium should indicate not more than 35 bacteria-carrying particles in 1 m^3 (1 per ft^3) of ventilating air.

2. During surgical operations the concentration of bacterially-contaminated airborne particles in the operating theatre averaged over any 5-minute period should not exceed 180 per m^3 (5 per ft^3), although it is recognised that for some special types of surgical operations, e.g., orthopaedic and transplantation procedures, higher standards of air cleanliness may be justified.

A certain division of opinion exists in respect to the best method by which this can be achieved. An improvement in the reduction of surgical sepsis over the last decade is probably due to some extent to the installation of plenum ventilation (Bourdillon and Colebrook, 1946; Blowers and Crew, 1960; *Lancet*, 1956, 1958, 1968). More recently the development of high and medium velocity laminar or linear flow ventilation and the high-input/high-exhaust enclosure has emerged (Charnley, 1964, 1970) and the surgical plastic isolator. (McLauchlan, 1974, 1976).

Plenum turbulant air flow system. A medium velocity system of this type is the method most commonly employed at present. If it is maintained and balanced correctly the system is reasonably efficient (coupled with good theatre discipline and correct protective clothing for personnel). Air at roof level is drawn by means of a fan through a series of filters, is humidified, cooled or warmed and forced into the operating theatre through high-level diffusers fitted into the walls or ceiling.

Filters must be changed regularly. Some installations incorporate a system of continuous-feed filters which move on automatically as they become clogged. Micro-organisms such as *Pseudomonas sp.* often multiply on cooling coils, eliminator plates and in water reservoirs of humidifying apparatus and may contaminate the air. The addition of bacteriocides to water reservoirs does not necessarily discourage the growth of bacteria and should therefore never be used. Humidification should preferably be by steam injection, although if this is not possible fresh soft water from spinning discs may be used. Easy access for routine cleaning of these components by maintenance staff is essential.

The air pressure in the operating theatre should be slightly greater than that outside the suite (Medical Research Council, 1962). The greatest pressure of air is always in the sterile preparation room followed by the operating theatre in which the pressure is only slightly less. The volume of air supplied to the theatre should maintain a pressure in the order of $+25\,Nm^{-2}$ to ensure that contaminated air does not enter from other areas. It is relatively easy to maintain an outward flow of air through the gaps around a closed

18 Operating Theatre Technique

Fig. 1.9 Diagrammatic arrangement of filtered/treated air flow in Medic modular operating theatre. (Medical Installations Company Limited.)

Fig. 1.10 Air flow pattern in medic modular operating theatre. (Medical Installations Company Limited.)

door. The difficulty arises when one or more doors are open, for it is not generally appreciated that providing temperature differences between rooms are within 1°C, an air flow of about 10 m³ per minute for each 1 m² (30 ft³ per minute for each ft²) of open doorway is needed to maintain an acceptable outward air flow. In practical terms a double door demands about 35 m³ (1,200 ft³) of air per minute and to allow for various other air leaks, the air volume to an average theatre should be between 45 and 60 m³ (1,500 and 2,000 ft³) per minute, providing 20 to 30 changes of air per hour at a velocity of between 3 m and 12 m (10 ft and 40 ft) per minute. *If several doors to a theatre remain open during operations this may seriously interfere with the outward-flow air pattern.* Approximately 10 per cent of the air volume will be provided by air flowing from the sterile preparation room (pressure + 35 Nm^{-2}) the operating theatre being its only outlet.

Extraction of air from the operating theatre is not mechanically aided. Air flows through the small gaps around closed doors and also spills via balanced flaps or valves set in the walls or lower part of doors. These flaps are hinged and weighted so that air is allowed to pass in one direction only – any tendency for a back-flow of air from the less sterile areas will cause them to close. When a theatre door is opened these flaps close and direct all outflowing air through the open doorway, thereby maintaining a degree of pressurisation.

The next highest pressure of air should be in the scrub-up (6 m³ or 200 ft³ per minute), anaesthetic (12 m³ or 400 ft³ per minute) and the clean circulation areas. Approximately 50 per cent of the air volume for the anaesthetic room flows from the operating theatre and 80 per cent of the supply in the scrub-up and clean circulation zone derives from the most sterile part of the suite. Extraction is again via gaps around doors and by balanced flaps from room to room. The pressure is in the region of +5 to +15 Nm^{-2}.

Only a small positive pressure of air ($+2.5$ Nm^{-2}) is needed in the protective zone, i.e. transfer section at the entrance to the operating department, recovery area and changing rooms. Virtually all the air is supplied by progressive flow from the sterile parts of the suite. Extraction here is again by balanced flaps except if there is a primary air-lock between the transfer and main hospital corridors. In this instance extraction can be by fan and should be in the order of 8 m^3 (260 ft^3) per minute. There is no mechanical input into the air-lock.

The lowest pressure in an operating department should be in the disposal area, disposal corridor and plaster room (-5 Nm^{-2}). Input is received only from the more sterile areas such as the operating theatre and extraction is by fan at approximately 15 m^3 (500 ft^3) per minute.

It was thought at one time that extraction of air at floor level helped to dissipate anaesthetic gases thereby avoiding an accumulation of flammable gases which could ignite under favourable circumstances. However, the zone of risk associated with flammable anaesthetics is now recognised as being an area extending for 25 cm around any part of the anaesthetic circuit or the gas paths of an anaesthetic apparatus; flammable gas mixtures escaping from anaesthetic breathing circuits rapidly dilute to a non-flammable level within a few centimetres of the point of escape (DHSS, 1971). A typical flow pattern for a theatre ventilation system is illustrated in Figure 1.7.

In the last decade research has indicated that there may be hazards to staff because of pollution of the theatre atmosphere by anaesthetic gases. In particular, current evidence points to a possible risk of spontaneous abortion amongst operating department staff. If is therefore important that no staff member is exposed to anaesthetic gases for at least the first three months of pregnancy. There may be other harmful effects from atmospheric pollution, although at present there appears to be no direct evidence to substantiate this. However, it is a sound principle of hygiene to take steps to reduce atmospheric contamination to the lowest practical levels.

There are two types of 'scavenging system' for the removal of anaesthetic gases in operating rooms; active and passive. The active system involves mechanical extract device, whereas with the passive system, a wall or ceiling terminal unit is provided for coupling to pipework to vent the expired gases either to the extract ventilation duct, or outside wall.

Care must be taken to check regularly the efficiency of the operating department ventilation. In addition to bacteriological sampling either by slit samplers or exposure of culture plates, the pressure differentials from room to room can be checked visually by tracing air-flows. This is performed by using a smoke test.

One method is to use glacial acetic acid and cyclohexylamine, holding the bottles close together with the tops removed. As the fumes rise from the bottles they mix and produce a smoke, enabling air currents to be traced. Alternatively an applicator, covered lightly at one end with cotton wool is dipped first into one bottle and then the other to create a flow of smoke. Any solution splashed on the skin should be washed off immediately.

Air currents should be checked at tops and bottoms of doors – both open and closed. If there is any backflow or air currents seem to flow from the less clean to the clean areas, this may indicate either a mechanical fault or that the filters are blocked and insufficient air is being forced into the suite.

An alternative to glacial acetic acid and cyclohexylamine is smoke generating tubes. In the United Kingdom these can be obtained from the Mine Safety Appliance Co. Ltd., Glasgow, E.3.

Laminar flow ventilation systems. These originate from developments in the construction of 'clean rooms' for the assembly of electronic components in the aerospace and electronics industry.

Advances in surgery have resulted in complex operations, many of which may take several hours; for example, orthopaedic or transplant procedures. This increases the problems in avoidance of particulate and bacterial contamination which is particularly important if the patient is receiving immunosuppressive drugs. Hence the need for ultra clean environments in operating theatres (Voda and Withers, 1966; Whitcomb and Clapper, 1966; U.S. Department of Health, Education and Welfare, 1967; Scott, 1970; Scott et al., 1971; Nelson, 1978).

The term 'laminar flow' refers to the passage of air through an efficient filter to remove inherent contamination, then moving it at a velocity such that it travels in a horizontal unidirectional form without any eddies or turbulance.

The fundamental difference between plenum turbulent ventilation and laminar flow can be summarised as follows. In the former, a downward displacement or turbulent flow of filtered air is created. Limitation on the liberation of contamination from within the room (e.g. shedding of bacteria-laden skin particles), is largely controlled by wearing special clothing such as Ventile/Scotchguard fabric, or non-woven fabric suits, and restriction on the movement of personnel. Pressurisation of the theatre prevents entry of air from outside, and thereby reduces the incidence of contamination from this source. Between 20 and 30 changes of air per hour at a velocity of between 3 m and 12 m (10 ft and 40 ft) per minute are provided by this system.

Laminar flow utilizes highly filtered air directed towards the operation area through a filter bank consisting of an entire wall (Fig. 1.11).

The volume of air passing through the filter bank moves initially at a velocity in the region of 21 to 33 m (69 to 108 ft) per minute making only a single transit over a given area. This reduces to about 18 m (59 ft) per minute at the periphery of the clean area. (Whyte et al., 1973, 1974; Nuegart, 1975). The volume and movement of air is sufficient to give 500–600 air changes per hour in the region of the operating site. When a solid object is encountered, the air flows round the object, interrupting the laminar flow only momentarily. Surgery is carried out in a uniform flow of clean air and contaminants are flushed away as they are released. For example; particles shed by the operating team are moved away by the air stream before they can drop on to the operation site.

The system incorporates High Efficiency Particulate Air (HEPA) filters which are 99·81 to 99·97 per cent efficient at the 0·5 m to 1·0 m and larger particle size, which is more than adequate to stop bacteria-carrying particles. Air returned to the periphery of the room, plus fresh air admitted through normal ventilation ducts is drawn back into the fans, first via a battery of pre-filters at the rear of the unit, and thence through the final HEPA filters. Most laminar flow units incorporate side walls which enable proper control and maintenance of the laminar air flow stream. Experiments have shown that these walls should extend for at least 1 metre from the filter banks, preferably more. (Whyte, 1975.)

Slight pressurisation of the operating theatre is maintained, as in the plenum system, to prevent injection of air from contaminated dresses outside the suite.

It is suggested that a disadvantage of some laminar flow systems may be the noise created by the fans and constant high velocity, horizontal flow of air which may prove trying to the operating team. However, unpleasant odours are quickly removed, the drying effect of the air stream prevents perspiration and the risk of contamination is reduced to a minimum. Regarding noise, it is claimed for one unit – the GEL-OT – that the noise level is between 54–55 dBA, and that users quite quickly become desensitised to the background hum (Boulton, 1976).

Sampling has shown that virtually no bacteria are allowed to settle in the ultra-clean area created by the laminar flow system. This compares with settling counts taken in an operating theatre with conventional ventilation, which have shown from 4 to 19 colonies per culture plate after only one hour's exposure.

High input/high exhaust enclosure. This was first developed by Mr John Charnley in

AIR STREAM PATTERN CAUSED BY AIRFOIL

LAF SYSTEM WITH BREATH EXHAUST IN USE

Figs. 1.11 and 1.12 GEL-OT Laminar air flow unit, showing air stream flowing in a horizontal direction across the operation site. (Gelman Hawksley Limited.)

Fig. 1.13 The Charnley-Howorth sterile enclosure in use. (Surgicair Division, Howorth Engineering Limited.)

Fig. 1.14 Howorth EXFLOW clean zone ventilation system. (Surgicair Division, Howorth Engineering Limited.)

1962. Since that time further improvements resulted in the Howorth Surgicair enclosure (Charley, 1973) and subsequently the latest EXFLOW clean zone unit, which does not require side walls.

The Charnley-Howorth enclosures are installed in an existing operating theatre to provide a highly filtered turbulent air flow at a velocity of 18 m (60 ft) per minute with up to 300 air changes per hour. The unit is fabricated from a metal frame with three transparent sides, and a fourth through which three quarters of the operating table and patient is made to enter. The fourth side is closed by sterilised curtains. Fans draw air from

Fig. 1.15 Charnley Body Exhaust System to reduce transmission of bacteria-carrying skin particles. (Surgicair Division, Howorth Engineering Limited.)

the operating theatre into the plenum chamber at the top of the enclosure. The air is discharged into the enclosure first through HEPA filters, and then through non-return valves and fabric sleeves which prevent entrainment of surrounding air. The flow of air passes out of the enclosive via gaps under the walls and is re-circulated after passing through the filter system (Fig. 1.14).

The enclosure is used in conjunction with the Charnley Body exhaust system which is specifically designed to remove body convector currents and exhaled breath of the operating team; a major source of operative infection. A surgical gown of Ventile/ Scotchguard or non-woven fabric (see Chapter 5), prevents the transmission of bacteria-carrying skin particles which are continually being shed by the operating team. Air from under the gowns is constantly extracted via the exhaust mask at 1·5 m^3 (5 ft^3) per minute, taking away shed skin scales and exhalations in addition to cooling the wearer, thereby preventing perspiration and reducing fatigue by continuous ventilation. A communication system integral with the mask is available enabling the team to talk to each other more easily, also to communicate with spectators outside the enclosure (Fig. 1.15).

The objective behind the enclosure is to isolate the surgical team from circulating personnel and spectators. The anaesthetist can remain outside the enclosure as illustrated in Figure 1.13. Separate packets of sterile instruments for each stage of the operation may be introduced through the open hatch at the foot end of the enclosure, without the contents coming into contact with the contaminated air. Alternatively, a convenient instrument technique can be employed.

The statistics of infection rates produced by Charnley (Table 1.1) indicate the development and apparent success of the system.

The EXFLOW Clean Zone Unit. Although the Charnley-Howorth enclosure offer considerable benefits in the reduction of operative infection the side walls, in certain operations, have been found restrictive. Merely to dispense with wall panels in a standard downflow system would cause entrainment of the contaminated room air around the periphery of the canopy.

To overcome this, Howorth have developed a unit which creates a clean air flow pattern which is centrally downwards and then radiates outwards in all directions, similar in shape to the open end of a trumpet. The central zone of this expotential air flow, which is over the target area (operation site), has a downward flow speed of 21 m (70 ft) per minute giving about 500 air changes per hour (Fig. 1.14).

This system prevents peripheral entrainment of contaminated air, and personnel and equipment moving towards the operation site must do so against the air flow. The body exhaust system is suitable for use with the EXFLOW unit.

Surgical plastic isolator. This is a development of the flexible film plastic isolator used in the veterinary field for producing bacteria-free animals by caesarian section (Trexler

Table 1.1 Comparative figures of infection rates at Wrightington Hospital

System	Year	Colonies/ Plate/Hr	Total number of operations	Infection %
Conventional theatre – exhaust ventilation	1959–1961	80–90	190	8·9
First prototype enclosure. Electro-static filter	1962	25	108	3·7
Second prototype enclosure. Howorth-donated system	1963–1965	1·8	1,079	2·2
Howorth permanent enclosure Mk I	1966–1968	0 (limit of accuracy)	1,929	1·5
Howorth permanent enclosure Mk I and Mk II	1969–1970 1971–1972	0 0	2,152 over 2,000	0·5 0·3
Howorth demountable system type DF10	1973–1976	0	over 4,000	0·3

IMPORTANT NOTE: Pre-operative 'umbrella' injections of antibiotics are **not** used at Wrightington Hospital. The figures above, therefore, reflect directly the effectiveness of the Charnley-Howorth enclosures.

et al., 1957). These veterinary isolators are simple sterile PVC bags with sleeves welded into their sides. The bag is stuck to the animal's abdomen and a caesarian section carried out, the bacteria-free young being delivered into the bag. The young are then maintained bacteria-free in a similar isolator inflated with sterile air.

The isolator developed for human surgery incorporates several sleeves for access to the operative field, and an air-supported entry port for instruments and sterile supplies.

The patient is prepared and draped in the usual way. The isolator bag is inflated with sterile air by a special blower and stuck to the operation area with special adhesive. Gloves for the surgical team are attached to appropriate blind ending sleeves.

The operation is carried out through an incision in the floor of the isolator. The impervious mechanical barrier acts as a containment system, only the wound being exposed in a completely sterile environment. It thus prevents airborne and direct contact cross infection during surgery (Silvester, 1978).

Humidity

As the air passes through the spinning water discs or steam humidifier in the ventilation plant its humidity is increased (Yates, 1967). The altered air must not be too dry and must have a humidity of between 50 and 60 per cent for optimum comfort and to lessen the tendency for static electricity formation.

Humidity is controlled by an electronic sensor switch situated in the operating theatre. An instrument called an hygrometer is available to measure this humidity level.

Heating

Combined with background heating, a ventilation system is a very satisfactory way of rapidly adjusting the temperature in the operating theatre.

Before entering through ceiling diffusers the air is passed over steam pipes within the duct. The amount of steam flowing through these pipes is controlled by an automatic mechanical valve which is operated by an electrical thermostat in the theatre. By adjusting this thermostat a reasonably constant temperature is obtainable, and in extreme variations of hot or cold weather rapid alteration of temperature is possible. The temperature of an operating theatre should be maintained at between 18·5°C and 22°C generally, *except* during hypothermia anaesthesia when it may be necessary to keep it below this level.

Background heating is best obtained by pipes or panels within the wall or ceiling. The heating provided by this source should be limited, for experience has proved that heating entirely by panels can be very oppressive particularly in the theatre. Another disadvantage is that it takes some time for pipes to heat up or cool down and therefore makes it impossible to vary temperatures rapidly.

Open radiators or pipes for heating the operating theatre are totally unacceptable; they are dust and bacteria traps.

Equipment and furniture

An operating theatre should contain only the minimum of equipment necessary for operating. Scrubbing and gowning-up should take place in a separate adjacent room. If due to old design these actions take place in the theatre they should be as far away from the operating areas as possible. Splashing is the most likely source of contamination whilst scrubbing up under these circumstances, and a careful watch on the water-tap pressure is advisable.

With pre-set tray packet systems for instruments, trolleys can be prepared in the operating theatre itself just before the operation starts. However, during a list or series of operations, and when a good deal of activity occurs (for example, positioning of the patient for a complicated operation), the sterile packets should be opened in the sterile preparation or lay-up room.

All theatre furniture must be of hygienic finish. Stainless steel or aluminium are ideal materials for trolleys, lotion bowl stands, etc., although nylon-covered mild steel is quite suitable where expense is of primary consideration.

Fig. 1.16 Surgical plastic isolator. (Vickers Medical.)

Small supplementary supplies e.g. sterile packets, strapping, lotions, etc., should be kept either in a recessed cupboard or on easily washable plastic laminate shelves in a corner of the room.

A wall desk 45·5 cm by 61 cm (18 in by 24 in) fitted under the X-ray viewing boxes will be found useful for writing up notes and swab registers, etc.

Adjoining the operating theatre are the anaesthetic, scrub-up, disposal and sterile preparation rooms. These must have adequate, wide connecting doors and be of the same hygienic finish as the operating room itself.

Anaesthetic room

The anaesthetic room is described in more detail in Chapter 10. Quietness is essential and it should be reasonably soundproof to minimise transference of general preparation sounds from the operating theatre. This important department must have adequate equipment which is maintained to a high standard and always ready for immediate use.

The post-anaesthetic recovery room associated with the operating department must be sited for convenient access of the anaesthetists. The services provided by this unit vary according to local requirements. It may be used for short-term recovery of patients after operation, indeed until they have recovered consciousness only. Alternatively it may be staffed to provide a 24-hour service and extended care after operation.

The scrub-up area

This should be sufficiently large to allow gowning and gloving in addition to scrubbing up. The wash basins can be either the conventional type a trough or an adjustable angled plate-glass sheet which channels water into a waterpipe.

Fig. 1.17 Three position 'scrubbing up' trough with foot operated tap and 'Nunk' liquid dispenser. (Northwick Park Hospital.)

The most important basic requirement is a wash basin of sufficient depth and height to minimise splashing the scrub clothes of those using it. Taps should be of the elbow- or foot-operated type, mixing hot and cold water into a single faucet and preferably controlled by a thermostatic mixing valve.

There should be a clock or other timing device fitted in a convenient position near to the wash basins. Individual clean nail brushes are supplied from a suitable dispenser which can be refilled with brushes afterwards and then autoclaved for terminal disinfection.

Scrub-up solution, e.g. PHisoHex, Betadine, etc., is supplied from dispensers, foot or elbow operated.

The gowning section must be located as far away from the wash basins as possible. Gown packets can be opened either on a suitable trolley or a cantilever shelf fitted to the wall and having a 15 cm (6 in) space at the rear to facilitate opening out the wrappings.

Adjustable shelves are suitable for storing packets of sterile gloves and gowns providing these are of a reasonable quantity. The basic stock should be kept in cupboards or preferably in the central sterile store.

Disposal room

This may also be called the sluice or sink room. Although basically its role is to handle the soiled instruments and dressings, etc., after operation, the extent depends on whether an HSDU or TSSU is available.

If an HSDU provides a full service, used trays of instruments may be simply overwrapped with the trolley drapes and returned to the centre for processing (Harvey, 1958; Bowie et al., 1963). In this case the disposal room will be utilised only for disposing of soiled linen and dressings. The room will require a suitable wash basin and slop hopper. It will probably be utilised also for cleaning equipment and storing cleaning apparatus for the operating room.

Where processing of instruments is done at operating theatre level the disposal room may be equipped with suitable work surfaces, cupboards for supplies, and ultrasonic cleaner and dryer.

It should be possible to dispose of soiled items without taking them through clean areas such as the sterile preparation or sterilising room (Fig. 1.18).

Sterile preparation room

This room serves only for the storage of sterilised instruments or drape packets, supply of lotions and other items which may be required immediately in the operating theatre, and preparation of sterile trolleys.

Other ancillary rooms

The surgeons', nurses, and technicians' changing rooms should be equipped with lockers or clothes racks for outside clothes. They should have showers and toilet facilities. As mentioned previously, planning of the department should arrange that personnel and visitors can change into protective clothing before actually entering the operating section.

A separate office should be provided for the operating department manager or supervisor, and in large departments, an office for the anaesthetic service also. These offices are best positioned near to the entrance of the department as they are often used for interviewing representatives and others.

Adequate storage facilities, particularly for bulky equipment, are essential. A central sterile store should keep the main bulk of sterile supplies for the various operating suites.

The department may include an X-ray darkroom, small laboratory, blood storage facilities, and rest rooms for the surgeons and staff to avoid the necessity of personnel entering the changing rooms except at the beginning and end of operating sessions.

STERILISATION

Sterilising facilities may be provided either limited, or sufficient for the sterilisation of all instruments and equipment needed. Where a pre-set tray system is supplied from the HSDU, CSSD or TSSU autoclaves are only needed for the dropped instrument.

Regretably some operating suites are *still* disinfecting their instruments by boiling; there is no place for this in a modern department. The time has now come to deplore such techniques for even in remote areas where finance is limited, instruments can be sterilised by steam, utilising a portable autoclave or pressure-type cooker.

Sterile saline or water

The most suitable methods of supplying this for use as hand lotion are sealed flasks prepared by the pharmacy or a continuous running water press (Bowie, 1956; Medical

Fig. 1.18 The disposal room of a four theatre department. In the foreground is a double-ended autoclave connecting with the sterile preparation room serving two of the theatres. This arrangement is repeated in the far background. In the centre are the ultrasonic cleaners and to the left of these, the supervisor's desk. (St James Hospital, Balham, London.)

Fig. 1.19 Theatre Sterile Supply Unit. Note washing machine and instrument drying cabinet on left; pre-set instrument trays being prepared on right. (Northwick Park Hospital.)

Research Council, 1959; Gordon, 1963; Tallett, 1963; Wells and Lynch, 1963; Howie and Kelsey, 1963; Medical Research Council, 1968). The multi-supply tank or water boiler cannot be guaranteed to produce a safe, sterile solution. Even if the process of sterilisation is adequate, it is virtually impossible to avoid recontamination when drawing off the solution. In addition the water sterilised in the tank at the best is chemically softened and certainly *not* non-pyrogenic.

This is described in greater detail in Chapter 6.

Fig. 1.20 Dispensing sterile lotion into hand lotion bowl.
(Royal Berkshire Hospital.)

Further reading on management useful in the operating department
BAKER, R. J. S. (1967) The Art of Delegation. *Journal of Royal Institution of Public Administration.*
BROWN, W. (1960) *Exploration in Management.* London: Heinemann.
DRUCKER, P. F. (1961) *The Practice of Management.* London: Heinemann.
GOWERS, E. (1970) *The Complete Plain Words.* London: Penguin.
JUDSON, A. S. (1966) *A Manager's Guide to Making Changes.* New York: Wiley.
REVANS, R. W. (1964) *Standards for Morale.* Oxford University Press.
SCHURR, M. (1968) *Leadership and the Nurse.* London: English University Press.
STEWART, R. (1963) *The Reality of Management.* London: Heinemann.
STEWART, R. (1967) *Managers and their Jobs.* London: Heinemann.

REFERENCES

ALPERT, S. (1973) Germ Free Research – *Biological Effects of Gnotobiotic Environments*, **87**.
BOULTON, C. (1976) Horizontal air-flow unit. *Nursing Times*, **72** (5), 197–8.
BLOWERS, R. and CREW, B. (1960) *Journal of Hygiene*, **58**, 427.
BOURDILLON, R. B. and COLEBROOK, L. (1946) *Lancet*, **i**, 561, 601.

BOWIE, J. H. (1956) *Lancet*, **ii**, 45.
BOWIE, J. H., CAMPBELL, I. D., GILLINGHAM, F. J. and GORDON, A. R. (1963) *British Medical Journal*, **ii**, 1322.
BUXTON HOPKIN, D. A. (1962) *Lancet*, **ii**, 245.
CHARNLEY, J. (1964) *British Journal of Surgery*, **51**, 195.
CHARNLEY, J. (1970) *Lancet*, **i**, 1053.
CHARNLEY, J. (1973) *Cleveland Clinic Quarterly*, **40**, 99.
COGWHEEL (1974) *Report of the Joint Working Party on the Organisation of Medical Work in Hospitals*. London: HMSO.
DEPARTMENT OF HEALTH AND SOCIAL SECURITY (1968) Article on Operating Departments. *Hospital Management*, September.
DEPARTMENT OF HEALTH AND SOCIAL SECURITY (1971) *Hospital Technical Memorandum No. 1*. London: HMSO.
DEPARTMENT OF HEALTH AND SOCIAL SECURITY (1976) Pollution of operating departments by anaesthetic gases, H.C. 76(38).
DOUGLAS, D. M. (1962) *Lancet*, **ii**, 245.
GORDON, A. R. (1963) *Nursing Times*, March 1, 353.
HARVEY, J. (1958) In *Medical Electrical Equipment*, p. 61. Edited by R. E. Molloy. London: Newnes.
HOUGHTON, M. and HUDD, J. (1967) *Aids to Theatre Technique*, 4th edn., chap. 1. London: Baillière, Tindall and Cassell.
HOWIE, J. W. AND KELSEY, J. C. (1963) *British Medical Journal*, **i**, 187.
Lancet (1956) Leading article. Ventilation of operating theatres. **ii**, 1197.
Lancet (1958) Annotation. Air contamination and layout of theatre suites. **i**, 203.
LEWIN (1970) *Report of a Joint Subcommittee of the Standing Medical and Nursing Advisory Committees on the Organisation and Staffing of Operating Departments*. London: HMSO.
MCKENZIE, N. (1971) *The Professional Ethic and the Hospital Service*, p. 5.
MCLAUGHLAN, J., PILCHER, M. F., TREXLER, P. C. AND WHALLEY, R. R. (1974) *Brit. Med. J.* **I**, 322.
Medical Defence Union/Royal College of Nursing Joint Memorandum (1977) Safeguards against wrong operations.
Medical Research Council (1959) Working Party, *Lancet*, **i**, 425.
Medical Research Council (1962) Operating Theatre Hygiene Subcommittee. *Lancet*, **ii**, 945.
Medical Research Council (1968) Aseptic Methods in the operating suite. *Lancet*, **i**, 763.
Medical Research Council, DHSS, Regional Engineers' Association (1972) Joint Working Party: *Operating Theatre Requirements*.
NELSON, J. P. (1978) *Hospital Topics*. September/October.
NUEGART, H. (1975) Sulzer Technical Review No. 1.
SALMON (1966) *Report of the Committee on Senior Nursing Staff Structure*. London: HMSO.
SCOTT, C. C. (1970) *Lancet*, **i**, 989.
SCOTT, C. C., SANDERSON, J. T. AND GUTHRIE, T. D. (1971) *Lancet*, **i**, 1288.
SILVESTER, J. C. (1978) *Nursing Times*, 1411, August 24.
TALLETT, E. R. (1963) *Lancet*, **i**, 489.
U.S. Department of Health and Education and Welfare (1967) May, Circular.
VODA, A. M. and WITHERS, J. E. (1966) *American Journal of Nursing*, **66**, 2454.
WELLS, C. and LYNCH, P. F. (1963) *Lancet*, **i**, 57.
WHITCOMB, J. G. AND CLAPPER, W. E. (1966) *American Journal of Surgery*, **112**, 681–685.
WHYTE, W., SHAW, B. H. AND BARNES, R. (1973) *J. Hyg. Camb.*, **71**, 559.
WHYTE, W., SHAW, B. H. AND FREEMAN, M. A. (1974) *J. Hyg. Camb.*, **73**, 61.
WHYTE, W., SHAW, B. H. AND BAILEY, P. V. (1975) *J. Soc. Environ. Eng.* Sept., 13.
YATES, J. (1967) *Hospital World*, **6**, 4, 5.
YEAGER, M. E. (1965) *Operating Room Manual*, 2nd edn, p. 3. London: Putnam.

2
OPERATING THEATRE LIGHTING AND ELECTROMEDICAL EQUIPMENT

The complexity of electromedical equipment used in the operating theatre has increased greatly during the past few years. Unless great care is taken in the maintenance and operating of this sophisticated equipment, potentially hazardous electrical situations can be created for patients and staff. Biomedical engineers and manufacturers have achieved a good deal in minimising these hazards, for example by developing 'earth-free' equipment where the patient is isolated electrically from earth or ground. Nevertheless, there must be an understanding by all working in the operating theatre of the principles involved and simple safety precautions to be observed.

The amount of electricity used in an operating department is often quite considerable, especially in a large unit, and provision is made for heavy loads.

The mains voltage supplied in the United Kingdom is between 220 and 240 V, 50 Hz, A.C. Emergency lighting is provided either from batteries at a low voltage, (12–24 volts) or by a supplementary generator which provides electricity at the standard mains voltage. In this case it is likely that the generator will supply a proportion of the electrical needs for the operating department through the normal wiring or additional separate circuits. It is important to ascertain the maximum loading from such a system. Upon mains failure, there could be a delay of up to 20 seconds before the generator comes into action. An automatic changeover switch is generally installed to ensure a temporary uninterrupted supply from batteries to the main operating light until the generator takes over (DHSS, 1974). Where special low voltage lamps are fitted exclusively for the emergency battery system great care must be taken to avoid interchanging with lamps used on the normal electricity supply.

In 1969 the Department of Health issued a recommendation that switches and socket outlets installed on the walls of operating theatres and anaesthetic rooms should *not* be of a sparkless type, regardless of the fixing height. A review of explosion incidents had shown that the danger is confined to anaesthetic breathing circuits and the area immediately surrounding expiratory or other leakage outlets from anaesthetic equipment. Tests carried out under typical working conditions showed that flammable gas concentrations exist only in an area extending for 25 cm from the points where leakage occurs and gases quickly dilute to a non-flammable level beyond this. Thus, ignition risks associated with wall switches and socket outlets is negligible under normal working conditions. This does not apply to portable electromedical equipment which is liable to be used close to anaesthetic equipment and switches on such equipment should continue to be of a gastight sparkless type.

A gastight sparkless switch consists essentially of a short glass tube containing a small quantity of mercury. When the switch is operated, the tube tilts, thereby causing the mercury to flow between two electrodes connected to the tube. Any sparks which do occur when the current begins to flow or is interrupted are contained within the glass tube and do not come into contact with the atmosphere. All of this mechanism is concealed behind a plate or metal case of the apparatus and is operated by an insulated knob or toggle switch.

The framework of electrical apparatus, including portable light fittings and electro-medical equipment, must be earthed directly through the earth pin of the plug mechanism. Electric flex to such apparatus contains three insulated wires—brown, blue and green/yellow. The brown wire is connected to the live terminal and the blue wire to the neutral terminal The green/yellow wire is always connected to the longer (earth) pin at the plug top at one end and to the metal frame of the apparatus at the other. (Previously the colour coding was red – live, black – neutral and green – earth). If a fault to earth occurs, the electric current has a safe passage to earth and not through an unfortunate person who may inadvertently touch the apparatus.

A nurse should not disconnect or reconnect any wiring, as this is the responsibility of the electrician, and if any electrical connection or wire is obviously loose the apparatus must not be used until thoroughly checked by the electrician.

Electric plugs

Standard 13 amp electric sockets are now provided in operating departments rather than special electric sockets. Standardisation enables any mains operated equipment to be used on the supply. This applies also to mobile X-ray apparatus; utilising 30 amp ring circuits, a special 13 amp *unfused* plug top connected to X-ray apparatus will only take high power from the circuit during a fraction of a second's exposure. This plug top is designed to accommodate the larger flexible cable provided on X-ray machines.

No moisture must be allowed to collect on the plug-tops pins. If this should occur the moisture must be dried off thoroughly before the plug is inserted. Apparatus should be disconnected from the socket by grasping the plug top and not the flex. The use of adaptors for interchanging plug tops of different sizes is not allowed, flexes can become frayed and connections loose.

THEATRE LIGHTING

When describing lighting equipment it is better to use the terminology usual with lighting engineers.

1. *Lamp.* This refers to the filament lamp.
2. *The Light Fitting.* Refers to the shadowless light fitting suspended from the ceiling, and includes the reflectors and the suspension gear. It also refers to mobile equipment, and is then described as a mobile light fitting or luminaire.
3. *The Light Field.* This is the task area, usually circular, illuminated by the light fitting.

The general lighting of the theatre may be provided by fluorescent tubes or filament lamps. These must be arranged to produce an even illumination with no glare, and are recessed in the ceiling, or alternatively in a dust-proof cornice surrounding the theatre at ceiling level.

The most important consideration, however, is the provision of a shadowless illumination of the actual operation area. This light fitting (or fittings) should be connected to a special switch incorporating an electrical relay which connects the emergency supply automatically upon mains or filament failure (Stevens, 1951; Smith, 1958).

Shadowless lighting is produced by directing the light on to the operation area (task area) from several angles to minimise shadows from the operator and his assistants.

Type of shadowless light fittings

Amongst the shadowless light fittings in common use are the single-reflector types, including the original scialytic with multiple mirrors, the metal reflector type and the multi-reflector type either contained in a single light fitting or set into a curved wall or in a domed ceiling at one end of the theatre.

The Scialytic Light Fitting. This consists of an optical lens, similar to a lighthouse lantern, surrounding a single lamp of 150 watts. Light rays from the lens are projected

Fig. 2.1 Scialytic operating light fitting with combined multi-reflector system. (Technical Lights & Equipment Ltd.)

on to a circle of mirrors which are set at 45 degrees to an imaginary perpendicular line running through the centre of the lens and which surround the inner circumference of the light fitting. These rays are then focused as a circular light field on the operation area.

Focusing of the light field is accomplished by sliding the lampholder up or down inside the lens. Release of a thumb screw at the top of the light housing will enable the metal tube (attached to the lampholder) to slide in or out of the supporting mount until the correct focus is achieved. This thumb screw must be retightened after focus adjustment. Alternatively adjustment of focus is controlled by a cam which is connected to a single external knob.

To focus, the operation table is raised to the height most generally used and the lamp position adjusted until the smallest possible spot of light illuminates the table. This should ensure that the light area will remain in focus as a spot when the table is raised or lowered between 15 and 23 cm (6 and 9 in) from this point to suit the individual surgeon.

The efficiency of this shadowless light, as with all light fittings, will depend to a large extent upon regular cleaning of the lens and mirrors. This should be the responsibility of the electrician, but care must be taken to ensure that the light is switched off before cleaning is commenced. Any harsh cleanser which may scratch the highly polished surfaces should not be used. Water or a window cleanser are quite suitable, followed by polishing with a soft, lint-free cloth.

Another factor affecting the efficiency is dimming of the lamp due to over-heating. As the light fitting is designed to be dust proof, ventilation is often poor. This will affect the life of the lamp, which sometimes needs changing before it actually burns out.

Shadowless light fittings may be fixed rigidly to the ceiling, but most are mounted on a swivel, counterbalanced arm or wires, which allow adjustment of position in relation to

Fig. 2.2 Sketch of the optical system in a scialytic light fitting.

Fig. 2.3 Sketch of optical system in metal reflector operating light fitting.

the operation area. It is possible also to mount the light on rails fixed to the theatre ceiling which allow movement across the theatre.

The Metal Reflector Light Fitting. This is basically the same as the scialytic lamp in respect of performance, but instead of mirrors the reflector consists of a concave, highly polished surface, either plain or made up of a number of facets. The lamp is situated at the central focal point and is adjustable in a similar manner to the scialytic type (Fig. 2.4).

A clear lamp should not be used in this type of light because it will give a small circle of highly concentrated light in the operating area. This light field may be only 5 or 7 cm (2 to 3 in) in diameter, and is generally too small and certainly very tiring to the

Fig. 2.5 One of four theatres in a multiple theatre department. Each has a Blin lighting system consisting of multiple spotlights. A viewing gallery for students and visitors is provided also. (St James Hospital, Balham, London.)

surgeon. Another important factor is that the depth of focus is very small and any adjustment in the operation table height will throw the light out of focus and produce poor illumination.

A pearl or opal lamp is more satisfactory for these reasons.

The larger the source of light *in the fitting*, the larger the diameter of the light field, and considerable adjustment of operation table height is possible before loss of focus occurs, thereby increasing the depth of focus. However, if this larger light source produces too much heat in the light field, the lamp may be surrounded with a heat-absorbing filter made from Chance glass. This filter absorbs most of the heat rays with only fractional reduction of the intensity of the light.

It must be remembered that the same considerations regarding the cleaning of reflectors apply as with other types of light fittings.

The Multi-Reflector Light Fitting. This has six to nine separate lamps in the light fitting instead of one lamp and special reflectors. These lamps are focused simultaneously on the operation area by manipulating a single knob fitted to the light housing.

The lamps used are smaller than those in the light fittings previously described. In one type of light fitting, the Hanalux (Fig. 2.6), they are of a lower wattage (40 W) and a lower voltage (24 V), and it is claimed produce a source of light which when used in conjunction with heat-absorbing filters is the best approximation to the colour of daylight possible with artificial lighting.

Although each lamp is of relatively lower intensity compared to the lamp in the single-reflector fittings, the cumulative effect of the six or nine lamps is very efficient, with the great advantage that should one lamp be inoperative the intensity of the light as a whole is only fractionally reduced.

The light field produced by the Hanalux Boston light fitting can be adjusted by a knob to between 16·5 cm (6·5 in) and 34·9 cm (13·75 in) in diameter. The maximum intensity of light at 16·5 cm (6·5 in) is approximately 90,000 lux and at 34·9 cm (13·75 in) diameter approximately 45,000 lux.

Provision can be made in this lamp for a television camera or alternatively an automatic camera which, combined with a built-in electronic flash mechanism, enables photographs to be taken during operation.

Another development in this field is the Castle/Daystar light fitting which produces a light in the region of 6,000° K approximating daylight colour (Fig. 2.8). The lamphead, measuring 101·6 cm (40 in) in diameter, incorporates six pod 30·5 cm (12 in) reflectors using incandescent quartz halogen lamps. The light is in focus at any distance from 76·2 cm to 152·4 cm (30 to 60 in) from the cover glass; the prime focus being 106·7 cm (42 in) from the glass providing a light field of about 40·6 cm (16 in) in diameter. The maximum intensity at the centre of the light field at this distance is 53,500 lux and 12,848 lux at the edges; a dimming device is provided to reduce this intensity by up to half.

The heat rise from the fitting is 1·67°C for each 10,700 lux of intensity, or 8·35°C for 53,500 lux of intensity. This is achieved by the following:

A dichroic coating on the reflectors creates a 'cold mirror' that separates heat from light transmitting 80 per cent of the infra-red energy up through the reflectors, whilst reflecting light energy downward;

Colour correcting cylinders cover each of the six lamps;

The skeletal configuration of the pod design takes advantage of upward air currents created by the infra-red rays being transmitted through the reflectors.

In the event of a mains electricity failure a 24 V emergency system composed of six 24 V quartz halogen lamps comes into operation. Illumination is focused over the entire area of the operation table, with shadow reduced light in the centre of the light field which will penetrate cavities. Readjustment of the focus may be required as the emergency lamps are off-centre from the main lamp.

Multi-Reflector Wall Lights. With these a shadowless effect is produced by mounting a number of 'spot' lights in the wall and ceiling surrounding the operation table. These lights (up to 40 in number) are permanently focused on one spot in the centre of the theatre and may be independently switched in sets of six or eight according to the angle from which the light is required (Fig. 2.5, page 37).

Fig. 2.6 A multi-reflector light fitting, the Hanalux Boston model with separate fibre-light satellite which gives a perfectly cool beam ideally suited to neurosurgery. (Siemens Electro-Medical/Surgical Group.)

Fig. 2.7 The newest version of a multi-reflector light fitting in the Hanalux range. Called the Amsterdam, this light has an optical system comprising of halogen lamps used in conjunction with a reflector system incorporating cold light mirrors, conversion filters and Fresnell lenses. The light colour variation range can be adjusted between approximately 5,200° K and 3,200° K. The illumination intensity is adjustable between 60,000 and 120,000 lux, with the illuminated field measuring between 20 to 30 cm in diameter. The light illustrated shows an additional centre cold spotlight with sterilisable sleeve. (Siemens Electro-Medical/Surgical Group.)

Changing operating light lamps

A spare lamp for the main light fitting and any mobile lights must always be easily available and placed in an accessible position. Lamp changing should be carried out by an electrician.

The light must **always be switched off at the wall switch** before attempting to change a lamp.

Generally speaking, the lamp may be reached either by a raised panel in the region of the electric flex entrance on the top of the light fitting or through a removable panel in the glass or plastic cover on the front of the fitting.

In the former case the panel may be removed by unscrewing one or two remaining thumb screws and turning the panel in a clockwise or anti-clockwise direction to free it from any retaining pins. The cover may then be detached together with the lampholder and fused lamp, or will provide access for removal of the lamp from the lampholder.

Fig. 2.8 Daystar shadowless light fitting. (Drayton Castle Limited.)

Access to the lamp through the glass or plastic cover at the front of the light fitting requires the release of three or four thumb screws, which allows the removal of the small central panel. There are no large modern operating light fittings requiring the removal of the complete front panel to reach the lamp. If the complete panel is ever removed for cleaning or other purposes the light fitting must be secured beforehand, as this will alter the counterbalancing and cause the whole assembly to spring upward towards the ceiling.

Where low-voltage or special lamps are used care must be taken to ensure that the correct lamp is fitted into the lampholder. A lamp should screw or plug into the holder easily and with no force. It should be remembered that certain lamps may be designed to burn efficiently in a particular position. A lamp which is suitable for burning in the portable 'spot' light fitting used mainly in a nearly horizontal position may burn out very quickly if used in the overhead vertical light, and vice versa. The cause of short life in a lamp may well be due to this reason as well as overheating which has been described.

Emergency lighting

The emergency lighting in the main overhead light fitting has already been discussed on page 33. These lamps come into operation automatically upon mains or fuse failure when the light is in use.

Emergency lighting should be tested regularly to ensure absolute reliability. During an emergency the supply must be switched off as soon as practicable and the use of unnecessary lights in the ancillary rooms carefully avoided. This will help to reduce the generator load, or 'drain' on batteries which are usually designed to give three or four hours' illumination on 'full loading'.

Sometimes mobile emergency light fittings are provided in the theatre. The apparatus generally contains a battery and trickle charger. This mechanism keeps the batteries continually charged and the light ready for immediate use.

Low-voltage apparatus

There is a large amount of apparatus in the theatre which uses a low-voltage current. To mention just a few, these include laryngoscopes, bronchoscopes, cystoscopes, head lamps and illuminated retractors (Smith, 1958). To some extent low voltage illumination is being replaced by fibre optics (page 308).

It would be very true to say that no other type of apparatus can cause so many problems as the low-voltage equipment. It often seems to go out of action just when needed, and unless a careful step by step check of the circuit is made, much time can be wasted. The efficiency of such apparatus depends to a great extent on regular checking of batteries, lamps and electrical contacts and this should be the responsibility of an electrician or trained technician. However, an understanding of simple circuit testing can contribute to better care of apparatus together with knowledge of simple circuit testing to trace faults.

A low-voltage circuit may be likened to a circle of electric current flowing from the positive terminal of a battery, along an insulated wire, through the lamp filament and along another insulated wire thus completing the connection to the negative terminal of

Fig. 2.9 The principle of series and parallel battery circuits.

the battery. Apparatus such as torches, cystoscopes, bronchoscopes, etc., often use the outer metal case as the electrical return path to the battery instead of a second wire.

Generally a low-voltage circuit for theatre use may range from 1·5 V for apparatus such as bronchoscopes to 10 V for a surgeon's headlamp. The electric current may be supplied from batteries or a transformer which reduces the mains voltage to the required level. A transformer may be a separate item of equipment or may be incorporated in apparatus such as the diathermy machine. Fibre light sources are discussed in Chapter 12.

In the case of batteries, two or more may be joined together either to give an increased voltage (series circuit) or prolong the period of supply (parallel circuit).

It is quite possible that when batteries or a transformer are working at full-power output the voltage given may be higher than that required for a particular lamp in an apparatus, and using a higher than necessary voltage may burn the lamp out immediately or reduce its life. It is usual in this case to introduce a rheostat into the circuit, which enables the voltage to be varied at will. The batteries or transformer may then be used for a variety of apparatus operating on different voltages.

A rheostat is an electrical resistance operated by turning a knob which when set at the required voltage reduces the slightly higher current to the required level. The rheostat should always be set at zero before switching on and connecting the apparatus.

Parallel lamp circuits

If any item of apparatus has more than one lamp it is usual to connect the lamps so that should one burn out the others will still illuminate. This is especially necessary in the case of an illuminated abdominal retractor which may have three or more lamps.

The basic method of connection can be illustrated with the example of a retractor with three lamps. Each of the lamps can be connected to the batteries by three separate sets of insulated wires. However, the most universal way is for each of the two wires leading from the battery or transformer terminals to be split into three, giving three positive and three negative wires. One positive and one negative wire is then connected to each of the lamps thereby allowing simultaneous illumination.

Care of apparatus

In order that a low-voltage circuit may operate satisfactorily all connections must be kept clean, dry and free from corrosion. After sterilisation, heat processed apparatus must be well dried before storing away. Good contact of the connections must be maintained and loose soldered contacts repaired immediately they are detected. Lamps must be securely screwed in position and the current source should, if possible, remain fairly constant. With batteries this means a careful watch for battery exhaustion.

Batteries left too long in a metal case tend to sweat, especially in humid atmospheres, causing corrosion and the discharge of power. All batteries not in actual use should be stored under dry conditions.

When a rheostat is connected in the power circuit it is preferable to switch on the full current slowly by commencing at nil volts and raising the current to the required level. This warms up the lamp filament before it receives the full current and increases its life considerably – a very important point as specialised lamps are often expensive and have a comparatively short life.

Checking a suspected faulty low-voltage circuit

This is a simple process if taken stage by stage, especially if a test lamp and battery are available. The test set consists essentially of a 1·5 V battery to which are connected two insulated wires, having rigid metal points at each of the two free ends, and a small low-voltage lampholder and lamp to which are also connected similar insulated wires. (A diagram of the circuit is shown in the Appendix.)

The battery is used for testing circuits and lamps, the lamp for testing faulty batteries. It is a simple matter for a carpenter to arrange these two items together in a box or on a movable board.

Irrespective of the type of apparatus tested (after connecting the apparatus correctly and switching on, as in the case of a laryngoscope, etc., it is found to be out of order) it is usually possible to check the faults as follows:

1. In the case of a transformer especially ensure that it is connected to the wall socket and is switched on correctly.

2. Check that the lamp is firmly screwed into position.

3. Check that all electrical connections appear to be in good contact and are not obviously broken. Where the apparatus has batteries in the handle, ensure that the inside of the case is free from any corrosion. Should there be corrosion, slight scraping of the contacts or tightening of loosened screws will usually suffice.

4. In the absence of a test battery try one or more new lamps in the lampholder or carrier. Small lamps can sometimes vary in size and length of the screw part. Should this be so, the centre contact at the base of the lamp may not reach the contact in the lampholder and it will appear that the lamp is out of order. These lamps should not be discarded as faulty until they have been tried with the test battery or in another lampholder or carrier.

Sometimes the centre contact of the lamp is made of a compressed coil of wire. Should the lamp not function in the apparatus but appear satisfactory on test with the testing unit, it may be advantageous to lengthen the contact by pulling out this coil of wire a fraction of an inch. When re-inserting the lamp be careful that the amount of lengthening is minimal, for if too much this contact may be pushed out of centre during screwing into position. This will then cause the wire to short-circuit across the inside of the lampholder, allowing the current to flow straight back to the battery or transformer and the lamp will still not light or may flicker.

5. If the lamp appears in order, check the batteries by connecting them with another apparatus known to be in working order, or use the test lamp, connecting it directly to the batteries. If the test lamp will not illuminate it is most probable that the batteries are exhausted.

6. Should the lamp still not function it is possible that the wires leading from the batteries or transformer to the lampholder or carrier may be broken somewhere within the insulation. These wires may be checked by connecting to other light carriers or lamps which are known to be in working order, or by using the test apparatus. The test is made by connecting the suspected faulty wires between the test battery and the two wires joined to the test lampholder.

ELECTROMEDICAL EQUIPMENT

The importance of earthing the metal framework of electrical apparatus has already been emphasised (page 34). This protects staff from shocks should an internal fault occur involving heavy electrical leakage or a direct 'line' to case (positive) connection. Unfortunately, earthing does not always give absolute protection to the patient, for if he is connected to 'earthed' electromedical apparatus it is possible under certain fault conditions for an electric shock to occur due to leakage current from another source or another instrument which has an undetected failure in its protective earth connection. This is particularly so where there is a direct intracardiac connection by means of a catheter (either liquid-filled or containing electrode wires, e.g. to an external pacemaker). The order of current which can cause disturbance to the pumping action of the heart, ventricular fibrillation and death, is discussed in papers by Green, Raftery and Gregory. The permissible leakage currents currently quoted from HTM 8 (i.e. less than 100uA) is classified much more completely in the draft IEC Document 62A (Secretariat) 10, ranging from 10 micro amperes to much higher values for permanently installed equipment. *Leakage is the term used in connection with a stray current present to some degree in every engineered electrical system originating from parts connected to the 'live' mains or other electrical energy source* (Hull, 1978).

The principal risk is when the earth connection to the apparatus is accidentally broken; the leakage current may find its way to earth (ground) through other equipment connected to the patient or through some earthed object which the patient may be touching. Another path to earth could be through an attending nurse or doctor, who touches the patient and allows the leakage current to flow through both patient and nurse or doctor.

Another risk associated with the previous one is when the patient is connected to two or more pieces of 'earthed' apparatus, *i.e. utilising separate electrical sockets*. Each instrument will possess a protective device such as a fuse or circuit breaker in the electrical supply system. If a fault occurs whereby the live cable comes into contact with some part of the earth system, either the metal framework of the instrument or elsewhere in the building, the patient could momentarily be at risk. This is because the fuse or circuit breaker does not interrupt the supply quickly enough to prevent electric currents flowing momentarily along the earth system and through the patient. An inter-earth current flows due to the voltage existing momentarily between two or more separate electrical sockets, via the earth wires, and the patient for the duration of the fault (Fig. 2.10).

Earth-free patient circuits

Although the above mentioned risks are rare they can be reduced further by various means including that of using equipment having 'earth-free' patient circuits. The electrical design of the inside of 'earth-free' equipment allows connections to the patient to be separated from earth. Consequently, the patient is on a 'floating' electrical circuit and

Fig. 2.10 Current through patient. Due to inter-earth resistance, momentary fault current and use of several earthed devices. (Figs. 2.10–2.15 reproduced with permission from Electrical Equipment Booklet – Patient Safety MO97–72 Northwick Park Hospital & Clinical Research Centre.)

not connected directly to the earth (Figs. 2.11 and 2.12). As a further explanation we can say that the inside of each apparatus is split into two halves – one half going to the patient and the other half obtaining electrical power and being connected to the hospital electrical supply. The equipment is so designed that an electrical failure would not be injurious to the patient. Completely 'earth-free' equipment is therefore safe for connection to the patient, both internally and externally. The patient and all attachments to equipment, are 'separated' from earth (Fig. 2.13).

It is possible that both 'earth-free' and 'earthed' equipment may have to be used on a patient at the same time. Although such a combination is not as safe as exclusively 'earth-free' equipment, the partial use of 'earth-free' equipment will still minimise danger of electric shock (Fig. 2.14).

Earthed patient circuits

If more than one piece of 'earthed' apparatus is connected to the same patient, e.g. 'earthed' diathermy machine and 'earthed' e.c.g. machine, it is possible for an inter-earth current to occur. To avoid this, external earth terminals should be fitted to each apparatus

Fig. 2.11 Basic earth-free equipment.

Fig. 2.12 Basic earthed equipment.

Fig. 2.13 All earth-free devices. Patient completely protected against current flow through body.

Fig. 2.14 Single earthed instrument with other earth-free devices. (Generally satisfactory intermediate standard but shock from live object is possible because of one direct earth.)

Fig. 2.15 Use of safety earth links. For two or more patient earthed instruments.

and when in use linked together with an approved safety earth wire which must be kept as short as possible (Fig. 2.15), this connects the patient to a common earth.

It is worth noting that when the expression 'earth-free' is applied to a diathermy machine it is relative; in a fault condition there is no danger of electrocution by external contact, but there is insufficient protection when intracardiac catheters are in place with intraventricular contact. A safety earth should be connected if other 'earthed' equipment is in use. In the more critical situation, therefore, diathermy machines should *not* really be regarded as 'earth-free'.

Safety precautions

Guidance and care are necessary to minimise the risk of injury to patients and staff when using electromedical equipment. Much of the preceding information follows the work of a Safety Committee formed at Northwick Park Hospital and Clinical Research Centre, Harrow, England. This multidisciplinary group consisted of doctors, biomedical and hospital engineers and nurses who meet to discuss developments in electromedical equipment and all aspects of electrical safety. The group formulated a safety guidance document (Northwick Park Hospital and Clinical Research Centre, 1972) and it is useful to reproduce the main points below:

Take care and think!

1. Do not place wet cloths, bottles of fluid or cups etc., on electrical equipment. Liquid seeping into the equipment could not only cause damage but also dangerous short circuits.

2. Never touch exposed pacemaker terminals, intracardiac catheters, or guide wires with one hand while making instrument adjustments or contacting electrically operated devices with the other hand. Wear rubber gloves when touching catheter connected metal fittings (except possibly in emergency).

3. Remove dried out saline solutions or jellies and always reapply the recommended amount of conducting material before placing electrodes on a patient.

4. Ensure that your hands are dry before touching the patient or electrical equipment; moisture allows more current to flow.

5. Disconnect from the patient any electrical equipment which is faulty.

6. Do not touch the patient and any kind of electrical equipment at the same time. You will provide the electrical link between the two, and there could be a fault.

7. Follow the manufacturer's instructions at all times.

8. If both 'earth-free' and 'earthed' equipment is in use, then some means of identification is necessary. A useful system is to apply green labels with appropriate wording and use green plugs for 'earth-free' and yellow labels and plugs for 'earthed' equipment. (This is the system used at Northwick Park Hospital.) Connect the *safety earth wire* provided between the *safety earth terminals* of all 'yellow label' equipment, when two or more of this type of apparatus are in use. This should be done before connection to the patient.

9. Ensure that electrical equipment is securely mounted so that it cannot be dislodged by the patient. Unexpected movement could cause breakage of wires, physical injury to the patient or even electrocution if the equipment is damaged.

10. Check all connections to the patient and equipment.

Look for:
>loose plugs
>kinks in wires
>worn or frayed wires
>electric cables touching hot surfaces.

Do not use mains extension cables and if in doubt call immediate attention to a suspected fault.

11. Take especial care with 'high power' apparatus, e.g. defibrillators, e.c.t. and diathermy machines. If misused, these can cause serious shock or burns to both patient and staff. *Never test* a defibrillator by power discharge when a synchroniser lead is connected to the patient – use an e.c.g. simulator for test purposes.

12. Use surgical diathermy 'indifferent electrodes' exactly as instructed by the manufacturers. The dry type of plate must make effective contact over a large flat surface of skin; separate small areas of contact could result in high-frequency electrical burns.

Monitoring equipment

Observation and recording a cardiac and respiratory function is called monitoring. A wide range of equipment and systems are available to monitor data such as electrocardiograph wave form, arterial pressures, venous pressures and heart rate, to mention just a few. It is beyond the scope of this book to describe these in detail and the reader who seeks this information will find a number of recommended books listed on page 65. However, the theatre nurse may be concerned in the use of some portable equipment; the safety precautions already enumerated in previous paragraphs are equally as applicable in the operating theatre as in the intensive care situation.

It is common now to manufacture modular equipment which allows maximum flexibility in deciding the range of the measurements to be undertaken. Various items of equipment are designed so that they can be interconnected and plug-in units allow the simple replacement of defective parts. The type of apparatus which the theatre nurse is most likely to meet is the cardiac monitor, single and multichannel with facilities for e.c.g. pressure wave forms and other cardiac parameters.

The cardiac monitor or electrocardiograph. This is an apparatus which records the electrical currents which are associated inseparably with cardiac contractions. As an electric

Fig. 2.16 Single channel non-fade electrocardiograph (e.c.g.) monitor with freeze facility for trace and digital heart rate display (Cambridge Medical Instruments Ltd.).

current is conducted readily through the body (for tissue fluids contain electrolytes, mainly chlorides of sodium and potassium in fairly high concentrations), the electrical currents generated by the heart are carried to the peripheral parts of the body. These can be conducted to the cardiac monitor or electrocardiograph via wires or leads connected to electrodes placed in contact with the skin; thus an electrical circuit is completed. The electrical currents are led from certain paired parts of the body surface, and any pair of

Fig. 2.17 Multichannel fibre optic recorder with facilities for direct write-out ultraviolet traces or high contrast photographic records. (Camtrace, Cambridge Medical Instruments Ltd.)

electrodes (or rather parts of the body to which they are attached), with their connecting wires are referred to as a 'lead'. Up to 12 pairs of leads may be used in diagnostic electrocardiography, but for monitoring purposes there are generally not more than 3 or 5 pairs.

Fundamentally the cardiac monitor of cardioscope consists of an electronic amplifier which amplifies the electrical currents of the heart and displays them, either as a trace on an oscilloscope or a continuous band of paper in a writing device. Figure 2.17 shows a six-channel fibre optic medical recorder offering a variety of recordings including echocardiograms, phonocardiograms, pressure wave forms, and apex and carotid pulse wave-forms. By an add-on unit the capacity can be increased to twelve channels. For teaching or other observation purpose an external monitor can be directly 'slaved' to both the monitor and recorder.

The basic characteristics of a cardiac monitor are:

1. Power supply; either from the electrical mains or batteries which may be rechargeable or replaceable.

2. Patient monitor cable dividing into three or five different coloured leads with terminals for connecting to the patient electrodes.

3. The oscilloscope screen (which may be green or covered with an orange filter) on which the e.c.g. trace or traces are displayed and may have an overlay grid scale.

4. A selector switch allowing the use of a number of channels (usually up to six) to select the most suitable trace.

5. Control knobs for height of trace (gain), brightness, focus, position and speed of trace (usually 12·5 mm, 25 mm and 50 mm per second).

6. Adjustable high/low alarm system which emits visual or audible signals if the heart rate exceeds above or below a pre-set range, e.g. 50 to 110 beats per minute.

Fig. 2.18   Normal e.c.g.

Fig. 2.19   Selecting the most suitable channel.

7. A recording device or pen writer which records the e.c.g. trace on a continuous band of paper, either at predetermined intervals, e.g. every 15 minutes, when the alarm system actuates or when a button is pressed. This device may be part of the monitor or added as an accessory when required. The monitor/recorder displayed in Figure 2.17 utilises a fibre optic footplate to enable instant ultraviolet tracings to be made on the recording paper. Inserting an alternative paper cassette provides a record on bromide paper.

The monitor requires some adjustment to achieve optimum viewing conditions. The theatre nurse should first seek a demonstration of the various controls and then adjust them one at a time until the action of each is fully understood. The brightness and focus control in particular may require adjustment; if the trace is surrounded by a ring as it travels across the screen it is too bright, the minimum amount of brightness acceptable should always be selected to avoid burning the screen of the oscilloscope. According to how long each configuration of the wave or complex is required on the screen, so the speed of the trace traverse is adjusted. Generally four to six configurations should be present on the screen as the trace travels across.

The channel should be selected so that the trace appears as a thin line rather than a fuzzy one which may obscure smaller waves. If necessary, the size of the waves may be increased by adjusting the gain control. So long as the waves are clearly identifiable, it is

Fig. 2.20 Limb electrode.

Fig. 2.21 Sites for chest electrodes.

Fig. 2.22 Chest electrodes positioned.

not generally important whether they are upright or inverted on the screen. Monitor observation is described further in Chapter 10.

Limb electrodes. These may be oblong brass plates 4 cm by 2 cm, slightly curved, plated with nickel or chrome. A screw socket is incorporated on the top side to which the lead is attached. The electrode is held in place by a band of rubber passing round the limb; one electrode is placed on each limb usually above the wrist or ankle. The leg electrode is positioned on the lateral aspect of the limb to avoid scratching the opposite leg with the screw (Fig. 2.20). Self-adhesive electrodes for limbs are available also.

Chest electrodes. These consist of small circular metal discs about 1 cm in diameter, mounted on a polythene disc and secured to the chest wall with non-irritant adhesive or adhesive tape such as Micropore (3M) or Dermacel (Johnson & Johnson). Usually three or four electrodes are used and positioned over the heart; the exact position of these is not critical and to some extent will be determined by the presence of surgical incisions and the best type of trace produced on the oscilloscope. Suitable sites are on or at either side of the sternum, below the nipples or below the clavicles (Figs. 2.21 and 2.22).

Care must be taken in the correct application of electrodes to the skin.

1. It is no use applying chest electrodes over hairy areas, this will prevent a good electrical contact; shave if necessary.

2. The skin must be cleaned thoroughly with ether meths or other solvent to remove traces of perspiration and grease.

3. Be certain that the surface of each electrode is perfectly clean and free from green corrosion; dirty electrodes should be cleaned with ether meths or methylated spirits.

4. A small quantity of a proprietory non-irritant jelly such as Cambridge (blue tube) should be applied to the contact surface of the electrode. With chest electrodes it is particularly important not to smother the electrode with jelly otherwise it may ooze on to the adhesive or fixing tape and prevent secure attachment to the chest with loss of good electrical contact. (Note: The electrically conductive pastes with a high salt content used for routine diagnostic electrocardiography are not suitable for long periods of monitoring. These pastes tend to produce skin reactions and excoriation over extended periods.) Alternatively, pre-jelled disposable electrodes may be used.

5. After attachment to the limbs or chest the electrodes connected to the leads and thence to the monitor. It is important to ensure that the leads of the monitor cable are secured to the limb, or chest with a suitable non-irritant tape, to avoid pulling the electrodes.

6. In the ward or intensive care situation, the electrodes are checked daily for correct position, security, cleanliness and irritation. If these are all satisfactory, and provided that the trace displayed on the screen is acceptable, the electrodes will be left undisturbed, although generally it will be found necessary to renew them after a period of five to seven days. An interference or absence of a trace may not be due to a faulty electrode. Assuming that the patient's condition is otherwise satisfactory, artifacts may occur with movement of the patient and it is better to check all connections and leads thoroughly before removing a suspect electrode. An artifact appears on the trace as irregularly interrupting spikes of varying height.

Peripheral pulsometers. These consist essentially of a photoelectric plethysmograph (which is a device for measuring peripheral blood flow in the earlobe or fingertip) a receiver and an amplifier. The plethysmograph is clamped to the ear lobe or held in contact with the tip of the finger by means of a Velcro strap. Signals are conveyed by a lead to the receiver/amplifier which may be mains or battery operated. The pulse rate per minute is displayed on a scale or meter and may be monitored also by a bleep from a built-in loudspeaker or buzzer.

Very careful positioning of the electrode is important, the plethysmograph is delicate and sensitive to movement artifacts. Care must be taken to secure the leads and avoid strain on the connections.

Cardiac pacing

The pacemaker is an apparatus which produces a series of electrical shock impulses to stimulate the heart ventricles to contract. Cardiac pacing is generally used for complete heart block although less commonly in the emergency situation it may be used for cardiac asystole applying the shock across the chest wall to cause contraction of the ventricles. In this situation, during surgery if the chest is open, the electrodes may also be applied directly to the heart. External pacing requires an apparatus capable of producing in excess of 20 V as compared to up to 9 V with internal pacemaking.

The apparatus is powered by replaceable mercury batteries or a rechargeable nickel cadium battery. It has a series of controls allowing adjustment of:

1. Pulse rate per minute, generally 30–160 although models are available with a range of 80–120 per minute.
2. Voltage 0–9 V.
3. Pulse width, i.e. duration, 1–2 milliseconds.
4. Selection of continuous or on demand impulses; continuous pacing impulses to stimulate the ventricles are supplied at a fixed or constant rate; the demand setting only supplies pacing impulses as they are needed, for example, if the heart beat is too slow. If the time interval between two QRS configurations is too long then the apparatus supplies a pacing impulse to cause ventricular contraction thereby increasing the heart rate. When the heart rate is faster than the selected rate on the pacemaker then no pacing impulses are produced.
5. Battery level indicator.
6. Terminals for the active and indifferent electrode leads.
7. A pulse output indicator in the form of a neon lamp and/or buzzer.

An insulated wire or endocardial catheter electrode is passed under local anaesthesia into a suitable vein in the arm or neck and from there, under X-ray control, through the right atrium to the right ventricle where the tip is wedged against the wall of the cavity.

Fig. 2.23 MP16 Demand/Continuous Pacemaker. (Cambridge Scientific Instruments Ltd.)

This forms the active electrode; the indifferent electrode consists of a wire loop buried subcutaneously near the skin incision. The two wires can then be connected to the terminals of the pacemaker apparatus.

With the epicardial technique, the electrodes are sewn onto the epicardial or outer surface of the heart exposed at thoracotomy. The wires are brought out through the chest wall for connection to the pacemaker.

Alternatively, the wires can be passed subcutaneously to the axilla and connected to a small battery-powered pacemaker buried beneath the skin. When the batteries become exhausted, the patient requires a further operation under general anaesthesia to replace the complete pacemaker; this however, does not need to be done very often; there are batteries having a life of up to 10 years. Developments have taken place in the production of nuclear powered pacemakers for implantation, which provide power almost indefinitely.

The impulses of a heart being paced if viewed on a cardiac monitor show that each QRS-T configuration, instead of being preceded by a P wave is now preceded by a pacing impulse (Fig. 2.24). The pacing impulse may appear as a narrow, bright vertical line immediately before each QRS-T configuration which is often wide and large but constant in shape. Points to note are whether the pacing impulse is present or absent; that the QRS-T shape is constant and immediately preceded by the pacing impulse; that the heart rate is correct and regular; whether any extra pacing impulses or QRS-T configurations are present.

Finally, it is important that theatre staff familiarise themselves with the type of pacemaker in use, particularly whether the power supply is from batteries or rechargeable cells, the method of adjusting controls and the method of attaching electrode leads, especially in the emergency situation.

Fig. 2.24 Pacing configuration.

Fig. 2.25 Ventricular fibrillation.

Defibrillator

This apparatus enables a single electric shock to be applied to the heart to correct ventricular or atrial fibrillation. The apparatus may be mains or battery operated with a facility to discharge the shock through the chest wall or via electrodes placed directly in contact with the walls of the heart.

When switched on, the difibrillator charges a condenser to a maximum energy of 400 J. The level of stored energy can be pre-set in steps between 15 and 400 J and this is released in a pulse having a duration of about 2·5 to 5 milliseconds. In the case of atrial fibrillation the defibrillator is coupled with an electrocardiograph so that the defibrillation discharge is delivered in synchronisation, normally 40 milliseconds delay after the peak of the R wave of the patient's e.c.g.

Although different makes of defibrillators vary slightly in the method of operation, basically the same technique is used. The following is a description of the method of using a Cambridge defibrillator; although instructions are printed on the control panel.

External defibrillation. The apparatus is equipped with electrodes which can quickly be withdrawn from the front for use. The controls associated with synchronised cardioversion (atrial fibrillation) are mounted behind the black lid on the front panel to avoid any possible confusion during emergency use of the equipment for ventricular fibrillation.

Fig. 2.26 Cambridge Defibrillator – Synchronised with external electrodes. (Cambridge Scientific Instruments Ltd.)

1. *Keep black lid shut.* Closing this lid automatically switches the machine from synchronised to emergency.
2. Apply electrode jelly liberally to electrode surfaces but avoid smearing on hands or from the electrode surface up on to the handle.
3. *Set output to 200–400 J for adult and 50–200 J for a child.*
4. *Apply electrodes firmly to patient,* one at the upper sternum and one over the heart apex; jelly must not be allowed to spread to make contact between the two electrodes.
5. *Instruct those present to stand well clear* of patient, bed and any connecting leads, etc.
6. *When stored energy meter reads required output, press prime button.*
7. *Press fire button on handle within 10 seconds,* this will discharge the shock to the patient and the apparatus will recharge immediately. If the defibrillator is not used within the 10 seconds period, the prime button must be pressed again in order to prepare the apparatus for use, this is a safety cut-out to avoid accidental discharge. After use switch off apparatus which effects a safe discharge of any stored energy.

Synchronised cardioversion. Open the black lid on the front panel of the apparatus and set switch to synchronise position.

1. *Connect the synchronisation lead from the e.c.g. monitor* to the three-pin socket which is normally covered by the black lid.
2. *Connect the e.c.g. to the patient in the normal way* and adjust gain so that the R waves not less than 1 cm high are displayed on the screen. Upward or downward waves are equally acceptable.

3. *Set output to required energy.*

4. The loudspeaker in the defibrillator will now bleep in synchronisation with each R wave.

5. Apply electrode jelly liberally to electrode surfaces as previously described.

6. *When stored energy meter reads required output*, press prime button.

7. *Instruct those present to stand well clear* of patient, bed and any connecting leads.

8. *Apply electrodes firmly to patient as previously described.*

9. *Press fire button* within 10 seconds of prime button and keep pressed until discharge occurs i.e. on the next synchronised bleep. After discharge the defibrillator will immediately recharge, but will not fire again until the prime button has been pressed.

After use, switch off apparatus, which effects a safe discharge of any stored energy. Clean the electrodes and return them to their storage space. If synchronisation defibrillation has been used, remove e.c.g. synchroniser lead and close black lid. Connect defibrillator to charger unit.

Again, a final point of importance; although defibrillation apparatus is designed for safe operation it is important that regular checks are made to ensure that it is in working order. Special testing devices are available to check the level of discharge between the two electrodes. A defibrillator is *not* a piece of apparatus to be stored away in some obscure cupboard and forgotten, because every second may count when it is needed during cardiac resuscitation. Its whereabouts must be known to *all* who work in theatre, and *all* must familiarise themselves with the correct method of operation of the particular apparatus in use.

Surgical diathermy

Surgical diathermy is a high frequency electric current. When this current is passed through the patient's body between two electrodes, the effect is to produce a concentration of current at the electrode being used by the surgeon. As the surgeon applies his 'live' electrode to the tissues, the current passes through the adjacent tissue cells and owing to their electrical resistance, heat is generated at this point. The effect is localised because the current from the 'live' electrode spreads out in the patient's body and travels to the 'indifferent' electrode which is a large electrode placed in contact with the patient's body. A high density of current occurs only immediately beneath the live electrode because further away (except under fault conditions) the current density is too small to have any heating effect.

When electro-section or cutting current is selected and used with a needle electrode, an arc is struck between the point of this electrode and the underlying tissues. The arc is very hot (in excess of $1,000°C$) and causes tissue cells to disintegrate instantly in front of the electrode which may be moved with a cutting effect.

Blood vessels which are cut may continue to bleed and it is necessary to apply the diathermy current specifically to the vessel to effect coagulation. The vessel is gripped with artery forceps and an electro-coagulation current is applied via the artery forceps until sufficient heat is generated to cause coagulation of the blood and arrest further bleeding.

Electricity direct from the mains could achieve coagulation of blood, but the current needed to do this at 50 Hz (the mains frequency) would cause intense activation of muscle, thereby preventing the surgeon from working. Also, such a current is likely to cause ventricular fibrillation (page 44) and probable death of the patient. A diathermy current operates at high frequencies and although about 500 mA (milliamperes) may be used, the current can pass through the tissues without activating muscles.

Diathermy machines generate currents within the range of 400 kHz (400,000 cycles per second) to 3 MHz (3,000,000 cycles per second). In one type of machine, the energy for diathermy is created by an electrical discharge across a spark gap. The spark generator produces 100 blocks of energy per second, the oscillating current being at about 400 KHz, but has a high harmonic content extending over a wide band of frequencies. (Fig. 2.27).

The valve generator machine usually produces bursts of energy 50 times per second, each burst oscillating at between 1·6 and 3 MHz per second (Fig. 27B and C). Usually the lower frequencies are suitable for coagulation and the higher frequencies more suitable for cutting of tissue. Such factors as the composition of the oscillating wave affect its working characteristics and are beyond the scope of this book.

These two systems may cause severe interference with certain electromedical recording apparatus. This is caused by the fact that both machines release their energy in pulses at 50 or 100 times per second which is broadcast through electric wiring and through the air. This frequency lies within the frequency reception band for such apparatus as e.c.g. and e.e.g. This means that even with efficient radio supression, e.g. mains electrical filters, the pulse repetition of the diathermy energy will be detected, amplified by the electromedical recording apparatus and obliterate any physiological data. A type of machine is now available which releases its energy either continuously, or at a frequency of 20,000 to 60,000 bursts per second (each of 1·75 MHz) which is outside the

Fig. 2.27 Oscilloscope traces of diathermy output.
A. Spark-generated diathermy, 100 bursts per second at about 400 KHz.
B. & C. Valve-generated diathermy, 50 bursts per second at between 1·6 and 3 MHz.
D. Valve-generated diathermy, modulated at 20,000 to 60,000 bursts per second at 1·75 MHz.
  (A. K. Dobbie.)

necessary frequency band for physiological instruments (Fig. 27d). This enables the use of electrical filters and screened cables to supress any possible interference (Figs. 2.28 and 2.29).

The essential working parts of a diathermy machine are two electrodes connected by heavy insulated wire to the terminals on the machine, the rheostat adjustment for current strength and the spark-free footswitch, which may have separate sections to control coagulation and cutting currents. Alternatively the coagulation and cutting currents may

Fig. 2.28 Diathermy machine (Eschmann Bros. & Walsh Ltd.) (1) Pilot lamp – fibreLIGHT (green). (2) ALARM indicator lamp – plate safety (red). (3) Socket for PLATE electrode cable. (4) Pilot lamp – electrosurgery (green). (5) Finger-switch – ACTIVE cable socket. (6) ON/OFF switch – electrosurgery. (7) Pilot lamp – SUCTION (green). (8) ON/OFF switch – SUCTION. (9) LP1/LP2 switch – fibreLIGHT lamp selector. (10) Vacuum control. (11) Jar selector lever. (12) Patient suction tube connection. (13) Suction jar. (14) Storage compartment (footswitch sockets within). (15) Bacterial filter. (16) Jar top and float assembly. (17) Jar release handwheel. (18) Vacuum guage. (19) FibreLIGHT on/off brightness control. (20) Fibrelight guide adapters. (21) COAGulation output control. (22) Pilot lamp – COAGulation (blue). (23) ON/OFF switch – BLEND. (24) CUTting output control. (25) Pilot lamp – CUTting (yellow).

be selected by turning a switch on the diathermy machine itself. There is usually a switch fitted to the machine to control the mains supply.

The live electrode which is used in the operating areas, is sterilised before connecting to the live terminal on the machine. There is a variety of different shaped electrodes ranging from a slender needle to a disc or ball-type point. These are connected to an insulated handle which is then coupled to the wire. Changing of these electrodes is made simple by the provision of a socket on the operating end of the wire.

The purpose of the indifferent electrode is to provide a surface of sufficient area to avoid any physiological effects at the site of application. This is because the indifferent electrode is in contact with hundreds or even thousands more cells than the live electrode which results in a correspondingly lower density of current in each cell. If the electrode is applied correctly, negligible heat is generated in this area.

The indifferent electrode at one time consisted of a lead plate wrapped in layers of lint soaked previously in a 15 to 20 per cent solution of salt. These electrodes are messy and inconvenient to apply to the skin. It has been known for diathermy burns to occur if the lint cover is either insufficiently damped at the outset, or becomes dried out during the course of an operation. Another disadvantage is that the strong solution of salt can cause a reaction to sensitive skin.

Fig. 2.29 Components (rear view) of diathermy machine illustrated in Fig. 2.28. (Eschmann Bros. & Walsh Ltd.)

Nowadays, the commonest types of electrodes are flexible metal plates. The thin flexible metal plate electrode can either be placed under the patient's body or carefully bandaged round the thigh to ensure even contact with the skin. It is unnecessary to use electrode jelly, though if a hairy site is chosen for application, shaving beforehand is advisable – the hair acts as an electrical resistance. If the patient's skin is dry, moistening with water or saline can be done with advantage before applying the plate. Care must be taken to renew a plate electrode which becomes buckled otherwise areas of irregular contact with the skin which result could allow points of high current density and risk of burns. The electrode is connected to the diathermy machine indifferent or earth terminal by a heavy insulated wire.

Another satisfactory type of electrode consists of aluminium foil half a thousandth of an inch thick backed with paper. A sheet of foil about 45·5 cm^2 (18 in) square is placed under the patient's body and connected to the insulated wire with stainless steel clips. It has the advantages that it is cheap, can be autoclaved and is transparent to X-rays. The foil electrode is particularly suitable for use with infants.

It is important that electrodes are connected correctly to the terminals on the diathermy machine. The connections being reversed will almost certainly result in diathermy burns to the patient; modern diathermy machines incorporate non-interchangeable connections to avoid this danger.

It is vital that the indifferent electrode remains in electrical continuity with the patient and diathermy machine. If there is a defect and a break in this continuity, the patient is exposed to grave risk of diathermy burns. Failure of the return path to the earth terminal of the diathermy machine causes the patient's body to rise to a high voltage when diathermy is used. If any part of the patient then makes contact with earthed metal or a large mass of metal, e.g. the operation table, then a burn is likely to occur at the point of contact. This is why special e.c.g. leads should be used in theatre; i.e. those which have a 10 kHz resistor moulded into the extremity of each lead which ensures that a diathermy burn cannot occur with any type of electrode.

To detect a possible break in continuity of the indifferent electrode connection, a monitoring system is usually incorporated in the diathermy machine. The wire connection from the indifferent electrode consists of two separate insulated wires. A low voltage electrical current is passed out to the plate electrode via one wire and back by the other thereby ensuring an earth return path for the diathermy current from the patient. Failure of one wire normally activates an audible alarm and may cut off the generation of a diathermy current.

As a precaution the patient should be protected by a **thick** layer of insulating material such as rubber sheeting if there is a danger of his coming into contact with metal parts of the table.

DIATHERMY MACHINE NOT WORKING

If a diathermy machine will not work when connected the following should be checked:

1. *After switching off at the wall socket*, check the wire leading from the plug top to ensure that there are no loose wires.

2. Ensure that the ON/OFF switch on the machine is correctly positioned; check with another socket.

If the machine will still not work consult an electrician. However, if an audible hum is made by the machine as it is switched on, but the current does not flow between the electrodes, the diathermy circuit should be checked:

1. *After switching off at the wall socket*, check that the electrode wires are connected correctly and securely to the machine.

2. Check that the insulated wires are still firmly soldered to both of the terminal connections in addition to the electrode handle and the plate connection. If a plate monitoring device is fitted, a broken indifferent electrode wire will be detected under 2 above.

3. Check that the metal connections are not corroded.

4. Check that the indifferent electrode is in good contact with the patient's skin.

Any further checks on the machine circuit are beyond the scope of theatre staff, and the electrician should be consulted.

The strength of current required depends upon the purpose for which diathermy is being used and on the type of machine. As a general rule maximum output is not usually needed, and for most cases one-third to a half of the maximum will often be sufficient. This current setting must of course be checked by the 'scrub nurse' assisting at the operation.

Surgical cautery

An electric cautery consists of a platinum wire loop or point which is raised to red heat by means of an electric current. This heated cautery point is then applied to the tissue area to cause coagulation.

The current may be produced by a low-voltage battery or transformer, although the transformer is preferable, as the output is more constant than that of a battery. The transformer has a rheostat knob which may be adjusted to alter the voltage applied to the platinum point. The cautery must not be used any hotter than at red heat, as too high a current will cause rapid burning out of the cautery point.

The cautery points, of which there is a varied selection, are mounted in a heat-resisting handle to which are connected two wires. These wires are then connected to the transformer *which must be switched off at the wall socket*. Sometimes a transformer has two sets of low-voltage output terminals, one set being marked *Lights*, the other set being marked *Cautery*. The cautery must not be connected to the lights terminals as this may overload the transformer and cause it to burn out. After connecting the wires the transformer may then be switched on.

CAUTERY APPARATUS NOT WORKING

If the cautery will not work check the circuit in the following order, *after switching off at the wall socket*:

1. Inspect the cautery points to see if they are broken, the most usual points of breakage being where the platinum wire joins the thicker mount.
2. Check through all of the electrical connections – cautery point to handle, handle to wire, wire to transformer terminals – to see if they are clean and not corroded. Corrosion may cause poor electrical contact and failure of the current to flow to the cautery point. Cleaning of the points on these low-voltage connections with a small piece of emery cloth is often all that is necessary.
3. Check that the cautery ON/OFF switch is correctly positioned.
4. See that the cable leading from the transformer to the plug socket has not been pulled away from its connections. This may be done by manipulating the cable a little to see if any wires are loose at the points of connection to the transformer and plug top.
5. Re-connect the transformer and switch on. If it still does not operate, the plug socket may be tested by connecting another item of apparatus, such as a portable light fitting which is known to be in working order.

Should this reveal that the socket is operating correctly, it is advisable to have the apparatus checked by an electrician.

Electric and pipeline suction units

These are a vital part of the theatre equipment for aspirating fluid, e.g. from the abdominal cavity or nasopharynx, etc.

The suction may be obtained with a portable machine or a larger central pump unit, connected by a pipe line system to wards and operating suites (Burns, 1958). With the pipe system coupling sockets are placed conveniently in the operating theatre, anaesthetic and recovery rooms, etc., for connection to a portable suction bottle unit in which aspirated fluids are collected (Fig. 2.30) (DHSS, 1972).

Portable suction machines are mainly of two types: (1) the high-vacuum rotary compressor pump, and (2) the reciprocating pump. The first type is most suitable for use in theatre and recovery room as it has the advantage of producing a good vacuum at a high rate of free air displacement, that is, rapid suction of large quantities of fluid. The second type is more suitable for ward use, for although the vacuum produced is reasonably

Fig. 2.30 Pipeline suction apparatus. (British Oxygen Company Ltd.)

Safety features

Several safeguards are included in the design of the suction controller and the receiver jar in order to prevent over-filling and contamination of the pipeline:
1. A tangential inlet tube in the receiver jar minimises frothing in the aspirated liquid.
2. A float valve in the receiver jar prevents transfer of liquid to the controller unit.
3. If the receiver jar is inadvertently re-assembled without the float valve, a secondary valve in the controller unit protects the mechanism and the pipeline from contamination.
4. A disposable filter of non-absorbent cotton wool is incorporated in the control unit.

Ease of sterilisation

All components which can become contaminated are easily disinfected, and afterwards re-assembly is simple and straightforward.

Before disinfection, equipment should be dismantled and all component parts cleaned thoroughly. The receiver jars, float valves and associated tubing are disinfected by soaking in a suitable antibacterial solution (e.g. Cidex).

The control unit should be disinfected with hydrogen peroxide using an ultrasonic nebuliser, or by using ethylene oxide.

Performance

High-Suction Controller Evacuates 1·5 litre receiver jar to 400 mmHg vacuum in under 4 seconds. Variable control from 50 to 500 mmHg vacuum.

Low-suction controller Evacuates 1·5 litre receiver jar to 140 mmHg vacuum in under 2 seconds. Variable control from 0 to 140 mmHg vacuum. Safety valve setting at 180 mmHg.

high the displacement of free air is much less, and the speed of suction is correspondingly reduced.

Any portable suction machines used in the operating theatre must have a spark-free switching mechanism and a flame-proof motor. All the well-known makes of rotary compressor or reciprocating pumps fulfil these requirements, and as the former are the most suitable for use in operating theatres they will be dealt with in more detail.

Fig. 2.31 High-vacuum rotary pump suction machine with change-over device between bottles. (Chas. F. Thackray Ltd.)

Although the various machines differ somewhat in design, they are basically similar in the method of fluid collection. The pump creates a vacuum in the glass suction bottle, into which the aspirated fluid is collected. This jar, which should be of 1·5 litre capacity for use in theatre, is provided with some method of quick release from its sealing cap. In some cases this will be a quick-release removable cap, and in others a method of securing the jar against a fixed metal cap which has a rubber washer or liner.

Incorporated in this cap are internal connections to the pump unit, and one or two external connections for suction tubing. Where two external connections are fitted, it is usual to have a selective tap to enable two suction tubes to be connected to the machine at once, e.g. one for the anaesthetist and one for the operation area. The tap is then positioned correctly for the suction tube in use at that particular time. Ideally, of course, it is preferable to have two suction machines for this purpose as both the surgeon and anaesthetist may require suction simultaneously.

In addition to the external suction tube connections a negative pressure gauge is fitted to the unit indicating the degree of vacuum, controllable by an adjacent screw valve. The

Fig. 2.32 Another type of high-vacuum suction machine. (Eschmann Bros. & Walsh Ltd.)

degree of vacuum obtainable with the rotary compressor vacuum pump is about 66 cm (26 in) of mercury, which is ideal for the rapid aspiration of large quantities of fluid. However, as in the case of suction required for neurosurgical and other delicate operations, this must be considerably less, about 13 cm (5 in) of mercury, hence the value of the adjustable screw valve.

To avoid the danger of foreign matter entering the pump unit should the bottle become overfilled an automatic cut-out is fitted at some point between the bottle and the pump. This generally consists of a float which rises as the bottle contents approach overflow and seals off the connection to the pump. A spare suction bottle is usually provided and some machines incorporate a quick change-over device between the two bottles (Fig. 2.31). The exhaust outlet from the pump should be fitted with a filter to prevent dissipation of contaminated air into the atmosphere. Modern rotary compressor pumps have an exhaust system which safeguards the machine to a certain extent in this respect, but nevertheless unnecessary strain should be avoided whenever possible.

The machine is mounted on strong antistatic castors and is connected with durable electric cable to a plug top.

POINTS TO OBSERVE WHEN USING SUCTION UNITS

1. The suction tubing must be of adequate bore to avoid blockage and collapse. The size will depend upon the tubing connections fitted to the machine and the suction nozzles used, but generally an antistatic tubing of 0·75 cm ($\frac{5}{16}$ in) bore and 0·3 cm ($\frac{1}{8}$ in) wall will suffice.

2. The tubing must be in good condition, without punctures and with a clean lumen.

3. The degree of suction required is regulated initially by compressing the tubing (after switching on the machine) whilst setting the adjustable valve at the necessary position, e.g. to maintain a suction of 25 cm (10 in) of mercury.

4. If the aspirated fluid 'froths up', the froth may be reduced by turning the suction tube connection tap so that the other unused connection is opened to the atmosphere, or alternatively opening fully the suction control valve. If this is not done, the froth may overflow and operate the cut-out mechanism prematurely.

5. The suction bottle must be emptied when the fluid reaches a pre-determined mark. If, by accident, it is overfilled thereby operating the cut-out, the machine is switched off, vacuum broken by opening the suction control valve and the bottle emptied before replacing and recommencing suction. If the cut-out is fitted in a separate chamber adjacent to the suction bottle, it may be necessary to empty this chamber before recommencing suction again.

6. Do *not* cause excessive strain to a suction pump by maintaining a constant high vacuum which occurs, for example, when the tubing is accidentally compressed or when the suction nozzle becomes occluded by contact with a towel.

7. After use, the bottle, cap, float and float chamber must be washed with an antibacterial agent (Chapter 6) and thoroughly dried. Movable taps, etc. must be lightly oiled at frequent intervals.

8. A final caution – do not leave a residual vacuum in the suction bottle after switching off. Possible cause: kinks in a coil of suction tubing wound round pegs fitted to the machine so that it is ready for emergency use. This may cause a back aspiration of oil from the vacuum pump with 'drying out' of the mechanism and consequent loss of efficiency. It is possible to lose half a pint, or more, of oil in this way.

REFERENCES

ARNOLD, V. F. (1958) In *Medical Electrical Equipment*, p. 177. Edited by R. E. Molloy. London: Newnes.
BURNS, J. T. (1958) In *Medical Electrical Equipment*, p. 229. Edited by R. E. Molloy. London: Newnes.
DEPARTMENT OF HEALTH AND SOCIAL SECURITY (1972) *Hospital Technical Memorandum No. 22*. London: HMSO.
DEPARTMENT OF HEALTH AND SOCIAL SECURITY (1974) *Hospital Technical Memorandum No. 11*. London: HMSO.
DOBBIE, A. K. (1969) *Biomedical Engineering*, 4, No. 5, pp. 206–216.
GREEN, H. L., RAFTERY, E. B. AND GREGORY, I. C. (1972) *Biomedical Engineering*, 7, No. 9, pp. 408–414.
HULL, C. J. (1978) *British Journal of Anaesthesia*, 50, 647.
Northwick Park Hospital and Clinical Research Centre (1972) Electrical Equipment Booklet. *Patient Safety* (M097–72). London: Holborn Press.
SAVAGE, B. (1954) *Preliminary Electricity for the Physiotherapist*. London: Faber.
SMITH, A. C. (1958) In *Medical Electrical Equipment*, p. 156. Edited by R. E. Molloy. London: Newnes.
SMITH, E. A. (1958) In *Medical Electrical Equipment*, p. 30. Edited by R. E. Molloy. London: Newnes.
STEVENS, W. R. (1951) *The Principles of Lighting*. London: Constable.

3
STATIC ELECTRICITY

From the previous chapter the reader will realise the importance of using spark-free electrical apparatus in the immediate vicinity of anaesthetic apparatus. Even if a great deal of attention is paid to the safety of electrical apparatus and the elimination of naked flames from the operating suite, explosion risks are not entirely obviated, for there remains the danger of a spark caused by static electricity (Vickers, 1978).

The extent of the risk of electrostatic sparks causing anaesthetic explosions was set out in a report from the Department of Health (1956). The report described an investigation of 36 anaesthetic explosions occurring during a seven year period, 1947 to 1954. Of these 36 accidents, 22 were almost certainly due to an electrostatic spark. The report recommended that antistatic precautions should be taken in all areas where anaesthetic apparatus employing a closed or partially closed breathing circuit is used with flammable anaesthetics. In the light of further experimental evidence, these recommendations have now been updated (DHSS, 1971a, b).

What is static electricity, how does it occur and why should it be of so much concern when anaesthetic explosions are relatively infrequent? (Well over three million anaesthetics are administered each year without an explosion mishap.) It is very true that the majority of operating department staff complete their careers without being witness to a single anaesthetic explosion. However, this is no excuse for overlooking simple precautions which will result in these small risks being almost entirely eliminated.

The generation of static electricity

The formation of this condition is a very simple matter and occurs whenever two dissimilar materials are separated. It is not necessary to cause friction, although this will increase the amount of static electricity produced. The surface of one material or object becomes positively charged and the other negatively charged, but to what degree depends not only on the briskness of separation of the surfaces (friction) but also on the ability of the material to absorb moisture readily from the atmosphere and in this way become antistatic for all practical purposes.

These charges of electricity can continue to build up an electric potential or pressure on the surface of the object until earthed or the object comes into contact with another object of a different potential. When this occurs the discharge of static between the two can cause a spark. It is as if the object stores up the static charge like a condenser and when earthed discharges the static as a spark which may be capable of igniting a flammable anaesthetic mixture.

Very high voltages can be created under favourable conditions, especially in a dry atmosphere, e.g., a person walking on a dry floor wearing ordinary rubber-soled shoes is capable of acquiring or being charged with a potential of 30,000 volts; the act of 'whipping off' a blanket lying on a rubber sorbo pad covering a trolley can produce a similar charge.

These dangers may be very real and steps which should be taken to minimise the formation of dangerous charges of static electricity are:
1. The elimination of materials which predispose towards the formation of static.
2. Allowing the charges to leak away as they are generated and before high potentials are built up.

1. STATIC FORMING MATERIALS

Some materials are more inclined to form static electricity than others. High on this list are most plastics and woollen blankets, which are a grave potential source of sparks.

The following list indicates the materials which may be found in the vicinity of an operating theatre. The order of the list shows that each becomes positively electrified when rubbed with any of the materials following, but negatively when rubbed with any of the materials preceding. The list also indicates that the further apart the materials are on the list the greater the charge produced upon rubbing together.

(*a*) Nylon
(*b*) Flannel and wool
(*c*) Viscose rayon
(*d*) Glass
(*e*) Cotton and linen
(*f*) Dry skin
(*g*) Wood
(*h*) Rubber
(*i*) Various plastics.

Of the materials listed, cotton, linen and viscose rayon are certainly ideal for theatre clothing and towels, blanket covers, etc., unless they have been specially treated to render them water repellent. They have to be quite dry to generate a charge under normal atmospheric conditions, as they readily absorb moisture. It is this property which makes them excellent for theatre use. The only blankets which should be brought into the operating theatre are those of the cotton cellular type, which do not predispose towards the formation of static electricity and are easily sterilised.

2. THE DISSIPATION OF STATIC CHARGES

If all objects were conductive to electricity and all floors conductive, static electricity would be dissipated as rapidly as it formed; unfortunately this is not so.

All ordinary rubber articles are very highly insulating and many items of theatre equipment are made from rubber, including sorbo trolley mattresses and wheels, macintoshes and tubing, etc. The use of ordinary rubber in the manufacture of these articles will prevent the leakage away to earth of any electrostatic charges which may form on the object. These charges will build up potential and leak away slowly unless they are earthed suddenly and dissipated as a spark.

The answer to this problem has been the discovery that, if during the manufacture of rubber, carbon black is finely dispersed through it the resultant rubber is electrically conductive to a degree, dependent on the quantities of carbon present.

This antistatic rubber has sufficient insulation to ordinary mains electricity, but does allow electrostatic charges to dissipate rapidly as they are formed. Unfortunately antistatic rubber is necessarily black, and in order to distinguish this rubber from other types all antistatic rubber components have a distinctive yellow mark.

The risk of an electrostatic ignition is now considered to be confined to an area extending for 25 cm around the anaesthetic gas circuit or gas paths. Flammable gas mixtures escaping from anaesthetic breathing circuits rapidly dilute to a non-flammable level within a few centimetres of the point of escape. All equipment used in this danger zone must be antistatic and all metal parts must be electrically continuous with the floor, e.g. by fitting antistatic castors or feet. All rubber must be antistatic and have effective contact with metal connections used in the breathing circuit of the patient.

Although plastics are regarded as highly electrostatic, it is not practicable to eliminate them entirely from anaesthetic apparatus. The degree of electrostatic risk depends upon the size of the component and whether, due to its position, an electrostatic charge may be formed by the component being rubbed or brushed against. Rotameters, for example, although consisting of some clear plastic parts, do not constitute a great risk due to their location. Plastic soda lime canisters, on the other hand, may be located where they can be brushed against with clothing very easily. In order to minimise a charge building-up on the surface of the canister it is prudent to incorporate an electrically conductive mesh, either buried in the plastic or in contact with the inner or outer surface. This mesh must be made electrically continuous with other antistatic components which are in discharge contact with the floor.

Antistatic polish applied to plastic has a limited effect. The polish is liable to get rubbed off and requires reapplication following cleaning or sterilisation.

As endotracheal tubes are moist in use they need not be made from an antistatic material. There is very little electrostatic risk associated with plastic transfusion tubing although the metal supports associated should have a satisfactory antistatic contact with the floor.

Diathermy quivers are intended to insulate a live electrode from possible shorting through towels or with metal/antistatic equipment. They should be made from either ordinary rubber or plastic; the electrostatic risk with these items is negligible.

The efficiency of antistatic rubber is calculated by measuring the electrical resistance in ohms. This ohmic resistance is in effect the degree of insulation to electricity, the higher the ohms figure, the more insulating is the rubber.

A normal high insulation rubber will have a high electrical resistance in excess of 1,000 million ohms (1,000 MΩ), whereas antistatic rubber in service should have a resistance not exceeding 100 MΩ (DHSS, 1971). This ohmic resistance is determined by measuring the amount of electricity which the rubber will pass under test.

Two insulated wire conductors, connected to a 500 V d.c. tester generator (Megger) are placed separately on two moistened areas of approximately 6·25 cm^2 (1 in^2), but 5 cm (2 in) apart, on the surfaces of the rubber being tested. By turning the handle on the tester a voltage of 500 V is generated and the amount of electricity passing between these conductors through the rubber will move a pointer on the tester scale, indicating the resistance in ohms.

There are many ways of testing various rubber objects and these are listed in the Department of Health circular (DHSS, 1971a) on static electricity.

The more common tests include the following:

(*a*) Rubber boots and shoes; the resistance is measured between the inside of the sole or heel and the under sole.

(*b*) Rubber tubing, etc.; the resistance is measured between spacings of every 1·5 m (5 ft) if the tubing exceeds this length.

(*c*) Furniture feet; the resistance is measured between the surface at the bottom of the cavity, and that normally in contact with the floor.

(*d*) Castors are tested by placing on a wet metal plate, and measuring the resistance between the plate and the metal framework of the trolley or hub of the wheel. When testing a castor fitted to a trolley, etc., the other castors should be insulated from the floor during the test.

(*e*) Sorbo pads or mattresses are tested by measuring the resistance between the top and underside, the electrodes being opposite.

(*f*) On thin sheeting the test areas should be on the same surface with approximately 50 mm (2 in) dry spacing between. (Measurements made through the thickness of thin sheeting are unreliable as they may be affected by small areas of conductivity.)

The recommended resistance limits for new equipment are as follows:

Anaesthetic tubing connecting machine to patient, per 1·5 m (5 ft) length: 25,000 Ω minimum, 1 MΩ maximum.

Mattresses or pads: 5,000 Ω minimum, 1 MΩ maximum.

Rubber boots and shoes: 75,000 Ω minimum, 10 MΩ maximum.

Castor tyres and other antistatic items: no lower limit but 10,000 Ω maximum.

The electrical resistance of some antistatic rubber items may increase with use. The maximum permitted electrical resistance of equipment in service is 100 MΩ and equipment exceeding this level should be replaced as having lost its antistatic properties.

All rubber operating theatre equipment, including tubing, sheeting, anaesthetic accessories, operation table mattresses, etc., should be made from an antistatic material and it is important to note that if the surfaces of these are damped, the electrical conductivity will be greater.

Antistatic Floors. If the surface of antistatic rubber is kept clean, the static charges will leak away to earth as they are formed, but the floor must also be antistatic. The efficient dissipation of static does depend a great deal on the provision of a suitable antistatic floor which has a resistance of not more than 2 MΩ new or less than 50,000 Ω in service measured between two separate electrodes placed 60 cm (2 ft) apart.

The most satisfactory materials for theatre floors from the antistatic aspect are *in situ* terrazzo or terrazzo tiles (DHSS, 1971a) laid upon a metal mesh. A direct-to-earth connection for antistatic floors has been found unnecessary. If the floor is laid correctly and has satisfactory antistatic properties, it is capable of equalising any electrostatic charges which are likely to develop on persons or objects which are in electrical contact with the floor.

Wood, linoleum or composition floors are not satisfactory in the theatre suite but antistatic PVC containing granules of carbon may be used. Damp mopping of the floor regularly during an operation list will increase the electrical conductivity considerably. Even if the surface dries rapidly, some moisture will be retained by the floor to a degree dependent on its composition, e.g. a tiled floor will be more absorbent than a PVC one.

3. HUMIDITY

A highly humid atmosphere is a deterrent to the formation of static electricity, but should not be regarded as a guarantee against it. Humidity is much less effective as an antistatic measure with plastics or synthetic fibres which have an inherent tendency to be moisture repellent.

The relative humidity in an operating theatre should be between 50 and 55 per cent, or compatible with comfort.

Steam 'wafting' into the theatre from a steriliser will not maintain a constant and equal humidity throughout the room.

The humidity should be maintained with special apparatus incorporated within the air-conditioning plant in the form of a humidifier, which has already been described in Chapter 1. This system can be automatic, being coupled directly to a hygrometer or may be controlled manually in conjunction with direct reading 'gold beater' hygrometers situated in the theatre and anaesthetic room. These hygrometers which indicate the relative humidity as a direct reading on a scale should be checked periodically against a wet/dry bulb thermometer.

Conclusion

The simple precautions necessary to minimise the possibility of an anaesthetic explosion being initiated by a spark of static electricity do not inconvenience the work of an operating suite.

All rubber components should be of antistatic rubber, tested regularly and renewed when the electrical resistance exceeds 100 MΩ.

Non-antistatic rubber or plastic components such as tubes, airways, etc., should be moistened inside and out before use.

No one should enter the theatre unless wearing antistatic shoes or boots and their clothes covered with a cotton or linen gown. This will reduce the amount of personal static electricity produced by walking.

All theatre outer clothing, etc., should be made of a relatively antistatic material, such as cotton or linen.

Woollen blankets must never be used, cotton cellular blankets are very suitable from an antistatic as well as a bacteriological aspect. Hot blankets are more likely to generate a static charge than cold or warm ones; in no case must a blanket be 'whipped off' a trolley.

REFERENCES

DEPARTMENT OF HEALTH (1956) *Report of a Working Party on Anaesthetic Explosions.* London: HMSO.

DEPARTMENT OF HEALTH (1971a) *Hospital Technical Memorandum* No. 1. *Antistatic Precautions: Rubber, Plastics and Fabric.* London: HMSO.

DEPARTMENT OF HEALTH (1971b) *Hospital Technical Memorandum* No. 2. *Flooring in Anaesthetic Areas.* London: HMSO.

VICKERS, M. D. (1978) *British Journal of Anaesthesia,* **50,** 659.

4
THE OPERATION TABLE AND POSITIONS USED FOR SURGERY

The modern operation table is an apparatus capable of adjustment to give a variety of positions for surgery. Some tables are designed for specific types of operations, but most are made as an all-purpose apparatus suitable for general use which can be adapted for specialised procedures by the addition of suitable accessories. The general operation tables illustrated are all-purpose tables which have raising, lowering, Trendelenburg and lateral tilting mechanisms for the table top; adjustable head and foot ends and a full range of accessories. The table top of each is covered with a sectional sponge rubber antistatic mattress, which is removable for cleaning.

Key
- Reverse Trendelenburg
- Trendelenburg
- Lateral Tilt left
- Lateral Tilt right
- Chair
- Breakback
- Up
- Down

Fig. 4.1   Mechanical-hydraulic five-section operation table. (Chas. F. Thackray.)

Figure 4.1 illustrates a mechanical-hydraulic five-section operation table proportioned to allow the majority of patients to be placed in position easily, so that their major points of articulation correspond to the four breaks in the table top. The table is controlled with a hand-held movement selector with push button controls for all major movements including, height, Trendelenberg and lateral tilts, flexion and chair position. The selector is mounted on a flexible cable allowing it to be used within an arc of 180° of the extreme head end of the table. To position the table, the required movement is selected by depressing the relevant button and pumping the foot pedal until the desired position is achieved.

Figure 4.2 illustrates an electro-hydraulic five-section operation table with telescoping spinal and femoral sections. The advantages claimed for this table are that each articulating section is in 'contour-correspondence' with the five anatomical regions. The table top has a head section, telescoping spinal section accommodating different lengths from the cervical spine to the lumbar arch, a pelvic section with a cut-out under the patient's perineum, a telescoping femoral section to ensure good popliteal flexion and a leg section. This adjustment allows precise positioning for patients short or tall; always with head on headrest, lumbar arch over table break, perineum over perineal cut-out and popliteal space over the knee break. The head section is movable from side to side through a 180° arc. Hydraulic control of height, Trendelenberg/reverse Trendelenberg, lateral tilt and flexion of the spinal and femoral sections are through a control head incorporating five levers which automatically return to a neutral position. The operation table is connected to an electric socket outlet with flexible cable and there is provision for emergency manual hydraulic control.

Fig. 4.2 Electrohydraulic five-section operation table. 1 = femoral-leg; 2 = pelvic-femoral; 3 = spinal-pelvic; 4 = head-spinal. (Drayton Castle Ltd.)

Figure 4.3 illustrates a heavy-base table similar to Figure 4.1, but the Trendelenburg tilt, lateral tilt and 'break back' or chair mechanisms are operated by one control knob and gear lever at the head end of the table. The back or kidney elevator is also controlled from the head end by a hand control. The accessories illustrated show lithotomy stirrups and shoulder rests. This operation table is illustrated as a neurosurgical chair in Figure 4.16.

Fig. 4.3 General operation table. Matburn 'break back' type. (Matburn Surgical Equipment Ltd.)

It is essential that all members of the theatre staff familiarise themselves with the operation table and its accessories which must be easily available and ready for immediate use. The whole apparatus must be maintained in good working order and checked before each operation list.

Fig. 4.4 The Kifa H3 operation table base is the latest version of the Kifa electro-hydraulic table. Everything is contained in the rectangular base – there is no remote pump unit or control panel built in the wall. The Kifa operation table top is interchangeable between the fixed base and a transfer trolley. This trolley is used to transport the patient between the changeover area and the operating theatre. It avoids unnecessary lifting for the patient is placed on the table top on entering the operating suite and remains on it until leaving.

Fig. 4.5 The Vac-Pac surgical positioning system consists of a set of five Vac-Pacs used to immobilise precisely the patient's body and extremities in any position desired. Each Vac-Pac is a soft, conductive plastic pad filled with a very fine granular material. An exhaust valve is attached. Before air is evacuated, the Vac-Pac is soft and can be moulded like a pillow around any part of the patient's body. When the patient is in the exact position desired, a vacuum tube is attached to the exhaust valve using pipeline suction (or any convenient vacuum source). As air is exhausted from the Vac-Pac, atmospheric pressure presses the granular filler together to form a solid mass. Within a few seconds the Vac-Pac becomes firm – almost like a plaster cast. The vacuum tube is then removed and the patient is held in perfect position. For re-use, the Vac-Pac can be returned instantly to its original soft condition by squeezing the valve and releasing the vacuum. (Howmedica U.K. Ltd.)

POSITIONS USED FOR SURGERY

Careful and correct positioning of the patient is very important, not only to provide good access for surgery but to prevent harm to the patient due to pressure, especially on nerves and bony prominences. These positions which are described can only be learned by repeated practical demonstrations, but the illustrations show essential points to be noted for various operations. The drapes have been omitted in order that these points are easily discernible (Jolly, 1950; Houghton and Hudd, 1967; Pearce, 1967; Ballinger *et al.*, 1972).

Supine or dorsal recumbent position

This and most of the following positions are demonstrated on a combined general and orthopaedic operation table which incorporates the majority of the features described already, plus accessories for orthopaedic procedures.

Fig. 4.6 Supine or dorsal recumbent position. Plaistow 'all purpose' operation table. (M.S.A. Ltd.)

The position is used for many operations, including those on the eye, ear, face, chest, abdomen, legs or feet, and with modifications is suitable for operations on the breast and arms or hands, which may be placed across the chest or extended on an arm table.

Operations on the flexed knee are performed by lowering the foot end of the table with the division between the centre and foot sections situated at the point of knee flexion. Alternatively the foot end of the table can be removed completely.

An anaesthetic screen can be used for this and other positions when it is desirable, for local anaesthetics, or to isolate the anaesthetist from the operative field (Chapter 9, Fig. 9.13).

Important points

1. The arms should be at the sides and secured by L-shaped arm retainers which are slipped under the mattress. This applies unless of course otherwise indicated by surgery or for transfusion. Alternatively the arms may be secured across the chest by pinning the operation gown around them.

2. Pressure points to watch and protect with folded towels or soft pillows are: the heels and the forearms where the arm retainer is in contact with the skin. A soft pillow behind the knees (which should be slightly flexed) will prevent hyperextension of the knee joints which may have painful consequences postoperatively.

Trendelenburg position

This position, a modification of supine, is used for intrapelvic operations, the object being to allow the intestines to displace away from the pelvic cavity by gravity towards the upper abdomen. They may then be packed off readily to leave easier access to the pelvic organs.

Fig. 4.7 Trendelenburg position.

IMPORTANT POINTS

1. The arms are at the sides and secured in the usual manner.
2. The flexion of the knees must be directly over the junction of the foot and central sections of the table.
3. Pressure points to watch and protect are: the heels, leg strap (folded towel between the strap and legs has been omitted from the illustration in order to show the heel pad), behind the knees and the shoulders.

The well-padded shoulder rests must be positioned to the point of the shoulders. On no account must they be placed at the root of the neck, because this would cause pressure upon the brachial plexus and result in paralysis. These rests must prevent the patient from slipping and becoming suspended by flexed knees, which would cause pressure on the lateral popliteal nerve.

Alternatively, well-padded pelvic supports or a Langton Hewer corrugated ribbed mattress (in direct contact with the patient's exposed skin) may be used to retain the patient in position. These avoid the danger of pressure on the brachial plexus.

Gall-bladder and liver position

This is another modified supine position which is used for operations on the gall-bladder or liver. The patient is positioned over the back elevator which is raised to produce extension, and thereby push the gall-bladder towards the anterior abdominal wall. One arm is shown extended on an arm table for transfusion. Alternatively the patient can be positioned over the hinged section of a 'break back' table which when flexed produces a similar effect.

IMPORTANT POINTS

1. Both arms may be secured in the usual manner, or one extended on an arm table as illustrated, but the abduction must not exceed 90 degrees to the body otherwise the brachial plexus may be stretched.

2. Pressure points to watch and protect are: the heels, behind the knees and at the point where the arm is extended from the table.

Fig. 4.8 Gall-bladder or liver position.

Lateral position of extension

This is used for operations on the kidney and chest, but may be modified slightly for operations on the hip. For the former operations the patient is positioned over the kidney

Fig. 4.9 Lateral position of extension for kidney and chest surgery.

78　　　　　　　　　　　Operating Theatre Technique

elevator which is raised to extend this region. Alternatively if an operation which incorporates a 'break back' is used, extension is achieved by positioning the patient over the division in the centre section before adjusting the angle of the table top.

For hip operations in the lateral position the patient lies on his side in a similar manner to that illustrated, but with no extension.

IMPORTANT POINTS

1. The upper arm is supported by a Carter Braine's arm support. The lower hand is placed at the side of the face and secured if necessary in the usual manner.

Fig. 4.10   Alternative lateral position of extension. (Eschmann Bros. & Walsh Ltd.)

Fig. 4.11   Lithotomy position. Alpha operation table. (Eschmann Bros. & Walsh Ltd.)

2. The underneath leg is flexed under the upper which is kept straight and secured to the table top with a padded bandage.

3. The patient is supported by pelvic and chest supports, which are well padded, and for additional security a bandage (padded strap or adhesive strapping) may be placed round the thighs and table top.

4. Pressure points to watch and protect are: the heels, between the legs, under the thigh retainer, upper and lower arms.

Lithotomy position

This is used for operations on the external genital organs, perineum and anal region. The buttocks project well over the edge of the table at the junction of the centre and foot section which is lowered or removed. The legs are flexed at the hips and knees, and raised with the feet supported in webbing slings suspended from the lithotomy poles. A douching funnel may be fitted below the perineal area.

IMPORTANT POINTS

1. The arms are secured in the usual manner.
2. The patient is first placed supine on the table and is then lifted down until his buttocks are at the edge of the centre section (foot section lowered or removed). *Both* legs are then flexed at the same time, abducted and secured by the webbing slings outside the poles.
3. Pressure points to watch and protect are: the forearms, buttocks and inner aspects of the thighs, which must be protected from pressure by the poles with pads of gamgee or sponge rubber. Note that the lithotomy poles are padded with sponge rubber to minimise still further any pressure on the patient's legs.

Breast and axilla position

This is the position for operations on the breast and axilla. It is a modified supine position, either with both arms extended and secured on arm tables, or one arm secured and the other on the affected side supported by a nurse (Chapter 5).

Fig. 4.12 Position for operations on the breast or axilla.

IMPORTANT POINTS

1. The extended arms must not be abducted more than 90 degrees to the body.
2. Pressure points to watch and protect are: the heels, behind the knees and at the point where the arms are extended from the table.

Neck position

This position is used for operations on the neck, especially thyroidectomy and tracheostomy. The patient is placed in the supine position with a pillow or sandbag under the shoulder blades, and the head is held by a nurse or assistant with the neck well extended. Alternatively, a padded horse-shoe provides a good support for the head in such operations. If local anaesthesia is being used, e.g., for tracheostomy, further restraint may be required and the patient is held by another assistant who immobilises him by the arms and thighs.

Fig. 4.13 Positions for operations on the neck.

IMPORTANT POINTS

1. The head must be held exactly in the mid-line with the chin upwards and the neck extended.
2. The arms are secured in the usual manner unless being restrained by an assistant.
3. Pressure points to watch and protect are: the heels, behind the knees, the arms where they are secured, between the shoulder blades, and the occiput if the operating time is lengthy.

Supine cranial position

This is used for frontal craniotomy and may be modified for parietal operations by rotating the head to one side. The patient's head is supported by a cranial support, and his thorax by the shoulder supports in conjunction with small pillows.

IMPORTANT POINTS

1. The degree of flexion or extension of the neck depends upon the surgeon's wishes and the most suitable position for maintenance of a clear airway.

2. The arms are secured in the usual manner (transfusions are generally administered via a vein in the foot during cranial operations).

3. Pressure points to watch and protect are: the heels, behind the knees, between the shoulder blades and the arms where they are secured.

Prone cranial position

This position is used for cerebellar operations and high cervical laminectomy. Some reverse Trendelenburg tilt is used and a padded strap placed round the thighs and the table top for additional security. The shoulders and thorax are supported by shoulder supports in conjunction with small pillows.

Fig. 4.14 Frontal cranial position (modified supine).

Fig. 4.15 Prone position for cerebellar and high cervical operations.

IMPORTANT POINTS

1. The degree of flexion or extension of the neck depends upon the surgeon's wishes and the most suitable position for maintenance of a clear airway.

2. The arms are secured in the usual manner.

3. Pressure points to watch and protect are: the feet (the toes must project either over the foot end of the table or a soft pillow sufficiently large to prevent them being compressed against the table top), under the strap, the arms where they are secured, and the shoulder supports which must be positioned to the points of the shoulders and not pressing on the root of the neck.

Sitting cranial position

This is a position for cerebellar cranial operations and high cervical laminectomy and is an alternative to that described in Figure 4.15. The patient is sitting and stabilised by the cranial support. The hands are placed in the lap and the body immobilised by securing the arms with body supports which are attached to the operation table at each side. These have been omitted in the illustration in order to show the position of the arms.

Fig. 4.16 Sitting position in neurosurgical chair. Matburn 'break back' table.
(Eschmann Bros. & Walsh Ltd.)

IMPORTANT POINTS

1. The weight of the patient must not be entirely supported by the cranial support. Body supports must be used to retain the patient in what would be a fairly comfortable position if he were conscious.

2. The degree of flexion of the neck depends upon the surgeon's wishes and the most suitable position for maintenance of a clear airway.

3. Pressure points to watch and protect are: the heels, behind the knees, the buttocks and the arms (which are protected by small pillows or folded towels).

Supine hip position

This is used mainly for nailing a femoral neck fracture, but is suitable for osteotomy, slipped femoral epiphysis, etc. The patient is in a supine position, with his pelvis supported by a supplementary table top which is translucent to X-rays and incorporates a slot for introducing anterior position film cassettes under the pelvis. The lower section of the table is removed, the feet are secured to foot pieces and traction applied to both legs. Counter traction is obtained against a perineal post fitted at the pubis. Body supports are needed only when lateral tilting of the table top is necessary in order to obtain greater exposure of the hip being operated on.

Two X-ray machines are positioned to obtain anterior and lateral position X-rays. The lateral film cassette is fitted into a holder at the side of the patient, corresponding to the hip being operated on. Any lateral tilting would be away from this side.

Fig. 4.17 Femoral neck fracture, position for nailing and other orthopaedic procedures. (Eschmann Bros. & Walsh Ltd.)

IMPORTANT POINTS

1. Both arms are placed across the chest or one is extended on an arm table for transfusion purposes.

2. The degree of abduction of the legs depends on the surgeon's wishes but must be adequate to allow positioning of the lateral X-ray machine. In the case of femoral neck fractures the foot on the affected side is usually internally rotated.

3. Pressure points to watch and protect are: where the feet are secured in the leather boot attachments, the buttocks (supported by a sponge rubber pad), the perineum, the arms and, if lateral tilting is used, at each body support.

Knee/elbow (rabbit) position

This is an alternative to lateral position (described under spinal puncture, Chapter 10) for lumbar laminectomy and removal of prolapsed intervertebral disc. The patient kneels with his head and arms supported on a pillow, and his body stabilised with body supports at each side of the table. For additional security a bandage or adhesive strapping may be placed round the thorax and table top.

Fig. 4.18 Knee/elbow (rabbit) position for laminectomy.

IMPORTANT POINTS

1. The pillow under the thorax and the retaining bandage may require adjustment in order that the patient's respiratory excursions are not impeded in any way. It may be necessary to use a pillow under the upper part of the chest and head only to leave the abdomen free for excursion.
2. The foot section of the table is lowered or removed, and the feet must project slightly beyond to avoid pressure on the toes.
3. Pressure points to watch and protect are: the insteps, between the thighs and the lower legs.

Jack knife position

One of the positions for rectal surgery or occasionally for lumbar laminectomy.

The patient should be placed in prone position with hips directly over the break in the foot section of the table. The arms should be flexed around the head of the patient and the lower part of the legs supported by a foot extension piece. The whole table is tilted into reverse Trendelenburg to the desired position.

IMPORTANT POINTS

1. A small pillow should be placed under the symphysis to avoid undue pressure and,
2. The patient's weight should be so balanced as to avoid pressure on the knees.

Fig. 4.19 Jack knife position for rectal surgery. (Drayton Castle Ltd.)

Endoscopy position

This is a modification of supine position. The head is raised slightly and the endoscope introduced into the pharynx. The head is supported by an assistant and the upper part of the table lowered. The endoscope is introduced with the head held in the degree of flexion or extension required by the surgeon. In the case of an oesophagoscope the head is lowered so that the oesophagus, pharynx and mouth are in a straight line. In the case of a bronchoscope the head is turned to the side opposite to that of the bronchus being examined.

Some surgeons use a Haslinger head support which enables these extension and flexion manoeuvres to be accomplished by turning a hand wheel.

REFERENCES

BALLINGER, W. F., TREYBAL, J. C. AND VOSE, A. B. (1972) *Alexanders Care of the Patient in Surgery*. St Louis: Mosby.
HOUGHTON, M. AND HUDD, J. (1967) *Aids to Theatre Technique*, 4th edn, chap. 4. London: Baillière, Tindall and Cassell.
JOLLY, J. D. (1950) *Operating Room Procedures for Nurses*, 3rd edn, London: Faber.
PEARCE, E. (1967) *Instruments, Appliances and Theatre Technique*, 5th edn. London: Faber.
YEAGER, M. E. (1966) *Operating Room Manual*, 2nd edn, chap. 3. New York: Putnam.

5
PREPARATION OF THE OPERATING THEATRE AND STERILE SUPPLIES

Preparation of personnel

No one should enter the operating section without changing into suitable protective clothing and operating theatre footwear such as canvas shoes, rubber boots or sandals reserved exclusively for the purpose. This rule must apply equally when there are no operations in progress, for outside shoes and ordinary clothing will carry contamination by bacteria into the suite (Ballinger *et al.*, 1972; Ministry of Health, 1959; Medical Research Council, 1968).

Personnel preparing for operations wear caps and masks in addition to suitable clothing and footwear. Ward staff and visitors are similarly attired during operations.

Research has proved that personnel should *not* take pre-operative showers. This apparently causes shedding of minute skin particles for a period of two hours afterwards, thereby increasing the risk of bacterial dissemination, particularly staphylococcus (Bethune *et al.*, 1965; Medical Research Council, 1968).

Surgeons, anaesthetists and male staff wear a poplin scrub suit which obviates the need for an additional gown when not assisting at operation. Although white is the traditional colour for this apparel, grey or blue is less tiring to the eyes. Green is acceptable also, but it does not provide any contrast between the clean and sterile fields. It is important to ensure that a person wearing a sterile gown is adequately covered. If the scrub suit is the same colour this makes it more difficult to observe.

Female personnel should wear a suit also, for it has been proved bacteriologically that suits minimise bacteriological dissemination compared with the standard dress in general use (Hill *et al.*, 1974; Mitchell and Gamble, 1974). Ideally the trousers and sleeves should have stockinette cuffs to restrain skin particles from axillae and perineum. The suit is best made from a closely woven poplin or fabric such as Ventile or Scotchguard (Speers *et al.*, 1965; Blowers and McCluskey, 1966; Le Bourdais, 1975); non-woven disposable material has also been proved of value (Mitchell *et al.*, 1978; Whyte *et al.*, 1978; Lidwell *et al.*, 1978). Alternatively, well-fitting dresses are better than gowns.

The hair should be covered with a closely fitting cap. This can be made from a short length of stockinette, secured at one end with a rubber band and worn like a ski-ing cap. There are specially shaped caps such as the Johnson 'J' or 'M' cap or those of the disposable paper or non-woven fabric type.

Masks are probably the greatest potential source of infection. The traditional mask of four to six layers of muslin offers very limited protection. When first worn it may be reasonably efficient but soon becomes saturated with moisture vapour from the wearer's breath.

The most efficient mask is of the high filtration disposable type of which there are several varieties. These masks should be moulded to facial contours and actually filter the respirations as compared to deflection with paper or cellophane insert types. It is claimed that such masks achieve a 98 per cent efficient filtration as compared with only 40 per cent with the muslin mask (Ford *et al.*, 1967; Furuhashi, 1978). Examples of these are the Bardic (C. R. Bard International Ltd.), the Aseptex or Filtron (3M) and the Surgine (Johnson and Johnson).

When removing a mask, care should be taken to avoid touching that part which has acted as the filter, for the hands can easily become contaminated with bacteria. Masks should be changed at least every operating session and should *never* be worn 'around the neck'. Mask 'wiggling' is also a potential source of infection (Schweizer, 1976).

Fig. 5.1 Poplin suit for theatre nurses.

Preparation of the operating theatre

Before an operating list, equipment is checked by the senior operating theatre nurse or the scrub nurse who also selects sterile packets, or may prepare instruments and special apparatus for sterilisation. Special attention is given to the operation table and accessories to ensure that these are correct and in working order. The shadowless light and other mobile light fittings are inspected for illumination and focus. All electromedical apparatus such as the diathermy and suction machines or pipeline suction set are switched on and tested as described in the chapter on electricity.

Anaesthetic equipment is checked by the anaesthetic nurse or technician, under the ultimate supervision of the person in charge. Vital inspection includes gas cylinders, soda lime canisters, lamps and batteries of laryngoscopes, etc., and the replenishment of drugs required by the anaesthetist.

The junior staff or auxiliaries are responsible for damp dusting all equipment particularly the shadowless light fitting and ledges, etc., within the suite, followed by cleansing of the floor before sterile trolleys are prepared (Minter, 1952). They should replenish supplies of sterile nail brushes, scrub solution, gown packets and supplementary items. The necessary number of bottles or flasks of sterile saline or water for hand-lotion bowls are placed in the warming cupboard until the correct temperature has been reached. Replenishment of bandages, strapping, splints and lotions, etc., should be arranged before the operation list commences.

Preparation of instrument trolleys

Instrument trolleys should be prepared *immediately before* an operation. It is a bad practice to prepare all trolleys required for a list in advance, for even if they are covered carefully, it is impossible to guarantee sterility when required later.

All surfaces of trolleys and tables which are to be used for setting out sterile instruments and apparatus should first be covered with a sterile impervious material before the application of sterile towels. This will prevent contamination of apparatus occurring should the sterile towels become soiled or wet. Suitable materials are disposable water-repellent paper sheets and proofed fabrics such as Ventile and Scotchguard.

After the instrument trays have been placed on the trolleys aseptically, the instruments are laid out by a nurse wearing sterile gown and gloves. It is a thoroughly bad practice for an 'unsterile' person to complete this arrangement using Cheatle transfer forceps, because of the great risk of contamination occurring when ungloved hands are moved to and fro over the sterile trolley. There is no place in a modern operating suite for use of sterilised forceps stored half submerged in a container of disinfectant.

Comprehensive sterile packets containing all the necessary equipment, and incorporating trolley drapes which fall into position as the packet is opened, will shorten the time taken for preparation and minimise bacterial contamination before operation (p. 101).

The scrub nurse

The nurse or technician acting as scrub nurse, scrubs up carefully, covers her operating theatre clothing with a sterile gown, and hands with sterile gloves. When scrubbing up, care must be taken to ensure that all parts of the hands and forearms are cleansed thoroughly, special attention being given to the nails and between the fingers.

It is important that no person should scrub unless he is free from upper respiratory infection and skin lesions. Cuts and abrasions or infected pimples can endanger the patient by increasing the possibility of infection.

Present-day opinion generally approves of a surgical scrub or wash which lasts no longer than five minutes. The conventional nail brush and soap technique is followed by a rinse containing 1 per cent Hibitane in methylated spirit. However, too much brushing tends to injure the surface of the skin and predisposes towards cross infection. It has been shown that the use of nail brushes can be limited to the nails only, providing a hexachlorophane solution such as PHisoHex, Disfex, or a povidone solution such as Betadine is used as a presurgical wash. Alternatively, polyurethane sponges impregnated with dehydrated hexachlorophane are available (Smylie *et al.*, 1959; Lowbury *et al.*, 1964; Yeager, 1966). This wash is carried out for three minutes only and leaves the skin covered with a film of hexachlorophane which persists for some considerable time. Hexachlorophane is alcohol soluble so that the final spirit rinse must be omitted. The hands must be dried with a sterilised towel before handling gown.

If brushes are used for scrubbing they should be a good quality nylon bristle with grooved plastic backs and of a size to fit the hand easily. They should be sterilised in metal dispensers that fit wall brackets and which permit the extraction of single brushes without contaminating the others.

Preparation of the Operating Theatre and Sterile Supplies

Fig. 5.2(A) When using ordinary soap the scrub-up or presurgical wash should last at least five minutes under running water. Less time is required when a hexachlorophane-containing soap solution (e.g. PHisoHex) is used. With these the forearms and hands are washed for one minute with a small quantity of the solution and then rinsed. (B) Particular attention is then paid to the nails, utilising either a sterilised nail-brush with light friction or orange-stick which is then discarded. (C) The main wash should occupy a further full two minutes and consists of reasonably vigorous massage of the hands and forearms up to elbow level with a mixture of solution and water as shown. Care must be taken to ensure adequate cleansing between the digits and skin folds. (D) Finally the hands and forearms are rinsed thoroughly under running water. The taps are turned off with the elbows and the hands kept in an elevated position to prevent water running down from the elbows. The hands and forearms should then be dried with a sterile towel before assuming the sterile gown and gloves. The hands must not be rinsed in spirit following this technique (Royal Berkshire Hospital, Reading).

As it is impossible to render the hands sterile, they must not come into contact with any part of the outside of the gown or gloves. The correct method of putting on gown and gloves in this way is illustrated. Nurses scrubbing up to assist at operations should keep their nails short and endeavour to avoid handling contaminated objects at all times, especially immediately before scrubbing up.

The scrub nurse is responsible for selecting, checking and arranging instruments required on the instrument table. She is responsible also for accounting for all instruments, needles and swabs or sponges at any stage of the operation, especially before any cavity is closed, and must inform the surgeon that these three items are correct, even though he may not ask. It is her duty also to prepare the ligatures and sutures, having them ready immediately when required.

A good scrub nurse will learn to anticipate a surgeon's needs, often having an instrument ready before being asked for it. Sometimes it may be necessary for the instrument nurse to act as surgeon's assistant in the absence of a house surgeon. The most advantageous way of placing the towels in position and assisting the surgeon are dealt with in a later chapter.

Fig. 5.3 Drying hands. (A) Both hands are dried with one towel. (B) The same towel is used to dry one forearm, taking care to avoid contamination of the hand. (C and D) The second towel is used to dry the other forearm. Nurse is wearing non-woven fabric disposable suit (Surgikos). (Royal Berkshire Hospital, Reading.)

The theatre runners or circulating nurses

In addition to the scrub nurse, one or two nurses or technicians are detailed to act as circulators. One nurse stays in the operating theatre, watching the scrub nurse and ready to bring anything she requires. Dispensing articles from sterile bags or packets, she replenishes sterile gowns and gloves on a sterile trolley or work top reserved for the purpose. It is incorrect for gowns and gloves to be removed from sterile containers by the hands of the operation team, even after the most thorough scrubbing.

The first circulating nurse also ties up the gowns, being careful to avoid touching any of the gown other than the tapes. She replenishes sterile warm or cold water in the lotion bowls and checks the swabs, displaying them on the counting rack in the required order.

The main duties of the second circulating nurse are to see that the instruments and trolleys are ready for the next case, and she should help in placing the patient on the operation table if a porter or technician is not available. She should also help the scrub nurse if the first circulating nurse has to leave the theatre, for on no account must it be left without one circulator.

Fig. 5.4 Correct method of putting on a sterile gown. (A and B) Ordinary gown without back panel. (C, D and E) The back panel which covers the unsterile tape is secured with the assistance of another 'scrubbed' person. (Royal Berkshire Hospital, Reading.)

It is impossible to define in a textbook the exact duties of circulating nurses. These duties will, of course, depend on the layout and system of particular operating departments.

All notes and X-rays relating to the patient must be available and it is the duty of the operating theatre staff to ensure that these are easily at hand.

The ward staff

Case notes and X-rays should be brought to the operating department by the ward nurse accompanying the patient. She must be able to answer the questions of the theatre nurse or anaesthetist regarding the pre-operative preparation of the patient, especially the premedication, the nature of the drug, the time it was given, whether urine has been passed and the time the patient last ate. After changing into protective clothing, ideally she stays with her patient as the anaesthetic is being administered. This may not always be possible in large operating departments, especially if there is a staff shortage on the ward. In this event, the ward nurse must convey all possible information regarding the patient to a member of the operating department staff at the point of check and transfer to the sterile area (MDU/Rcn, 1977).

Fig. 5.5 Showing open method of putting on sterile gloves. (A) The packet containing the gloves is first peeled open by the circulating nurse. (B) Powdering the hands – away from the sterile gloves. (C) Inserting first hand, holding by inside of cuff only. (D) Inserting second hand; glove on first hand in contact with *outside* of second glove only. (E) The cuff of the second glove is pulled over the stockinette sleeve. (F) The remaining cuff is pulled over the stockinette sleeve.

Preparation of the Operating Theatre and Sterile Supplies 93

Where the operation table is easily mobile, and in a busy operating suite where two or more tables are available, the patient may be placed on the table in the anaesthetic room or in the transfer area. In this case the positioning may be accomplished in the anaesthetic room before entering the theatre, thus avoiding unnecessary disturbance in sterile areas. This system is applicable also with the Swedish Kifa operation table described in Chapter 4.

An unconscious patient should remain in the recovery area at least until his reflexes return. If, for some reason, the anaesthetist authorises the return of a patient not fully conscious to the ward, he must be accompanied by a competent nurse and a tray, containing a mouth gag, tongue forceps, box-wood wedge, vomit bowel, swabs and a small towel. The patient's gown and blankets (preferably cotton) should be ready to cover him when leaving the theatre. Handling the unconscious patient is dealt with in Chapter 10.

Fig. 5.6 Closed glove technique. (A) The hands are not pushed beyond the stockinette cuffs. (B) The left-hand glove is grasped *through* the left sleeve. (C) The glove is flipped over the wrist and (D) grasped by the second hand (through the gown sleeve). (*cont'd*)

94　Operating Theatre Technique

Details of the operation, together with any special instructions regarding the patient's post-operative care, are conveyed to the ward sister either by the ward nurse who has stayed in theatre, or by the nurse designated to return with the patient after operation. These instructions should be written down to ensure accuracy.

Swab checking and operation register

It is essential to adopt safeguards against failure to remove swabs, etc. from patient (MDU, Rcn., 1977). Whatever system of swab or sponge checking is in force, it should be the practice to record the check in a register or on a record sheet attached to the patient's notes. The system, of course, will vary according to the method of checking, but it is necessary to state the total number of swabs used during an operation and to have the signatures of the scrub nurse and the circulating nurse, one of whom should be

Fig. 5.6 (cont'd)　(E) After stretching the cuff the glove is pulled over the sleeve and (F) the hand is forced through the stockinette cuff into the glove. (G) The second glove is put on in a similar manner except that one side of the cuff can be grasped with the already gloved hand and (H) the right hand is forced through the stockinette cuff into the glove. (Figs. 5.6 and 5.7 reproduced by courtesy of the Pioneer Rubber Co. Ltd., U.S.A.)

a registered nurse. Any mistakes made in this register must be rectified immediately by re-writing the whole entry before recording the next swab check (Fig. 5.8).

All swab checking systems, however efficient, are dependent to a great extent on the human elements, but certain precautions will help to avoid accidental discrepancies in the actual count.

No Loose Swabs should be allowed in the theatre, with the exception of those used by the anaesthetist which are dyed a distinctive colour. Swabs needed for dressings must be packed in fixed numbers in a dressing packet and are not introduced into the sterile area until required. Swabs used for operation are made into packets also and are checked very carefully both before and after they are used.

Fig. 5.7 Method of gloving a second person. (A) The cuff is stretched over the fingers of the helper, thumb of glove downwards and (B) the hand is forced through the stockinette cuff and into the glove.

A nurse should *never* bring an unsterile or loose swab into the operating theatre for any purpose. For wiping a surgeon's brow a small towel should be used, whereas for the mopping of a small area of bloodstained or soiled floor a clean mop or cloth is preferable. Similarly, a circulating nurse should *never* remove a swab from the theatre without permission of the scrub nurse. It is often the odd swab removed or introduced accidentally which is the cause for concern during a count.

Swab Location. This is very important and any swab which is packed into a wound and left in position for any period must have a suitable length of tape or thread attached to one corner, e.g. tonsil swabs 15 cm by 2·5 cm (6 in by 1 in). This tape or thread is clipped with a haemostat and indicates the presence of a swab.

The swabs must be prepared from gauze which contains a continuous strand of barium (Raytec, Chex, etc.) and if there is any doubt regarding a missing swab, an X-ray can be taken before the wound is closed. The presence of a swab is indicated by the X-ray shadow of a barium strand. This is, of course, an additional safeguard and should not replace an efficient swab-checking system.

Large quantities of swabs may be used during a major procedure and even with the most careful swab count, with numbers reaching three figures, theoretically it is possible to lose a complete packet of swabs. There is a further safeguard, available commercially, which minimises this possible danger.

Date	Name	Hosp. No.	AGE	Ward	Operation	Surgeon Assistant	Anaesthetist Assistant	Instrument Nurse/Assistant	Circulating Nurse/Assistant	Time On	Signature	Time Off	Signature	Serial Number
1.3.79	John Brown	Z3265	22	A2	Laparotomy	Mr Jones / Dr Stevens	Dr Green / Dr Fells	S/N George	S/N Broad	—	—	—	—	1001
1.3.79	Mavis South	D2323	39	B3	Herniorraphy	Mr Jones / Dr Stevens	Dr Fells	ODA Smith	S/N Brown	—	—	—	—	1002
1.3.79	Michael West	B5679	56	A2	Varicose Vein Stripping	Dr Stevens / Dr Howe	Dr Fells	S/N George	S/N Broad	—	—	—	—	1003
1.3.79	Jack Dunn	C1212	62	E1	Arthroplasty of Hip	Mr Bones / Dr Oseous	Dr Hard / Dr Tims	S/N Ward / S/N Evans	ODA Smith	—	—	—	—	1004
1.3.79	William White	A2215	20	E1	Menisectomy	Mr Bones / Dr Oseous	Dr Hard	S/N Evans	ODA Smith	11.30	ODA Brown	11.50	ODA Brown	1005
														1006
														1007
														1008
														1009
														1010

Fig. 5.8 Sample page from a swab and instrument check register which records application of tourniquets also.

Mölnlycke of Sweden market pre-packed swabs incorporating a check mark on the outside of the packet. This check mark, which indicates the quantity of swabs contained within the packet can be torn into two halves. One half is retained by the scrub nurse and the other displayed in the swab check area. When the count is made, in addition to checking the number of swabs, the upper and lower halves of the check marks are compared to confirm the number of packets of swabs in use.

If Mölnlycke swabs are not available it is simple to modify the method to personal needs. Several colours of luggage type labels may be used and these are purchased with a perforation running across the centre. The number of swabs (i.e., fives) should be marked on each section together with a serial number. At operation it is simple to compare the serial numbers of each half during the swab check procedure.

Most operating departments have a special operation register into which details of the operations are entered each day. This book usually contains details of the patient, operation, surgeon and assistants, anaesthetist, anaesthetic and sometimes the name of the scrub nurse.

Fig. 5.9 The Mölnlycke check system for swabs, showing the two-part check label. (Mölnlycke Ltd.)

The preparation of dressings

At one time preparation of dressings or swabs was usually the duty of the theatre staff. Nowadays manufacturers' pre-prepared dressings are available in sizes to suit all requirements.

Swabs or sponges are prepared from gauze which may be cotton or rayon, both materials having excellent absorbency. The gauze must contain a continuous filament of X-ray opaque barium (Raytec, Chex, etc.). Available also are X-ray opaque sheets of foam cellulose which have a very high absorbency, and are very useful for abdominal packs and minute ophthalmic mops when cut to a suitable size.

Although the sizes of swabs vary enormously according to the type of operation and individual preference of the surgeon, there are some average types and sizes which are in common use.

Large Abdominal Packs. These can be made 46 cm (18 in) square, from about 36 layers of gauze. These should be stitched around the edges, and a short length of tape attached to one corner. A pair of haemostats is clipped to this tape which is left protruding when the packs are placed inside the abdomen. Soiled packs should not be washed for re-use. It has been proved that laundered packs predispose towards abdominal adhesions, probably due to detergent or soap residue.

Large Swabs or Sponges. These may be made as a pad 23 cm by 7·5 cm (9 in by 3 in) containing about 24 layers of gauze when folded, and 23 cm by 46 cm (9 in by 18 in) containing four layers when opened out. These sizes may be varied more or less as required but it is better to standardise to one size of large swab in a particular unit. Alternative sizes range from 15 cm by 10 cm to 23 cm by 23 cm (6 in by 4 in to 9 in by 9 in).

Small Swabs. These range from 5 cm square to 7·5 cm by 10 cm (2 in square to 3 in by 4 in), having about 16 layers. The important point is to ensure that there is sufficient difference of size between these and the larger types in use, to avoid any confusion during the swab checking procedure at operation.

Swabs and Packs. These should be bundled in fixed numbers (fives) by tying with thread, a narrow bandage, rubber bands or lightly stitching together. These bundles are

Fig. 5.10 (A) The empty package with attached upper half of check mark is handed to the circulating nurse. The lower half of the check label is retained in the sterile area, the empty package and upper half of the check label is handed to the circulating nurse. (Mölnlycke Ltd.) (B) When swabs are checked, the lower halves of the check marks are compared with the upper parts hanging with the swabs and a total count made of used and unused swabs. (Mölnlycke Ltd.)

checked by a second person before packing and are checked again by two persons before the operation commences. Manufacturers now supply swabs and packs already bundled in fives. (MDU/RCN, 1977).

Anaesthetic Swabs. These must be made smaller than those in general use and coloured gauze prepared by the manufacturers is available for this purpose. The size of swabs required will vary according to individual preference but a 2·5 cm (1 in) square swab is usually adequate.

If the dyed gauze is not available it may be made simply by dyeing white gauze with a weak solution of brilliant green, gentian violet, Bonney's blue or proflavine. The gauze is then dried before making into swabs. Throat packs for the anesthetist should also be made from dyed gauze 5 cm (2 in) wide by 3 m to 6 m (3 yd to 6 yd) long, depending on the thickness of gauze.

Rolls of gauze 7·5 cm or 11·5 cm (3 in or 4½ in) wide by 3 m or 4 m (3 yd or 4 yd) long made by folding 23 cm (9 in) wide gauze with a barium filament into three or two respectively are often used for packing off cavities, e.g., during gall-bladder operations or as a pack prior to the secondary suture of a septic wound. These may be used also for bandaging amputation stumps, to obtain even pressure over a skin graft although, for these purposes the gauze should not contain a radio-opaque filament.

Wool Balls, or Pieces of Gamgee. For the application of skin antiseptic, wool balls, or pieces of gamgee about 10 cm (4 in) square, are very useful for they seem to hold the skin antiseptic better than the conventional gauze swab. Although these materials are not generally used in the operation area, they must be accounted for within the swab check.

Fig. 5.11 Dissection swabs, wool ball, 'taped' swab and patties or 'bits'.
1. Compressed cotton dental rolls for dissection swabs.
2. Wool ball covered with tubular gauze.
3. 'Taped' swab with barium strand.
4. Patties made from cottonoid.
5. Pattie or 'bit' made from ribbon gauze rolled into suitable size.

It is advisable to cover the wool balls with a thin layer of gauze or a short length of tubular bandage knotted upon itself. This is especially useful when adhesive substances such as gum mastic are being used which would otherwise cause wisps of wool to adhere to the skin. These firm compact pads held in a sponge forceps form an ideal sponge for cleansing contaminated wounds.

Alternatively, polyurethane sponge cubes 4 cm (1½ in) in size are very suitable for applying skin antiseptic and withstand sterilisation quite well.

Small Dissection Swabs, 'Bits', 'Pledgets' or 'Patties'. These are used during general surgery, thoracic surgery, neurosurgery and vascular surgery.

1. Compressed dental cotton-wool rolls 9 mm by 2·5 cm (⅜ in by 1 in) securely clamped in the jaws of a haemostat may be used as dissection swabs. These require very careful checking at operation as they conflict with the radio-opague checking concept.

2. 'Bits' or 'pledgets' are prepared from pieces of Raytec, Chex, etc., gauze folded to form a mop about 1·25 cm (½ in) square.

3. 'Patties' are made from B.P.C. cotton-wool or lintine. A piece of cotton-wool about 2·5 cm (1 in) square is moistened and stitched with a length of strong black radio-opaque thread. After autoclaving these fluff out into a suitable size.

Lintine or 'Cottonoid' is supplied in sheets 31 cm by 7·6 cm (12 in by 3 in), which are cut into suitable sized 'patties'. These are stitched with a length of black thread, care being taken to avoid using actual knots to secure it in position. Knots and rough surfaces will damage delicate nerve tissue, and it is for this reason also that the 'patties' must be moistened slightly at operation.

All these small mops are made into bundles of 5 or 10 and are checked carefully before and after operation.

Wool Rolls. If required sterile these are cut to suitable size and re-rolled loosely before packing into the packets. If a high vacuum/high-pressure autoclave is available they need not be rerolled.

Sterile Bandages of all materials, especially crêpe, are frequently required and may be packed into a separate dressings packet or container. A tightly wound bandage cannot be completely sterilised because the steam will not penetrate into the actual centre of the bandage, however the outer layers coming into contact with the dressings are sterile, and are therefore preferable to non-sterile bandages.

ENT and Ophthalmic Dressings. These are prepared and generally kept in separate packets containing suitable dressings for the eye and ear, including fast-edge bandages, ribbon gauze, and eye pads made from best quality cotton-wool, covered each side with cotton bandage.

Operation linen

Operation towels, sheets and gowns are made from a strong close-weave material such as balloon fabric or repp, or a disposable non-woven fabric (paper), and may be white, although green, blue or grey is more restful to the eyes of the operation team.

It is better to minimise the number of towel sizes in an operating suite and generally three or four sizes and types will suffice. The average towel for covering a trolley should measure at least 122 cm (48 in) square, although a trolley measuring 122 cm (48 in) by 61 cm (24 in) will require an oblong towel measuring 183 cm by 152 cm (72 in by 60 in). This enables easier packet preparation by using one towel for the trolley drapes even if the trolley sizes are large.

For towelling lower limbs, these larger size towels 183 cm by 152 cm (72 in by 60 in) will be found useful also and will reduce the number of towels required to the minimum.

For abdominal surgery, there may be a preference for a large sheet measuring about 213 cm by 183 cm (84 in by 72 in) and having a longitudinal reinforced slit 31 cm (12 in) by 10 cm (4 in) placed centrally and slightly towards one end. This holed sheet or towel may be utilised also for operations in the lithotomy position, or a lateral thigh operation such as the insertion of a Smith-Peterson nail. The addition of two bag-shaped leg covers stitched to the edges of suitable holes, 30 cm (12 in) from each side of the central slit in a holed towel, obviates the need for extra towels to cover the legs in lithotomy position.

Gowns are made with long sleeves for the operation team and short sleeves for personnel who are not scrubbed up. They should be made with an overlap of material at the back which, when tied correctly, covers the unsterile tapes. This is especially useful if the surgeon turns his back to the operation area as may happen during intra-abdominal manipulations.

All linen materials should be kept in a good state of repair and examined for tears, etc., before packing in the packets or containers.

The preparation of packets

Most hospitals now use a sterile packet system. Separate linen or paper packets of sterile materials and instruments are prepared for individual operations, a fresh set of packets always being opened for each operation.

The outdated 'drum' system should now be condemned, for the risk of bacterial contamination due to ill-fitting shutters and lids is considerable. In addition, the use of a multi-item container for unwrapped items cannot guarantee sterility indefinitely especially if it remains open for a considerable period of time during an operation list. There is a version of the metal drum available called the Wessex Casket (see Chapter 6) which consists of a metal box incorporating high efficiency bacterial filters in the top and bottom panels. These filters are permeable to steam and the casket is suitable for sterilising trays of instruments. Even this is now of doubtful technique for the reasons given above.

Small items may be double wrapped and sterilised in a Bri-pac (Smith and Nephew) or Permapak (Luxan) box. The container then acts only as a dust cover until the inner packets are removed for use.

Small Towels. These are folded or rolled into a convenient size. A 'criss-cross' method of packing in boxes permits efficient air removal and steam penetration and is preferable to packing the articles in unbroken columns.

Large Towels or Abdominal Sheets. These are packed in a similar manner but it will be found advantageous to fold them in such a way that, when opened at operation, they are conveniently arranged for easy 'towelling up'.

This is accomplished (see illustrations) by folding the towels lengthways in sections about 23 cm (9 in) wide from each side to the centre. The 23 cm (9 in) wide finished folds are then folded again in 23 cm (9 in) sections equally from each end to the centre, making a folded towel about 23 cm (9 in) square which is a convenient size for packing. Towels folded in this way are less liable to become contaminated, especially in the centre, when opened out by two persons at operation.

Gowns. These are folded inside out in three or four folds, care being taken to contain all the tapes within the folds. The gowns are then rolled or folded equally from each end to the centre (see illustrations). This will ensure that when the gown is opened at operation, whichever end is grasped the gown will only unroll halfway and avoid touching the floor.

Macintoshes. In the operating theatre these have now been replaced either with a water-repellent disposable paper item or fabric such as Ventile and Scotchguard which can be laundered and re-proofed.

These items can be packed and sterilised in a similar manner to fabric towels or drapes.

Gloves. These are supplied presterilised in peel-open packets. Alternatively, if re-processing is unavoidable or special types of gloves are in use they may be put in individual packets which are placed in outer paper bags or Bripac/Permapak boxes.

Dressings and Bandages. These, including materials such as gauze and wool, are packed loosely and sterilised under the same conditions as towels and gowns.

Sterile packet systems

These methods have supplanted the use of drums and caskets. In principle they are quite simple and mean the preparation of sterile supplies either in parcels or sealed bags, the contents of which are used for one procedure only. Any supplies remaining are discarded for re-sterilisation and a fresh packet opened for the next procedure.

There are a number of different methods of packing sterile supplies, each has its advantages and disadvantages but basically all the items required for an operation are prepared together either in one or several packets, i.e., items required for an abdominal operation could be prepared as a comprehensive single set or divided into the various components as separate packets.

In the latter instance, one would contain the requisite number of gowns and small hand towels, a second rubber gloves, a third the requisite towels or drapes, swabs and gauze packs, etc., and a fourth the instruments and steam-sterilisable ligatures.

Fig. 5.12 Four stages of folding a large towel.

The packets are covered with a material which enables sterilisation to take place, acting also as a barrier to bacteria during the periods of storage before use. Amongst suitable wrapping materials are linen, crêpe paper and non-woven fabrics.

No material is ideal for wrapping all items and although it is desirable to standardise to the most suitable, two or three types may need to be utilised according to requirements. The correct gauge of linen or paper must be selected for wrapping fabrics and instruments. Paper manufacturers in the United Kingdom now conform to a Department of Health specification in respect of sterilising wrapping papers. Items must always be double wrapped to prevent contamination after sterilisation or during opening of the packet (Allen, 1965; Speers and Shooter, 1966; Medical Research Council, 1968).

Irrespective of whether the packets are prepared in a Hospital Sterilising and Disinfecting Central Sterile Supply Department unit or the Operating Suite, basic techniques are similar. Space would not permit a description of all methods in use but there are several which are more generally approved, i.e., the comprehensive Edinburgh Pre-Set Tray system prepared in a Theatre Sterile Supply Unit; modified forms of the Pre-Set

Tray system; separate drape and instrument sets and supplementary items in paper and nylon.

The Edinburgh Pre-Set Tray system (in brief)

The most logical and time-saving method is to prepare all the requirements in one comprehensive packet. This is not a new idea for it has been in use for many years particularly in the United States but there are several problems associated with the

Fig. 5.13 Four stages of folding a gown.

method. Some difficulty may be experienced after sterilisation in completely drying out a packet containing a large number of instruments combined with drapes. This is specially so in the High-vacuum/High-pressure autoclave and is due to excessive condensate forming on the instruments during the steam phase.

Secondly, unless the correct packing procedure is carried out, instruments tend to become displaced during handling and transit and this is inconvenient when the packet is opened for use.

Research conducted by the Royal Infirmary at Edinburgh revealed that if instruments and drapes are packed and sterilised on solid aluminium trays of 12 s.w.g. or 14 s.w.g. weight, there is sufficient residual heat left to vaporise this excess condensate during the drying phase.

The trays are made to conform in width and depth to the British Standard High-vacuum/High-pressure rectangular autoclaves, i.e., 66 cm by 66 cm (26 in by 26 in). The size of the trays are such to allow setting out of instruments and drapes in the order of their use. The largest size 61 cm by 61 cm (2 ft by 2 ft) is adequate for a major surgery set, the medium 61 cm by 31 cm (2 ft by 1 ft) for smaller sets and the smallest 31 cm by 31 cm (1 ft by 1 ft) is designed for other supplementary items. Full details of tray specifications are given in the Appendix.

The Edinburgh trays are ideal, particularly when a considerable number of instruments are needed in a surgery set. However, they are not absolutely essential and smaller heavy-gauge aluminium press-out trays about 4 cm (1½ in) in depth may be utilised as an alternative.

Theatre Sterile Supply Unit

This can be part of the Hospital Sterilising and Disinfecting Unit, Central Sterile Supply Department, or built adjacent to the operating suite. It is basically the same layout as any CSSD which handles the processing of ward instruments and dressings. It

Fig. 5.14 The work area of a central sterile supply department. Clean hoist to the operating theatres is in the background. (Northern General Hospital, Sheffield – Telegraph and Star Studios.)

should have a soiled truck unloading area; processing area for soiled instruments and which includes mechanical and ultrasonic washing machines; a tray assembly area; supplementary pack assembly area; soft goods supply storage area; prepared pack and tray holding area; sterilising area; processed stores area and administrative areas. Linen repair and inspection facilities may be incorporated in the unit or may form part of the hospital laundry services.

At Edinburgh a minimal amount of sterile instrument sets are stored in the operating suite. Each afternoon preceding elective surgical sessions, the operating department manager provides the service unit with a list which details surgical supplies required for each operation. General-use instrument sets are kept in the TSSU sterile store and delivered as required, while sets used in a specific theatre (e.g. cardiothoracic) are kept in the sterile storage area of the user theatre. The used sets are returned immediately to the Sterile Supply Unit, for processing and resterilisation. The operating suite does, of course, maintain a fixed stock of supplementary instrument packs for emergency use and linen packets including sterile gowns, swabs, dressings and other small items.

At the end of the operation, prior to folding over the linen covers of the trays used ready for removal from the operating theatre, the scrub nurse should dispose of any

Fig. 5.15 Dismantling the instrument trays (instruments are put into basket for washing). (ASSA Training Handbook for Sterile Supply Assistants.)

contents of gallipots, separate the used and unused instruments, collect used knife blades, broken glass vials, ligature packets and non-traumatic suture needles in a foil dish or other protective packet before placing in the paper disposal bag.

The used trays, salvaged drapes and dressings, empty hand basins, plastic bag containing the soiled swabs and the stapled paper laundry bag are collected and returned to the Theatre Sterile Supply Unit. On arrival in the unit the laundry, swab and disposal bags are marked with a serial number designated for the operation so that the bags can be identified later if an instrument is found to be missing. These are placed in the laundry-holding section until the instruments have been processed and re-set on the tray or trays used during the operation. If the loss of an instrument is not detected at the off-loading bench it certainly will be detected while the instruments are being re-set. When the instruments have been re-set and it is clear that the numbers are correct the laundry bag, disposal and swab bags are disposed of in the appropriate manner (ASSA, 1975).

Fig. 5.16 The drapes have been fixed to the tray and the assistant assembles instruments and utensils. (ASSA Training Handbook for Sterile Supply Assistants.)

Salvaged dressings and drapes are returned to the supply storage area and the tray with its linen covers is disassembled. Special instruments such as scissors, skin hooks and amputation knives are separated from the general instruments and washed separately. The remainder of the instruments are loaded into baskets for processing in the washing machine. Unused instruments are generally loaded into a separate basket and the used instruments into as many further baskets as may be required. Jointed instruments should be opened widely and those such as probes and nerve hooks which might drop out of the basket during washing can be clipped or thrust through plastic sponges to keep them within the basket.

There may be several instrument baskets per surgical operation and if the trays arrive at the service unit in rapid succession from different operating theatres, it is important to be able to distinguish instruments used at one operation from those used at another. The Edinburgh Royal Infirmary have devised a labelling system to overcome this difficulty.

Above the tray off-loading bench there is a board on which hang groups of four metal discs. The discs are marked with the operating theatre number and the serial number of the particular operation on the list. As each basket is loaded with instruments, an appropriate disc is hooked on to the rim of the basket and is left there till the instruments have been removed from the basket for re-setting at the end of the processing line. The tray checker removes the discs after checking the re-set tray. The discs are then returned to the board for further use.

Whilst the instruments are being processed the large trays are cleansed with a suitable solution such as spiritous Hibitane 0·05 per cent and then transferred to the tray assembly area on to a 61 cm by 61 cm (2 ft by 2 ft) trolley. Two layers of fabric covers, one blue and one green are arranged over both the tray and the trolley. (The different colours are to differentiate between the cover handled by the circulating nurse and the cover handled by the scrub nurse wearing sterile gown and gloves.) These covers are pushed down into the tray by a mould of appropriate size for the tray; and a spring-retaining cord is stretched over the covers into the gutter round the upper aspect of the tray.

After the instruments have been washed, ultrasonically cleansed, dried and inspected they are set out according to the particular arrangement (Fig. 5.16). The instruments are checked by two persons against a list (Fig. 5.17). A set of swabs and fabric drapes are placed over the instruments to retain them in position during transit and sterilisation (Fig. 5.18) and the covers are folded over as illustrated (Figs. 5.19, 5.20). After sterilisation, the trays are held in the processed stores area until required. If prolonged storage is necessary after sterilisation an additional plastic dust cover is used.

A modified Pre-Set Tray system

The 61 cm by 61 cm (2 ft by 2 ft) special tray is ideal, particularly when large instrument sets are needed, e.g. major laparotomy. As stated previously, if no H.S.D.U. is available the system is quite suitable for preparation and sterilisation within the operating suite. However, the autoclaves may be too small to take the large size tray and the alternative medium size, i.e., 61 cm by 31 cm (2 ft by 1 ft) may be inadequate for an average general set, or perhaps neither of these trays may be easily available. In these circumstances the Pre-Set Tray system can be introduced utilising any convenient deep aluminium tray, providing it is of sufficient gauge to retain enough residual heat for drying the instrument set during the post-steam cycle. Alternatively, cardboard or polypropylene trays may be used although prolonged drying may be necessary.

Basically the method is similar to the Edinburgh system but as the trays generally do not have the special double gutter to accommodate the spring-retaining cord one layer of fabric cover is placed *outside* the aluminium tray (Figs. 5.23E to J).

Separate drape and instrument sets

The Pre-set Tray system is only suitable when there are sufficient instruments to allow adequate time for processing and sterilisation. When this is impossible, the alternative is to sterilise the instruments separately and then add these to a suitable operation packet.

All the swabs, and drapes, are prepared in a linen or paper packet. The method of folding is basically the same as that described under the modified tray system. Packet covers should consist of not less than two layers of fabric which act as a trolley drape also.

Fig. 5.17 Two persons check the instruments against the list. (ASSA Training Handbook for Sterile Supply Assistants.)

Suitable fabrics include Repp, Ventile and Scotchguard (which are water-repellent and can be re-proofed in the hospital laundry (Brigden, 1964), see Appendix). In addition, there should be a plastic or paper outer wrap if the packet is to be stored for longer than a few hours.

Instrument trays can be wrapped as in Figures 5.23K to Q or placed in a Wessex casket and this is preferable to open trays, which require the use of Cheatle transfer forceps.

Supplementary items

Single instruments and other supplementary items such as orthopaedic implants, additional packets of swabs, etc., can be packed into small packets or paper bags. Rigid containers can be used for some instruments and for steam sterilisation are made from cardboard or polypropylene. Except for Wessex caskets, metal containers are generally only suitable for the dry heat process.

Fig. 5.18 Swabs and drapes are added to the tray. (ASSA Training Handbook for Sterile Supply Assistants.)

Packets are prepared similar to those described previously utilising a diagonal method of folding the two layers.

Paper bags can either be heat-sealed or have a plain folded top. In the former case the Kraft bag incorporates a heat-sensitive adhesive band inside the open end (Thermotop). After the contents have been placed inside, the open end is sealed by squeezing between the heated jaws of a special heat-sealing machine. The bag generally has a small panel of heat-sensitive ink which changes colour after the packet has been sterilised. If this has

Fig. 5.19 Inner wraps folded. (ASSA Training Handbook for Sterile Supply Assistants.)

not been provided a small piece of 3M indicator tape should be affixed to the bag for the same purpose. (3M indicator tape is in the form of dark stripes which appear on the surface of the tape if it has been through the sterilisation process. No 1222 is designed for steam sterilisation, No 1226 [Indair] is for dry heat and No 1224 [Indox] is for ethylene oxide.)

Folded top bags are prepared as illustrated and the folds held in position with a small piece of 3M indicator tape. The cardinal rule with paper bags is that two must always be used. The outer bag acts as a dust cover during storage so that when the inner is opened in the operation area, the possible dissipation of dust is avoided (page 118).

Polypropylene Containers are tubular in form with a perforated lid. When the items have been packed inside the tube, the perforated lid retains a two-layer paper filter which permits passage of steam but acts as a barrier to dust and bacteria during storage. The lid is sealed on with a band of 3M indicator tape.

Metal Containers are generally made from aluminium in the form of tubes or boxes. They are most suitable for dry heat sterilisable items such as osteotomes, special knives and syringes, etc., and as sterilisation is by conduction of heat the container can be sealed before processing.

Fig. 5.20 Outer wraps folded over the contents and sealed with heat sensitive tape. The set is identified by writing the name of the set on one length of tape. (ASSA Training Handbook for Sterile Supply Assistants.)

Sterilisation and storage

Sterilisation of packets is dealt with at great length in the following chapter. After sterilisation a piece of cellulose tape imprinted STERILE may be applied to the packet and stamped with the date of autoclaving. Alternatively, the date can be marked on the 3M indicator tape used to secure packet folds. This date is a guide to turnover rather than sterility.

The packets should be stored in a clean dry environment until required. If this is in the Hospital Sterilising and Disinfecting Unit and the storage is likely to be prolonged for more than a few hours, the packets should have an outer dust cover made from plastic or paper. In a properly air-conditioned operating department normally it should be unnecessary to have dust covers but the packets must be stacked carefully in rotation of sterilisation date. This ensures that none are stored for too long a period.

Fig. 5.21 Trolley loaded with theatre trays placed in sterilisation chamber. (ASSA Training Handbook for Sterile Supply Assistants.)

Packets which usually require some form of dust cover within the operating suite are items such as orthopaedic implants or specialised instruments used infrequently. In this case, if the item is small enough, Bri-pac or Permapak boxes are very suitable and enable quite a number to be stored in a small area.

A high standard of cleanliness is necessary in packet storage areas. Shelving or cupboards should be damp-dusted regularly with a suitable anti-bacterial agent (e.g., spiritous Hibitane 0·05 per cent).

Preparation for operation

The outer cover of the packet is opened by hand (Fig. 5.25A), care being taken to avoid contamination of the inner packet which is opened by the scrub nurse as illustrated. With the Pre-Set tray very little additional preparation is needed with the exception of a few supplementary items (Figs. 5.25H, 5.26 and 5.27).

Fig. 5.22 Sterilised sets on 'cooling racks'. (ASSA Training Handbook for Sterile Supply Assistants.)

Where separate drape and instrument packets are in use these are opened aseptically and transferred to the main trolley by the scrub nurse. Items in rigid tubes or paper bags should, preferably, be removed with sterile forceps by the scrub nurse (Fig. 5.26D) although they can be dropped on to a sterile surface with care.

Gown packets should be opened only to the inner layers, which are left folded for opening by the instrument nurse just before gowning up. Gloves are dispensed from individual paper bags as required (Fig. 5.5A, page 92).

Using this type of packet system, even during busy operation lists, the preparation time of trolleys is shortened considerably. Only one trolley need be prepared, the next instrument packet is opened as the next operation is ready to start. This ensures minimal bacterial contamination and reduces the rush or tension which previously tended to be present during preparations in the operating theatre.

The care of instruments and apparatus

After use the instruments should be cleansed carefully with a stiff brush under running cold water. Alternatively, an ultrasonic cleanser or mechanical washing machine

Fig. 5.23 *The modified pre-set tray system.* (A) aluminium tray placed on outer piece of blue Ventile. (B) Green trolley drape in position over aluminium tray, wooden former pushes drape flat, which is then held in position with a cord and spring. (C) Major basic instruments set out. (D) Swabs and drapes placed over instruments. This helps to retain them in position during sterilisation and handling afterwards.

(cont'd)

may be used combined with a suitable detergent solution, e.g., Neodian, Lab-brite. The process should include a cycle of cold water followed by a detergent wash and finally a very hot rinse 83°C (Fig. 5.28). Staff must be adequately protected by wearing aprons and rubber gloves.

If excessive contamination has occurred, e.g. following a septic operation, it is better to autoclave them for four minutes at 134°C before processing. However, during subsequent cleansing the instruments must still be regarded as potentially infected due to the debris adhering.

Instruments should be dried hot soon after removal from the washing machine, ultrasonic cleaner or a hot detergent solution such as 0·5 per cent cetrimide. After cleaning and drying they should always be examined carefully each time for defects, i.e., loose rivets and screws, cracking of forceps' jaws, lack of apposition between grooves and, in cutting instruments, blunt cutting edges, etc.

Debris inside joints may be removed by applying a little silicone solution such as M.S.A. 550 or instrument Lube, and 'working' the joint, which will create friction and express most dirt particles. If silicone is used the instrument must be re-washed before sterilisation.

Fig. 5.23 (*contd.*) (E) Rear part of green trolley drape folded to the front and then turned back on itself. (F) Front part of green trolley drape folded towards the back and then folded back on itself. (G) Second side fold of green trolley drape. (H) The outer blue piece of Ventile is folded as previously described.

(*cont'd*)

Sharp Instruments. These should be handled with very great care. The cutting edges of fine cataract knives, scalpels, osteotomes and gouges, etc., must not be damaged. These instruments must be dried thoroughly after use to avoid rusting, as they are often manufactured from carbon steel.

The cutting edges of knives, etc., may be examined by viewing the edge under a strong light. A sharp knife edge will appear black, but if the edge appears as a broken or continuous white line, the knife is blunt and should be discarded for resharpening.

Scissors. These should have even edges and secure rivets. Good quality scissors require only occasional sharpening, in any case the scissors remain semi-closed during sterilisation, thereby protecting the edges.

Fig. 5.23 (*cont'd*) (I) The final side folds of the blue Ventile. (J) The completed major basic instrument set ready for sterilisation. (The contents, date packed and initials of tray assembler and checker are written on the 3M autoclave tape with felt pen magic marker). (K) *Instruments packed separately to drapes*; a fracture and bone set which is wrapped in three layers, fawn and blue Ventile and Sterilwrap crêpe paper. A diagonal method of folding is used with corners turned back for easy aseptic opening at operation. The first front fold, fawn Ventile. (L) The second side fold.

(*cont'd*)

Suture Needles. These are generally available now as disposable but, if for reasons of economy, re-use is necessary, they must be washed thoroughly after use, special attention being paid to the needle eye. Rust marks should be removed with fine steel wool and soap, following which the needles are carefully dried. They are sterilised by dry heat or autoclaving (utilising a piece of anti-rust paper) after packing in paper envelopes.

Fig. 5.23 (*cont'd*) (M) Tucking in the final fold, fawn Ventile. (N) The blue Ventile layer is folded in a similar manner. (O) The final paper layer folded diagonally as before, first side fold. (P) The front paper fold. (Q) The completed packet ready for sterilisation. This paper layer is required only if the packet is being sterilised outside the operating suite. Note the packet is tied with cotton tape and a piece of 3M indicator autoclave tape has been applied.

Needles having blunt or rough edges should not be kept for further use and must be discarded.

Syringes and Hypodermic or Serum Needles (Non-disposable). These are rinsed thoroughly after use. Care must always be taken to remove blood from the inside of barrels and needles otherwise it will be impossible to sterilise them. An ultrasonic cleanser or good non-pyrogenic detergent such as Neodian, Lab-brite, etc., should be used, and the needles checked for blockage by passing a stilette through.

Fig. 5.24 *Supplementary items in Kraft paper bags.* (A) Folded top – first diagonal folds. (B) Second fold. (C) Final fold which is held in position with (D) a piece of 3M autoclave tape.

Fig. 5.25 *Opening sterile packets at operation.* (A) The outer crêpe paper layers are opened, utilising the turned-back diagonal corners. (B) The inner blue layer is also opened by the circulating nurse, fold one.

(*cont'd*)

Glass/metal special syringes are always dismantled before sterilisation; the different degrees of expansion between the metal and glass will cause cracking of the barrel. *All glass* syringes are sterilised assembled in the dry-heat oven or infra-red apparatus, and unassembled in the autoclave, as in the latter case it is possible that sufficient moist heat will not reach the piston of an assembled syringe.

With the exception of syringes having interchangeable barrels and pistons, care must be taken to avoid the exchange of components. Manufacturers generally engrave corresponding numbers or letters on the pistons and barrels to ensure correct assembly. Incorrect assembly may result in an ill-fitting piston.

If the syringes are to be sterilised by the dry-heat method, after cleaning they should be carefully dried inside and out with acetone or ether before *very lightly* lubricating the piston with sterile liquid paraffin or silicone solution. Silicone solution is preferable if the syringes are sterilised assembled as it obviates the risk of pistons becoming jammed in the barrel. They may then be sterilised in packets, metal containers or glass tubes.

Fig. 5.25 (*cont'd.*) (C) Opening the second side fold. (D) The final blue fold which exposes the innermost fawn wrapped package. (E) The scrub nurse lifts out the inner package (which contains a hand lotion bowl set complete with bowl stand drape). (F) Grasping the topmost part of the drape, the scrub nurse lowers the bowl and drape into the lotion bowl stand.

(*cont'd.*)

Some special instruments such as cystoscopes, laryngoscopes and other endoscopic apparatus are made heat-sterilisable today, but manufacturers' instructions regarding sterilisation should be followed carefully. Endoscopes may be disinfected by 'pasteurisation' or sterilised, or in a chemical solution, e.g., Cidex, Hibitane 0·5 per cent. Sterilisation can be achieved by formaldehyde at subatmospheric steam pressure, or ethylene oxide vapour can also be used if suitable apparatus and bacteriological control is available (Medical Research Council, 1968).

After use, endoscopes are cleansed carefully, first under cold running water, and then in a hot detergent solution, special attention being given to the inside tube. A cotton-wool swab on a metal probe or a pipe cleaner will be found useful for cleaning and drying the inside of an endoscope. After drying, the instruments are lightly lubricated, inspected for

Fig. 5.25 (*cont'd.*) (G) The drapes are opened to cover the lotion bowl stand, (H) exposing the hand lotion bowl which is then filled with sterile water or saline. (Fig. 1.20, page 31). (I) *Opening the pre-set tray of instruments*; removing the autoclave tape after checking that it is the correct set and has been autoclaved. (J) The blue layers are opened by the circulating nurse.

(*cont'd.*)

general defects, including the lamps and lamp carriers which are tested before putting them away (see Chapter 13).

Non-disposable rubber drainage or suction tubing is washed through with cold water after use. The lumen of suction tubing can easily become blocked with hardened blood and debris caused by inefficient cleansing and repeated sterilisation. To avoid this, the tubing should be rolled between the hand and a board, or stretched in sections to dislodge any particles adherent to the lumen wall. The tubing is then flushed by attaching it to a pressure nozzle or tap and forcing cold water through it.

Following this, the tubing is washed with hot detergent solution and hung up to dry partially before sterilisation.

In most operating theatres a stock of assorted sterile drainage tubes is kept ready in plastic or paper packets. Special drains, such as Marian's suprapubic tubing for draining the bladder, may be sterilised with the instruments when they are likely to be needed during an operation.

Non-disposable Rubber Catheters are cleansed as tubing, being rinsed through from the 'eye' end. After detergent washing and drying, the surface of a catheter must be

Fig. 5.25 (*cont'd.*) (K) The inner green trolley drape is opened by the scrub nurse, the side folds. (L) The front fold of the trolley drape. (M) The rear fold is opened, note the front fold already opened protects the sterile gown of the scrub nurse as she stretches over the trolley.

examined for irregularities or deterioration and if found, the catheter should be discarded. A smooth surface is essential to avoid trauma to the delicate urethral mucosa.

Some catheters have an inflatable cuff or obturator bag which should always be tested before and after use.

Non-disposable Plastic Drainage Tubing and Catheters. Those made from vinyl resins (vinyl Portex), nylon, polythene, polypropylene, silicones and polycarbonates, are cleansed in a similar manner to rubber.

Fig. 5.26 *Supplementary items in a rigid autoclavable polypropylene tube.* (A) The autoclave tape is removed. (B) Removing the perforated lid, paper filters still in position. (C) Lifting off the paper filters, taking care not to touch the top sterile edge. (D) The contents of the tube are taken with sterile forceps by the scrub nurse.

This type of tubing should be sterilised only when needed or stored dry in sterile packets. Many catheters are now supplied disposable and sterile in a packet.

Reusable Solution Rubber Gloves. These should be washed thoroughly in cold water before removing from the hands. They should be washed again in cold water to ensure complete removal of blood stains.

If the gloves have been used for a septic case they should be discarded. Following a clean case, they are scrubbed inside and out with a detergent solution.

The gloves are then dried either by hanging up until the outside is dry, turning, and then repeating the process, or rubbing each side with a towel whilst holding them on a warm surface.

Each glove is then tested for perforations by inflating with a foot pump, twisting the wristband so that the palm and fingers are under air pressure and plunging below the surface of a fluid (Williams *et al.*, 1966). Following this the sound gloves are finally dried and lightly powdered inside. Industrial methylated spirit may be used as the testing fluid to facilitate easy drying.

Gloves with perforations should be discarded as resistant tetanus spores may remain in the patch of a rubber glove.

Tests have shown that granulomata may form in wounds if a talcum glove powder is used. Talc deposition in the wound may occur if the surfaces of gloves are inadequately wiped before operation, or if a glove should become punctured during use.

Talc-free absorbable powders containing basically either starch or magnesium are less likely to cause this complication, although by 1965 the sixteenth case of starch granuloma had been reported (Bates, 1965). If this type of powder is used (Biosorb, K285, Diastol) the minimum should be applied to the inside of the gloves only (British Medical Journal, 1973).

Fig. 5.27 *Supplementary items in folded top paper bags.* (A) 3M autoclave tape removed, opening first folds. (B) Utilising gusset to open remaining folds of bag. (C) Contents removed with sterile forceps.

After powdering, the gloves are grouped in sizes, each cuff being folded over about 6·5 cm (2½ in). They are packed as pairs in separate paper or linen bags having two compartments, one for each glove. A small green or similarly dyed swab should be placed just inside the palm of each glove to ensure adequate penetration of the steam.

Fig. 5.28 Helpex automatic washing machine for instruments and apparatus. The machine drum rotates in both directions, repeatedly plunging the moving items into a heated washing solution. Rinsing is accomplished by repeated immersion in hot water, cold water and, if desired, distilled water. Drying is accomplished by centrifuging to throw off water droplets, at the same time introducing a blast of hot (or cold) air. The cycle is controlled automatically by a punched card control system shown top left. (Siemens Medical Group.)

A small quantity of powder is required for use with each pair of gloves to lubricate the hands. This may be contained in small cellophane bags which are filled with about one teaspoonful of powder and placed *with the end open* in one compartment of the glove packet. Alternatively it is possible to purchase one brand of glove powder already packed in small sterilisable paper packets (Biosorb).

Regent, Velvex, Pioneer, etc. surgeon's disposable rubber gloves are also available. These are made from a latex rubber and are supplied presterilised together with a suitable glove powder. They are designed to be used only once for surgery but afterwards following decontamination, may be utilised in the wards and departments for non-sterile procedures.

Gum Elastic Catheters. These are rarely used as they are easily damaged and require very careful handling. They are cleansed in the usual manner, and after use *may* be submerged vertically in a suitable anti-bacterial agent such as Cidex or Hibitane 0·5 per cent. Ureteric catheters should be syringed through with a fine needle and syringe before resterilising and the lumen must be filled with the solution by means of a syringe and needle. Alternatively, subatmospheric steam/formaldehyde may be used to sterilise these types of catheters.

Sterilisation by heat is always more reliable, and if this is difficult it may be advisable to consider using catheters made of a heat sterilisable material. It is for this reason that the latest forms of plastic are being found very useful for catheters and bougies.

REFERENCES

ALLEN, S. M. *et al.* (1965) *Lancet,* **ii**, 1343.
BALLINGER, W. F., TREYBAL, J. C. AND VOSE, A. B. (1972) *Alexander's Care of the Patient in Surgery.* St. Louis: Mosby.
BATES, B. (1965) *Annals of Internal Medicine,* **62**, 335.
BRIGDEN, R. J. (1960) *The Nylon Packet System of Sterilisation.* London: Nursing Mirror.
BRIGDEN, R. J. (1964) *Nursing Times,* December 11.
BETHUNE, D. W., BLOWERS, R., PARKER, M. AND PASK, E. A. (1965) *Lancet,* **ii**, 458.
BRITISH MEDICAL JOURNAL (1973) **ii**, 502.
FALK, H. C. (1942) *Operation Room Procedure for Nurses and Internes,* 3rd edn, pp. 24, 83. London: Putnam.
FORD, C. R., PETERSON, D. E. AND MITCHELL, C. R. (1967) *American Journal of Surgery,* **6**, 787.
FURUHASHI, M. (1978) *Bulletin Tokyo Medical Dental University,* **25**, 7.
HILL, J., HOWELL, A. AND BLOWERS, R. (1974) *Lancet,* **ii**, 1131.
LE BOURDAS, E. (1975) *Dimensions in Health Services.* **52**, (2), 27 (Toronto).
LIDWELL, O. M., MACKINTOSH, C. A. AND TOWERS, A. G. (1978) *Journal of Hygiene, Cambridge,* **81**, 43.
LOWBURY, E. J. L., LILLY, H. A. AND BULL, J. P. (1964) *British Medical Journal,* **ii**, 531.
MEDICAL RESEARCH COUNCIL (1968) Aseptic methods in the operating suite. *Lancet,* **i**, 763.
MEDICAL DEFENCE COUNCIL AND ROYAL COLLEGE OF NURSING (1977) *Joint Memoranda on Safeguards to Remove Swabs,* etc.
MINISTRY OF HEALTH (1959) *Report on Subcommittee on Staphylococcal Infection in Hospitals,* p. 35. London: HMSO.
MINTER, S. (1952) *Theatre Technique for Nurses,* pp. 2, 10. London: Nursing Mirror.
MITCHELL, N. J. AND GAMBLE, D. R. (1974) *Lancet,* **ii**, 1133.
MITCHELL, N. J., EVANS, D. S. AND KERR, ANN. (1978) *Lancet,* **i**, 696.
SMYLIE, H. G., WEBSTER, C. V. AND BRUCE, M. L. (1959) *British Medical Journal,* **ii**, 606.
SPEERS, R. AND SHOOTER, R. A. (1966) *Lancet,* **ii**, 469.
SCHWEIZER, R. T. (1976) *Lancet,* **ii**, 1129.
WÄLLENBERG, E. AND JÄRNHALL, B. (1956) *Svenska Läkartidningen.* **53**, 2578.
WHYTE, W., HODGSON, R., BAILEY, P. V. AND GRAHAM, J. (1978) *British Journal of Surgery,* **65**, 469.
WILLIAMS, R. F. O., BLOWERS, R. AND GARRARD, L. P. (1966) *Hospital Infection – Causes and Prevention.*
YEAGER, M. E. (1966) *Operating Room Manual,* 2nd edn, p. 18. London: Putnam.

6
STERILISATION

An understanding of the methods adopted for the sterilisation of materials used in an operating theatre is one of the most important aspects of theatre technique.

The main method sterilisation (i.e. the destruction of all micro-organisms and spores) is by heat. However, gamma irradiation is being used for the sterilisation of catgut, catheters and bulk dressings, although at present the equipment required is not practical for general hospital use (Jefferson, 1958; Darmady et al., 1961).

Disinfection (i.e. the destruction of all micro-organisms except spores) can be achieved by pasteurisation, sub-atmospheric steam and chemicals. The addition of formaldehyde to the sub-atmospheric steam process will effect sterilisation.

A great deal of research and many tests have been made regarding the minimal times and temperatures for sterilisation by a particular method. Times and temperatures quoted allow a margin of safety and are based upon bacteriologists' recommendations.

Bacteria and their destruction

We should recall our knowledge of the bacterial structure in order to appreciate fully its destruction.

A simple bacterium consists mainly of a cell wall surrounding protoplasm, which is a suspension of proteins in a solution of organic substances and salts.

One of the easiest ways of destroying bacteria is to upset the equilibrium of the protoplasm. The simplest and surest way is to apply heat to cause some irreversible protoplasmic change within the bacterial cell. This coagulation of protein depends to a great extent on the quantity of water contained by the bacteria. Vegetative bacteria contain about 80 per cent water, and as a result their protein coagulates readily at a relatively low temperature, and they are easily destroyed by five minutes' boiling (Perkins, 1956a). However, some bacteria contain within their protoplasms, oval or spherical bodies which will survive boiling. These bodies are called spores and our aim must be to destroy all bacteria and their spores during sterilisation.

The effect of moisture on the coagulation temperature of proteins bears a relationship to the temperatures at which bacteria are destroyed. Moist heat is a more efficient sterilising agent than dry heat, and when moisture is present bacteria are destroyed at much lower temperatures and shorter times than when moisture is absent.

When dry heat is used for sterilisation the process is primarily one of oxidation. Bacteria exposed to hot air may be dehydrated greatly before the temperature can rise sufficiently to cause death by coagulation. It is for this reason the death by dry heat is regarded as a slow burning up process or oxidation.

It is inadvisable to refer to the destruction of bacteria at a certain point (thermal death point) (McCulloch, 1945). A more accurate term refers to the combination of temperature and time (thermal death time); the higher the temperature the shorter the time. Generally speaking, a temperature of 121°C at 1·05 kg per cm^2 (103·4 KN/m^2, 15 lb per square inch [p.s.i.]) of pressure steam for 15 minutes, will kill the most resistant spores. This timing commences only *when the correct temperature of steam has reached* **all** *parts of the materials being sterilised*. It is therefore considered necessary to allow a safety margin of time equivalent usually to about double the thermal death time to ensure adequate penetration of packets. However, *it is necessary to conduct individual tests to determine the penetration time with a particular type of autoclave and packet*.

Sterilisation by dry heat requires much higher thermal death times. As bacteria show a marked resistance to dry heat, a temperature in the region of 160°C and an exposure of one hour are essential. This exposure period of one hour does not, of course, include the period of time necessary for all parts of the load to reach the temperature of 160°C.

Although dry heat is destructive to rubber and fabrics, it can be used for the sterilisation of glassware and instruments, such as fine knives, made from carbon steel which may otherwise rust if exposed to moist heat, and where sterilisation of surfaces only is required.

The effect of chemicals on bacteria is rather a complex action which varies with the nature of the chemicals used. A chemical reaction occurs between the bacteria and the chemical, being dependent on several factors including temperature, chemical strength, resistance of the organism and, most important, the duration of free contact between the two. The chemical effect can be one of oxidation, halogenation, poisoning of vital enzymes, hydrolysis and coagulation.

METHODS OF STERILISATION (GENERAL PRINCIPLES)

HEAT STERILISATION

1. Autoclaving (steam under pressure).
2. Dry heat.
3. Steam/formaldehyde (at sub-atmospheric pressure).

HEAT DISINFECTION

3. Steam at sub-atmospheric pressure.
4. Pasteurisation.
5. Boiling.

COLD STERILISATION

6. Gamma-irradiation.
7. Ethylene Oxide.
8. Ultra-violet light radiation.

COLD DISINFECTION

9. Various chemical solutions.

Heat Sterilisation

1. Autoclaving

This is by far the most efficient method of sterilisation for materials that will stand up to heat and moisture (Medical Research Council, 1968).

The highest temperature that can be reached by boiling water in an open vessel is 100°C. With increased pressure, the water can be raised to much higher temperatures before it boils, e.g., at a pressure of 0.35 kg per cm^2 (34.47 kN/m^2, 5 lb p.s.i.) the temperature reaches 105·5°C; at 0·7 kg per cm^2 (68·95 kN/m^2, 10 lb p.s.i.). 115°C; and at 1·05 kg per cm^2 (103·4 kN/m^2, 15 lb p.s.i.) the temperature will reach 121°C, etc.

High pressures of steam, however, are not the only consideration for efficient sterilisation, as a pressure may be due to a mixture of air and steam with a relatively low temperature (McCulloch, 1945). It is the high temperatures that really matter but, in addition, the steam should be at a point where it has just changed from water into steam (phase boundary steam) (Walter, 1948). In this condition the steam not only has an increased temperature in relation to the pressure (sensible heat), but when it condenses on a cold surface (the materials being sterilised) a great deal of extra heat (latent heat) is given up. The latent heat absorbed by the materials being sterilised is more important for the destruction of bacteria than the sensible heat.

This steam heating of fabrics being sterilised by a process of condensation is relatively rapid (McCulloch, 1945), as compared with dry-heat sterilisation, which is slow, heat being conducted from one instrument to another and from one container to the next, etc.

The physical process of heating the fabrics to the sterilising temperature can be described as follows:

In a sterilising chamber (autoclave) which has been well exhausted of air the steam entering promptly fills the free spaces surrounding the load. As steam contacts the cool outer layers of the fabrics a film of steam condenses, leaving a minute quantity of moisture in the fibres of the fabrics. Air contained in the fabric interstices, being heavier than steam, is displaced by gravity in a downward direction, and the latent heat given off during the process of condensation is absorbed by that layer of the fabrics.

The next film of steam immediately fills the space created when the first film condensed into water, and it does not condense on the outer layer of the fabrics but penetrates into the second layer, condenses and heats it. This process continues until the whole load is heated through, and no further condensation occurs, the temperature within the packet or drum remaining at that of the surrounding steam.

If initial air elimination from the chamber is not good it will be difficult for the steam to displace air from the interstices of the fabrics, due to the small difference in density between the air pockets in the packets or drums, and the air that has gravitated below the load to the bottom of the chamber. This means that the pocketed air and steam may eventually mix, but it will be impossible to attain a sterilising temperature which is equivalent to that of the surrounding steam without prolonged exposure. A procedure involving a double- or multi-vacuum technique helps to extract this air and thoroughly heat the load before sterilisation commences. Exceptions to this rule are instruments, which require only one pre-vacuum, as the air displacement from these loads is comparatively rapid if they are packed correctly.

In the Gravity Displacement Autoclave after a partial vacuum of about 500 mm of mercury has been created, (an absolute pressure of 250 mmHg (32·8 kPa; standard atmospheric pressure being 760 mmHg), steam is admitted to the chamber and applied to the load until the selected temperature/pressure has been reached *in the chamber*. (Very low pressures are generally quoted with reference to the perfect vacuum.) Air from the interstices of the fabrics which has been displaced into the lower part of the chamber, but has not been discharged by the special thermostatic condensate release valve, is extracted by a second vacuum. A second application of steam displaces most of the remaining air pockets and thoroughly heats the load throughout to the surrounding steam temperature.

In the high-vacuum/high-pressure autoclave where an electric pump is used to obtain a vacuum, all air may be extracted in one operation, or there may be a series of pre-vacuums and steam pulsations before the sterilising cycle. This breaks down any small airpockets and results in a final pre-vacuum of about 0·5 to 1 mmHg (65·82 to 131·7 Pa).

It will be observed that the steam used for sterilisation of materials must have a certain temperature and pressure in order to be optimally effective. Furthermore, the steam must reach all parts of the load and unless packets or boxes are prepared very carefully, adequate penetration cannot be ensured. Materials should be packed with good spacing between the articles, with folds placed vertically to allow steam to pass easily in a downward direction through them, any tendency to force too many items in one packet or box being avoided. It should not be necessary to compress the box contents in order to close the lid, neither must a linen or paper packet be wrapped tightly to fit in an inadequate size of cover.

Unless a pre-set tray is used, utilising heavy-gauge aluminium trays (p. 103) it is difficult to sterilise large quantities of instruments with bulky drapes. The unequal rate of condensation between the fabrics and instruments will require an extended drying cycle.

Arrangements for the correct supply of steam and maintenance of the apparatus is not a responsibility of the nurse, but if dressings are wet or damaged when removed from the autoclave there is something wrong with the apparatus or its operation and the engineer should be consulted.

Sterilisation by autoclaving (application of methods)

Most hospitals use 'mains' steam (supplied from the boiler house) to operate autoclaves which are generally of two types, (1) the downward- or gravity-displacement type, and (2) the modern high-vacuum/high-pressure type. For hospitals without a mains steam supply, autoclaves are available that generate their own steam either by electricity or gas, and they are used in a very similar manner to the mains steam models.

The gravity-displacement autoclave

Working pressure is 1·05 kg to 2·11 kg per cm^2 (103·4 to 206·8 kN/m^2) 15 lb p.s.i. to 30 lb p.s.i., vacuum is 380 to 508 mmHg (50 to 66·54 kPa) via an ejector valve. It consists basically of a circular or rectangular metal chamber, surrounded by a hollow jacket of a similar material, being designed to withstand pressures of steam in excess of those in use. A suitable door, also designed to withstand high pressures of steam, and controlled by a single hand wheel, is fitted to one or both ends. The autoclave may be installed between two rooms, the materials to be sterilised being placed in the chamber from one room (the soiled side), and removed from the other (the clean side).

Steam reaching the autoclave from the boiler house is usually at a much higher pressure than required. A reducing valve reduces this pressure of from about 5·55 kg per cm^2 (551·6 kN/m^2, 80 p.s.i.) to the level required and prevents any greater pressure of steam entering the autoclave than the maximum pressure at which it is designed to operate.

TO STERILISE

1. The inner chamber is loaded with packets or boxes which are placed in such a way that free passage of steam through the material is possible. This usually means placing the packets or boxes on their sides so that the steam passes through the folded layers. As steam is lighter than the air which is displaced it should enter the chamber at the top, pass through the load, and be discharged at the bottom through the thermostatic release valve.

2. The door is securely closed with the bolts 'well home' and must not be opened again until the sterilisation is complete and the chamber pressure gauge reads zero.

There are two important gauges that are fitted to an autoclave, one recording the jacket pressure and one the chamber pressure. The pressure in the jacket may be kept on all day, but that in the chamber rises only when the appropriate valve is opened. Another essential accessory is the provision of a thermometer in the steam condensate release or discharge line, and when the correct temperature in relation to the pressure used has been reached by this thermometer the sterilisation cycle is commenced.

Fig. 6.1 Diagram of a steam-pressure steriliser of the gravity air displacement type. (J. M. Bowie – by kind permission.)

3. The first cycle is an initial vacuum, which is created and held for about 5 minutes, followed by the admittance of steam to the chamber. When the selected temperature/pressure has been reached *in the chamber*, a second vacuum is created and also held for 5 minutes (except for instruments). On the gravity displacement autoclave there is a limiting factor to the greatest degree of vacuum obtainable. With some types, fitted with a powerful ejector, this may be in the region of 457 to 508 mmHg (60 to 66·54 kPa), but the average vacuum does not usually exceed 380 mmHg (50 kPa).

4. In the second cycle the steam is admitted to the chamber again and raised to the selected temperature/pressure. For dressings, gowns and instruments, etc., in packets and boxes a temperature/pressure of 126° C, 1·41 kg per cm^2 (137·9 kN/m^2, 20 p.s.i.) is maintained for 30 minutes. Instruments on open trays should be sterilised at 130° C, 1·76 kg per cm^2 (172·3 kN/m^2, 25 p.s.i.) for 6 minutes.

During this second steam cycle the holding time is correlated to the temperature indicated by the thermometer in the discharge line, which is always the coldest part of the chamber. During the period of sterilisation this thermometer must register one of the

Fig. 6.2 Record of sterilising temperature showing double-vacuum technique.

following temperatures and the holding time from this point must be *not less than the time period stated*:

> 134°C for 3 minutes.
> 130°C for 4 minutes.
> 125°C for 8 minutes.
> 121°C for 12 minutes.
> 115°C for 18 minutes.

This is the temperature and time at which all parts of the load must be held and *it is advisable to increase the time by 50 per cent of that stated to ensure absolute safety*. The appropriate composite holding times and temperatures listed in Table 6.1 allow this margin of safety.

5. The steam is released from the chamber, and the materials, with the exception of gloves, are dried in a vacuum for 40 minutes to one hour. Gloves need only 6 minutes drying from the time the vacuum reaches 380 mm (50 kPa), providing the gloves are packed in individual *paper* bags before placing in the packets or boxes.

The moisture remaining finely distributed in the dressings, etc., during the period of sterilisation is at the same temperature as the surrounding steam. As soon as the pressure is reduced and the steam exhausted, this moisture flashes into vapour by virtue of the residual heat in the fabrics and from the surrounding hot jacket, the temperature of which are above boiling point. The real drying process therefore consists of getting rid of this steam vapour as fast as it forms.

This constitutes the final cycle of sterilisation, and with an efficient autoclave using steam at phase boundary point it should not be necessary to suck in air, which may be contaminated, except to break the vacuum. The air required for breaking the vacuum must be well-filtered, to avoid recontamination of the load, using a release valve incorporating a high-efficiency filter such as one made from glass fibre or ceramic material. This filter should be disinfected during the steam cycle by allowing free steam to permeate through it.

6. After the correct period of drying the autoclave is switched off, the vacuum broken, *and when the chamber pressure gauge reads zero*, the door is opened. The operator should be wearing a clean overall and wash his hands before unloading the chamber; the batch number should be applied to packets and boxes as they are unloaded.

STERILITY TESTS

It is a good practice to use some form of test material placed in the packets or boxes to indicate adequate sterilisation.

Chemical indicator tubes (Browne's tubes) are reliable if stored in a cool place and these should be placed in the centre of packets and boxes before sterilisation.

The fluid contained in these tubes changes colour when the correct sterilising procedure has been accomplished (Howie and Timbury, 1956; Howie, 1961; Knox, 1961; Kelsey, 1967). The change can be compared with that of the traffic signals, from red, through yellow to finally green, when the correct temperature and time have been attained. It is important to store these tubes at a temperature of less than 21°C, otherwise there may be a variable degree of premature chemical reaction, resulting in inaccurate readings when used for test purposes.

Browne's tubes are manufactured in four different types, covering the sterilisation of articles in gravity displacement autoclaves, high-vacuum/high-pressure autoclaves, dry-heat ovens and dry-heat conveyor ovens. These four types are:

Type One: Black Spot, for testing the sterilisation of dressings, gowns and gloves, etc., in the gravity displacement autoclave. Safety is indicated after 10 minutes at 125°C or approximately 6 minutes at 130°C.

Type Two: Yellow Spot, for testing all articles in the high-vacuum/high-pressure autoclave. Safety is indicated after 3·5 minutes at 130°C.

Type Three: Green Spot, for testing syringes, glassware and instruments, etc., by the dry-heat process in a dry-oven. Safety is indicated after one hour at 160°C.

Type Four: Blue Spot, for testing sterilisation by the dry-heat process in an infra-red conveyor oven. Safety is indicated after 45 minutes at 160°C.

In all cases the tubes are operative over a range of temperatures and times. A lower temperature must be compensated by a longer exposure, and vice versa.

In some operating departments a separate box or packet is used, into which are placed some of the indicator tubes, and after being processed in the lower portion of the autoclave this is opened immediately If the tubes have not changed colour correctly several other packets are opened aseptically, their tubes checked, and if the liquid is amber or red the batch is re-sterilised and a fresh tube used after the functioning of the autoclave has been checked.

Other chemical test indicators are available including Steamclox (a card with segments which change from pink to green according to time/temperature reached), and Diack controls, a tube containing a chemical tablet which changes colour in a similar manner.

Although these chemical test-tubes indicate the correct working of the autoclave they do not actually show the lethal effect of the sterilising procedure. Bacteriologists therefore prepare a test packet containing usually the spores of an organism of the thermophil group such as *Bacillus stearothermophilus*, which is extremely resistant to heat, and this may be placed in a packet or drum before sterilisation. After exposure to the sterilising process, the packet is returned unopened to the bacteriologist for examination. However, bacteriological tests of an autoclave are not necessary for routine use and should be restricted to use as an occasional check on sterilising efficiency for the test takes up to three days to complete.

Another method of checking whether adequate temperatures are being attained by all parts of a load is by the use of thermocouples or electrical thermometers (Howie, 1961). These thermometers are placed in various positions within the packet or drum, and are connected to a control panel via wires which are contained in fibre-glass insulation. These wires pass either between the door gasket and its seating or for preference a special nipple in the chamber wall (especially applicable to high-vacuum/high-pressure autoclaves) and are placed in position before the door is closed. The temperatures may be checked at any time during the period of sterilisation and rate of steam penetrating to various parts of the load is clearly shown.

A very important addition to the autoclave is a time chart recording the sterilising procedures. This chart will indicate the vacuum, temperatures and relative times of each sterilising load, and is a reliable check for the operating theatre or service unit-supervisor, who is often unable to supervise every sterilising load. Once the correct temperatures and timings have been decided, any variation by the autoclave operator is easily observed and the record chart is permanent for future reference. Recordings of pressure only are of no value as they do not indicate the temperatures attained, owing to the variable degree of mixture with air.

The high-vacuum/high-pressure autoclave

This works at a pressure in the region of 2·25 to 2·46 kg cm^2 (220·59 to 241·3 kN/m^2, 32 to 35 lb p.s.i.) and a temperature of 134°C to 136°C. A high-vacuum pump removes air from the chamber before sterilisation down to an almost complete vacuum of 0·5 to 1 mm 1 Hg (65·82 to 131·7 Pa). The process is controlled automatically.

Although in earlier models of this apparatus attempts were made to obtain a high vacuum in one stage, it has been found that utilising a vacuum pump only will not achieve a vacuum much lower than 20 mmHg (2·67 kPa). This was followed by steam at 134°C for 3 minutes, a post vacuum of varying degree and admission of filtered air to the chamber. This type of cycle did not give consistent results for they often depend upon how the chamber was loaded and the kind of materials being sterilised.

Research has shown that a pre-vacuum/steam pulsation technique will achieve a much better removal of air from the autoclave chamber before sterilisation (Bolton, 1966; Knox and Pickerill, 1967). Basically, steam pulsation technique consists of allowing a charge of steam to enter the chamber after an initial high vacuum has been drawn, then following this by another vacuum draw and repeating the process to give two or more steam pulses. The logic is that any residual air is diluted each time and replaced with water vapour; each steam pulse and vacuum draw resulting in repeated reduction of air content without reducing the total pressure in the chamber. The high-vacuum/high-pressure autoclave relies upon a pre-vacuum stage which reduces the air content in the chamber to 1 mmHg (131·7 Pa) or less.

With negligible air in the chamber and some pre-heating of the load, penetration of steam into the items being sterilised is very rapid. High temperatures in the region of 134°C are reached very quickly and an exposure to this temperature for 3·5 minutes will ensure sterility. It is important though, as mentioned previously, that all parts of the load must reach this temperature before timing commences. For automatic control of process a simple and accurate means of measuring the partial air pressure (pre-vacuum) and a load simulator which simulates the conditions within the packet or cardboard box are required. This obviates the need for a thermocouple within the load to control the process.

Depending on the size of autoclave chamber the total cycle in this type of autoclave is from 25 to 35 minutes. The chamber can be fully loaded with soft packets providing a few centimetres of space is allowed between the load and the chamber wall. An angled condensate plate can be fitted underneath each shelf on which pre-set trays are being sterilised. These slope downwards to one or other side of the chamber in order to prevent drips of condensate from the lower surface of a tray above wetting a tray below (Fig. 5.21).

THE CYCLE OF OPERATION

For a high-vacuum/high-pressure autoclave, this can be summarised as follows.

After loading the chamber and closing the door:

Stage 1. Pre-vacuum. The air is removed from the chamber by a vacuum pump and controlled steam pulsations. The vacuum achieved should be in the order of 0·5 to 1 mmHg (65·82 to 131·7 Pa) (Fig. 6.4).

Stage 2. Sterilisation. Steam is admitted to the chamber and when all parts of the load have reached a temperature of 134°C this is maintained for 3·5 minutes (Fig. 6.5).

Stage 3. Drying. Achieved by an adequate post vacuum, checked periodically by a test packet of huckaback towels which when removed from the autoclave, unfolded and allowed to cool are not sensibly damp (Fig. 6.6).

Stage 4. Breaking the Vacuum. This should be completed within 3 minutes, through a glass fibre or ceramic type filter (Fig. 6.7).

The chamber is unloaded and the packets date stamped together if desired with the batch number of that particular load. Pre-set trays should have a plastic dust cover applied, especially if they are to be stored for more than a few hours. This cover should be applied only after the trays have cooled off.

Fig. 6.3 (ASSA Training Handbook for Sterile Supply Assistants.)

The setting before the cycle commences
When the door closing action is complete the pointer on the cycle indicator moves to pre-vacuum, i.e., the cycle begins.

Pressure Gauges
Absolute pressure gauge records vacuum attained (in mmHg).
Temperature gauge records the temperature reached and held during sterilisation.
Chamber (compound) pressure gauge records the vacuum condition and steam pressure.
Jacket (compound) pressure gauge records the pressure maintained in the jacket.

Fig. 6.4 (ASSA Training Handbook for Sterile Supply Assistants.)

Pre-vacuum period
   The air is being drawn from the chamber and contents (load). Removal of air is assisted, for example, by intermittent bursts of steam into the chamber when a vacuum is being drawn.

Fig. 6.5 (ASSA Training Handbook for Sterile Supply Assistants.)

Sterilising period
   The chamber is filled with steam under pressure. The actual sterilising time begins when the correct temperature and pressure have been reached.

Fig. 6.6 (ASSA Training Handbook for Sterile Supply Assistants.)

Post-vacuum period
Steam is removed from the chamber and condense moisture from the load. Vacuum drawn is recorded on the pressure gauge.

Fig. 6.7 (ASSA Training Handbook for Sterile Supply Assistants.)

Filtered air is drawn into the chamber to eliminate the vacuum and equalise the inside and outside pressure.

STERILISER FUNCTION TESTS

These should be performed daily and the two most effective are the Bowie/Dick indicator tape test and the chamber vacuum leak test. The high-vacuum/high-pressure autoclave is a complex piece of machinery. Machines should have built-in safeguards which interrupt the sterilisation cycle if faults occur but this is not always so and the autoclave may appear to function correctly when in fact it is not.

A possible fault relates to inadequate extraction of air from the chamber during the pre-vacuum cycle. It may be due to a faulty pump but equally because air has leaked back through faulty door-seals or valves. This means that steam can penetrate the load only slowly and in an irregular way, which may result in unsterile packets.

The Bowie/Dick Indicator Tape Test. This test is a means of determining the efficiency of air removal from the steriliser chamber during the pre-vacuum cycle. It does not indicate directly that sterilisation is achieved, but that air removal has been adequate to allow sterilisation to take place at 134°C for 3·5 minutes or 126°C for 12 minutes. In practice this is very simple. A standard test pack is made up consisting of 36 huckaback towels, 0·6 m^2 (6 ft^2), (complying with B.S.I. 1781.TL.5) folded and forming a stack 25 to 28 cm (10 to 11 in) high (Bowie, 1961; Bowie *et al.*, 1963, 1975; Morris and Everall, 1975). In the centre is placed a piece of paper 30 cm (12 in) square to which has been fixed a cross of 3M indicator tape No. 1222, such as is widely used for sealing packets, indicating they have been autoclaved. Alternatively, a sheet consisting entirely of the basic indicator tape material can be used. The towels should be washed initially before using and whenever they become soiled or discoloured. Between tests they are unfolded and hung out to air for at least one hour.

The test pack is placed in an autoclavable cardboard box (Bripac/Permapak) or wrapped in fabric or paper. It is now placed by itself in the autoclave and subjected to a standard sterilising cycle. Care must be taken to ensure that the 'Holding' or 'Sterilising' time does not exceed 3·5 minutes at 134°C or 12 minutes at 126°C. If the automatic cycle is set for

Fig. 6.8 (left)   Tape showing a satisfactory result with uniform colour change.

Fig. 6.9 (right)   This is an unsatisfactory result – the colour change is irregular and incomplete in the centre.

a longer holding time this must be cut short, for the purposes of the test, to 3·5 minutes, by using the manual control. Should there be any doubt about this the engineer should be asked for advice.

When the cycle is finished the pack is removed and the paper with the tape is examined. After a satisfactory run the tape will show a colour change *which is the same*

Fig. 6.10 High-Vacuum/High-Pressure autoclave with steam generator. (British Steriliser Ltd.)

at the centre as the edges. If the tape at the centre is paler than it is at the edges, it means there was a bubble of air there and the steriliser was not working correctly. If this happens, the autoclave must be taken out of service immediately until the fault has been rectified.

Unless the test is carried out exactly as described it may not be truly reliable. In particular the following points should be noted.

Fig. 6.11 Graph showing hi-vac cycles. (British Steriliser Ltd.)

1. The more air there is to remove, the more exacting will be the test and that is why the test pack is used by itself in an otherwise empty chamber.

2. The exact colour change shown by the processed tape may depend upon the storage conditions of that tape. The important thing is whether the *same colour change* occurs at the centre and the edges.

3. The contrast in colour change from centre to edge will be reduced to an unreadable level if long 'holding' periods are used. That is why the *'holding' period must not exceed 3·5 minutes at 134°C.* Even an extra minute or two may seriously affect a comparison of results.

4. *Because of this it is very important to realise that if an autoclave fails to pass the Bowie/Dick test as described, it cannot be made safe merely by increasing the 'holding' time until a uniform colour change is produced. Such a steriliser is in urgent need of skilled attention.*

5. The Bowie/Dick test is relevant only to high-vacuum/high-pressure autoclaves. It is valueless in downward displacement autoclaves.

The Vacuum and Leak Test (instrumentation required). In order to carry out this test the autoclave requires additional instrumentation fitted, which is capable of measuring small variations in the degree of vacuum attainable within the chamber. Most autoclaves already incorporate the necessary instrumentation as follows:

1. The control camshaft is modified so that a position can be obtained manually directly subsequent to the 'pre-vacuum' position, when all valves on the camshaft are

closed. This position has a location cam and a significant reference mark on the camshaft position indicator, known as the *'leak test'* position.

2. A 0 to 100 mmHg (0 to 13·17 kPa) absolute pressure gauge (tolerance ± one per cent F.S. reading) is mounted on the front panel, and connected via a manual valve directly beneath it in series with an electrical solenoid valve (normally closed to the chamber by the shortest route in copper pipe of a least 0·6 cm (0·25 in) diameter, in such a way that the pipe will drain into the chamber.

The solenoid is operated by a micro-switch actuated by the control camshaft so that the valve is opened only when the camshaft is in the 'pre-vacuum' and the 'leak test' positions.

3. A toggle switch is mounted on the front panel adjacent to the absolute pressure gauge. This switch is wired in series with the coil of the vacuum pump motor contactor, so that the contactor may be de-energised and the motor stopped.

Fig. 6.12 High-vacuum/High Pressure autoclave of the fixed base design which incorporates a vertical cylindrical chamber lifted by means of compressed air cylinders.

The goods to be sterilised are placed in the cardboard containers or, in the case of pre-packed theatre trays, on a special frame, and these are loaded on a roller track and transported automatically to the processing position under the vessel. This is lowered and the cycle commences.

When the cycle is complete the vessel is raised and the sterilised goods are moved automatically on to a roller track at the rear and the next container takes its place.

The automatic equipment is fitted with a reliable device to prevent the vessel descending until the containers are properly positioned. Similarly, should there be no containers available for sterilising the machine will cease to operate until more are made available. (Sanderson Sterilisers Limited.)

4. A Smith's or similar 0 to 30 minutes timer is useful mounted on the front panel adjacent to the absolute pressure gauge.

5. An extra outlet may be fitted in parallel with, and adjacent to the absolute pressure gauge, so that the gauge can be calibrated regularly against either a standard gauge or mercury column.

Note: Any other method may be used provided that the chamber is isolated by the valves which are normally used during a process, so that they are tested for leakage.

The recommended post-vacuum pressure should be less than 50 mmHg (6·56 kPa absolute pressure) and it is possible to modify the camshaft in such a way that the solenoid valve to the leak test gauge can be opened and the post-vacuum pressure checked.

From this rather technical description of the instrumentation required the reader may imagine that the actual test is equally complex. This is not so for the vacuum and leak test can be conducted effectively by any supervisor of an operating suite or operating theatre service unit.

Method of performing the test (autoclave instrumentation as described):

1. Close and lock the door with the chamber empty. The steriliser must be on manual control.

2. Turn the control cam-shaft to '*pre-vacuum*' position and open manual valve beneath the absolute pressure gauge.

3. When the pressure indicated on the absolute pressure gauge is less than 20 mmHg (2·627 kPa), turn the control camshaft to '*leak test*' position, and wait 10 seconds for the vacuum valve to close.

4. Turn the toggle switch to the '*off*' position and wait until the needle on the absolute pressure gauge starts to return.

5. When the gauge needle starts to return, take a reading, set and start the timer for 10 minutes. When the timer reaches zero take another reading on the absolute pressure gauge.

6. Close the manual valve beneath the absolute pressure gauge and turn the toggle switch to '*on*'.

7. Rotate the control camshaft to '*post-vacuum*' position and hold for 4 minutes. Note the reading on the absolute pressure gauge and rotate control camshaft once again to the '*break-vacuum*' or '*off*' position. Finally where applicable, press the automatic *re-set* button and with the control camshaft in the '*off*' position, the door may be opened.

The test can be deemed a failure if the vacuum fails to reach 20 mmHg (2·627 kPa), or the leak at stage 4 is greater than 10 mmHg (1·317 kPa) in 10 minutes. If this result is observed, skilled engineering assistance must be obtained and the cause of the fault investigated immediately.

The high-vacuum/high-pressure autoclave is a very effective method of steam sterilisation, providing regular efficiency tests and maintenance are instituted. It may not be possible to perform the vacuum and leak tests due to the appropriate instrumentation being non-existent. However, the Bowie/Dick Test must be carried out daily as described and will provide a reliable means of assessing the efficiency of the autoclave.

2. Dry heat (in the form of hot air)

This can be used for sterilising many items, but is destructive to linen and rubber or plastic articles, etc. (Perkins, 1956b).

Certain articles can be sterilised easily and safely, including non-disposable syringes, glassware, needles, mechanical drills (especially the compressed air types), fine knives and other delicate instruments that will withstand this dry heat but not the wet methods. Very suitable containers for sterilisation and storage can be made from aluminium tulle-gas boxes after they have been emptied. Larger items can be folded in sheets of aluminium foil, but care must be taken not to compress the packets unduly as puncture of the foil may occur.

A special electric oven is used, designed to achieve a uniform temperature in all parts of the apparatus. There are two types: (1) the gravity-convection type, and (2) the mechanical-convection type.

The Gravity-Convection Type

This is limited to a small size, usually not exceeding about 0.027 m^3 (1 ft^3), has heaters in the base and sides, and relies upon air circulation according to the slight temperature differences of various parts of the chamber. Heated air rises and cooler air descends, being displaced by it. As the warm air ascends it gives off some of its heat to the load and at the same time the descending cool air is warmed as it passes over the heaters. The warm air now rises, the cool air descends again and the process is repeated, setting up gravity convection currents.

The Mechanical-Convection Type

This utilises a motor blower to circulate the air.

The heater bank is contained in a chamber on one side, and separated from the working chamber by a perforated diffuser wall. An adjustable air inlet opens into the heater chamber directly in front of the heater bank and motor blower. Air is drawn through the air inlet over the heaters and is forced into the working chamber through another diffuser wall on the opposite side of the chamber. As the warm air gives off some of its heat to the load it passes back into the heater chamber, mixes with the incoming fresh air, and the process is repeated. This good circulation of warm air ensures even and rapid heating of the load being sterilised.

With both types of dry-heat sterilisers, *when all parts of the load* have attained the required temperature of $160°$C, timing is commenced and should consist of at least one hour's exposure. The period necessary for even heating to be achieved varies considerably with the capacity of the oven, type of load and the containers in which the articles are packed. With the gravity-convection steriliser, articles packed in aluminium boxes may require a total exposure of up to two and a half hours, and needles in glassine envelopes one and a half hours. With the mechanical-convection steriliser this time can usually be reduced to one and a half hours and 80 minutes respectively. However, individual tests must be made with a particular oven using suitable Browne's tubes, green spot, stearothermophilus spore papers, and where possible a check by the engineer with thermocouples or electrical thermometers placed in the centre of the load.

Non-disposable glass syringes can be sterilised by dry heat. The syringes are carefully cleansed with cold water, then Neodian, Lab-brite, etc., or an ultrasonic cleaner, followed by acetone or ether to remove fat, etc., and the barrels are finally *very lightly* lubricated with a silicone solution. They are packed into containers which may be sealed before placing in the dry-heat steriliser. A useful container is one made as an aluminium tube, with a metal cap sealed in position over the open end. It is possible to demonstrate a tidal movement of air out of, and subsequently into, containers using this type of seal during the sterilisation process, and at the end of the cycle. As the remaining sterile air in the container cools and contracts, a tidal flow of air occurs from the oven into the container.

Table 6.1 Sterilisation by heat
A. Steam autoclave, gravity or downward displacement type

Materials Being Sterilised	Initial Vacuum (Twice) Degree	Initial Vacuum (Twice) Holding Time	Initial Steam Cycle Pressure	Initial Steam Cycle Temp.	Sterilising Steam Cycle Pressure	Sterilising Steam Cycle Temp.	Sterilising Steam Cycle Holding Time	Final Vacuum (Drying) Degree	Final Vacuum (Drying) Holding Time	Total Cycle (Approx.)
Gowns, towels, dressings, etc.; in paper, or linen packets	300 mmHg (39·47 kPa) to 250 mmHg (32·8 kPa)	5 min (each time)	1·41 kg per cm², (137·9 kN/m², 20 p.s.i.)	125°C	1·41 kg per cm², (137·9 kN/m², 20 p.s.i.)	125°C	30 min	300 mmHg (39·47 kPa) to 250 mmHg (32·8 kPa)	40 min	90 min
					1·76 kg per cm², (172·3 kN/m², 25 p.s.i.)	130°C	25 min		30 min	75 min
Metal instruments on open trays, ligatures, etc.	Not needed		Not needed		1·76 kg per cm², (172·3 kN/m², 25 p.s.i.)	130°C	6 min	Not needed		7 min
Metal instruments with minimal wrappings, ligatures, etc.	Not needed		Not needed		1·76 kg per cm², (172·3 kN/m², 25 p.s.i.)	130°C	6 min	450 mmHg (59·2 kPa)	1 to 2 min	9 min
Metal instruments, ligatures, etc., in packets with normal wrappings	300 mmHg (39·47 kPa) to 250 mmHg (32·8 kPa)	5 min (once only)	Not needed		1·76 kg per cm², (172·3 kN/m², 25 p.s.i.)	130°C	15 min	300 mmHg (39·47 kPa) to 250 mmHg (32·8 kPa)	7 to 10 min	27 to 30 min
Rubber gloves. (With gloves in upper part of chamber)	300 mmHg (39·47 kPa) to 250 mmHg (32·8 kPa)	5 min (once only)	1·76 kg per cm², (172·3 kN/m², 25 p.s.i.)	130°C	1·76 kg per cm², (172·3 kN/m², 25 p.s.i.)	130°C	6 min	450 mmHg (59·2 kPa)	5 min	30 min
			2·25 kg per cm², (220·59 kN/m², 32 p.s.i.)	134°C	2·25 kg per cm², (220·59 kN/m², 32 p.s.i.)	134°C	3 min	450 mmHg (59·2 kPa)	3 min	20 min
Intravenous fluids	Not needed		Not needed		0·7 kg per cm² (68·95 kN/m², 10 p.s.i.)	116°C	60 min	Gradual exhaust of steam from chamber	..	
					1·05 kg per cm², (103·4 kN/m², 15 p.s.i.)	121°C	45 min			

Table 6.1 Sterilisation by heat (*contd.*)
B. Steam autoclave, High-vacuum/High pressure type

Materials Being Sterilised	Initial Vacuum	Sterilising Steam Cycle	Final Vacuum (Drying)	Total Cycle
Gowns, towels, dressings, metal instruments etc., in packets or boxes	Approximately 0·5 to 1 mmHg (6·58 to 13·17 Pa)	3½ min 134°C	5 to 10 min	Approximately 25 min

C. Dry-heat steriliser

Articles Being Sterilised	Period
Syringes, compressed air drills, some types of electric drills and saws, powders, osteotomes, etc.	With efficient circulation of hot air these should be exposed for a period of 60 minutes when the temperature has reached 160°C in all parts of the load. This may mean a total cycle of between 1¼ to 2¼ hours, or more.

D. Pasteurisation

Articles Being Disinfected	Period
Endoscopes (cystoscopes, etc.)	Maintain in a hot-water bath at 75°C for 10 minutes (ensure they are completely covered and allow time for water to regain temperature when cool endoscope is added to the bath). Process in subatmospheric steam/formaldehyde autoclave at 82°C for 90 minutes, total-cycle approximately 2½ hours.

If containers are removed from the oven before cooling occurs, there is a possibility that unsterile 'room' air could be entrained. For this reason it is advisable to keep the oven door shut until the thermometer or recording pen indicates that the internal temperature has dropped to 50°C.

Fig. 6.13 Dry-heat steriliser. (Laboratory Thermal Equipment Ltd.)

Heat Disinfection

3. Sub-atmospheric steam pasteurisation/formaldehyde sterilisation

Whilst the two previous methods are practical and effective ways of sterilising most fabrics and instruments, there is still the problem of heat-sensitive articles such as plastics and optical devices. Previously there were only two cold methods that could be relied upon to kill spores, gamma irradiation (impracticable in most hospitals) and careful bacteriologically controlled ethylene oxide gas. Alder and Gillespie at the Bristol Royal Infirmary had been using steam at 90°C to disinfect blankets for several years

(Alder et al., 1966). They were impressed with the minimal damage to most items that were disinfected. Further experiments resulted in a technique that is applicable to the pasteurisation of heat-sensitive instruments.

In a modified autoclave, steam under sub-atmospheric pressure at temperatures below 90°C will rapidly kill non-poring organisms after the air in the chamber has been removed by a high-vacuum pump. Most bacterial spores are killed also but a small proportion are very resistant. *If formaldehyde vapour is added to the steam, it can destroy all spores and effect sterilisation.* Low-temperature steam, and low-temperature steam/formaldehyde cycles can be incorporated in one and the same autoclave.

Fig. 6.14 Graph of low temperature/formaldehyde method. (British Steriliser Ltd.)

THE CYCLE OF OPERATION

Low-temperature steam formaldehyde sterilisation can be summarised as follows: After loading the chamber and closing the door:

Stage 1. Pre-vacuum. A flush of steam is drawn by the vacuum pump through the surrounding jacket and the chamber whilst the pressure is reduced to approximately 380 mmHg (50 kPa). At this point the jacket pressure is held steady and the pump continues to evacuate the chamber until a pressure of about 50 mmHg (6·56 kPa) is reached. This is maintained for 10 minutes to effect complete air clearance from both the chamber and the load.

Stage 2. Sterilisation. A predetermined quantity of formalin is automatically delivered into the chamber from an externally fitted dispenser or container. The valves of the autoclave are so arranged as to admit about 55 ml of formalin per 100 litres (1 ml per 292 cm^3) of autoclave chamber capacity. The formalin first enters a heated vapouriser where it is converted to steam and gaseous formaldehyde before passing into the chamber. At the same time there is a controlled injection of steam which allows the chamber pressure to rise into equilibrium with that of the jacket at about 380 mmHg (50 kPa). Once this equilibrium pressure is reached (82°C saturated steam temperature), continuous pressure waves of steam, followed by condensation, are applied within the upper and lower absolute pressure limits of 380 mmHg and 330 mmHg (50 kPa and 43·42 kPa). These pressure waves occurring at approximately once every 90 seconds, promote penetration of the formaldehyde vapour into all parts of the load.

In order to maintain the formaldehyde concentration in a sub-atmospheric cycle, the chamber must remain virtually closed. This does produce a problem of the extraction of condensate which is formed during the decompression phase of each pressure wave. The removal of condensate is achieved through an automatic condensate release valve fitted in the chamber drain. Duration of the pasteurisation stage is normally in the order of 90 minutes and this is determined by bacteriological check of a standard load.

Stage 3. Flushing. The pressure is once more reduced in the chamber by means of the vacuum pump and a continuous flush of steam is applied. Pumping and steam flushing is carried out at an absolute pressure of about 50 Torr (28 in Hg, 711 mmHg) and this ensures that most of the formaldehyde is removed from the chamber and the materials being pasteurised. This stage lasts for approximately 12 minutes.

Stage 4. Drying. A final reduction of pressure to 30 Torr (29 in Hg, 737 mmHg) or less, achieves drying of materials over a period of approximately eight minutes.

Stage 5. Breaking the vacuum. Filtered air is admitted until atmospheric pressure is reached in the chamber. This generally takes about two minutes.

Penetration tests. Lengths of narrow bore tubing form difficult test pieces; they are realistic, easy to prepare and to standardise and are readily included with any routine run. A useful method is to infect the lumen of a 2·7 m length of 3 mm bore plastic tubing with spores of *B. globigii* and *B. stearothermophilus*. These are processed in the laboratory in the normal manner and in some instances it has been found that the pasturisation cycle can be reduced to between 60 and 75 minutes and still maintain effective destruction of spores.

One such device is the Northwich Park Hospital test helix (Line and Pickerill, 1973). This consists of stainless-steel tubing 3 mm bore by 455 cm length with a gas-tight capsule for the spore strip at one end. The capsule is in two parts which fit together against an O-ring seal and secured by a knurled ring. The device enables use of more easily handled standard spore test strips rather than liquid suspensions introduced into the lumen of a tube. It has been found that the helix is a more efficient test for penetration of formaldehyde vapour.

Chemical tests are available to check routinely the penetration of formaldehyde vapour. They do not replace the periodic spore tests.

The Browne formaldehyde test consists of a square of white paper, enclosed in a small envelope of thin transparent plastic, which is permeable by steam and formaldehyde vapour. The paper gradually turns red as the vapour reaches it; the tint depending on the duration of exposure and the concentration of the vapour.

It is recommended that a test-piece is placed on the outside and in the centre of each pack. The outside test indicates the pack has been through the sterilisation process; the inner test piece should be examined when the pack is opened, and if found not to have reached the control tint, the goods should be rejected.

The following are some of the items suitable for disinfection by this method: nylon, Terylene, Acrilan and rayon fabrics; polyurethane; teflon tubing; perspex; silicone rubber; anaesthetic equipment such as endotracheal tubes, valves, connectors etc.; cystoscopes and other endoscopic instruments having electrical systems (low-voltage); catheters and tracheostomy tubes, etc.

4. Pasteurisation in water

Pasteurisation of endoscopes is carried out simply by immersion for 10 minutes in water at a temperature of between 75°C and 85°C (Francis, 1959). A thermostatically controlled water bath is used and even non-boilable instruments withstand this treatment very well. It is in practice as effective as boiling and will destroy vegetative bacteria very rapidly.

Fig. 6.15 Miniclave portable low-temperature/low-pressure steriliser. (Chas. F. Thackray.)

Undoubtedly it is preferable to the use of chemicals if autoclaving is contraindicated and the sub-atmospheric steam method is unavailable (Medical Research Council, 1968).

5. Boiling

The boiling of instruments should be regarded as a means of disinfection only; it does not kill spores. This technique has no place in a modern hospital, nor indeed even under extremes of isolation. If a small portable autoclave is not available then an ordinary domestic pressure cooker will be an acceptable alternative.

Cold Sterilisation

6. Radiation

Generally limited to sterilisation on a commercial scale there are two methods in general use, gamma irradiation from a Cobalt 60 source and electron bombardment from a linear accelerator (Mackenzie, 1966).

Fig. 6.16 Portable autoclave (Little Sister) which can be operated from a standard 13A power socket. (Surgical Equipment Supplies Ltd.)

The usual dose is in the region of 2·5 M, rad. and the technique is highly successful for most disposable items which require sterilisation only once. Degradation and ageing does occur when sterilising some materials so care is taken to select those suitable for irradiation.

The Cobalt source is the most economical process if it can be kept running the full 24 hours. It has greater penetrating power than the linear accelerator which is more suitable for thin packets such as catgut, scalpel blades, needles, etc.

An irradiation sterilisation service provided by the Atomic Energy Authority at Wantage, Berkshire, England is available to hospitals. This service consists mainly of contract sterilisation although arrangements can be made to process a small number of items. The user is required to adhere to certain methods and sizes of packets. Full details are available from Irradiated Products Ltd., Denchworth Road, Wantage, Berks., England.

7. Ethylene Oxide

Ethylene oxide is suitable for sterilising heat labile articles. It is a method now well established in the United States, Germany, Switzerland and France; although in the United Kingdom until about 1965 ethylene oxide gas was limited to commercial processes. Use at hospital level has been minimal due to concern in respect of its toxicity and explosive characteristics and also the difficulty of controlling the efficiency of the process.

Ethylene oxide, known as a gas since 1859, has been used as an industrial disinfectant for over forty years and was introduced as a clinical sterilising agent in 1949 by Philip and Kays. The chemical acts by alkylating the proteins of micro-organisms thereby upsetting their equilibrium. If the process is applied correctly, this reaction is irreversible and reanimation of the alkylated germ is prevented.

The gas is an epoxide and unfortunately besides being an extremely efficient alkylating agent it has the ability to ignite with an exothermic reaction which has on a number of occasions blown whole factories into the air. This explosive polymerisation can be avoided, firstly by mixing ethylene oxide with an inert gas such as carbon dioxide, and secondly, by employing a sterilising process which extracts most of the air from the chamber before the introduction of ethylene oxide (Fischer, 1971). One process uses pure ethylene oxide under a constant vacuum so that it is impossible for the gas to leak out and mix with air (Weymes, 1966).

Fig. 6.17 Sterivit Automated Ethylene Oxide Steriliser at Hallamshire Hospital, Sheffield. Applied for sterilising used cystoscope in rate volume.

A word of caution on safeguards to prevent explosions; cylinders of ethylene oxide stored in the liquid phase must be fitted within 2 to 2·5 metres (6 to 8 feet) of the steriliser served to avoid the possibility of separation. If separation and a leak in the line occurs, air may be drawn into the chamber with ethylene oxide to form a highly combustible mixture.

Initially care must be taken in cleansing instruments and apparatus that all visible protein material is removed; although a high pressure process (Sterivit) has been proved to have the ability to penetrate even salt encrusted spores e.g. when inactivating Statens Seruminstitut *B. subtilis* dried on pure quartz sand (Leo Pharmaceutical Products, Denmark, 1971, personal communication). The articles being sterilised must be dry, for if they are wrapped in polythene film whilst still wet, they will remain wet after sterilisation. The most suitable packing material is low-density 300 gauge polyethylene or nylon

Table 6.2 Disinfection by chemicals, anti-bacterial agents in common use, dilutions. (The minimum period of immersion unless otherwise stated is 10 minutes.)

Chemical or proprietary preparation	CLEANSING AND DISINFECTION					DISINFECTION		
	Linen bowls, etc. (%)	Heavy contamination inanimate objects (%)	Burns, wounds, initial pre-surgical skin preparation (%)	Pre-surgical hand rinse (%)	Final pre-surgical skin preparation (%)	Anaesthetic apparatus (masks, tubes, etc.) (%)	Endoscopes electrodes, cables and lamps (%)	Metal instruments (osteotomes, etc.) (%)
PHENOLIC GROUP								
(Sudol) Aqueous	1	2	..	..	..	..	..	2
(Printol) Aqueous	1·25	3	..	..	..	..	..	3
(Printol D) Aqueous	1	2	..	..	..	..	..	2
(Hycolin) Aqueous	1	1·5	..	..	..	..	..	1·5
(Stericol) Aqueous	1	2	..	..	..	..	..	2
(Clearsol) Aqueous	1	2	..	..	..	..	..	2
Chloroxylenol								
(Pure Dettol) Aqueous	5	..	5	5	..	5	..	..
Chlorhexidine Gluconate								
(Hibitane, 5 per cent concentrate) Aqueous	0·5	..	1	..	..	0·5	10	..
Industrial methylated spirit	..	..	..	1	10	..	..	10
SYNTHETIC DETERGENTS								
Cetrimide B.P.								
(CTAB Cetavlon) Aqueous	1	..	3	1	..	1	..	..
(Savlon Hospital concentrate) 15 per cent Cetavlon 1·5 per cent Hibitane Aqueous	0·5	..	3 to 1	..	..	0·5	10 (20 min)	10 (20 min)
Industrial methylated spirit	..	..	..	3	..	..	10	..
Benzalkonium Chloride								
(Roccal, 10 per cent concentrate) Aqueous	0·5	..	10 to 5	1	..	0·5	10	..
Industrial methylated spirit	..	..	..	1	..	..	..	10
HALOGENS HYPOCHLORATES*								
(Sodium Hypochlorate)	1	..	..	..	..	..	..	..
(Chloros)	1	..	..	..	..	..	..	..
Iodine								
2 per cent in industrial methylated spirit	..	..	..	..	Undiluted	..	..	..
POVIDONE-IODINE								
(Betadine) antiseptic Surgical scrub	..	..	Undiluted	Undiluted	..	..	..	..
FORMALDEHYDE								
Activated Glutaraldehyde (Cidex) solution effective for 14 days after activation. 20 minute exposure to destroy pathogens	..	..	..	..	..	†	†	..

Items marked thus † are suitable for disinfection by that particular method. * not suitable for metal surfaces.

film; used as one of two layers which are rapidly penetrated by ethylene oxide, moisture and heat under the appropriate controlled conditions.

An essential part of the sterilising process using ethylene oxide is the maintenance of adequate humidity (70–80 per cent) *with effective moisture distribution throughout the load*. Humidification should be achieved automatically by the steriliser and there must be fail-safe mechanisms to monitor this and any other parameters of the process. Some authorities recommend that adequate humidity can be achieved by preconditioning the items to be sterilised, holding them in a room at 50–60 per cent humidity for several hours before sterilisation. This method is somewhat haphazard as compared to automatic humidification in the steriliser.

The Sterivit apparatus (Fig. 6.17) utilises a 15 per cent ethylene oxide, 85 per cent carbon dioxide mixture under pressure and with controlled humidity. There are a range of chamber sizes available between 25 litres and 2,000 litres, although one with a capacity of 100 to 500 litres (0·382 to 0·496 m^3) will be adequate for most requirements of a hospital-based on CSSD or HSDU. The larger chambers are used mainly for sterilising bulky items of equipment such as complete ventillators or cardiovascular bypass machines. The sterilising process is automated as follows:

1. The steriliser is loaded, the door closed and start button activated.

2. The first stage consists of raising the temperature in the chamber to 55/60°C. A pre-vacuum is drawn and the chamber pressure reduced to approximately 70 Torr; at the same time steam is introduced to create a humidity of 70 to 80 per cent. This stage takes 20 to 25 minutes depending on the size of chamber.

3. Ethylene oxide 15 per cent with 85 per cent carbon dioxide is introduced from a gas cylinder directly into the chamber until a pressure of 3·87 kg per cm^2 (379 kN/m^2, 55 p.s.i.) is reached. This achieves an ethylene oxide concentration of 1,200 mg per litre of chamber capacity, and exposure is maintained for 60 minutes.

4. A post-vacuum of approximately 70 Torr is drawn and held for 25 to 50 minutes depending upon the size of chamber. During this time air is drawn through a high efficiency filter and through the chamber to 'rinse' out ethylene oxide residues from the load. (Note: some other non-pressurised processes require extended periods of exposure for sterilisation; these may be between 1 and 4 hours. Under these circumstances elimination of toxic residues is proportionally more difficult, and takes a longer time. Residues extracted from the chamber must be vented to outside the building.)

The total cycle of the Sterivit process depends on the size of chamber; at the lower end of the scale the 25 litre chamber steriliser takes 100 minutes, the largest chamber of 2,000 litres capacity takes 160 minutes for the whole process.

Practically all materials except metals absorb differing amounts of ethylene oxide. Under normal conditions the desorption of ethylene oxide is a slow process and for this reason many authorities recommend that, after sterilisation, goods should be stored on an open shelf for at least 24-hours and sometimes as long as four days before use. This is to allow elimination of the toxic residue by natural diffusion to atmosphere.

Using the high pressure method of sterilisation coupled with a short exposure and adequate post-vacuum the amount of depth of absorption of ethylene oxide can be reduced (Fischer, 1971). Furthermore, the high diffusion coefficient of the additive carbon dioxide, and the low concentration of a 15 per cent ethylene oxide mixture helps to reduce the problem still further. By an adequate post-vacuum, powerful filtered air-rinse under vacuum and elevated temperature, the ethylene oxide residues can be reduced to a negligible level. Under these circumstances a 24-hours shelf life before use should ensure desorption of any remaining residues.

A precaution worth taking following any ethylene oxide process is to take care that apparatus is not used with saline or blood products before it has been flushed with oxygen or sterile water. In these circumstances even a minute amount of ethylene oxide residue can react with the chlorine radicle to form chlorohydrates, the toxicity of which is not entirely understood at present. For similar reasons articles which have been sterilised by gamma irradiation should not subsequently be resterilised by ethylene oxide. This is the only instance when such precautions are necessary (Boger, 1976).

With ethylene oxide there are no means at present of adequately monitoring the actual ethylene oxide concentration at any given point during sterilisation. For this reason it is necessary to rely upon bacteriological controls. A method in common use is Oxoid prepared *B. stearothermophilus* on filter paper and *B. subtilis* (var *globigii*) 10^6 on aluminium strips prepared to the method of Beeby and Whitehouse (Cunliffe, 1966). Envelopes containing up to ten of these strips are placed at different points in the steriliser chamber and within all articles where it is considered that penetration could be a problem. The strips are incubated overnight and if no growth is apparent, the steriliser load is released for use after the 'airing' period.

Under careful preparation and control the spore test described is a good method of monitoring sterilisation. A simpler test utilising earth spores emanates from Denmark. The Danish State Serum Institute test consists of *B. subtilis*, first immersed in a solution of 0·9 per cent NaCl and then dried on pure quartz sand. The sand is then packed in a paper envelope which is used for test purposes in the normal manner. This is a very severe test due to the presence of salt (in contact with the spore) which tends to inactivate ethylene oxide. In practice it could be regarded as more appropriate to the working situation as many items may not be adequately precleansed.

A chemical indicator can be included with each packet to indicate to the user that it has been through the ethylene oxide process; it is not a direct indication of sterility. A gas indicator green tape with yellow stripes is available. This changes shade after exposure to ethylene oxide (Index No. 1224). Chemical sachets or impregnated filter papers can be prepared in the laboratory and these change colour after being exposed to the gas (Colquhoun, 1969).

Examples of heat-labile equipment suitable for sterilisation by ethylene oxide are: cardiac catheters, endoscopes (including cystoscopes), cryoprobes, aortic grafts, ophthalmic instruments, plastic and rubber tubing, senoran evacuator, Sengstaken tubes, Bird's respirator.

8. Ultra-Violet Light Radiation

This is a form of surface radiation with light having a wavelength of 2537 Ångstrom units. It is suitable only for sterilising surfaces as its penetration is poor. Amongst its uses is the sterilisation of small items such as bone chips, grafts and blades.

Ozone liberated by the process may prove objectionable, especially during sterilisation of air. High intensities of light are required and unless care is taken by personnel, overexposure to ultra-violet radiation may result.

Cold Disinfection

9. Chemical solutions

We now emphasise the term *disinfection* in preference to *sterilisation* because under normal conditions chemicals cannot be relied upon to kill spores. It is a method that is used only when sterilisation by heat is impracticable and is ineffective unless the chemicals can reach all parts of the articles, which *must* be free from debris, blood and pus, i.e., as in ethylene oxide sterilisation (McCulloch, 1945; Perkins, 1956b; Sykes, 1958).

It must be realised that although fairly short periods of contact with certain chemicals will ensure the destruction of bacteria these short periods refer only to articles with smooth surfaces, such as scalpels. If an instrument has rather intricate parts or joints, some time will be required for the chemical to penetrate into the indentations or joint surfaces.

If the chemical is used in combination with heat the period for disinfection will be reduced. The importance of using heat for sterilisation whenever possible cannot be over-emphasised.

Many new chemicals are now in use in the operating theatre, but the lists on page 152 includes also some of the older and well-established ones. In all cases the instrument must be thoroughly rinsed before use to remove chemical traces which at high concentrations may prove irritant to body tissues.

The phenol and coal-tar derivative group

Carbolic acid (or phenol in its pure state) and cresol with soap (lysol) are now not used as a disinfectant because there are many derivatives that are more effective and less dangerous to use.

The effect of phenols and its derivatives are not clearly understood but it is thought they act by coagulation and lytic tissue effects on the bacteria. Their action seems to be dependent on selective concentration at all surfaces with desaturation of proteins and increase in cell permeability.

SUDOL

This is a clear soluble disinfectant of the lysol type with somewhat reduced corrosive hazards and a germicidal potency generally twice that of Lysol B.P. For general disinfectant purposes in potentially heavily contaminated situations, e.g., infected linen and floors, the dilution is 2 per cent. For surface disinfection when the contamination is light, e.g., walls, tables, trolleys, etc., the dilution is 1 per cent, which falls within the range of 'in-use' dilutions recommended by Kelsey and Maurer in 1967. Rubber gloves must be worn.

PRINTOL

A clear soluble disinfectant with a phenolic base but rather less corrosive than the lysol type. Its dilution in heavily contaminated situations is 3 per cent but for routine surface disinfection this can be reduced to 1·25 per cent (Kelsey and Maurer, 1967).

PRINTOL D

Similar to Printol except that it incorporates a detergent system which increases its capacity to reach the source of infection through dirt and organic contamination. Dilutions of 2·5 per cent for heavy contamination and 0·75 per cent for routine surface disinfection (Kelsey and Maurer, 1967).

For the disinfection of infected linen the manufacturers recommend a dilution of 0·5 per cent for four hours with Printol or Printol D.

HYCOLIN

This is a balanced combination of synthetic phenols which are less corrosive than lysol. It is used for general purposes at a dilution of 1 per cent and this should be increased to 2 per cent for heavy contamination.

CLEARSOL

Contains 40 per cent of phenols consisting chiefly of the powerful xylenol fraction and a mild detergent system. Suitable for general disinfection at a recommended dilution of 1 per cent.

These five synthetic phenolic disinfectants are effective against all common Gram-positive and Gram-negative organisms including *Pseudomonas aeruginosa* (*pyocyanea*). They are compatible with anionic and non-ionic substances such as soaps, anionic detergents, etc.

CHLOROXYLENOL (DETTOL)

This is a relatively non-toxic non-irritant antibacterial agent which is active against most organisms, including the streptococcus, but rather less active against certain Gram-negative organisms. The destruction of spores is somewhat doubtful.

Dettol antiseptic contains 4·8 per cent chloroxylenol and 9 per cent terpineol, and is used at a dilution of 5 per cent for general disinfection purposes, 10 minutes being the minimal period of immersion recommended for disinfection.

It is not advisable to bring chloroxylenol preparations, especially strong solutions, into contact with plastics as they tend to cause deterioration of the material.

CHLORHEXIDINE (HIBITANE)

This well established antibacterial agent has proved to be of great use. Single or infrequent applications to the intact skin of any strength solution will not cause irritation, but repeated applications of a 1 per cent solution may eventually give rise to erythema. The dilutions in common use should not give rise to any irritation of the user's skin (Rose and Swaine, 1956).

Hibitane Hospital Concentrate 5 per cent is a solution of 5 per cent chlorhexidine gluconate, and an aqueous dilution of 0·5 per cent of the concentrate is used for the surface disinfection of inanimate objects, such as bowls, tables, etc. This dilution of Hibitane concentrate is equivalent to 0·025 per cent effective concentration of the antibacterial agent, chlorhexidine gluconate.

For the prophylactic treatment of wounds a Hibitane concentrate dilution of 1 per cent in water (0·05 per cent effective concentration) is used; for pre-surgical skin disinfection, 10 per cent dilution in 70 per cent industrial methylated spirit (0·5 per cent) with an added dye such as geranine or methylene blue (Lowbury, 1961); for the *emergency* pre-surgical disinfection of heat-labile instruments, which are immersed for a minimum of 10 minutes before use, a dilution of 10 per cent of Hibitane concentrate in 70 per cent industrial methylated spirit (0·5 per cent); and for the final pre-surgical rinse of hands (unless pHisoHex is being used), 1 per cent dilution of Hibitane concentrate in 70 per cent industrial methylated spirit (0·05 per cent). *Dilutions given in brackets always refer to the effective concentration of the antibacterial agent.*

The Hibitane concentrate is generally supplied coloured a distinctive red, and is effective against a wide range of Gram-positive and Gram-negative organisms. Although as with other antibacterial agents, blood slows down the bacterial activity of Hibitane, it is claimed that a dilution of 0·4 per cent (0·02 per cent) in 50 per cent blood, considerable bactericidal effect is retained. At the dilutions in common use Hibitane cannot be relied upon to kill spores, but it appears quite comparable with other similar antibacterial chemicals. Except in the greater dilutions it is not compatible with soaps and should not intentionally be combined with these.

HEXACHLOROPHANE

This is an antibacterial agent which can be combined with soap in a proportion of usually 2 per cent (Gould et al., 1957; Lowbury, 1961). Pre-surgical washes called pHisoHex and Disfex are available and enable the scrub-up time to be reduced to three minutes. The method of use has already been described in the previous chapter.

Hexachlorophane is more effective against Gram-positive than Gram-negative organisms, but its main value lies in the regular use of a solution or soap containing the chemical. If the surgeons and theatre staff use pHisoHex, Disfex or hexachlorophane soap regularly it has been shown that the bacterial flora of the skin is reduced, and it is quite possible to rely upon a three-minute pre-surgical wash under these conditions (Smylie et al., 1959). However, as the effect is cumulative, it may require repeated applications before its action is effective. But care must be taken not to use hexachlorophane preparations for regular total body bathing; there is a possible risk of toxicity from absorption of hexachlorophane into the blood stream (Scowen, 1972).

Synthetic detergent disinfectants

The quarternary ammonium compounds are surface-acting detergents or amines which are derivatives of ammonium chloride. They are bacteriostatic in high dilutions, although their activity is affected by the type of water used for dilution, or contact with anionic-type soaps. Hard, acid or iron-rich water reduces their bacteriocidal activity.

These compounds are effective against most Gram-positive organisms, but not against Gram-negative organisms, especially *Pseudomonas Aeruginosa* or tubercle bacilli.

CETRIMIDE B.P. (C.T.A.B. CETAVLON)

This is in effect an antibacterial detergent. It is not compatible with soap, but used in a dilution of not less than 0.5 per cent possesses very useful detergent properties which may be applied to the cleansing of contaminated wounds.

Although the higher concentrations are necessary for detergency, its antibacterial properties extend down to 0.2 per cent and at this dilution cetrimide may be used for the general washing of equipment such as bowls, etc.

Cetrimide has been combined with chlorhexidine to increase its antibacterial action against Gram-negative bacteria and this preparation is available, known as Savlon Hospital concentrate, which is supplied as a concentrated solution containing 1.5 per cent chlorhexidine gluconate and 15 per cent cetrimide.

The dilutions of Savlon Hospital concentrate are as follows:

For general antibacterial purposes, such as washing equipment, an aqueous dilution of 0.5 per cent Savlon Hospital concentrate is used; pre-surgical rinsing of hands or the preliminary treatment of burns and clean wounds, 1 per cent aqueous dilution of the concentrate; for contaminated or dirty wounds, 3 per cent aqueous dilution of the concentrate; for the *emergency* disinfection of heat-labile instruments which are immersed for a minimum of 10 minutes before use a dilution of 10 per cent of the concentrate in 70 per cent industrial methylated spirit may be used.

BENZALKONIUM CHLORIDE (ROCCAL, ZEPHIRAN)

This is similar in action to the other quaternary ammonium compounds. The B.P. solution contains 50 per cent w/v of benzalkonium chloride; Roccal (Bayer) contains 1 per cent benzalkonium chloride and Roccal concentrate (Roccal 10X) contains 10 per cent. If used at a dilution of not less than 0·5 per cent it has very useful detergent properties which may be utilised for the cleansing of contaminated wounds (Spalton, 1951). Its antibacterial properties extend down to 0·025 per cent for irrigation of the bladder, but for general purposes the greatest dilution is not less than 0·5 per cent.

For pre-surgical skin preparation and the cleansing of contaminated wounds, the aqueous dilutions should be between 1 and 0·5 per cent effective concentration respectively. A 70 per cent industrial methylated spirit may be substituted as the diluent for pre-surgical skin preparation when a more rapid action is desired. When full detergency is not required, a dilution of 0·5 per cent aqueous (0·05 per cent) is quite adequate for antibacterial purposes, and this dilution should be used for the general disinfection of inanimate objects such as bowls or linen etc.

For the final pre-surgical rinse of hands a dilution of 1 per cent (0·1 per cent) aqueous or in 70 per cent industrial methylated spirit should be used, and at this concentration there should not be any undue irritation to the user's hands.

Roccal or Zephiran can be used for bladder or urethral irrigation in the dilution of 0·05 per cent (0·005 per cent), but for retention lavage this dilution must be increased to 0·025 per cent (0·0025 per cent).

Halogens and halogen compounds

The most widely used of these are the hypochlorites and iodines. Chlorine-based compounds act mainly by oxidation and the liberation of its odours may be objectionable. Iodine acts directly by iodination and oxidation, being able to change into the vapour-state readily.

SODIUM HYPOCHLORATE

This is an effective anti viral disinfectant for inanimate objects. As a solution giving 1 per cent available chlorine it can be used for surface application such as floors, and soaking infected linen. It should not be used for instruments or steel holloware as Chlorine damages the surface. Commercial preparations include Chloros and Stericol which are supplied as a concentrated solution requiring dilution before use.

IODINE

Iodine is very insoluble in water and therefore is generally combined with alcohol. As a 2 per cent solution in industrial methylated spirit, combining readily with organic material this is still regarded by many as the ideal pre-surgical skin preparation. It is certainly the most lethal to bacteria of all preparations used for this purpose, but unfortunately it does produce an occasional skin irritation which is disturbing for the patient. If a wound is very heavily contaminated and there has been a lengthy delay of the patient's admission to hospital the use of an iodine pre-surgical skin preparation may be indicated.

POVIDONE-IODINE (BETADINE)

This is a non-stinging, non-staining, film-forming, water-soluble iodine complex (Marr and Saggers, 1964). It is not irritating to skin and mucous membranes and unlike iodine tincture can be safely bandaged or applied as a compress. It is a topical disinfectant that retains the unique, non-selective microbiocidal activity of iodine, without the undesirable side effects mentioned above. It kills all organisms including spores and has a more prolonged action than ordinary iodine. Its brown colour can easily be washed off skin as well as cotton, wool and silk and its action is unimpaired by blood, serum, pus or soap.

Betadine is available as an aqueous antiseptic solution which is used undiluted for pre-operative skin preparation and as a surgical scrub. The latter contains a suitable detergent and forms a rich lather which is non-staining and non-irritating.

Formaldehyde

Although formaldehyde is a very powerful and effective disinfectant, its use for pre-surgical disinfection is largely falling into disrepute unless combined with sub-atmospheric steam. Disinfection failures in formalin cabinets have been described for many years and it is doubtful whether the formalin vapour penetrates the lumen of catheters even with control of the humidity in the cabinet. The use of formalin combined with sub-atmospheric steam, has been described on page 147.

ACTIVATED GLUTARALDEHYDE

This is a 2 per cent aqueous solution buffered to a pH 7·5–8·5 by the addition of 0·3 per cent sodium bicarbonate.

Cidex is a commercial preparation of glutaraldehyde containing an anti-rust agent. Vegetative bacteria and tubercle bacilli are killed in 20 minutes and some spore-forming species are killed in 10 hours at 20° C (Spalding, 1963; Stonehill et al., 1963; Medical Research Council, 1968).

The solution is suitable for disinfecting lensed instruments such as cystoscopes and other types of endoscopes providing the instrument is clean and partially dismantled. It is also suitable for anaesthetic masks etc.

The in-use dilution is slightly irritant to skin and mucous membranes and severely irritant to the eye. All instruments should be rinsed thoroughly in sterile water before use in surgery.

Once activated long life Cidex solution is effective for four weeks.

Note: Bacterial contamination of dilute solutions such as cetrimide and chlorhexidine and even phenolics can occur under certain circumstances. For this reason cork enclosures or cork liners in screw-cap bottles should not be used as cork appears to nourish and protect organisms. Contamination can occur also with the practice of 'topping up' half-empty bottles or of refilling stock bottles without resterilisation. Another cause may be due to the use of unsterile solutions or glassware or the transfer of bacteria to bottles during use (e.g., from the fingers of nurses contaminated while handling infected articles or patients).

Bottles of disinfectant solutions should be date-stamped and used in rotation. Stocks must be kept at a minimum, and the points made above observed. (Medical Research Council, 1968).

Many hospital authorities have established a policy to limit the number, variety and variations in dilutions of disinfectant in general use. Such a policy ensures that the most effective chemical is chosen and lends itself also to economy.

APPLICATION OF METHODS

It is important to remember that the easiest and most effective method of sterilisation is by moist heat, and whenever possible is the method of choice. If an antibacterial agent is used, a thorough pre-cleansing is as vital as the application of the chemical which should always be given sufficient time to penetrate to all parts of the instrument.

Anaesthetic Apparatus. After careful cleansing, inside and out with soap and water or a chemical detergent such as Neodian or cetrimide, rubber face masks, rebreathing bags, corrugated tubes, airways, endotracheal or bronchial tubes should be immersed in 0·5 per cent aqueous Hibitane or Savlon for a minimum period of 10 minutes. Alternatively they should be immersed in Cidex solution for a similar period of time. A rebreathing bag or corrugated tubes should be hung up to dry, care being taken to ensure that the inside of the bag and corrugations are thoroughly dried. The airways and endotracheal or endobronchial tubes may be dried by placing them on a towel covering a warm surface.

Ideally corrugated tubes, 'Y' pieces, Heidbrink valves and some rubber airways and endotracheal tubes, etc., should be autoclaved after a thorough cleansing, but it is inadvisable to treat the vinyl plastic variety in a similar manner as they tend to become opaque. Before autoclaving a 'cuffed tube' the cuff or obturator bag must be empty. A method of disinfecting ventilators is described in Chapter 10, page 261.

Bougies, Catheters, etc. These are dealt with under the appropriate headings, e.g., metal, plastic and rubber.

Electrical Apparatus. Quite a large proportion of electrical apparatus used in surgery is now manufactured suitable for sterilisation by heat. Care must always be taken to observe the manufacturers' instructions regarding a particular instrument as it is possible for some parts to be heat sterilisable and others not.

A large proportion of electrical leads and illuminated retractors are now made autoclavable, but after use they should be dried very thoroughly to minimise corrosion. Those not sterilisable by high temperatures should be immersed in a 10 per cent aqueous solution of Hibitane (0·5 per cent), for a minimal period of 30 minutes, sterilised by ethylene oxide or alternatively subjected to the sub-atmospheric steam/formaldehyde process.

Diathermy or cautery electrodes may generally be autoclaved. If heat sterilisation is contraindicated, *emergency* disinfection may be effected by immersing them in a 10 per cent aqueous solution of Hibitane (0·5 per cent) or Cidex for a minimal period of 10 minutes.

Several of the more modern electric bone drills and saws may be autoclaved complete; in most cases, however, only the outer motor cover or the flexible drive is sterilisable in this way. The cable must be covered with a sterilised cotton sleeve before use and care taken to ensure that no moisture has collected on or near electrical contacts.

Generally speaking, electric lamps are damaged by heat and should therefore be sterilised ideally by ethylene oxide, or immersed in a chemical antibacterial agent such as 10 per cent aqueous solution of Hibitane (0·5 per cent) or Cidex.

Endoscopes. The same rules apply to endoscopes, including cystocopes, bronchoscopes, oesophagoscopes, etc., but extra care must be taken with optical attachments such as telescopes, lenses and lighting attachments.

A rapid increase of pressure of steam may cause cracking of the optical attachments, although in practice with modern apparatus this complication is minimised. Similarly breakage may occur if a hot endoscope is cooled too rapidly in cold water before use. Sometimes only the sheath of an endoscope is heat sterilisable, and if the optical/lighting system is required sterile it must be processed by sub-atmospheric steam/formaldehyde, ethylene oxide, or immersed in a 10 per cent aqueous solution of Hibitane (0·5 per cent) vertically for a minimal period of 10 minutes. On no account must instruments containing lenses come into contact with any alcohol-based solutions; it will dissolve the lens-mounting cement.

Pasteurisation of endoscopes is carried out simply by immersion for 10 minutes in a boiler thermostatically controlled at 75°C–85°C instead of 100°C, and it is enough to destroy vegetative bacteria very rapidly. Undoubtedly this is preferable to the use of chemicals when higher temperatures are contraindicated.

Metal Ware. This is sterilised by autoclaving at 134°C, 2·25 kg per cm^2 (220·59 kN/m^2,

32 p.s.i.) for six minutes, little or no drying being necessary. Alternatively the articles are contained within a packet and sterilised with the drapes (p. 104).

Glassware. Generally all glassware may be autoclaved if certain precautions are taken and steam can reach all surfaces of the glass. To avoid breakage it is advisable to pre-heat the articles being sterilised by placing them in the autoclave chamber beforehand.

After sterilisation glassware should be allowed to cool slowly, thereby avoiding cracking which may occur if the articles are cooled too rapidly. Glassware should not be sterilised together with metal instruments as the latter can cause unnecessary breakages. Dry-heat sterilisation is the method of choice for all glassware.

Linen. Gowns, caps, masks and operation drapes are packed into linen, paper or nylon packets or Bripac/Permapak boxes. These are sterilised at 126°C, 1·41 kg per cm^2 (137·9 kN/m^2, 20 p.s.i.) for 30 minutes or 134°C, 2·25 kg per cm^2 (220·59 kN/m^2, 32 p.s.i.) for three and a half minutes.

Lotions. Normal saline and sterile water for hand lotion use should be prepared as individual glass bottles of $\frac{1}{2}$ or 1 litre capacity, which are autoclaved so that the temperature of each container is maintained at 115°C, 0·7 kg per cm^2 (68·95 kN/m^2, 10 p.s.i.) for 30 minutes. (British Pharmacopoeia, 1973).

The holding period of sterilisation depends upon a number of factors which include type of autoclave, capacity and load, i.e., $\frac{1}{2}$ or 1 litre bottles. This period should be determined initially by a thermocouple recording the temperature reached inside a bottle of water at the centre of the load. Subsequently the temperature/holding period is checked either by an integrated thermocouple or a black spot Browne's tube suspended in one of the filled bottles. The holding period selected for a load of mixed $\frac{1}{2}$ and 1 litre bottles must be that suitable for the latter.

When sterilising bottles of liquid in an autoclave certain precautions must be taken. The metal caps must have a well-fitted rubber washer which is renewed regularly; a pre-vacuum is drawn and steam admitted to the chamber gradually; and after sterilisation the steam pressure must be reduced over a period of about 30 minutes, otherwise the liquid may boil violently and the bottles burst. *A post-vacuum must not be drawn.* At this stage some autoclaves incorporate a special fluid cycle with spray cooling after sterilisation whilst (Howie and Timbury, 1956) maintaining pressure of air in the autoclave chamber. This avoids bursting of bottles.

After sterilisation the caps of the bottles are sealed with *sterile* cellulose tape or a plastic seal. Once a seal on a sterile bottle has been broken, the stopper removed and the contents exposed to the air, a *sterile* label does not indicate sterility of the contents. Saline or water from a sterile bottle or flask must not be used for injection, infusion or washing of sterile instruments unless the seal of the bottle is unbroken at the time of use.

Once opened and not used, such bottles should be regarded as contaminated and must be discarded. Bottles such as the Matbick type incorporate their own seal.

Metal Instruments. These are divided into the heat sterilisable and non-heat sterilisable types.

The heat sterilisable metal instruments are made generally of stainless steel which will not rust if the instruments are dried after use. Such instruments, including scissors, dissecting and artery forceps, metal bougies and catheters, etc., may be sterilised on open trays in an autoclave for six minutes at 130°C, 1·76 kg per cm^2 (172·3 kN/m^2, 25 p.s.i.).

Non-autoclavable instruments made from carbon steel, such as solid scalpels, twist drills and osteotomes, etc., are better sterilised by dry heat or ethylene oxide.

In the dry-heat process of sterilisation the instruments are exposed to a temperature of 160°C for one hour *plus* additional time necessary to allow heat penetration to all parts of the load. This additional period ranges between a half and one and a half hours.

In an emergency a 10 per cent Hibitane (0·5 per cent) solution in industrial methylated spirit will disinfect metal instruments in a *minimum* period of ten minutes, providing that the chemical has access to all parts.

Nail Brushes. These should be autoclaved at 130° C, 1·76 kg per cm^2 (172·3 kN/m^2, 25 p.s.i.) for six minutes, or 134° C, 2·25 kg per cm^2 (220·59 kN/m^2, 32 p.s.i.) for three and a half minutes. The most satisfactory method is to autoclave the brushes in a metal brush dispenser and keep them in the dry state until needed. A separate clean brush is then used for each person.

The best method for reprocessable suture needles is to prepare the needles as sets in paper bags and sterilise by the dry-heat method or autoclaving. Using the latter method, a small piece of vapour phase inhibitor anti-rust paper should be included with the needles when packing; this applies also to steam sterilisation.

It is very important to ensure that debris is not lodged in the eye of a suture needle or at any point along the shaft before sterilisation. Suture needles are difficult to clean; ideally pre-sterilised disposable suture needles should be used.

Rubber Goods. Some of these, including non-disposable tubing, drainage sheeting, catheters and certain endotracheal and endobronchial tubes can be autoclaved providing the drying cycle is not prolonged.

Macintoshes are treated with an antibacterial agent such as 0·5 per cent aqueous Hibitane, and if heavily contaminated should be autoclaved.

Powders. The only satisfactory method of sterilising powders to avoid clumping is by dry heat or gamma irradiation. These are available commercially, ready-sterilised.

Plastics. Most non-disposable plastics in common use in the operating theatre may be sterilised by wet heat, but care must be taken as at boiling-point and above they become softened and easily damaged.

Polyvinyl chloride (vinyl Portex, both translucent and ivory Magill variety) and polythene tubing, etc., should be sterilised in ethylene oxide or pasteurised in sub-atmospheric steam/formaldehyde. Most polyvinyl tubing can now be purchased ready sterilised.

Nylon tubing can be sterilised by this method also, but due to its high melting-point 200° C steam sterilisation as recommended for metal instruments can be employed.

Plastic tubing should never be shaken upon removal from a water pasteuriser as it is then very brittle and may break at the point where it is secured with bandage.

It is important to ensure that there are no kinks or air bubbles in the tubing during pasteurisation and it is preferable to fill the tubing with water beforehand. Kinks in the tubing will result in flattened sections and air bubbles with inefficient disinfection of the lumen. Plastic tubing which has flattened sections or irregularities following sterilisation can often be returned to its original shape and section by re-heating and then cooling rapidly whilst maintaining the desired position.

The use of other items of plastic equipment in the theatre is rather questionable due to the danger of static electricity formation (Chapter 3), but all inanimate objects such as arm supports and translucent X-ray cassette holders for fracture tables, etc., are disinfected with a 1 per cent aqueous solution of Hibitane or Savlon before and after use. Other antibacterial agents which may be used for this purpose are Roccal and Bradosol at their recommended dilutions. The usual type of materials used for these articles are perspex and fibre glass.

Suture Materials. Most ligatures and sutures available in foil or plastic sachets are presented as sterile peel-open overwrap packets. Unopened inner sachets can be disinfected by immersion in a suitable fluid recommended by the manufacturer for a minimum period of 30 minutes before use.

Plastic envelopes containing sterile non-boilable catgut are stored in a fluid supplied by the catgut manufacturers which consists basically of isopropyl alcohol.

Monofilament Nylon and Silkworm Gut. These are generally sterilised with the instrument sets but can be autoclaved separately in packets at standard autoclave temperatures and times.

Braided, Twisted, Plated, and Floss Silk, Nylon, or Linen Thread, etc. These are wound on to metal, nylon or glass ligature reels and are autoclaved. Sterile peel-open packets containing various sizes of nylon, silk and linen thread.

Metal Wire, Mesh and Suture Clips. All are autoclavable before use as described under metal instruments. They may be stored in dry sterilised boxes or packets, but in the case of Cushing's or McKenzie's ligature clips these may be included in the set of instruments.

REFERENCES

ALDER, V. G., BROWN, A. M. AND GILLESPIE, W. A. (1966) *Journal of Clinical Pathology*, **19**, 83.
BOGER, W. (1976) *Hospital Topics*, Sept/Oct. 12.
BOLTON, J. (1966) *British Hospital Journal*, May 13, 867.
BOWIE, J. H. (1961) *Sterilisation of Surgical Materials. Symposium.* London: Pharmaceutical Press.
BOWIE, J. H., KELSEY, J. C. AND THOMPSON, C. R. (1963) *Lancet*, **i**, 586.
BOWIE, J. H., KENNEDY, M. H. AND ROBERTSON, I. (1975) *Lancet*, **i**, 1135.
British Pharmacopoeia (1963) p. 396.
COLQUHOUN, J. (1969) *British Hospital Journal*, July.
CUNLIFFE, A. C. (1966) *Proceedings Central Sterilising Club*, April 29–30th.
DARMADY, E. M., HUGHES, K. E. A., MURT, M. M., FREEMAN, B. M. AND POWELL, D. B. (1961) *Journal of Clinical Pathology*, **14**, 55.
FISCHER, E. (1971) Meeting on ethylene oxide sterilisation, University of Wales, September 6th.
FRANCIS, A. E. (1959) *Proceedings of the Royal Society of Medicine*, **52**, 998.
GOULD, B. S., FRIGERIO, N. A. AND HOVANESIEN, J. (1957) *Antibiotics*, 7, 457.
HOWIE, J. W. (1961) *Journal of Clinical Pathology*, **14**, 49.
HOWIE, J. W. AND TIMBURY, M. C. (1956) *Lancet*, **ii**, 669.
JEFFERSON, S. (1958) *Radioisotopes*, p. 278. London: Newnes.
KELSEY, J. C. AND MAURER, I. M. (1967) *Public Health Laboratory Service Bulletin*, **26**, June.
KNOX, R. (1961) *Journal of Clinical Pathology*, **14**, 13.
KNOX, R. AND PICKERILL, J. K. (1967) *British Hospital Journal*, December 15th.
LINE, S. J. AND PICKERILL, J. K. (1973) *Journal of Clinical Pathology*, **26**, 716–720.
LOWBURY, E. J. (1961) *Journal of Clinical Pathology*, **14**, 85, 88, 89.
MCCULLOCH, E. C. (1945) *Disinfection and Sterilisation*, 2nd edn. London: Kimpton.
MACKENZIE, S. (1966) *British Hospital Journal*, September 16, 1733.
MARR, M. S. AND SAGGERS, B. (1964) *Nursing Times*, June 12.
MEDICAL RESEARCH COUNCIL (1945) *The Sterilisation, Use and Care of Syringes.* War Memo. No. 15. London: HMSO.
MEDICAL RESEARCH COUNCIL (1959) Working Party. *Lancet*, **i**, 425.
MEDICAL RESEARCH COUNCIL (1968) Aseptic methods in the operating theatre. *Lancet*, **i**, 763.
MORRIS, C. A. AND EVERALL, P. H. (1975) *Lancet*, **i**, 923.
PERKINS, J. J. (1956a) Bacteriological and surgical sterilisation by heat. In *Antiseptics, Disinfectants, Fungicides, Chemicals and Physical Sterilisation.* Edited by C. F. Reddish. New York: Lea and Febiger.
PERKINS, J. J. (1956b) *Principles and Methods of Sterilisation*, p. 163. Springfield, Ill.: Thomas.
RENDELL-BAKER, L. (1970) *Hospitals*, October.
RENDELL-BAKER, L. AND ROBERTS, R. B. (1970) *Current Researches in Anesthesia and Analgesia*, November.
ROSE, F. L. AND SWAINE, G. (1956) *Journal of the Chemical Society*, **4**, 4422.
SCOWEN, (1972) *Report of U.K. Committee on the Safety of Medicines, 'Hexachlorophane'*, February.
SMYLIE, H. G., WEBSTER, C. V. AND BRUCE, M. L. (1959) *British Medical Journal*, **ii**, 606.
SPALTON, L. M. (1951) *Chemist and Druggist*, November 24.
SPALDING, E. H. (1963) *Association of Operating Room Nurses' Journal, U.S.A.*, May/June.
SYKES, G. (1958) In *Disinfection and Sterilisation*, pp. 170–339. Edited by McCulloch. London: Kimpton.
STONEHILL, A., KROP, S. AND BORICK, P. M. (1963) *American Journal of Hospital Pharmacy*, 20, 458.
WALTER, C. W. (1948) *The Aseptic Treatment of Wounds.* New York: Macmillan.
WELLS, C. AND WHITWELL, F. R. (1960) *Lancet*, **ii**, 643.
WESSEX INSTRUMENT CASKET, Feature article. *British Hospital Journal*, March.
WEYMES, C. (1966) *British Hospital Journal*, September, 1745.

7
LIGATURE AND SUTURE MATERIALS

A suture is a stitch used in surgery to approximate living tissues or structures until the normal process of healing is complete.

A ligature is a suture used to encircle a blood-vessel to arrest or control bleeding.

Ligatures and sutures are divided into two main groups: the absorbable and the non-absorbable. The absorbable are digested and absorbed during the process of healing. This group includes natural materials such as catgut and collagen, synthetic materials such as polyglycolic acid and living sutures fashioned from tendons or fascia. The non-absorbable group remain permanently in the tissues after the process of healing is complete. This is especially useful when the tissues are weakened and require reinforcement for some considerable time after operation, as in the case of herniorrhaphy. This group includes natural materials, such as silkworm gut, and man-made fibres of the nylon or polyester type.

Table 7.1 Categories of ligatures and sutures

Absorbable Ligatures/Sutures
- A. Natural: catgut, collagen, living tissue
- B. Synthetic: Polyglycolic acid

Non-absorbable Ligatures/Sutures
- A. Natural: Silkworm gut, Silk, Linen, Cotton
- B. Synthetic: Polyamides, Polyesters, Polyoletins
    - I Polyethylene
    - II Polypropylene

Metallic Wire

Adhesive Tape Closures

Catgut

The most generally used material in this group is surgical catgut, which is substantially pure collagen prepared from the submucosal layer of the first third of the small intestine of government-inspected sheep (Forrester, 1975).

The preparation of surgical catgut is controlled by the Department of Health. All manufacturers must reach very high pharmaceutical standards laid down by law before their product can be marketed.

THE PREPARATION OF SURGICAL CATGUT

Before export to this country the excised intestine is mechanically cleansed at the abattoir, and 'casings' of 16 to 18 mm diameter are frozen for transport.

On arrival at the catgut laboratories the intestines are rapidly thawed and slit longitudinally into three or four ribbons (Fig. 7.1). Batches of ribbons are then thoroughly scraped under a water spray to remove muscle and fatty material. The process is called sliming.

The ribbons of gut may be treated also in several baths of an alkaline solution to remove the fat by saponification.

Fig. 7.1 Splitting New Zealand milk lamb intestines into ribbon. (Ethicon.)

According to the diameter of the gut required, two or more ribbons may be spun together into strands before drying under tension followed by polishing the surface of the strands.

This dried catgut is now known technically as raw *plain* catgut. After sterilisation this catgut would be absorbed in muscle tissue in approximately 5 to 10 days, or about a quarter of that time in the peritoneum or serous membrane.

In order to prolong the time of absorption in the tissues and reduce irritation (Postlethwait, 1969), the raw catgut can be hardened or chromicised by immersing the strands in a chromic salt solution bath. As chromic salts are normally colourless, it is usual to add colour to this bath to indicate visually the difference between *plain* and *chromic* catgut.

The degree of hardness depends upon how long the catgut is immersed in the chromic salts. The most generally accepted degree today is medium chromic catgut which, under normal conditions, will persist in the tissues from 15 to 20 days, or a quarter of that time in the peritoneum and serous membrane.

Fig. 7.2 Machine sliming to remove fatty material from sheeps' intestine. (Ethicon.)

Fig. 7.3 Spinning multiples of ribbon into raw surgical catgut. (Ethicon.)

Each of the strands is then graded carefully into about eight standard metric sizes ranging from 0·75 to 5 (6/0) to size 2). (*The ligature or suture sizes quoted first refer always to BPC metric gauge, the sizes in brackets are the old equivalents. The metric size approximates the diameter of the strand in millimetres × 10.*) The full range from thinnest to thickest is 0·75 (6/0), 1 (5/0), 1·5 (4/0), 2 (3/0), 2·5 (2/0), 3 (0), 4 (1), 5 (2). These strands also undergo a tensile strength test over a surgeon's knot, and must reach a minimum BPC breaking load, as follows:

Size	BPC minimum breaking load (tensile strength)	Typical tensile strength supplied
0·75 (6/0)	0·07 kgf*	0·34 kgf
1 (5/0)	0·15 kgf	0·64 kgf
1·5 (4/0)	0·35 kgf	1·04 kgf
2 (3/0)	0·65 kgf	1·72 kgf
2·5 (2/0)	0·85 kgf	2·58 kgf
3 (0)	1·25 kgf	3·54 kgf
4 (1)	2·20 kgf	4·53 kgf
5 (2)	3·0 kgf	5·55 kgf

*kilogram force

Fig. 7.4 Electronic gauging of finished catgut strands before polishing. (Ethicon.)

After dividing the finished catgut into convenient lengths of 76 cm (30 in) or 1·52 m (5 ft), it is either wound on to card formers, plastic formers or coiled into a suitable size for the container. Sterilisation is effected by exposing the catgut to gamma irradiation or electron bombardment after it has been packed and sealed.

Before this process of sterilisation, which is carefully controlled by laboratory tests, the catgut is packed either in plastic envelopes or aluminium foil packets containing a solution similar to purified industrial methylated spirit. The plastic packets are heat

Fig. 7.5 Finished sutures being placed in foil packets before sterilisation. (Ethicon.)

sealed, and the aluminium foil packets sealed with a special process. This is done under clean conditions as sterilisation follows afterwards.

Packets of catgut are generally presented in a sterile peel-open overwrap outer cover.

THE SIZES OF CATGUT IN GENERAL USE

This will depend a great deal upon the requirements of a particular surgeon. The tendency, however, is for the finest possible size to be used in all cases, and with the continual improvement of tensile strength the sizes in common use are much finer than those used in previous years.

For the ligation of small blood-vessels 2 or 2·5 (3/0 or 2/0) *plain* catgut is generally sufficient. Large blood-vessels and pedicles, such as those requiring ligation in gynaecological surgery, require a stouter *chromic* catgut, size 4 (1) or thicker.

The suture of stomach or bowel in the adult necessitates using size 2·5 or 3 (2/0 or 0) *chromic* catgut, whereas a child needs 2 (3/0) for these tissues.

In an adult the peritoneum and muscle can be sutured with *chromic* catgut sizes 4 or 5 (1 or 2), a child will require at least a size smaller, 3 (0).

Fig. 7.6 (above left)   The peel-open overwrap packet which contains the suture packet. (Ethicon.)

Fig. 7.7 (above right)   Plastic peel-open overwrap packet. (Davis & Geck.)

Fig. 7.8 Opening an aluminium foil catgut pack. (A) The packet is held with the thumbs together on either side of the notch. (B) Tearing open along the dotted line. (C) Removing the suture. (Ethicon.)

If subcutaneous tissue is sutured a size 2 or 2·5 (3/0 or 2/0) *plain* catgut is preferable, especially in the case of a subcutaneous suture for thyroidectomy.

Some surgeons will use *chromic* catgut throughout an operation, but if *plain* catgut is used it is important that this is not introduced as a suture (or ligature) into the peritoneum due to rapid absorption, except in very special circumstances decided by the surgeon, e.g., in the urinary tract.

Fig. 7.9 (A) Removing catgut from foil packet. (B) Stretching catgut by hand to remove kinks. (C) Stretching catgut with forceps to remove kinks. (D) Threading a suture needle with forceps.

THE HANDLING OF SURGICAL CATGUT

At operation the circulating nurse peels open the outer overwrap cover. The inner packet is taken by the scrub nurse using long sterile forceps.

A plastic envelope is opened first by shaking the contents to one end of the packet and then tearing across from the 'V' cut or cutting across the other end whilst holding over a kidney dish to catch the fluid contained.

An aluminium foil packet is opened by tearing across the V-cut at one side of the packet. Care must be taken not to squeeze the packet as this done, for fluid may be sprayed out under pressure and may cause damage to the user's eyes.

1. The catgut is removed from the tube or packet with sterile forceps, together with the size label which is useful for reference, especially when several sizes are in use.

2. In general surgery, the catgut is removed from the packet and each end of the strand grasped with the gloved hands and stretched slightly to remove the kinks. In orthopaedic surgery this operation *may* have to be performed using forceps, care being taken to ensure that the catgut is not crushed with the forceps except at the end of a strand. A crush mark in the centre of a ligature or suture may cause it to break during handling.

3. The material is then cut up into suitable strands for ligatures or sutures which are threaded on to needles either by hand, or for orthopaedic operations by using a non-touch technique. The material should be threaded from within the curve of the needle outwards, leaving one end about 5 to 10 cm (2 to 4 in) long. The material may be locked in the eye of the needle either by passing through a second time in the same direction or by tying a single knot. If it is frequently necessary to have a locked suture, it is preferable to use a special needle such as the Paterson or spring-eye needle, which locks the catgut without passing it through the eye a second time or tying a knot.

Fig. 7.10 Non-traumatic sutures, catgut and silk.

Even with Paterson eye or spring-eye needles two strands of catgut always pass through the tissues. This creates unnecessary trauma, especially when suturing delicate tissue.

The use of non-traumatic sutures is now well established and this obviates the disadvantages of doubling the suture when using a needle having an eye.

Non-traumatic sutures are manufactured by fusing the suture material into a needle designed with one end hollowed.

Catgut is very suitable for use in non-traumatic needles, and is supplied as prepared general closure intestinal or plastic sutures, sizes 4 to 1 (1 to 5/0) on various shapes and sizes of needles.

Catgut ligatures and sutures must not be left exposed for any length of time. Ideally the ligature or suture is only removed from the tube or packet just before required, but if prepared previously it must be kept covered with a small sterile towel.

It is very important to ensure that catgut is *not* soaked before use, as this causes the material to swell and increases the speed of digestion in the tissues. Passage once through the tissues will lubricate the suture sufficiently for use. If the surgeon insists on pre-moistening the catgut, it may be drawn *very gently* through a moistened glove or swab.

Care must be exercised when handling catgut to avoid fraying, as this will weaken the strand considerably and may cause the breaking of a suture line post-operatively.

Living sutures

These are tissue sutures obtained from the patient himself.

The most usual are strips of fascia lata used in Gallie's herniorrhaphy and obtained from the lateral aspect of the thigh. In one method the strips of fascia 0·5 cm by 18 cm (¼ in by 7 in) approximately are obtained through a long thigh incision, following which the fascial defect and skin are sutured. It is possible also to remove these strips via two small incisions using a fasciatome, but in this case the fascial defect is not sutured.

The fascial strips are secured on a large-eye Gallie's needle either by locking the fascia through itself or stitching with separate silk sutures before being darned into position over the hernial defect.

Tendons may be used in a similar manner also, the plantaris tendon of the leg being suitable as its removal results in minimal interference with function.

Collagen tape

Reconstituted chromic collagen tape (Ethicon) is intended as a substitute for autologous and homologous fascia used in various repair operations.

Its advantages over the patient's own fascia, or over beef fascia are that it avoids an operation on the leg to obtain fascia lata; it ties easily without the need of secondary sutures; it is stronger than fascia of similar mass; and it contains no extraneous tendinous material as that found in beef fascia.

In ophthalmic surgery collagen tape can be used as a frontal muscle sling for the correction of blepharotosis or ptosis. Ptosis may be congenital or senile but generally it is acquired by accident which severs either the levator muscle or the third cranial nerve, or by the invasion of the muscle by a tumour.

In other branches of surgery it can be substituted where fascia would normally have been used. In repair of lacerations of the liver for example or in nephropexy, the breadth of the suture is an advantage with these extremely soft tissues. Collagen tape can be inserted with a suitable needle such as Gallie's or Wright's.

Collagen tape is supplied in lengths of 60 cm (24 in) by 3 mm (⅛ in) in width.

Synthetic absorbables

Dexon

For many decades the only absorbable suture in general use was catgut. In 1970, a synthetic absorbable material became available for the first time under the trade name Dexon and this product is now well established as an alternative to catgut. (Anscombe, Hira and Hunt, 1970; Davis and Geck, 1971; Miln, O'Connor and Dalling, 1972.)

Dexon is a synthetic polymer of glycolic acid, a naturally-occurring substance. It is absorbed in tissues essentially by hydrolysis and not digested by proteolysis as are gut and collagen. The material is developed by extrusion as fine strands which are then braided to form a uniform gauge thread. Tests have shown a minimal absorption in tissue at 15 days, maximum absorption at 30 days and essentially complete resorption after 60 to 90 days after operation.

A polyglycolic acid suture is extremely inert and causes minimal tissue reaction (Edlich et al., 1974). Size for size with catgut it is stronger, is fray resistant and does not become slippery in use. The BPC gradings of breaking load in kgf over a surgeon's knot can be summarised as follows:

Size	Typical tensile strength supplied
0·75 metric (6/0)	0·44
1 ,, (5/0)	0·82
1·5 ,, (4/0)	1·3
2 ,, (3/0)	1·8
2·5 ,, (2/0)	2·8
3 ,, (0)	4·5
4 ,, (1)	5·9

The material is handled in precisely the same manner as cutgut. The main contra-indication is that it should not be used where extended approximation of tissues must be maintained; a non-absorbable material is more suitable for this purpose. As with all sutures, care must be taken with respect to drainage and closure of infected wounds. Dexon requires special care in placing the first knot; it will not slip and 'snug' down under additional throws. The first throw is always placed exactly where required and knots tied in this way remain secure. Dexon is not suitable for resterilisation at hospital level.

Although Dexon is used mainly for deep sutures it can be used as a conventional skin suture or as a subcuticular closure. This technique is particularly suitable for cosmetic surgery where minimal tissue reaction is essential.

NON-ABSORBABLE LIGATURES AND SUTURES

Materials in this category may be divided into two classes, those manufactured from natural raw materials and those which are entirely synthetic, being prepared in the laboratory. Non-absorbable sutures are not generally used in an infected wound as they may cause sinus formation.

Natural Materials

Silkworm gut

This is obtained from the glands of the silkworm killed before it is ready to spin its cocoon, and is drawn out into monofilament (one strand) threads of varying diameters, measuring about 25 to 36 cm (10 to 14 in) in length and of a slightly roughened surface.

The material lacks flexibility and is difficult to tie and its use is largely superseded by the introduction of synthetic monofilaments.

Silk thread

A material, white or black in colour, which may be either twisted or braided from numerous gossamer strands, supplied on spools of 25, 50 or 100 metres. Generally silk thread is now supplied on sterilisable nylon or polypropylene spools. If wooden spools are supplied it should always be rewound on to metal, nylon or polypropylene spools before sterilisation, for if left on wooden spools the expansion of the wood will stretch and weaken the material.

Armour Suture Laboratories supply braided silk already wound on a spool contained in an autoclavable ligature egg.

The sizes vary from very fine 0·75 to 6 (6/0 to 4) or even stronger. These sizes must comply with the minimum BPC breaking load. The minimum breaking load in kg force, over a surgeon's knot, braided silk are as follows:

Size	BPC minimum breaking load	Typical tensile strength supplied
0·3 (8/0)		
0·75 (6/0)	0·20 kgf	0·30 kgf
1 (5/0)	0·40 kgf	0·64 kgf
1·5 (4/0)	0·75 kgf	0·95 kgf
2 (3/0)	1·3 kgf	1·54 kgf
2·5 (2/0)	2·0 kgf	2·3 kgf
3 (0)	3·0 kgf	3·27 kgf
4 (1)	4·5 kgf	4·58 kgf
5 (2)	6·0 kgf	6·40 kgf
5·5 (3)	7·0 kgf	—
6 (4)	8·0 kgf	—

The very fine sizes from 0·3 (8/0) virgin silk and 0·75 to 2 (6/0 to 3/0) are useful in vascular and nerve anastomosis, ophthalmic surgery, plastic surgery and intestinal suturing; 2·5 to 4 or 5 (2/0 to 1 or 2) for general ligatures or sutures; and up to size 6 (4) or more for large pedicles such as haemorrhoids, etc.

It is important to use serum-proofed silk to reduce capillary attraction, which is the peculiarity of a plaited or braided material. The capillary attraction which a non-serum proofed material has is rather dangerous, as bacteria may lodge in the minute spaces of the braiding, becoming a permanent source of irritation and wound infection.

Where many silk sutures are required during the operation either non-traumatic, ready-needled sutures are used, or alternatively it is advantageous to thread the needles beforehand and autoclave ready for use. The appropriate needles are threaded with various sizes of silk and are stitched loosely on to a pad before sterilisation. In this method very great care must be taken to check the total number of needles both before and after operation.

Linen thread

A ligature or suture which is prepared from linen flax and is used in a similar manner to catgut. Many surgeons use it for ligatures and sutures of the viscera, muscle and skin.

The thread is available ready sterilised in packets containing up to 50 cut strands (Ethicon) and wound on autoclave spools (Armour). The standard colours are cream/white or black.

The tensile strength of linen must comply with the minimum BPC breaking load over a surgeon's knot.

Size	BPC minimum breaking load
0·75 (6/0)	0·30 kgf
1 (5/0)	0·60 kgf
1·5 (4/0)	1·25 kgf
2 (3/0)	1·9 kgf
2·5 (2/0)	3·0 kgf
3 (0)	4·0 kgf
4 (1)	6·3 kgf
5 (2)	8·2 kgf

Cotton thread

Originating from cotton plants the fibres are usually twisted rather than braided. It has a limited use, mainly for fine ligatures, for the tensile strength of cotton is the least of all sutures available. It does, however, gain about 10 per cent in strength during sterilisation at the expense of some shrinkage. For this reason cotton should be prepared as cut lengths and not wound on to spools.

A combination of cotton and polyester fibre in black or white is available under the trade name of Ethicot (Ethicon).

It is supplied in sizes 3/0 to 1, with a minimum breaking load in kg force over a surgeon's knot of:

Size	Breaking load
2 (3/0)	0·79 kgf
2·5 (2/0)	1·7 kgf
3 (0)	2·6 kgf
4 (1)	3·4 kgf

Ethicot is serum-proofed and non-capillary.

Synthetic Non-absorbables

Polyamides—Nylon

This was the first synthetic plastic suture material which was developed during the 1939–45 war and it is obtainable in two main categories – monofilament and multifilament or braided.

THE MONOFILAMENT VARIETY

This is a single strand of nylon, generally blue in colour, which is similar to silkworm gut and may be used as such, but has a smoother surface.

It is supplied in sizes ranging from 0·75 to 5 (6/0 to 2) which must comply with the minimum BPC breaking load in kg force over a surgeon's knot.

Size	BPC minimum breaking load (tensile strength)	Typical tensile strength supplied
0·75 (6/0)	0·25 kgf	0·37 kgf
1 (5/0)	0·50 kgf	0·73 kgf
1·5 (4/0)	1·0 kgf	1·13 kgf
2 (3/0)	1·6 kgf	1·63 kgf
2·5 (2/0)	2·7 kgf	2·77 kgf
3 (0)	3·5 kgf	3·67 kgf
4 (1)	5·5 kgf	5·58 kgf
5 (2)	7·0 kgf	7·43 kgf

The material can be obtained in several lengths, from 36 to 102 cm (14 to 40 in), the shorter length for skin sutures and the longer length for the nylon darn in herniorrhaphy, or for suturing muscle.

The finest sizes are suitable for plastic face sutures, whereas the strongest are more applicable for 'through-and-through' abdominal tension sutures. A monofilament nylon suture must be cut at least 10 mm ($\frac{3}{8}$ in) long, as slight slipping of the knot may occur under certain conditions.

Nylon as a single strand is relatively inert, can be safely used in the presence of infection (Moloney et al., 1950; Everett 1970; Edlich, 1974), and may be left in the tissues with very little unfavourable reaction occurring.

THE BRAIDED VARIETY

This can be compared to braided silk and is used in a similar manner. The sizes available range from 1·5 to 6 (4/0 to 4) and the same tensile strengths as braided silk apply. There are generally only three colours available: white, black and green, which do not refer to a particular size but are only preferential colour choices. It is supplied on autoclavable spools (Armours).

The material is available also ready sterile in packets and as sterile non-traumatic sutures. Braided nylon, like monofilament, is often used for hernia repair and may be prepared as a nylon mesh which is stitched over the hernial defect.

Sizes 1·5 to 2·5 (4/0 to 2/0) are used for plastic surgery, skin sutures or fine intestinal sutures; 2·5 to 4 (2/0 to 1) for ligatures and general muscle sutures; and 5 to 6 (2 to 4) for herniorrhaphy or large pedicle ligatures.

Polyesters (terylene)

Polyester fibre is supplied as a braided material and is marketed surgically under several trade names, including Ethibond (Ethicon), Dacron (Davis and Geck) and Arbralene (Armour). Ethibond (green in colour) is coated with polytetramethylene adipate

Fig. 7.11 Linen thread and braided materials, mersilene, nylon and silk; monofilament nylon.

(polybutylate) to ensure smoothness and handling with no risk of flaking or fraying. Dacron is available in white or blue thread and Arbralene in white or black.

Sizes in common use are 1 to 2·5 (5/0) to 2/0) for plastic, skin, ophthalmic, or intestinal sutures and ligation of small vessels; 3 to 5 (0 to 2) for muscle sutures and stout ligatures. The materials available are serum proofed and are handled in a similar manner to braided silk, braided nylon, or linen thread. Polyester is also used for the fabrication of cardiovascular prostheses, e.g., bifurcated aortic grafts.

Polyolefins

Linear polyethylene

Under the trade name Dermalene (Davis and Geck), linear polyethylene is available as a monofilament suture. It has excellent tissue tolerance and foreign body reactions are considerably reduced.

Dermalene is blue in colour and has a low elasticity with a soft pliable feel and minimum stretch. It knots firmly with a double knot and has a reduced tendency to slip. Its main use is in vascular anastomoses, plastic surgery and other procedures which require exceptionally inert sutures.

Sizes available are 1 to 2 (5/0 to 3/0) either with or without needle attached.

Polypropylene

Monofilament polypropylene, coloured deep blue, is available under the trade name Prolene (Ethicon). The material is extremely inert, stronger than monofilament nylon in most sizes and very malleable; it will crush and deform easily upon knotting. This knot-holding characteristic is superior to other synthetic suture materials.

Care must be taken not to resterilise Prolene more than three times by standard autoclaving, otherwise loss of strength will occur.

The material is available in sizes 0·2 to 5 (10/0 to 2), with or without needles. Prolene is suitable for any instance where a non-absorbable suture is required.

Metallic wire

Suture wire is prepared mainly from three metals – non-toxic 18/8 stainless steel SMO or EN 58 J, the alloy tantalum and silver.

All these may be obtained as a single-strand suture and the first two as several strands, either twisted or braided, known as multifilament wire.

The multifilament wire is more flexible and less likely to kink during handling. The sizes are graded either as BPC metric or S.W.G. (Standard Wire Gauge). The former vary from 0·5 to 9 (7/0 to 7), and the latter gauge from fine 40 S.W.G. to stout 18 S.W.G.

Surgical suture wire is used mainly today in orthopaedics and thoracic surgery. For tendon sutures sizes 0·5 to 2 (7/0 to 3/0) or 40 S.W.G. to 30 S.W.G. are suitable, whereas a stouter wire of sizes 3 to 9 (0 to 7) or 29 S.W.G. to 18 S.W.G. would be needed for wiring fragments of bone in apposition.

It may be used also for closing an abdominal incision in the obese or carcinomatous patient, for oesophageal anastomosis, closure of a chest incision or as a mesh in the repair of hernial defects.

It is very important that wires made from different metals are not used in contact with each other in the tissues, as a reaction may occur resulting in corrosion (Chapter 23).

Fine wire is used for threading tonsil, nasal and aural snares.

LIGACLIP ™
LIGATING CLIPS & APPLIERS

The system
Appliers and cartridges are colour-coded; selection therefore is fast and accurate. Each clip is formed and locked in the applier when the applier is inserted in the cartridge. Cross-locking action between serrations in the applier and the clip keep the clip locked in the applier, without slipping, twisting or dropping out, until the occlusion is made. There's no need for the scrub nurse and the surgeon to grasp the appliers by the handle to maintain tension during transfer.
Result: no lost clips, no lost time.

Clips
are made of physiologically inert tantalum, packaged in sterile, autoclavable Nylon cartridges. Spring pressure between the clip and the shoulders of the cartridge prevent the clip from falling out. Only six clips to a cartridge means no waste, and it is seldom necessary to sterilise leftovers.

Spring locking action between applier handle and retaining pin provides further security.

The appliers
are made of surgical stainless steel and are colour-coded to match the clips. Sturdily made, they will work reliably even after hours of hard use.

Colour-coding by size
Both cartridges and appliers are colour-coded.
Blue—small; white—medium; yellow—large.

Fast no-ring pick-up
The clip is formed—and locked in place—when the applier is inserted in the cartridge. There's no need to hold the rings during loading.

Secure no-ring transfer Nor is there any need for the scrub nurse—or the surgeon—to maintain ring tension during transfer, since the clip is locked in the applier. No lost clips—no lost time. Transfer is fast, positive, sure.

Fig. 7.12 Ligaclip vascular clips. (Ethicon.)

Metal clips (ligature)

Ligatures of flattened silver or tantalum wire are used in neurosurgery and chest surgery for arresting haemorrhage from small vessels or compressing nerve endings by clipping them. One variety is known as Cushing's or McKenzie's clips and are V-shaped, being prepared with a special cutting clamp which bends and cuts the wire in one operation.

The small V-shaped clips, each arm being about 0·45 cm ($\frac{3}{16}$ in) long, are stored on a stand or galley, and are removed with special forceps, being handed in the forceps to the surgeon. The wire, clamp, galley and insertion forceps are sterilised together by autoclaving.

The clips are very useful for ligating small vessels which are too small or inaccessible for hand ligatures.

Commercially prepared and sterilised clips are available in small, medium and large sizes (Ligaclip, Ethicon). The insertion forceps and cartridges are colour-coded for easy identification.

Metal clips (suture)

These are metal clips, having two sharp points which, when the clip is closed, grip the edges of a skin incision. They are generally used to approximate a wound which heals quickly, e.g., in the region of the neck. They may be used also to close an abdominal incision or thigh incision in conjunction with tension sutures.

The two main types in use are Michel and Kifa. Both are loaded on to special insertion forceps, but the Kifa has two projecting lips on its upper surface which allow easy removal after healing has taken place. When these lips are squeezed with forceps the clip open quite easily.

Fig. 7.13 Michel and Kifa skin suture clips. 1A. Insertion and removal forceps (Kifa). 1B. Suture clips (Kifa). 2A. Insertion forceps (Michel). 2B. Clip galley loaded with clips (Michel). 2C. Suture clip (Michel).

Fig. 7.14 Some uses for Steristrip skin closures. (Surgical Products 3M United Kingdom Ltd.)

Adhesive skin closures (for skin)

These are microporous strips of tape which employ a chemically inert, synthetic adhesive that adheres firmly, is virtually non-irritating and removes easily and painlessly. Steristrip skin closures are sterile strips of Micropore surgical tape pre-cut to specific sizes, used for a variety of purposes including primary closure of wounds, as an adjunct to suture, and the following suture removal.

The technique of application is described in Chapter 9, page 220.

REFERENCES

Anscombe, A. R., Hira, N. and Hunt, B. (1970) *British Medical Journal*, **57,** 108.
Davis and Geck (1971) *Proceedings of a Symposium on Polyglycolic Acid Sutures.*
Edlich, R. F., Panek, P. H., Rodenheaver, G. T., Kurtz, L. D. and Edgerton, M. T. (1974) *Journal of Biochemical Materials Research Symposium*, **8,** 115.
Everett, N. G. (1970) *Progress in Surgery (Basel)*, **8,** 14.
Forrester, J. C. (1975) *Nursing Mirror*, Jan 16th, p. 48.
Miln, D. C. O'Connor, J. and Dalling, R. (1972) *Scottish Medical Journal*, **17,** 108.
Moloney, G. E., Russell, W. T. and Wilson, D. C. (1950) *British Journal of Surgery*, **38**, 52.
Postlethwait, R. W. (1969) In *Repair and Regeneration.* McGraw-Hill: New York.

8
STORAGE AND HANDLING OF LIGATURE MATERIALS AND ASSOCIATED INSTRUMENTS

As a continuation of the previous chapter, we must now consider the storage and handling of ligature materials and associated instruments. Formerly, these would have been described as part of the 'ligature trolley', which consisted mainly of metal and glass dishes for the storage of sterilised instruments in an antibacterial solution. Nowadays, the use of such 'solution' storage techniques is obsolete; emphasis has already been given in Chapter 6 to the importance of heat sterilisation and the dry storage of sterilised items.

Fig. 8.1   A selection of ligature and suture requirements.

1. & 2. Dissecting forceps, non-toothed.
3. Scissors, stitch.
4. Carless suture scissors.
5. Kilner needle holder.
6. Fine needle holder.
7. Mayo needle holder.
8. Catgut suture – general closure with needle attached.
9. Catgut ligature.
10. Suture needles of appropriate size and shape (see Fig. 8.7).
11. Nylon – monofilament.
12. Linen thread.

Virtually all sizes and types of ligatures, sutures, scalpel blades and needles etc, can be purchased presterilised. Those items which are more convenient to process at hospital level can easily be presented in sterile packets or boxes (Brigden, 1962). All such sterile supplementary items are stored in dispensers or other suitable containers on trolleys, shelves or in cupboards in the sterile preparation room.

Storage and Handling of Ligature Materials and Associated Instruments

If ligature materials, e.g. braided materials such as silk and polyester, are sterilised at hospital level, they should be prepared as cut lengths or wound onto cards or metal or nylon spools before sterilisation, either with the set of instruments or in packets. (Wooden spools swell during sterilisation and cause damage to the material by stretching it.) The spools may be contained in ligature eggs which are marked with the size of material; ligature material is available already prepared in this way (Armours).

Fig. 8.2 Storage of sterile requisites in clean utility or sterile preparation room.

1. Boxes of ligature and suture requirements stored in dispenser.
2. Sterile scalpel blades in dispenser.
3. Supplementary sterile instruments in packets.
4. Preset trays of sterile instruments.
5. Heated cabinet for lotions.
6. Lotions stored at room temperature.

Wire may be stored on metal spools also, but if possible these should be of a larger size to avoid rather small loops of wire which would otherwise tend to kink during the preparation of sutures. Manufacturers also prepare wire lengths and sutures, packed in sterile packets, and these are of special use in tendon repair. A Pulvertaft wire suture for tendon repair is available wound on a card, but this must be sterilised before use.

In many operating theatres, scalpel handles, probes, fine dissecting forceps, Michel and Kifa suture clips, suction nozzles etc. are sterilised in packets as supplementary items. These are used in conjunction with ligature requirements and are stored as described previously.

Under clean, dry, storage conditions an intact packet will keep the contents sterile. However, freshly sterilised items should always be positioned behind those already in store and by doing this the use of outdated products should be avoided.

The ligature storage trolley, shelves or cupboards should be given a thorough clean each week. Packets must be inspected for integrity and replaced if there is any doubt in respect to seals or surface.

General ligature requisites

SUTURE NEEDLES

These are made from plated carbon steel or martensitic stainless steel and occasionally austenitic stainless steel (Chapter 23). The stainless steel needles are to be preferred as they do not rust or snap easily as may the carbon steel variety. The small extra cost is amply compensated for by these two advantages.

Fig. 8.3 Sterile disposable suture needles in peel-open packet (Steriseal Ltd.).

All needles fall into two principal classes: cutting needles and round-bodied needles.

1. *Cutting Needles* have sharp edges, are often triangular in section, and cut a track as they pass through the tissues. They are only used on strong tissue which will not be unduly damaged, such as fascia, muscle tendon and skin. The edge of cutting needles must be sharp, and they must be examined regularly for wear, being discarded when worn as the cost of resharpening would exceed the cost of replacement.

2. *Round-bodied Needles* cause less damage and do not actually cut the tissues, but make a puncture which closes very easily afterwards. They are used for suturing delicate tissue such as mucous membrane, fat and intestine.

Almost any style or shape of suture needle may be obtained as a non-traumatic variety; needles into which the catgut or other suture material is fused. This avoids the double thickness of material which is always present when it has been threaded through a needle eye. Round-bodied, non-traumatic needles are used for the closure of intestine, stomach, the ducts of glands, blood-vessels, and for the suture of nerves or any delicate tissue which may become traumatised during suture with conventional needles. Cutting, non-traumatic needles are used in plastic surgery for the suture of the face and other areas of skin, to minimise scar formation. They are used sometimes also for tendon suture, or for conjunctival and corneal suture in ophthalmic surgery.

Fig. 8.4 Set of general closure needle packs.

Fig. 8.5 Needle pack. The outer pack is peeled open (Fig. 8.3) and the inner blister illustrated is transferred to the sterile field.

Fig. 8.6A and B The needles are fixed in a set pattern onto a loose foam pad. Examples of general and gynae closure sets. (Steriseal Ltd.)

Suture needles are further subdivided into straight, curved, half-circle, five-eighths circle, and special shapes or types.

Straight Cutting Needles. Size 6·5 to 10 cm (2¼ to 4 in) in length, are used for skin sutures. The most common type are called Simm's abdominal needles.

Straight Round-bodied Needles. These are usually the fine intestinal type. Sizes 5 to 7 are used for intestinal suture or as a fixation needle during nerve and tendon suture. In the latter case, the degree of pull required (upon the proximal and distal segment of the nerve or tendon) to allow approximation of the cut ends, is maintained by passing a round-bodied needle through each segment, and this prevents retraction during suture. (An alternative would be to use silk 'stay' sutures for this required pull.)

Curved Cutting Needles. These are used mainly for the suture of skin. Sizes 10 (small) to 20 (fine) are used on a needle holder, and those 2/0 (large) to 9 (medium) are used by hand (hand needles).

These needles may be obtained in normal or fine gauge, depending upon the wishes of the surgeon, but needles used in the region of the face should always be the very finest possible.

Fig. 8.7 Selection of suture needles in general use.

1. Straight triangular cutting needles (Simm, skin).
2. Half-circle triangular cutting needles (muscle tendon, fascia, etc.).
3. Curved triangular cutting needles (skin).
4. Five-eighth-circle round-bodied and lance-point needles (Moynihan, for peritoneum and muscle respectively).
5. Fascia needle (Gallie).
6. Half-circle triangular cutting needle (fistula).
7. Reversed cutting-edge needle (Hagedorn).
8. Curved triangular cutting needle (non-traumatic, for eye and plastic surgery).
9. Trocar-point needles (Mayo, for muscle and pedicles, etc.).
10. Half-circle round-bodied needles (peritoneum, fat, etc.).
11. Round-bodied fish-hook needles (Symond, for hernia repair, etc.).
12. (*Top*) Curved round-bodied needles (peritoneum, intestine, fat, etc.).
12. (*Bottom*) Straight round-bodied needles (intestine, transfixion ligatures).

Amongst special curved cutting needles the ophthalmic types deserve individual description. These are very fine needles ranging from size 1, which is about the size of a 16 curved cutting needle, to size 6, which is a quarter of that size. There are, of course, special needles such as the Stallards which is a flattened section corneal needle and others which have reversed cutting edges, etc.

Some surgeons use ordinary cutting needles for the suture of tendons, but most express a preference for the non-traumatic type, such as the Pulvertaft, or multi-filament wire suture. The Pulvertaft is a single strand, fine 40 S.W.G. stainless steel wire, (0·5 metric/7/0) fused into a size 18 curved or straight cutting needle, and is supplied wound on a card which can be sterilised by autoclaving, or dry heat. The multifilament wire suture is welded in to one end of a similar size needle and packed ready sterilised in a plastic or foil packet. Both of these sutures are available as a single-armed (one needle) or double-armed (two needles) assembly.

Fig. 8.8 An autoclaved suture pack, opened out for use.

Half-circle Cutting Needles. These are used mainly for the suture of fascia and muscle tendon. Sizes 10 (small) to 20 (fine) are used on a needle holder and sizes 2/0 (large) to 9 (medium) are generally held in the surgeon's hand. Special needles of this type are: the fistula, which are coarse, strong needles; and Lane's which have rather a large eye in comparison to the gauge, which is very useful for threading silk up to size 2/0.

The fistula needles range from size 3/0 (large) to 4 (small), and the Lane's from size 1 (small) to 4 (fine), the larger size being equivalent to a size 17 ordinary half-circle needle.

The Five-eighths Circle or Fully Curved Needle. This is generally of the Moynihan variety. These needles resemble a five-eighths circle as their name implies, and are based upon the idea that nearly every surgical stitch when tied, approximates a circle very closely. In consequence, the more closely the track of the needle follows this, the more evenly will the tension be applied to the tissues.

These Moynihan needles may be round-bodied or cutting edge, which are used for suturing peritoneum or fat, and muscle tendon respectively. The round-bodied type is conventional, but the cutting needle has a flattened lance point, which is rather spear-shaped.

There are three sizes, small 8·2 cm ($3\frac{1}{4}$ in), medium 10 cm (4 in) and large 11·4 cm ($4\frac{1}{2}$ in), with a smaller round-bodied size about 3·8 cm ($1\frac{1}{2}$ in), for intestinal suturing.

Special Shapes and Types. Mayo, Symond's round-bodied fish hook, Hagedorn's reversed, and Gallie's fascia needles are the most popular, all of which are held in a needle holder for use.

The Mayo Suture Needle. This needle (for catgut), having a large square eye, is a very strong needle used extensively in gynaecology and obstetrics, or where excessive leverage may occur, e.g. during the repair of a hernia.

There are two varieties, the round-bodied and the trocar point (cutting), sizes ranging from 1 (medium) to 4 (small).

Symond's Fish Hook and Hagedorn's Reversed. These are both fish-hook in shape and are used for inaccessible suturing. The Symond's needle is round-bodied and the Hagedorn's has a reverse flattened point.

Sizes vary from 1 (large) to 10 (small), size 6 being useful for hernia repairs.

Gallie's Fascia Needle is a very broad, flattened needle, with a large eye and a lance point. A strip of fascia lata may be threaded on to this needle and used in hernia repair operations.

There are only three sizes, the most commonly used being small 3·8 cm ($1\frac{1}{2}$ in); the other two sizes are medium 4·5 cm ($1\frac{3}{4}$ in) and large 5·7 cm ($2\frac{1}{4}$ in), all of which are half-circle in shape.

It should be pointed out that the sizes of general needles, i.e., curved cutting needles, etc., vary only a little from one size to the other. The nurse will find that many surgeons use alternate size needles in which the difference of size is easily discernible, e.g., 2, 4, 6, 8, 10, etc.

Bonney Reverdin Needles are special needles which in effect incorporate their own needle holder.

These needles have an eye near to the point which is open on one side. A small, slender shutter may be slid along the handle to close this eye after the suture material has been inserted into it. The closed needle is passed through the tissues first; then the eye is opened; the suture material gripped; the eye closed, and the needle is withdrawn, pulling the suture material through the tissues to complete the stitch.

The finer varieties are used by plastic surgeons, e.g., for the repair of a cleft palate, but the most commonly used are the coarser varieties, favoured by gynaecologists, e.g., for uterine suturing.

Scalpel blades and handles

The Bard Parker scalpel handle permits the fitting of various sizes and shapes of scalpel blades according to the wishes of the surgeon.

There are six sizes of scalpel handles on the market at present; they are, sizes 3, 4, 5, 9, 3L and 4L. Of these the nurse will find that sizes 3, 4 and 5 are the most generally used.

Sizes 3 and 4 are the general purpose handle of medium length; size 5 is a long fine handle, useful during laminectomy, etc.; size 9 is a short fine handle of special use in plastic surgery; sizes 3L and 4L are long general purpose handles of application for deep cavities. The latter three sizes are only recent additions to the range.

Of the Paragon, Swann Morton, Gillette and similar ranges, the most popular sizes of scalpel blades are 10, 11, and 15, which fit handles 3, 3L, 5 and 9; sizes 20, 22, 23 and 24 which fit handles 4 and 4L.

Of the Gillette range, sizes A, B and C fit handles 4 and 4L; size D fits handles 3, 3L, 5 and 9.

Most manufacturers are now packing their scalpel blades in grease-free packets, such as the Vapour Phase Inhibitor or metal foil pack. The packet is designed as a sterile peel-open type with the blade ready for use. Individual packets of blades are presented in dispenser boxes which can be stored in a suitable rack.

Most skin-graft knives now incorporate disposable blades available in a sterile peel-open packet. If they are supplied unsterilised these may be coated with a light oil before wrapping in their protective paper cover. This oil should be removed before sterilisation, by soaking in a little trilene or ether, after which the blades should be lifted out and dried carefully. This should not be done in a confined space owing to the vapour liberated.

Skin graft blades can be sterilised by dry heat or alternatively by steam providing they are wrapped in vapour phase inhibitor anti-rust paper.

Solid scalpels

Most of these instruments are made from carbon steel because of the difficulty of obtaining a really good edge with stainless steel.

Under this heading come orthopaedic scalpels, cartilage knives, tenotomy knives, bistouries, etc.

ORTHOPAEDIC SCALPELS

These vary in size from a small 2·5 cm (1 in) blade to a 23 cm (9 in) amputation knife and are either straight or bellied in shape. The edges of these should be inspected regularly after use for bluntness, as described in Chapter 5. They are used where there is a risk of breaking a detachable blade, e.g., excising fibrous tissue at a fracture site.

Swann Morton have produced a disposable solid type blade and handle, which is similar to the Bard Parker knives but does not snap easily and may be used in all cases where a solid scalpel is required.

CARTILAGE KNIVES

These are rather a small type of solid knife, the three most popular being the Munro, Smillie and Fairbank.

The Munro has a long handle, with a short blade and a slender stem between the blade and the handle. The Smillie knives have a chisel-type point and are made as a set of three; two with concave edges, one curved for the right and one for the left, and a straight chisel blade for use with a special retractor. The Fairbank knives are made as a set of two; one curved for cutting to the right, and one curved for the left. They have a small blunt probe point with the cutting edge at one side only and are used mainly for meniscotomy as opposed to meniscectomy (Fig. 23.98).

TENOTOMY KNIVES

These are long and slender, being used for dividing a tendon through a small puncture wound. They either have one or two cutting edges, generally with a sharp point. Amongst the most popular are the Parker's double cutting-edge spear-type point, the Jones' single cutting edge and the Adam's set of seven shapes, including blunt and sharp-pointed varieties. There are too many types for individual description, as some surgeons arrange the sharpening of their knives to suit individual tastes.

BISTOURIES

These are knives which are generally used in conjunction with a special probe or guard for the division of ligaments or fibrous bands of tissue, etc., e.g., during a strangulated hernia operation.

Although there are bistouries with sharp points, the most generally used are those having a probe point which ensures that the cutting is only with the side edge of the knife.

All these knives can be sterilised by dry heat.

Scissors

Although it is better to sterilise those scissors in common use together with the general instruments, it is common practice to store at least the special types of scissors in autoclaved packets.

Scissors may have both points sharp, both blunt, or one sharp and one blunt. They are made from martensitic stainless steel or plated carbon steel, although the latter are not often used in the operating theatre, except perhaps for cutting dressings.

Scissors having both points sharp are generally used for removing sutures, or are of a special type such as fine iridectomy scissors. They may be straight, curved on flat or angled on flat and are mostly of the fulcrum lever principle, although some special iris scissors such as the De Wecker's have a special spring cross action, enabling the surgeon to use them between his forefinger and thumb. It is very useful to reserve ordinary stitch scissors for use on the ligature trolley during the preparation of ligatures and sutures, so that they do not become mixed with the scissors reserved for the surgeon. Scissors having both points sharp and with serrated edges are available for cutting cartilage, used almost exclusively by the plastic surgeons. Stitch scissors are useful also for cutting fine wire sutures not stouter than 30 S.W.G.

The majority of scissors used for dissection have both points blunt or rounded and are available straight, curved on flat or angled on flat. The most popular are the Mayo scissors or modifications of this pattern, the most usual sizes being from 13 to 20 cm (5 to 8 in) in length. In addition to dissection, these scissors are often used for cutting ligatures and sutures, although it is better to reserve a separate pair for this purpose, to give the surgeon the advantage of scissors used exclusively for dissection.

Although Mayo scissors may be obtained in lengths up to 23 cm (9 in), when a long fine pair is required, the surgeon will often prefer a pattern such as the Metzenbaum, McIndoe 18 cm (7 in) or similar. If he requires a heavier pair, his choice may include Nelson's or Mile's which are made in lengths up to 28 cm (11 in), and as straight or curved on flat blades. These longer scissors are of special use in thoracic surgery.

A short fine pair of scissors for use in plastic surgery, peripheral nerve or tendon surgery would be the 13 cm (5 in) Kilner or Strabismus scissors, both available as straight or curved on flat blades. The Kilner's scissors have flattened, fine points, which made them very adaptable for skin dissection.

Scissors having one sharp and one blunt point are useful for cutting dressings although they may be reserved for use by the assistant when he is cutting ligatures and sutures. Some dressing scissors are made with a blunt platform extending from the tip of the lower blade. This facilitates the introduction of the lower blade under a dressing or bandage, and prevents injury to the patient's skin.

In orthopaedic theatres it may be necessary to store a variety of probes, drills, osteotomes, and gouges, etc., in sterile boxes or packets. The difference between the various types is described in Chapter 23.

Suture clips

These are generally loaded on to a special galley which also forms part of an approximation forceps (Fig. 7.13). The insertion forceps are grooved for the Michel-type skin clips, but are, in addition, bowed for the Kifa type to accommodate the projecting lips.

Drainage tubes, catheters, syringes, and hypodermic needles

A selection of these may be stored in autoclaved packets or purchased ready sterile from the manufacturer.

The handling of ligature and suture materials

It is very bad practice to prepare ligatures and sutures for several operations at the beginning of an operation list. Materials so prepared have to be stored on a 'stock' trolley and even with the greatest care it is impossible to guarantee sterility.

A separate, small, sterile trolley may be used as an operation ligature trolley for each case, but it is a more convenient procedure to use a corner of the instrument trolley, placing the prepared materials between two small sterile towels. It is preferable that these towels be of a different colour to the general drapes so that they serve to isolate the ligatures, etc., from the rest of the trolley.

Fig. 8.9

1. Endotracheal suction catheter.
2. Short polyvinyl suction drain.
3. Long polyvinyl suction drain with connector.
4. Foley type catheter in rigid container.
5. Foley type catheter in peel-open plastic pack.
6. 'T' tube drain in peel-open pack.

The scrub nurse collects her requirements with long handled forceps from the packets opened by the circulating nurse, placing them into a kidney dish.

The scrub nurse may prepare several ligatures and sutures at the commencement of the operation but should avoid having too many exposed, especially if the operation is a long one. The length of a ligature should not generally exceed 31 cm (12 in); a continuous suture length ranges between 46 and 61 cm (18 and 24 in), and an interrupted suture length should be between 31 and 46 cm (12 and 18 in).

If the surgeon insists upon a non-touch technique being used, the scrub nurse must handle all ligatures and sutures with forceps, taking great care to avoid crushing the material, especially catgut.

The handling of catgut has been dealt with in Chapter 7. If the surgeon is using a braided material such as silk or polyester, and he requires the suture locked in the eye of the needle, the material will have to be knotted once upon itself. Doubling braided materials through the needle eye is not satisfactory as they tend to slip. Ideally, of course, a non-traumatic suture or a Paterson eye needle should be used.

Fig. 8.10 (A) Peeling open a sterile scalpel blade foil packet. (B) Scrub nurse removing sterile scalpel blade from peeled-open packet. (C) Ligature packet in heat-sealed Kraft paper bag. First the bag is nicked, then ... (D) ... torn across without touching the torn edge ... (E) ... the packet is opened utilising the side gussets and the scrub nurse removes the inner sterile packet with forceps.

When tension sutures are being prepared, using thin rubber or plastic tubing to prevent 'cutting in' of the suture after tying, the needle is threaded and a 2·5 cm (1 in) length of tubing passed over the needle point and slid into position overlying the material in the eye. This will prevent the suture material (especially monofilament nylon) from becoming unthreaded, and will simplify positioning the tubing before the suture is tied. The surgeon will require two pairs of artery forceps for each tension suture to secure the ends until he is ready to tie them, after the muscle has been sutured.

Only the end of a needle holder's jaws must be used to grip a needle which is held at a point one-third from the eye and two-thirds from the needle point, the only exception being a fish hook and Gallie's fascia needle. These are gripped at a point about one-quarter from the eye.

Gripping the needle in the one-third/two-thirds position ensures that the surgeon can pass the needle the maximum possible distance through the tissues without further adjustments and with the least possible risk of it snapping at its weakest point, which is near the eye.

When preparing a needle and holder for a right-handed surgeon, the nurse holds the instrument in her right hand and grips the needle with its point facing her left hand. The procedure is reversed for a left-handed surgeon and when the needle is to be used vice versa.

Some needle holders have a cranked handle, and when viewed sideways it will appear that the jaws are at a lower level than the handle. The needle should be gripped so that when it is in the correct position for use the cranked handle is above the level of the jaws and not vice versa when viewed sideways. Suturing of fairly superficial tissues and skin is easier when using this type of needle holder, as the cranked handle remains above the level of the skin even if the jaws are below. This means that the surgeon is able to hold his hand parallel to the skin instead of at an angle, and so avoids obscuring his view of the suture line.

REFERENCE

BRIGDEN, R. J. (1962). Sterile Packets for Implants and Special Instruments. *Nursing Mirror*, March 30.

9
DRAPING OPERATION AREAS AND ASSISTING THE SURGEON

Although it is the ultimate responsibility of the surgeon to ensure that the operation area is correctly draped following skin preparation, this is frequently left to an experienced member of the operating theatre staff.

Furthermore, another doctor usually acts as the surgeon's first assistant, but there are occasions when a theatre nurse has to act in this capacity. This is especially so in the smaller hospital, where the medical staff is limited in number, but it must be fully understood that the duties of theatre staff do not normally include those of first assistant.

Preparing the operation area

1. ELECTIVE PROCEDURES

In most cases the first pre-surgical skin preparation is performed in the ward. This generally consists of cleansing the operation site and surrounding area, followed by careful shaving. It is claimed that shaving the operation site on the day before operation is a bad practice, since minor abrasions of the skin may encourage the growth of organisms and actually produce papillitis or dermatitis. There are opposing views on this hypothesis, but a controlled cross-infection study carried out by a nurse, suggested there were advantages in shaving the operation site 18 hours before operation (Linton, 1974). The first preparation may also include the application of a non-irritant skin antiseptic and sterile towels. This only applies, of course, to cases where there are no open wounds, for these generally require surgical toilet under anaesthesia.

In theatre, the sterile towels are removed and the operation area is painted with the antibacterial agent of choice, i.e., alcoholic Hibitane 0·5 per cent, alcoholic iodine 2 per cent, or Povidone iodine, etc. Application of this antiseptic should commence first at the site of incision, continuing in ever widening circles or squares, until a sufficient area has been covered. A second application of antiseptic, using fresh swabs, is made after the first has dried (Public Health Laboratory Report, 1965; Medical Research Council, 1968).

It is essential to paint a much larger area than required for the purpose of operation (Ginsberg *et al.*, 1967; Hamilton Bailey, 1967; Ballinger *et al.*, 1972). This should extend at least 15 cm (6 in) beyond the area isolated by the sterile towels or drapes, to allow manipulations or readjustment of towels during operation.

When the operation site is near the genitals or anus, the application of a skin antiseptic should be towards this area which is painted last. The swab used for this purpose must always be discarded after passing over the anus.

Suggested minimal areas of preparation for various operations are listed in Table 9.1.

2. CONTAMINATED WOUNDS

Any open wound must have a thorough toilet under anaesthesia before applying the usual skin antiseptic.

Sterilised nylon bristle nail brushes and an antiseptic detergent such as aqueous Savlon 3 per cent are ideal for this purpose. To assist efficient cleansing of a limb, a large, sterile, shallow tray is placed under the wound area and used as a douche tray.

At least two brushes must be available for this procedure, the first being used for the initial cleansing of skin for a wide area surrounding the wound, and the second in a separate bowl of solution for the wound itself. During initial cleansing, the wound is covered with a sterile swab or towel and it is at this stage that any hairs are shaved away.

Table 9.1 Areas of skin preparation in ward and theatre

Area of Operation	Area of Preparation
Skull	Entire skull, forehead, ears and neck.
Face	Entire face and neck and if necessary including the ears. For eye operations the eyebrows *may* be shaved off, and the lashes are cut with petroleum jelly smeared scissors. This is not necessary if Steridrape adhesive incise drapes are used.
Chest—	
Supine	From mid-abdomen to shoulders and neck, extending laterally round loins and thorax, on both sides.
Lateral	From mid-abdomen to shoulders; including the lateral aspects of the thorax and loins on the affected side and extending over the spine.
Abdomen	From the nipples to the upper part of the thighs, extending laterally round abdominal wall and pelvis, on both sides; including the genital region.
Genital region	From the umbilicus to mid-thighs, extending laterally round the pelvis and including the genital and anal regions.
Anal region	The upper part of both thighs, the buttocks, genital region and lower part of the abdomen.
Spine	From the shoulders to the upper part of the thighs, including the anal region and extending laterally round the loins and thorax.
Hand, forearm and upper arm	From the finger tips to the elbow (or shoulder for upper arm).
Foot and ankle	From the toes to knee level for full circumference of the limb.
Lower leg and knee	From the toes to mid-thigh for full circumference of the limb.
Hip and thigh	Whole of the leg, buttocks, and genital region; extending up to the level of the ribs; and over the lateral aspect of the abdomen on the affected side.

Although a certain amount of care should be exercised when cleansing a wound, to avoid damage to exposed nerves, etc., it is very important to remove as much debris as possible. The sterile nylon brushes will be found useful for this, but large fragments of foreign materials or damaged tissue and blood clots which cannot be removed by gentle brushing should be left for removal by the surgeon.

After a thorough toilet, the area is dried with a sterile swab or towel, and skin antiseptic applied before placing the drapes in position.

When a general anaesthetic is not practicable, the surgeon will administer local or regional anaesthesia following minimal cleansing and before wound toilet is commenced.

Draping the operation area

The operation area must be draped to allow free access for the surgeon, but the towels should be so arranged that manipulations do not expose any unprepared skin areas (see Figs 9.6 to 9.12).

A sterile water repellent sheet (e.g., Ventile fabric or disposable material) should be placed in position first, to prevent contamination should the sterile drapes become damp or soiled.

Methods of towelling or draping are essentially practical procedures, depending upon the wishes of the surgeon, the area, and sizes of towels available. In this chapter we must therefore confine ourselves to general observations, and use these as a basis for practice.

ABDOMINAL OPERATIONS

Four pieces of water-repellent drape may be draped to surround the incision area. One piece of fabric should always be placed in position over the pubic area first, followed by a piece on each side and another one over the chest.

However thorough the preparation is, the skin surface will not remain surgically clean indefinitely. If the operation lasts for more than half an hour or so, the patient will begin to perspire resulting in surface contamination from organisms within the sweat pores. In order to minimise this contamination the skin may be covered with a piece of self-adhesive plastic sheet, Steridrape (polyethylene), Vi-Drape (PVC), Opsite (polyurethane), which is stretched over the operation area and with a sterile swab, is smoothed flat from the centre to the periphery. This ensures positive adhesion and avoids air bubbles being trapped beneath the sheet.

Fig. 9.1 Upper abdominal operation, applying the skin antiseptic in ever-widening squares.

Fig. 9.2 A water repellent drape is positioned over pubic area.

Fig. 9.3 Four pieces of water repellent drape in position, application of plastic sheet. The protective backing is removed from the self-adhesive Steridrape, Vi-Drape, or OpSite as shown, taking care to ensure the sheet is kept under tension to avoid creases.

Steri-Drape

Surgical Drapes examples

- Covers wide area, obviating the use of permeable cloth draping materials near the incision
- X-ray and eye transparent
- Eliminates need for injurious towel clips
- Lint-free, sterile operation area

Size: 60cm x 45cm
Adhesive Area: 50cm x 45cm

Size: 38cm x 41cm
Adhesive Area: 28cm x 41cm

Steri-Drape 2 incise drapes

Fig. 9.4 Steridrape incise drape for abdominal surgery.

- Provides effective colostomy dressing
- For use in laparoscopy, circumcision, thyroid procedures.

Size: 41cm x 41cm
Adhesive Area: 10cm x 12.5cm
Aperture: 6.3cm dia.

Aperture Drape

Fig. 9.5 Steridrape aperture drape.

- Protects wound edges from drying infection, and retractor abrasion
- Isolate infected areas, perineun, contaminated sites and gowns.

Size: 46cm x 30cm
Adhesive Area: 46cm x 3cm

Towel Drape

Fig. 9.6 Steridrape surgical towel drape.

Steri-Drape™ 2
Surgical Incise Drapes

Position drape over patient with liner face down. Grasp liner from underneath and begin peeling liner back.

Peel back liner material, folding liner upon itself. DO NOT REMOVE LINER COMPLETELY. Leave last fold adhered to adhesive area.

Using folded liner as a "handle bar," stabilize drape over patient. With a folded sterile towel, press and smooth drape to skin, first along planned line of incision. Remove liner completely and incise directly through sterile STERI-DRAPE Surgical Drape.

Steri-Drape™
Surgical Towel Drapes

After cutting STERI-DRAPE Surgical Towel Drape in half, unfold the drape. Reach across the surgical site and apply adhesive edge parallel to planned line of incision.

With one hand, slowly peel away protective liner. Use other hand to press adhesive to skin. Repeat procedure for applying other half of drape to opposite side of planned line of incision.

After incision, tuck ends of Towel Drape over wound edge to extend sterile field into peritoneal cavity.

APPLICATION TECHNIQUE

Fig. 9.7

3M and Steri-Drape are trademarks

Fig. 9.8

Figs 9.7 and 9.8 Application technique for Steridrape Surgical Incise and Towel Drape. (Surgical Products, 3M United Kingdom Ltd.)

200 Operating Theatre Technique

Fig. 9.9 The plastic sheet applied to the abdomen and smoothed into position with a swab from the centre to the periphery, to avoid air bubbles being trapped underneath. (The incision is made through the plastic sheet on attached skin.)

Fig. 9.10 The lower extremities are covered with a large drape.

Draping Operation Areas and Assisting the Surgeon 201

Fig. 9.11 A second large drape is placed over the chest and head (a wire screen may be used to isolate the anaesthetist and provide clear access to the patient's airway).

Fig. 9.12 'Holed' abdominal sheet positioned over previous drapes, towel clips applied.

The incision is made through the plastic sheet and underlying skin.

The entire area may then be draped with a large abdominal sheet having a central aperture, or four/five towels positioned as previously described. This arrangement appears the neatest, and prevents the side towels from slipping down.

The patient's arm or arms abducted on an arm support for transfusion or other purposes, should be covered with small towels before commencing the abdominal draping.

A metal wire frame fitted to the operation table head, and draped with the upper part of the abdominal sheet, may be used to isolate the anaesthetist from the sterile areas. It also prevents the drapes from covering the patient's face and obscuring a clear observance of his appearance. The frame is of special use when the patient is conscious and a local or spinal anaesthetic has been administered. Care must be taken, however, to avoid the

Fig. 9.13 Anaesthetic screen at operation table head. (If the patient is broad, soft pads will be required between the patient's arms and screen uprights.)

patient's arm coming into contact with the metal frame, especially if diathermy is being used as this could result in accidental burns (Fig. 9.13).

If a plastic sheet has not been applied to the skin during draping, after the incision has been made, small skin or surgical towel drapes may be applied to the skin edges. These should be of the plastic type and not 'tetra towels', which soon become soiled with blood and lose their protective value.

THORACIC AND KIDNEY OPERATIONS

Several small pieces of water repellent fabric and standard towels are draped similarly to abdominal operations, leaving the area of incision exposed.

LIMB OPERATIONS

It is important that the drapes are secured to withstand any manipulations of a limb during operation.

In addition to small towels, some larger, about 152 cm (5 ft) square, should be available – two for a lower limb, and one for an upper limb.

Only the incision area of the limb should be exposed during operation, unless of course multiple incisions are necessary as for the ligation of varicose veins. Towels may be used to cover the unrequired skin areas, but a sterile stocking made from stockinette or calico stitched at one end is less bulky.

It is very important that all parts of a limb (including the foot) which will be subject to handling by the surgeon must be painted with skin antiseptic.

In orthopaedic surgery, Steridrape, Vi-Drape or OpSite are generally applied to the skin thereby providing a drape through which the surgeon makes his incision.

Fig. 9.14 Draping the lower limb.

(A) Application of skin antiseptic.   (B) Piece of Ventile positioned over other leg.

(cont'd.)

A sterile water repellent sheet must be placed under the limb before the towels and should extend well about the operation site. For operations on the lower extremities, this means from the foot end of the operation table to mid-thigh, or higher if necessary. When one leg is involved, the water repellent sheet covers the other completely. In the case of upper limb operations, it should cover the arm table and extend well up to the axilla. With the arm across the chest, the water repellent sheet is placed, extending from lower abdomen to axilla.

After covering and overlapping the water repellent sheet with towels, a 'shut off' towel is used to isolate the prepared from the unprepared areas of the limb. This towel is placed under the limb and crossed over on the opposite side, to be secured with a towel clip or clips.

Fig. 9.14 (cont'd.)

(C) Lower large drape which completely covers unaffected leg.
(D) After application of a small piece of Steridrape, Vi-Drape or OpSite to the incision area the lower part of the leg is wrapped in a sterile towel.
(E) A calico bag is placed over the wrapped leg to retain towel in position, this may be bandaged or clipped.
(F) Draping is completed with another large sheet placed over the upper part of the patient. This procedure is suitable for a meniscectomy or similar operation on the knee.

(A) The under drape is positioned over the unaffected limb and secured with the self-adhesive edge.
(B) A large utility drape is used to wrap the operative leg which is then covered with stockinette.
(C) The perineum is covered with a split sheet which has a self-adhesive edge to ensure complete isolation.
(D) A large drape is used to cover the upper half of the patient.
(E) Draping completed; anaesthetist's screen covered.

Fig. 9.15 Draping a hip using Barrier* disposable surgical drapes (SurgiKos, Division of Johnson & Johnson Ltd.).

*reg. trade mark.

The Neurosurgical Sitting Position. This position with the head flexed and immobilised by a cranial support, requires first a sterile water repellent sheet and towel placed across the shoulders extending from neck level to cover the chair back.

The draping is then completed as previously described, but the towels are draped first over an instrument table positioned just in front of the patient's forehead, and then over transfusion stands at each side of the operation table (Fig. 9.17, p. 207).

SPINAL OPERATIONS (INCLUDING LAMINECTOMY, SYMPATHECTOMY, DECOMPRESSION, EXCISION OF PILONOIDAL SINUS, ETC.)

The Prone Position. A patient placed in the prone position (or the knee/elbow flexed rabbit position), for lumbar, sacral, or mid-thoracic approach, may be draped as for abdominal operations, utilising the 'holed' water repellent sheet and towel.

High Cervical Areas. These can be draped similarly, but in addition the head should either be isolated with antiseptic barrier towels, or covered first by using the two-towel technique described for ENT operations. The cross-over point of the towels should be at the occiput.

Pieces of sterile cotton-wool tucked in at each side of the neck will prevent soiling due to blood trickling down during operation.

Lateral Position. These should be draped similarly to thoracic procedures, using four separate water repellent sheets and towels.

Steridrape, Vi-Drape or OpSite can be applied as for an orthopaedic operation.

EAR, NOSE AND THROAT OPERATIONS

In all cases the upper part of the head and hair may be draped in almost the same way.

Two opened towels and a water repellent sheet are placed under the patient's head, the upper towel is crossed over a point above the operation area and secured with a towel clip, i.e., for operations on the eyes, at a point in the centre of the forehead; for operations on the mouth or nose, at a point over the nose bridge after covering the closed eyelids with a sterile swab, etc.; and for operations on the ear, superior to the ear on the affected side.

This method of draping will ensure that the hair is always covered and, in addition, the sterile towel underlying, cover the area beneath the head.

The draping is completed by covering the lower part of the patient with a sterile water repellent drape and one or more towels extending from just below the operation area. For operations on the eyes or ears, the lower half of the face, including the nose, should be covered; for those on the mouth or nose, the lower drapes extend from the chin.

OPERATIONS ON THE NECK

The head is covered as above, but the towel is crossed over at the centre of the chin.

A pad of sterile wool can be tucked in at each side of the neck to absorb any blood which may trickle down during operation. This is followed by a sterile water repellent sheet across the chest and one or more towels to cover this and the lower extremities.

The use of towel clips to secure towels in this region is often avoided, due to the difficulty of applying towel clips to the chin for it is very irritating to find that these clips frequently pull away during the course of operation. The alternative is to use three or four monofilament nylon sutures at each point and these cause very little trauma. The sutures are cut out before removing the drapes.

Fig. 9.16 Operating microscope used for ENT and eye surgery showing method of draping with a sterile plastic sleeve. (Carl Zeiss [OberKochen] Ltd.)

OPERATIONS ON THE EYE

The hair is covered as for ENT operations, but the towel is crossed over the forehead just below the hairline. The draping is completed by covering the lower part of the patient with a sterile water repellent drape, extending from just below the operation area. A special incise drape (Steridrape) may be applied to exclude virtually all surrounding areas from the operation site. This eliminates the need for clipping eye lashes and extends the sterile field up to the eyeball itself.

Ear
(A) A circulating assistant lifts the patient's head off the table. The 'scrub' nurse or surgeon lays two drapes on the table under the head, which is then lowered on to the drapes.
(B) The uppermost drape is folded over the patient's head in turban fashion, to cover the hair. It is secured with a towel clip, and the head is then turned to leave the operative ear uppermost.
(C) An adhesive fenestrated drape is unfolded. The paper covering the adhesive on the underside of the drape is then removed, and the drape placed over the head such that the ear is exposed through the fenestration. The drape is pressed firmly around the ear to ensure adhesion.
(D) and (E) A large patient drape is placed on the patient; it is then partially unfolded to the side and the backing paper removed from the adhesive strip, being at the patient's head end. The upper end of the drape is unfolded and fixed to the upper drape using the adhesive strip.

Fig. 9.17 Draping procedures for head and neck (Barrier disposable drapes—Surgikos, Division of Johnson & Johnson Ltd.).

Draping Operation Areas and Assisting the Surgeon

Neck

(F) A circulating assistant lifts the patient's head off the table. The 'scrub' nurse or surgeon lays two drapes on the table under the head, which is then lowered to the drapes. The uppermost drape is folded over the patient's head and mouth, in turban fashion.

(G) A large patient drape is placed on the patient; it is then partially unfolded to the side and the backing paper removed from the adhesive strip, being at the patient's head end.

(H) The upper end of the drape is unfolded and fixed firmly to the chest, well within the 'prepped' area.

(I) A large utility drape is cuffed for approximately 15 cm (6 in).

(J) The cuffed utility drape is secured, along the side of the throat, using towel clips as follows:
The towel clips are positioned inside the cuffed fold. One towel clip secures the drape to the head towel; another secures it to the large patient drape. The procedure is repeated on the other side; additional towels may be placed around the throat to define the incision area.

CRANIAL OPERATIONS

These often last a long time and it is important that the drapes remain secure and sterile throughout the whole period. Furthermore, unless great care is taken, soiling of the towels after incision involves the risk of contamination from the underlying skin.

Supine or Prone Position. This requires a sterile water repellent sheet to be placed under the head first.

Self adhesive plastic sheet (Steridrape, Vi-Drape or OpSite) may be applied to cover the scalp (Fig. 9.16). The closed eyelids must be covered with sterile eyepads.

Fig. 9.18 Final drapes for cranial operation.

The anaesthetist must have access to the patient's airway during operation and further drapes should always be placed with this in mind. A sterile water repellent sheet extending from the scalp and across the chest is draped over a large instrument table or wire screen placed about 31 cm (12 in) above the patient and at shoulder level.

The final towel is placed around the head, first draped over the water repellent sheet (covering the instrument table or wire screen), and then over transfusion stands at each side of the operation table (Fig. 9.17).

This method of draping will ensure complete isolation of the anaesthetist from the operation area, and by forming a tent over the patient provides good access to the patient's airway and lower extremities.

PERINEAL OPERATIONS (VAGINAL, RECTAL, CYSTOSCOPY, URETHRAL OPERATIONS, ETC.)
IN THE LITHOTOMY POSITION

The first stage is placing a sterile water repellent sheet under the buttocks. This is important, as it prevents contamination from the lower part of the operation table which would otherwise become rather wet during the course of the operation.

A 'holed' water repellent sheet or plastic adhesive drape is used to isolate the operation area from surrounding unprepared skin and this is followed by a special drape having two lateral leg 'bags' stitched to either side of a central slit. The central slit is adjusted around the operation area and the 'bags' cover both legs and operation table stirrups. The upper and lower ends of the 'holed' towel cover the abdomen and lower end of the operation table respectively.

Alternatively, a small towel may be placed over each leg and stirrup, followed by a standard 'holed' towel with its slit over the operation area, and sides secured around each leg and stirrup.

A sterile douche tray may be added after the drapes have been positioned correctly.

Synchronous combined excision of the rectum performed simultaneously from the abdominal and perineal route by two surgeons, requires complete draping of the two areas. This is achieved by using a drape as previously described, but having a slit which will extend from the anus to the umbilicus. A small towel is placed to cover and isolate the genitals.

Many surgeons operating in the perineal region appreciate a towel draped as a trough between the patient and themselves. One edge of this towel is secured just below the operation area and to the towel covering the leg and stirrup on each side, the other edge being clipped to the surgeon's gown. This method will prevent dropped instruments from slipping to the floor and will provide the surgeon with a 'shelf' for his swabs, etc., if he should so desire. Alternatively a narrow table placed transversely may be used and is placed in position before draping.

Assisting the surgeon

It would be very presumptous to even suggest that the technique, of assisting the surgeon either as first assistant, second assistant or scrub nurse, can be learned from a book. This, like draping the operation area, can be perfected only by careful practical study under the experienced surgeon or theatre superintendent. There are, however, certain basic points which are fairly universal and common to assisting in general.

THE SCRUB NURSE

The development of logical thinking plus a silent technique, whereby metal instruments may be picked up or put down with minimal noise, cannot be over-emphasised (Ginsberg et al., 1967; Willingham, 1971).

The instrument or Mayo trolley is prepared by laying out only those instruments which will be required in the early stages of the operation. These instruments are replaced with others when necessary and as the operation progresses. The instrument trolley should not be crowded as this only leads to confusion, especially at a later stage of the operation.

It is important that the instruments should always be laid out in the same order, not only for tidiness, but because many valuable seconds can be lost searching for a vital instrument. A standard method of preparation of this and other trolleys used in the operation area will reduce delays, especially during critical periods.

Steri-Drape™ 2
Surgical Incise Drapes

APPLICATION TECHNIQUE

Orientation markings may be applied to the dried, prepped skin.

Position drape over scalp with liner face down. Grasp liner tab from underneath and begin peeling back.

Peel back liner material, folding liner upon itself as you go along. DO NOT REMOVE LINER COMPLETELY. Leave last fold adhered to adhesive area.

3M and Steri-Drape are trademarks

Using folded liner as a "handle bar," stabilize drape over scalp. With a folded sterile towel, press and smooth drape to scalp, first along planned line of incision. Remove liner completely and incise through sterile drape surface.

Fig. 9.19 Application technique for Steridrape used in neurosurgical operations. (Surgical Products, 3M United Kingdom Ltd.)

Draping Operation Areas and Assisting the Surgeon

(A) A small towel is 'cuffed' to protect gloved hands, and is then tucked underneath the patient's buttocks.
(B) Lithotomy legging is unfolded with the foot piece uppermost, the gloved hand is positioned inside the protective cuff, and
(C) the legging is slid over the patient's leg and lithotomy pole. This procedure is repeated for the other leg.
(D) Lithotomy sheet is placed folded, with the lithotomy fenestration over the operation area. It is then first unfolded downwards to cover the 'flexed' lower part of the table, and then the remainder of the sheet is unfolded towards the patient's head.
(E) The white protective patch covering the adhesive surrounding the fenestration is carefully peeled off, and the edge of the sheet pressed down firmly to ensure adhesion to the skin, thereby isolating the operation area.

Fig. 9.20 Draping for lithotomy position (Barrier disposable drapes—Surgikos, Division of Johnson and Johnson Ltd.).

The majority of surgeons appear to prefer the order of instruments whereby those required first are placed on the right-hand side of the instrument trolley facing them. This is, of course, a very flexible rule and must be adapted to suit the needs of a particular surgeon, but once established should be strictly adhered to.

The suggested order of instruments would be: at the front of the trolley from right to left, scalpels, dissecting forceps, scissors, artery forceps; at the back of the trolley, retractors, tissue forceps, etc., and any special instruments which may be required at that particular time. If the trolley has a raised edge, the handles of the instruments should project slightly over this edge. Accidental contamination of these projecting instruments is unlikely as the Mayo trolley should be positioned well within the sterile operation area. Some people will disagree with this statement, but it is much easier to pick up an instrument, silently and correctly, when placed in such a manner.

Instruments having sharp points, such as scissors and scalpels, etc., must be placed with their cutting edges or points away from the surgeon.

Soiled instruments should be cleansed before replacing them on the instrument trolley.

Fig. 9.21 Preparing the Mayo trolley.

(A) First a piece of water repellent material tucked under the tray edge to secure.
(B) The Mayo bag is slid over the tray. This ensures a sterile surface underneath and in the vicinity of the upright as well as the upper surface of the tray.

A small wire basket clipped to the front of this trolley is useful but is more applicable to thoracic and vascular surgery, where it is essential to remove blood clots from instruments before re-use.

Sharp instruments (indeed any instruments) must not be left lying on drapes covering the patient. If the surgeon requires the scalpel conveniently at hand, it should be placed in a small kidney dish and may be held by an assistant.

When passing instruments, they are placed firmly into the surgeon's hand, and it should not be necessary for him to reach for them. Most instruments such as artery forceps, tissue forceps, towel clips, scissors, etc., are always handed in the closed position, on the first ratchet when that is applicable. An instrument should always enter the surgeon's hand so that it may be used without further adjustment. With artery forceps, especially of the curved type, this means the point at the correct angle required by the surgeon, viz., generally upwards.

Self-retaining retractors are also handed for use in the closed position; but self-retaining bone clamps, dissecting forceps, and multiple joint cutting forceps should generally be open when handed to the surgeon.

These are, of course, only a few of the many instruments which the nurse will handle, but it is her duty to determine the correct way to handle a particular instrument *before* operation.

Naturally, the method of passing instruments will depend upon the way in which the surgeon is accustomed to taking them, i.e., if a surgeon extends his hand for a scalpel with the palm uppermost, the scalpel is placed with the blade horizontal, pointing towards the instrument nurse and with its cutting edge facing in the same direction as the extended finger tips. As he closes his fingers on the handle, the cutting edge will be in the correct position for use.

The non-touch technique of passing instruments is now virtually obsolete for it is logical that as the surgeon handles the instruments with his gloved hands there seems no reason why the scrub nurse should not do likewise. However, in orthopaedic surgery care should be taken to avoid touching sterile implants or the points of instruments with the gloved hands.

The preparation and threading of suture needles has been dealt with in the previous chapter, but we must now consider the correct way of handing the prepared suture to the surgeon.

If the needle has been mounted on to a needle holder, this instrument should be handed to the surgeon so that as he takes it, the needle is facing in the correct direction for immediate use. A right-handed person will require the needle facing his left hand, and a left-handed person vice versa. The long end of the suture material is held by the nurse either with her fingers or with forceps, whichever is applicable, until the assistant takes over or the surgeon has completed his first suture.

A large curved or hand needle is held by its mid-shaft, between the index finger and thumb, with the eye facing the nurse and the point towards the surgeon. A straight needle is held between the index finger and thumb but with the eye facing the surgeon and the point towards the nurse. Presenting the needle in this way will allow the surgeon to complete his first suture without further readjustment.

Ligatures may be handed to the surgeon in ligature eggs, grasped between forceps or the fingers. In the first case, the surgeon will lift the ligature egg from the nurse's extended palm. Care must be taken to ensure that there is sufficient ligature material protruding from the egg, for if it is too short it may slip back through the hole and require re-threading. After use, the egg is returned to the instrument nurse by dropping it back into her hand.

In the second case, a length of ligature material grasped between forceps should not exceed 31 cm (12 in) the surgeon using the 'instrument tie' with forceps in each hand.

When ligatures are tied by hand, the nurse must ascertain with which hand the surgeon is accustomed to tying. If he uses a left-hand tie, the nurse should face the surgeon, holding the ligature taut, with one end in her right hand and the centre in her left. He will generally take the ligature with his right hand, so that the short end is ready for grasping with his left. This procedure is, of course, reversed for a right-hand tie.

The most important point regarding *all* instruments is that they must be given a rapid final check before handing to the surgeon or his assistant. Special attention is paid to adjustable screws, ratchets, scalpel blades, their edges, and any moving parts on a particular instrument. Although instruments should always be checked by a responsible person before sterilisation, this rapid final check should *never* be overlooked.

The position of the scrub nurse in relation to the surgeon is dependent upon his wishes, and also the area and type of operation. The most logical place is that facing him, for in this position she can follow the surgeon's movements, anticipating his requirements.

Steri-Drape™
Special Ophthalmic Drape

APPLICATION TECHNIQUE

Clean and dry area around eye. Hold eyelids open with retractors.

Remove protective liner covering adhesive. Press adhesive surface to eyelids and brow. Unfold drape. Smooth adhesive securely to area. Adhesive will not adhere to moist cornea or conjunctiva. Withdraw retractors.

Lift plastic film away from the cornea and cut from lateral to medial canthus with a scissors.

Tuck loose flap of drape film under eyelid, isolating lid and lashes. Insert solid blade of speculum to secure flap in place.

Complete placement of speculum. Fixation sutures may be inserted at this time.

3M and Steri-Drape are trademarks

Fig. 9.22 Application technique for Steri-drape used in ophthalmic procedures. (Surgical Products, 3M United Kingdom Ltd.)

Some surgeons, however, prefer the scrub nurse a little to the side and behind their operating hand which is extended back as the instruments are required.

It is very difficult to make hard and fast rules regarding this, but readers will find the following to be of general application.

For operations on the face, neck, chest, abdomen or thighs, with the surgeon standing at the right-hand side of the operation table, the nurse should be opposite his right hand and with the instrument trolley at her left. A surgeon standing at the left-hand side of the operation table will require the scrub nurse opposite his left hand and her trolley at the right.

During operations on the lower limbs the nurse may adopt a similar position as above, or stand at the foot of the operation table facing the surgeon, and with the instrument trolley in front of her.

When a surgeon is at the operation table head, i.e., during craniotomy, the best position for the scrub nurse is opposite his right hand with her instrument trolley or neurosurgical table placed over the patient. If the surgeon is left handed the position may be reversed.

A similar position is adopted at the other end of the table when the knee is flexed over the foot end of the table which is lowered or removed, as during excision of torn meniscus.

An operation performed on the arm table is best served by the nurse standing behind her instrument trolley, facing the patient, and with the surgeon at her right or left, with his assistant opposite.

Fig. 9.23 An abdominal operation correctly draped, showing relative positions of surgeons and instrument nurse, etc. (Northwick Park Hospital, London.)

Occasionally the nurse will be compelled to stand behind and a little to the side of the surgeon owing to the nature of the operation. This is often necessary, for example, during Smith Petersen pinning for fractured neck of femur, where X-ray apparatus occupies considerable space normally required by the instrument nurse.

Whichever position is adopted, the nurse should always be able to observe the surgeon's movements and be capable of handing him his instruments with the minimum of inconvenience (Pearce, 1967).

Finally, it is the duty of the scrub nurse to keep a very careful check on the instruments, needles and swabs or packs, etc., used in the operation, and she should be able to account for *all* at any stage of the operation. She should always inform the surgeon of their correctness before being asked, and must obtain acknowledgment in every case.

THE SURGEON'S FIRST ASSISTANT

Occasionally it becomes necessary for a member of the nursing staff to act as first assistant.

The purpose of an assistant is to help the surgeon as required, and it is only he who can decide to what extent this assistance is necessary. As the practical knowledge of his assistant increases, so the surgeon will permit him or her to assist more fully. It must be understood that the assistant's duties are to follow the surgeon's wishes exactly, and to perform only those actions which the surgeon expects or are duly requested.

This obvious statement is, of course, only a repetition of that made at the beginning of this chapter, for we must realise that a good assistant is trained in a particular surgeon's ways and methods by practical guidance, and certainly not from a book. The following suggestions are meant as a basis for the embryo assistant, but will be of some help to those who may be called upon suddenly to assist the surgeon.

The assistant either faces the surgeon, standing at the opposite side of the operation table, or is placed at the surgeon's side opposite to the place occupied by the instrument nurse or second assistant.

The main duties of a first assistant are to keep the operation field unobscured and free from blood, either with a suction tube or gauze swabs, using with the latter a 'dabbing' action rather than wiping which may disturb minute blood clots and increase bleeding. Where excessive bleeding is anticipated from the incision, the surgeon may require pressure to be applied at each side of the wound as the incision is made. This applies particularly to operations on the cranium, due to the vascularity of the scalp.

If the assistant is permitted to apply haemostats to severed vessels, care should be taken to grasp only the vessel and a minimum of surrounding tissue with the forceps tip. Excessive tissue clamped with a vessel will require an unnecessarily stout ligature with consequent risk of slipping, and furthermore, resultant necrosis of the tissue may affect healing.

Whenever possible the surgeon will apply forceps to vessels after dissection from surrounding tissue and before division. He will apply his forceps across the vessel first, followed by the assistant who places his in close proximity. The vessel will be divided by scissors or if the forceps are very close, with a scalpel.

During ligation of a vessel the forceps are held by the assistant in such a manner that they may be re-applied immediately should the ligature slip. After the litature has been placed around the forceps, the handle is depressed, and the points elevated towards the surgeon, avoiding excessive leverage. It should not be released until he indicates (usually by saying 'off') and care must be taken to do this comparatively slowly in order that the first hitch of the ligature may be tightened on the vessel.

Deep vessels do not generally permit the elevation of forcep points, but they should always be directed towards the surgeon unless he indicates to the contrary.

When cutting a ligature the scissors are held by the thumb and third finger, with the index finger extending along the shanks to the joint, thereby steadying the instrument. As far as possible, the scissor points only are used for cutting, for if the whole length of the blades is used, more than the ligature may be divided, possibly with disastrous results. Ligatures should be cut fairly short, about 13 mm (¼ in), except for the larger vessels which the surgeon will indicate.

In order to avoid the contamination of clean instruments the used instruments should always be returned to the instrument nurse, and not dropped on the drapes covering the patient or on the instrument trolley.

Incise drapes or surgical towel drapes may be applied in various ways but the best method is illustrated in Figures 9.1–9.5 (page 196). The use of fabric skin or tetra towels is now an outdated practice because they soon become soaked with blood and lose their protective value.

Fig. 9.24 Following the surgeon's suture
(A) Simple continuous suture.
(B) Simple continuous suture—'non-touch' technique.
(C) Continuous 'blanket' suture, 'non-touch' technique.

Deep retractors are placed by the surgeon and should *not* be removed by the assistant unless he or she is requested to do so. Superficial retractors, on the other hand, require some alteration of position during the initial dissection and a good assistant will, if the surgeon permits, learn to follow him in this respect without any effort on the surgeon's part. The retractors will be moved to provide the surgeon with the greatest possible access in the particular area which he is working but this is dependent on the degree of retraction permissible.

The care with which a retractor must be used cannot be over-emphasised and undue force must be avoided owing to the trauma which can result. The surgeon will decide the degree of retraction possible and this must not be exceeded, the tendency being for the retractor to be *held* and not *pulled*.

Steri-Strip™
SKIN CLOSURES
Basic preparation and application techniques

1. Clean and dry skin for at least 2½ inches around the wound, making sure to remove skin oil or exudate. For best results, use a sponge moistened with either alcohol or saline followed by a firm wipe with a dry sponge. A thin coat of Tr. of Benzoin may be helpful in certain cases. Be sure gloves are dry before handling the tape.

2. Grasp package tabs and peel back.

3. With sterile precautions remove card, break on perforated line and tear off the card tab. Remove strips as needed.

4. At midportion of the incision, apply one-half of the first strip up to one wound margin and press firmly into place.

5. Appose skin edges exactly using fingers or forceps. Press the free half of the tape firmly into place.

6. In large wounds apply additional strips at intervals in the same manner. This eases separation stress and facilitates wound edge approximation.

7. Should the skin surfaces become moist with perspiration, blood or serum, wipe dry with sponge before applying the next strip.

8. Complete the closure with additional strips spaced approximately ⅛ inch to allow for drainage.

9. If, as sometimes happens in large wounds, the skin has gapped under the first strip or two due to initial stress, remove these strips and reapproximate the wound edges with fresh strips.

Note: The correct application of STERI-STRIP Skin Closures requires careful attention to instructions. As in all suturing, ease of application can be attained with STERI-STRIP Closures only after several uses.

3M and Steri-strip are trademarks

Fig. 9.25 Method of preparing skin and application of Steri-strip skin closures. (Surgical Products, 3M United Kingdom Ltd.)

1. **Redistribute stress.** Apply additional strips approximately ¼ inch from and paralleling the wound (ladder pattern) to redistribute the tension. This variation gives added protection against unusual disruptive stress.

2. **Action areas.** For wounds over joints, or in other areas where motion may cause "scissoring" of apposed edges, a criss-cross application gives greater security.

3. **Unusual laceration.** With V-shaped lacerations, the point of the V is anchored with the forceps and strips applied across both legs of the V.

4. When applying Surgical Dressing, or any other dressing, make sure it completely covers the ends of the tape strips.

Contraindications. When proper steps of application and follow-up are observed, no anatomical regions (except those extremely limited in size) are contraindicated.

3M and Steri-Strip are trademarks

Fig. 9.26 Steri-strip application variations. (Surgical Products, 3M United Kingdom Ltd.)

Any form of retractor used in the location of a delicate organ such as the liver or lungs, requires some form of pack or swab between it and the organ concerned. A pack should never be obscured by a retractor without the knowledge of the surgeon and instrument nurse, and the assistant should ensure that used packs and swabs are returned to the scrub nurse rather than dropped on to the floor, to assist her in the location of packs and swabs after the operation.

Small swabs or sponges should not be removed from sponge-holding forceps by the assistant, owing to the danger of these swabs being mislaid, especially when large quantities are being used. It is the duty of the scrub nurse to change these swabs when necessary so that a very careful check can be made of the total in circulation.

Any swabs or sponges used as packs must have a tape attached which is always visible and must have a haemostat clipped to it.

Soiling of the drapes which can occur when opening the bowel, etc., is avoided by using additional towels or packs just before the incision is made. These may be a distinctive colour, often red, and are placed to isolate the bowel from the general drapes. Instruments used for the procedure should remain on these towels or in a separate kidney dish, and are discarded with the towels when the bowel closure is complete.

Fig. 9.27 Types of sutures.

1. The blanket or continuous locked suture.
2. Continuous suture and method of using perforated buttons to support tension sutures.
3. Continuous mattress suture.
4. Interrupted mattress suture.
5. Figure-of-eight sutures around pins.
6. Method of placing first and second half-hitches in the square or true knot.
7. The square knot reinforced by third half-hitch.
8. The Halsted interrupted mattress suture.

(From *Manual of Operative Procedure*. Ethicon Sutures Ltd.)

The surgeon and his assistant change their gloves before concluding the operation and whilst the soiled drapes are being removed.

Hot saline packs prepared by the scrub nurse are replenished when necessary, unless the surgeon indicates that a particular pack should remain in position. This maintenance of moisture and warmth is particularly applicable to exposed bowel which should be kept covered whenever possible.

Sutures are cut in a similar manner to ligatures, but a continuous suture requires the assistant to follow the surgeon, keeping each loop taut as it is made.

After the first knot has been tied, the continuous suture should be held about 8 cm

(3 in) from the first loop, pulling the strand a little towards the side of the incision. As the surgeon passes his needle through the tissues and makes each loop, the strand is released. It is then grasped again and the loop held taut, the process being repeated until the surgeon has sutured the entire length of the wound. The degree of tension varies but should be sufficient to prevent each loop slipping, without drawing the tissues together tighter than required by the surgeon.

Fig. 9.28 Types of sutures.

1. Purse-string suture around open stump.
2. Closing stump by Cushing stitch.
3. Methods for ligation of pedicles with anchored ligatures.
4. Interrupted Lembert inverting stitch.
5. Continuous Lembert stitch.
6. Two methods of continuous over-and-over closing sutures.
7. Subcuticular suture for closure of skin incision. Perforated buckshot used to anchor suture.
8. Interrupted skin sutures – multiple needle technique.

(From *Manual of Operative Procedure*. Ethicon Sutures Ltd.)

Where a non-touch technique is operable, this procedure must be performed with forceps, preferably of the non-toothed variety or those specially designed for the purpose. Care must be taken to avoid crushing the material, for if this occurs in the middle of a strand, it may break during suturing or at some stage post-operatively.

Certain continuous sutures, such as the blanket type, require the assistant to hold the material in the correct position for the surgeon to catch each loop with minimum delay. Various methods are illustrated.

Skin sutures are cut at least 13 mm (½ in) long for subsequent removal. Tension sutures, or those retaining drainage tubes are always left longer than those used for general closure, for easy identification. A different colour of suture material is also very useful for these special sutures which are often removed at different intervals to the skin sutures.

Fig. 9.29 Types of sutures.
(A) Variety of methods for securing the ends of completed continuous sutures. Technique for securing ends of both double and single sutures demonstrated. Note method of dividing suture to avoid double thickness of knot.
(B) Method of beginning subcuticular suture by placing square knot lateral to incision. Method of ending suture at opposite end of incision.
(C) Alternate method for the completion of subcuticular continuous suture by placing a holding knot around end of subcuticular suture.
(D) Methods of placing transfixing ligatures to prevent slipping.
  1. Transfixing ligature of pedicle.
  2. Method of placing transfixing ligature in vessel.
  3. Tying transfixing ligature of omentum or of hernial sac.
(From *Manual of Operative Procedure*. Ethicon Sutures Ltd.)

Adhesive skin closures are a method of closing skin incisions which is gaining popularity. Many surgeons use Steri-strip skin closures either alone or as an adjunct to suture. Since 1962, the technique has been used for thousands of major surgical procedures such as appendectomies, thoracotomies and orthopaedic procedures. The non-reactive nature of the tape and adhesive backing makes the material very suitable for plastic procedures such as skin grafts and the secondary closure of infected wounds.

Success of the technique is dependent upon careful adherence to the method of application which is illustrated in Figures 9.25 and 9.26.

THE SURGEON'S SECOND ASSISTANT

This duty is frequently delegated either to a nurse or dresser who requires experience before assisting in the capacity of instrument nurse or first assistant. During major operations it may be essential to have a fully experienced person in this position.

Generally the second assistant helps the first by holding extra retractors and performing the duties which the surgeon may indicate.

Fig. 9.30 Insertion of Michel suture clips.

The correct application of dressings may be supervised by the first assistant, although this task is completed by the scrub nurse, except in special circumstances.

The infected case

Extreme care must be taken to avoid cross infection following an infected operation (Medical Research Council, 1968). Of special importance are the precautions to be taken when dealing with Australia antigen positive patients; staff are particularly at risk in this instance (Waterson and Batterson, 1977; Hackshaw and Hackshaw, 1975).

Patients who are suspect carriers of Hepatitis B (serum hepatitis, Australia antigen positive) include those with liver disease, patients in renal units, drug addicts, the tattooed, patients who have received repeated blood transfusions, and those on immunosuppressive drugs. The virus is present in blood, saliva, urine, faeces, bile and vomit, and staff should avoid contact with any of these.

The most important principle is to ensure that all staff realise that special care must be taken when carrying out procedures during an operation. Only the minimum number of staff should be allowed in the room and all personnel should wear caps, masks, glasses or protective goggles, disposable gowns, gloves and plastic overshoes. The following outlines the basic procedures that should be adopted:

Patients should be brought to the operating department on their bed, or on a trolley covered with water repellent disposable sheets. The patient should be taken directly into the theatre, *not* through the anaesthetic room. After operation recovery should take place in the theatre *not* in the post-operative recovery area. After the patient has entered, folded towels

Fig. 9.31 Removing soiled gown and gloves (Royal Berkshire Hospital, Reading).

(A) To protect scrub suit and arms from contamination with bacteria which is present on outside of gown; the gown is peeled off one side of body, using the opposite hand, and the inner side of the gown is turned outward.

(B) The outer side of the soiled gown is turned away from the body, keeping elbows flexed and arm away from the body, so that the soiled gown does not touch the arms or scrub suit.

(C) To prevent outer surface of gloves from contaminating hands, the gloved fingers of one hand grip the outer surface of the cuff and pulls off the glove inside out.

(D) and (E) To prevent contamination of the ungloved hand, the person grasps the inner part of the cuff and pulls the remaining glove off the hand.

soaked in sodium hypochlorate 1 per cent solution should be placed inside all doors. Except in emergency, from this moment no one is allowed to enter or leave the room.

Preparations before operation include the removal of extraneous equipment and furniture from the theatre, but retaining sufficient supplementary items such as suture materials and strapping etc. to avoid unnecessary 'fetching' during operation. Adequate supplies of formalin 10 per cent solution and sodium hypochlorate 1 per cent solution should be available.

Instruments should be transferred from the pre-set tray or packet onto a trolley covered with disposable drapes. The tray, linen drapes and wrappers are returned to the HSDU; all drapes should be disposable whenever possible.

Several buckets lined with plastic bags are required, and these, together with an enamel tray placed on a plastic sheet should be partially filled with hypochlorate solution. The buckets are for used syringes, broken glass, scalpel blades etc., and the tray is for swabs which, if a check is required, can be laid out in order for counting.

Suction traps should be fitted between all suction lines and the machine or vacuum terminal unit. These are discarded for destruction after operation. If blood is spilt at any time, it must be wiped up immediately with a paper towel soaked in hypochlorate solution.

Yellow labels should be available for identifying specimens. The specimen containers, after closing, should be wiped over with hypochlorate solution and then, with *clean* gloved hands dropped into a plastic bag which is then sealed.

After operation, the scrub nurse, still wearing gown and gloves, carefully bundles up the drapes and other disposable items and places them in their respective plastic bags, then waxed lined bags which are stapled by another person wearing clean gloves. This person then labels the bags with yellow stickers and removes them for disposal.

Instruments are soaked in formalin 10 per cent for three hours before sending in sealed bags to the HSDU for terminal heat disinfection and cleaning. (Hypochlorate should not be used as it damages the surface of metal objects.) Used items collected in hypochlorate solution are similarly left soaking for three hours, and then placed in appropriate bags, sealed, labelled and sent for destruction. If any ordinary linen has been used and is not blood stained, it is soaked in hypochlorate solution for three hours before sending to the laundry as infected linen. Linen which is blood stained must be incinerated.

The scrub nurse removes her gown and gloves, taking care not to contaminate her hands. Staff, still wearing gowns and gloves, clean the equipment and theatre thoroughly using hypochlorate solution. The theatre should be left for an hour before further use.

Afterwards, all personnel involved, either in the operation or cleaning the room, should leave their contaminated clothing and overshoes in appropriate disposal bags at the door, stepping into a clean gown before going to the changing rooms to shower and obtain clean theatre clothing.

REFERENCES AND FURTHER READING

BAILEY, H. (1967) *Demonstrations of Operative Surgery*, 3rd edn. Edinburgh: Livingstone.
BALLINGER, W. F., TREYBAL, J. C. AND VOSE, A. B. (1972) *Alexander's Care of the Patient in Surgery*. St. Louis: Mosby.
GINSBERG, F., BRONNER, L. S. AND CANTLIN, V. L. (1967) *A Manual of Operating Room Technology*. Philadelphia: Lippincott.
HACKSHAW, M. AND HACKSHAW, J. E. (1975) *Nursing Times*, October 16, supp. IX.
LINTON, J. (1974) Occasional Papers. *Nursing Times*. July 4, 11, 18.
MEDICAL RESEARCH COUNCIL (1968) Aseptic Method in the Operating Suite, *Lancet*, **i**, 763.
PEARCE, E. (1967) *Instruments, Appliances and Theatre Techniques*, 5th edn. London: Faber.
PUBLIC HEALTH LABORATORY REPORT (1965) *British Medical Journal*, **i**, 1251.
WATERSON, S. AND BATTERSON, P. (1977) *Natnews*, January, 8.
WILLINGHAM, J. (1971) *Operating Theatre Techniques*. English Edition.

10
ANAESTHETICS AND THE ANAESTHETIC ROOM

Anaesthesia is a complex, highly developed science.

So vast is this clinical field that it would be quite impossible to describe in this chapter all the equipment and techniques which are available today. For further information the reader is advised to consult a textbook dealing specifically with anaesthesia.

The anaesthetic nurse, assistant or technician must familiarise themselves with the basic principles of apparatus and the use of drugs in the particular theatre in which they work. It would be wrong to suggest that it is necessary to know all the mechanisms of anaesthetic apparatus, or all the effects and complications of certain drugs, but an intelligent and sensible understanding of the basic principles involved is essential in order to give efficient assistance to the anaesthetist.

The maintenance of anaesthetic apparatus is the task of an expert, and the anaesthetic assistant should not tamper with complicated mechanisms about which he or she knows nothing, for it is the anaesthetist's ultimate responsibility to ensure that the apparatus is working correctly before use. However, minor servicing described in this chapter can easily be accomplished by the experienced anaesthetic assistant in co-operation with the anaesthetist. The anaesthetic nurse or technician who has a natural aptitude for dealing with things mechanical may obtain further information from the technical booklets applicable to a particular anaesthetic machine.

The anaesthetic room, general layout

In Chapter 1 we learned that the anaesthetic room should be of the same hygienic construction as the theatre and preparation room. Where there are several anaesthetic rooms in a multiple theatre suite, the construction, equipment, and layout of each should be identical whenever possible. Equipment should not be interchanged between rooms, and to avoid this it is important to ensure that adequate replacements are available.

All anaesthetic rooms should contain dust-proof cupboards, having an adequate number of wide shelves with an impervious surface and, if possible, glazed doors. Equipment stored in these cupboards is laid neatly on the shelves, labelled and in order (Fig. 10.1). All items must be clearly visible and *always* kept in the same place. Items such as laryngoscopes should be duplicated as they are known to fail at crucial moments. Unless absolutely essential, the cupboards should not be used as a store for general replacements. Various sizes of endotracheal tubes, etc., may be kept separate by storing them, complete with their connectors, in individual paper bags. These plus laryngoscopes and other equipment are conveniently stored in a dispenser (Fig. 10.3) which also has provision for holding anaesthetic masks on pegs. This prevents damage to the mask cushion. In this way, equipment can be arranged ready for immediate use, and the preparation of special trolleys is simplified.

Separate locked cupboards are required for scheduled and controlled drugs, and the keys carried by the anaesthetic nurse or sister on duty. These cupboards may also contain the register used for recording controlled drugs administered to the patient in theatre. It is the legal obligation of the anaesthetist to enter all use made of controlled drugs, the name of the patient and quantity used. Drugs for immediate use may be stored in a locked drawer fitted to the anaesthetic machine. Provision should be made to secure the anaesthetic machine to a wall when left unattended.

Fig. 10.1 Anaesthetic room storage units at the Royal National Orthopaedic Hospital, London. (Cuxson Gerrard Ltd.)

A small wash basin with elbow-operated mixing taps and requisites for 'scrubbing up' should be provided in the anaesthetic room. This basin should be positioned away from areas in which sterile trolleys are being used.

An adequate suction machine or pipe line suction device must be available, together with a suction tube and selection of suction nozzles and catheters with connectors of proper size. This should be in addition to the general theatre suction machine and unless being used by the anaesthetist in theatre, is always kept ready in the anaesthetic room, as the timely use of suction machine can be life-saving on occasions. (A suction device working off the oxygen cylinders on the anaesthetic machine is to be deplored. There is the danger that the oxygen may be used up very quickly and result in anoxia from lack of oxygen in inspired gases unless the device is connected exclusively to its own cylinder. This danger is obviated if piped gases are in use.)

A dispenser should be provided containing a selection of disposable sterile syringes in sizes ranging from 2 ml to 20 ml, hypodermic and intravenous needles.

Fig. 10.2 Floor plan of a typical anaesthetic room, similar to that depicted in Fig. 10.1. (Cuxson Gerrard Ltd.)

Fig. 10.3 The Gerrard-Reading anaesthetic equipment dispenser for airways, face masks, endotracheal tubes, connections, laryngoscopes, etc. (Cuxson Gerrard Ltd.)

In addition to general diffused lighting, which should be colour corrected, a small manoeuvrable spotlight, wall or ceiling mounted, is useful during intravenous procedures.

Two trolleys about 46 cm (18 in) square are necessary for the exclusive use of the anaesthetist for transfusions and local anaesthetic techniques.

At least two transfusion stands should be available; a Martin transfusion pump (Fig. 10.4) to enable rapid transfusion of blood should be fitted to one, or ideally to each of the stands, to supplement the pumping device of plastic recipient sets.

Fig. 10.4　The Martin transfusion pump. (Eschmann Bros & Walsh Ltd.)

Essential equipment always ready for use should include a sphygmomanometer, stethoscopes, cardiac arrest set and transfusion sets. Access to a tracheostomy set, a defibrillator and monitoring apparatus is essential (Chapter 3).

All movable equipment is positioned suitably for the anaesthetist's convenience and when the most advantageous arrangement has been made, should remain unchanged to avoid confusion.

Types of anaesthesia

Although methods of anaesthesia can broadly be grouped into several main types, it is important to realise that they are not separate entities, for each may be and often is used in conjunction with the others.

The main types are given below. (Note. The names of drugs when given first time refer to the *British Pharmocopoeia* nomenclature, those following in brackets refer to the brand names.)

1. General anaesthesia, induced by inhalation of gases or the vapour of volatile liquids which vaporise readily at normal room temperatures. These include:

Nitrous oxide. Stored in cylinders in a liquid form, under pressure, often referred to simply as 'gas'. Nitrous oxide is a weak anaesthetic agent of which high concentrations (50–60 per cent) are used in conjunction with other anaesthetics and oxygen.

Cyclopropane. A potent gas stored in cylinders in a liquid form and used only in low concentrations (15 per cent). It is flammable and explosive and therefore must not be used in the presence of cautery or diathermy.

Ether. A volatile liquid which has a wide margin of safety in use although prolonged inhalation can cause post-operative vomiting and depression, has an unpleasant, irritant smell, is flammable and explosive when mixed with oxygen.

Halothane (Fluothane). A volatile liquid which is neither flammable nor explosive. Its characteristics include lack of irritation of the respiratory tract; effectiveness in low concentration; rapid recovery after administration; absence of side effects such as vomiting.

Methoxyfluorane (Penthrane). Similar to halothane but vaporises less readily; induction and recovery are slower, has analgesic properties in low concentration.

Trichloroethylene (Trilene). A blue coloured liquid with a relatively slow rate of vaporisation. Trilene has a predominantly analgesic effect and is used to supplement other gaseous anaesthetics. Used alone as a 0·5 per cent mixture in air it can be administered in small amounts in childbirth to relieve pain without loss of consciousness, must not be used in a closed circuit as it is incompatible with soda lime.

2. General anaesthesia induced by the intravenous administration of drugs such as the short acting barbiturates. The most commonly used in this class are thiopentone sodium (Pentothal, Intraval), methohexitone sodium (Brietal); and non-barbiturates such as propanidid (Epontol) a very short acting agent, ketamine hydrochloride (Ketalar), and Althesin a steroid anaesthetic agent. Epontal is very suitable for use in accident and dental departments.

Other drugs, although they may not necessarily be anaesthetics in themselves, are often used intravenously in combination with those listed above. Drugs in this class include analgesics such as pethidine, phenoperidine (Operidine), pentazocine (Fortral) and papaveretum; 'competitive blocker' muscle relaxants such as curare (Tubarine), gallamine triethiodide (Flaxedil), pancuronium bromide (Pavulon) and toxiferine (Alloferin); depolarising muscle relaxants such as suxamethonium (Scoline); hypotensive agents such as trimetaphan (Arfonad) and pentolinium (Ansolysen). In addition there are antidotes and stimulants which are discussed on page 266.

3. Local anaesthesia induced by surface application, local infiltration, regional nerve block and epidural or subdural spinal injection of drugs such as procaine (Novocaine), lignocaine (Xylocaine), amethocaine (Decicaine), prilocaine (Citanest), bupivacaine (Marcaine) and cinchocaine (Nupercaine). Cocaine is used for surface application only, e.g., ophthalmic surgery.

4. Induced hypothermia is a state of lowered body temperature produced by physical cooling of patients who are under the effect of a general anaesthetic, and the so-called lytic cocktail of which the most important element is chlorpromazine (Largactil, Megaphen).

5. Neuroleptanalgesia is a state of indifference and insensitivity to pain induced by the intravenous administration of a potent analgesic drug combined with a tranquilliser, e.g. phenoperidine (Operidine) or fentanyl (Sublimaze) combined with a butyrophenone tranquilliser such as droperidol (Droleptan) or haloperidol.

The patient is easily rousable with a normal blood pressure and when awakened remains quiet. He is in a state of apathy and mental detachment in which he is mildly sedated and uncaring about his surroundings.

Preparation for anaesthesia

1. The gas cylinders and soda lime canister, etc., on the anaesthetic machine are checked by an experienced anaesthetic nurse or technician (if permitted to do so), and reserves of these, together with bottles of halothane (Fluothane), trilene and ether are kept nearby.

2. The anaesthetic nurse also sets out instruments and apparatus required by the anaesthetist. She or he prepares trolleys and trays when necessary for open ether, intravenous anaesthesia, endotracheal intubation, and local, regional or spinal analgesia.

The anaesthetic machines

Although there are many varieties of anaesthetic machines, the principles involve the supply of anaesthetic gases to the patient, either alone or in conjunction with the vapour of volatile anaesthetic agents. Most operating theatres are now supplied with piped gases, but nevertheless each machine must be fitted with oxygen and nitrous oxide cylinders for emergency use in case of failure of piped gas supplies.

Anaesthetic Gas Cylinders are coloured in accordance with a British Standards Institute code. Oxygen cylinders are painted black with a white top and O_2 printed in black;

Fig. 10.5 Pin index system.

A. Pin index cylinder yoke, retaining clamp rotated hooked in position. Note neoprene washer surrounding gas inlet and two projecting pins just below. These pins correspond to the position of the two holes in the cylinder valve. The distance between the pins varies according to the type of gas in use, i.e., oxygen, nitrous oxide, carbon dioxide or cyclopropane. This prevents incorrect coupling of cylinders to the machine.

B. Oxygen cylinder with pin index (flush type) valve. The upper hole is the gas outlet which fits over the inlet on the cylinder yoke. A gas-tight union between the two is accomplished by applying *hand pressure* only to the screw on the retaining clamp shown in B which is rotated to hold the cylinder in position. (BOC Medishield.)

nitrous oxide are blue with N_2O printed in black; cyclopropane are orange, with C_3H_6 printed in black; and carbon dioxide are painted grey with CO_2 also in black.

These colour codings, together with some others which are *not* generally used on anaesthetic machines, are described on British Oxygen Company charts.

Regulators are attached to each cylinder to reduce the high-pressure gases, thereby making delivery easily adjustable through individual rotameters which control the amount of gases flowing into the machine and to the patient. There is a cylinder contents gauge either for each cylinder, or fitted between two cylinders of the same gas. Nitrous oxide gauges do not accurately give an indication of quantity until virtually empty, i.e., pressure is constant as long as there is liquid nitrous oxide in the cylinder.

Before connecting a new cylinder, after the protective cap has been removed, the valve should be opened momentarily to expel any dust which may have lodged in the valve seating. Failure to observe this may cause grave damage to the delicate gauges on the machine. The procedure is known as 'cracking the cylinder'.

Modern anaesthetic machines incorporate cylinders which have valves of the 'pin index type', which cannot be connected to the incorrect regulator. The washer between the cylinder and cylinder yoke or regulator yoke must be changed regularly, as it becomes worn.

The cylinder valve must be centred correctly with the cylinder yoke or regulator yoke, and the holding screw turned carefully into its location on the back of the valve, using *hand pressure* only. A leak at this point when the valve is opened usually indicates a worn or absent washer or the gas cylinder being connected to the wrong pin index yoke (Fig. 10.5).

With the male fitting type of valve, used for large oxygen and compressed air cylinders, the bullnose regulator or reducing valve is screwed into the valve seating by hand, and is further tightened with a spanner unless it carries an 'O' ring seal in which case it should be tightened by hand only. If a leak is apparent which cannot be cured by tightening the hexagon nut, the regulator should be replaced at the earliest opportunity, after trying another cylinder. Sometimes a leak may be due to a damaged cylinder valve seating.

Important. On no account must *any* grease be used on cylinders, regulators or connections, for the friction produced by the gas may ignite the grease and cause an explosion. Cylinder capacities and pressures are listed in the Appendix.

Varieties of anaesthetic machines

There are many different types of anaesthetic machines. Fundamentally, these machines consist of three main groups: (1) a semi-closed circuit Boyle's type to which can be added a closed circuit; (2) similar to (1) but incorporating a ventilator; (3) a self-contained carbon dioxide absorption circle (closed) circuit. For purposes of clarity the basic characteristics of a Boyle's type anaesthetic machine will be described followed by specific reference to particular models.

BASIC BOYLE'S TYPE ANAESTHETIC MACHINE

These machines are designed to use pipeline gas supplies; plus reserve cylinders or just cylinder gas supplies. For pipeline gas supplies the machine is connected to the pipeline outlet by flexible rubber hoses incorporating self sealing Schrader connectors. In addition the machines are generally fitted with two nitrous oxide cylinders, two oxygen cylinders and one carbon dioxide cylinder. The extra gas and oxygen cylinders are reserves. There may also be provision for cyclopropane (C_3H_6), but the gas cylinder should be removed from the machine when not in use to eliminate the fire/explosion hazard due to its explosive properties.

The high-pressure gases pass through regulators or reducing valves to the rotameters and thence into a common supply tube either direct to the patient, or are diverted through the halothane (Fluothane), trilene or ether vaporiser, and thence to the reservoir bag. From this bag the gases are carried via the corrugated rubber tube, angle piece and face mask or endotracheal tube to the patient (Fig. 10.6). Adjustment of an expiratory valve situated between the corrugated tube and the face mask enables expiration and excess gases to escape.

Regulators or reducing valves on anaesthetic machines are usually of the Adam's or endurance type, and they reduce the high gas pressures to 344 to 689 mB,* 34·47 or 68·95 kN m^2, 5 or 10 p.s.i. See Appendix, page 778, for details of medical gas cylinder contents.

This enables easy delivery of the gases through individual high-pressure rubber tubes or soldered metal tubes to the control flowmeters (rotameters).

A separate regulator is used for each gas cylinder. An aneroid gauge attached to the regulator indicates the pressure of the cylinder contents.

Rotameters have now superseded other forms of flowmeters for anaesthetic use, due to their greater accuracy.

A rotameter is an accurately made conical glass tube containing a 'float' or 'bobbin' which rises and rotates as the flow of gas increases. The flowmeter must be set perfectly vertical, otherwise the float will not spin round. If not vertical, friction will be caused between the float and the glass wall, and the reading will be inaccurate. A non-spinning float usually requires the flowmeter to be realigned and cleaned by the maintenance engineer.

Rotameters are individually calibrated according to the type and quantity of gas used. These calibrations are shown in the Appendix.

With the exception of cyclopropane, the flow of gases is controlled by a fine adjustment needle valve on the rotameter. Cyclopropane is generally controlled directly from the cylinder by a special key, circular being the safest to avoid accidental jarring when in use.

The three or four rotameters are grouped together, feeding gases into the machine. The oxygen flowmeter is always placed at the extreme left of the 'flowmeter bank', followed by the cyclopropane, carbon dioxide and nitrous oxide on the extreme right. An oxygen bypass lever supplies emergency oxygen when an increased flow of pure oxygen is required.

Vaporisers are of two types:

(A) The standard Boyle type with an unknown percentage of vapour delivered which changes with time of use and many other factors too numerous to control.

(B) The thermo-compensated type with a known percentage of vapour delivered within various ranges of temperature and gas flows.

The Boyle type. This incorporates a valve or slotted drum which allows the anaesthetist to divert a portion or all of the fresh gases above the surface or through the volatile anaesthetic agent before passing to the patient. The proportion of gases not diverted into the vaporisers passes directly to the patient.

The gases enter the vaporiser via a U-shaped tube over which there is positioned a plunger holding a cylindrical hood. This plunger may be lowered over the open end of the U-tube to increase the vapour concentration. When preparing the machines this plunger must be kept up, except when filling the bottles with anaesthetic agent. It is then lowered to cover the U-tube to prevent liquid entering this tube, which would lead to a dangerously high concentration of vapour.

*milliBar.

Both the ether and trilene vaporisers on the Boyle's machine are practically identical, the only difference being that the trilene bottle is smaller. The ether vaporiser utilises copper tubing to prevent decomposition of ether by sunlight.

The vaporisers are situated outside the closed circuit – this is known as V.O.C. (vaporiser outside circuit) and in no circumstances do the patient's respirations pass through it.

The vaporisers are filled with anaesthetic agent through the filler cap, a small plastic funnel being found very useful for the purpose. The trilene bottle should not be filled above the 100 ml (4 oz) level and the ether above the 150 ml (6 oz) level. Ether or *any* anaesthetic must be put into the bottle either by the anaesthetist *only* or *directly under his supervision*.

Fig. 10.6 A semi-closed circuit (diagrammatic).

Trilene is dyed blue, ether is colourless and with the advent of halothane (Fluothane) which is also colourless very great care must be taken to avoid mistakes.

Before the anaesthesia is commenced, the control levers of the vaporisers are placed in the closed position and the plungers set at their highest level.

The thermo-compensated type. This type, e.g., Fluotec, has replaced the standard vaporiser for the modern tendency is to use vaporisers producing known concentrations. With these vaporisers known percentages of halothane can be added to the fresh gases of any standard continuous flow anaesthetic apparatus. The patient's respirations are not diverted through halothane as dangerously high concentrations would result.

With the Fluotec Mark 3 any concentration of halothane (Fluothane) between 0·5 per cent and 5 per cent can be chosen by rotating a calibrated control dial to the appropriate setting. The delivered concentration of the anaesthetic is almost independent of the following factors which have an important effect on the performance of a Boyle's vaporiser.

1. Room temperature variation
2. Cooling of the liquid by evaporation

Fig. 10.7 The 'Off' position of the Fluotec vaporiser shown diagrammatically.

Fig. 10.8 Showing the Fluotec vaporiser in the 'On' or any calibrated position.

Key to Figs 10.7 and 10.8.
A Fresh gas inlet.
B Fresh gas channel.
C Rotary valve.
D Main cover.
E Thermostat.
F Channel from vaporising chamber.
G Gas outlet to patient.
H Port to vaporising chamber.
J Port from vaporising chamber.
K Control knob.
L, M, N Combined filler drain plug.
O Channel to vaporiser.

3. Duration of use
4. Level of the liquid
5. Variation in the total flow of fresh gases
6. The effect of shaking
7. Pressure fluctuations due to use of ventilators.

Variable factors 1, 2 and 3 are compensated for by a thermostat (bi-metallic strip) fitted in the vaporising chamber. This corrects for these variables within a range of 18°C–35°C.

The vaporising chamber is designed so that the calibration is constant from full to almost empty, i.e., while there is still just a trace of liquid visible through the level window (factor 4).

Factors 5 and 7 are compensated by a special type of gas control which ensures accurate results at fresh gas flows between 2 litres to 10 litres per minute. (Channel F, Fig. 10.8.)

Factor 6 is compensated for by a series of wicks which ensures complete saturation of

Fig. 10.9 (Left) Pin safety system for anaesthetic volatile liquids. (Right) Diagram of system fitted to Fluotec vaporiser. (Cyprane/Fraser Sweatman Incorporated).

Key:
1 Outer tube, pin safety unit.
2 Inner tube, pin safety unit
A Fresh gas inlet.
B Fresh gas channel.
C Rotary valve.
D Main cover.
E Thermostat.
F Channel from vaporising chamber.
G Gas outlet to patient.
H Port to vaporising chamber.
J Port from vaporising chamber.
K Control knob.
L Combined filler drain plug.
M Retaining screw.
N Blank plug in filler socket on vaporiser.
O Channel to vaporiser.
P Displaced air channel when filling.
Q Combined filler/drain unit on vaporiser.
R Drain tap.
S Drain socket and displaced air channel when draining.

Fig. 10.10 Fitting the pin safety cap and unit to bottle of anaesthetic liquid.

Fig. 10.11 The pin safety system adaptor/plug is fitted into the filler socket (after removing a blank plug N) making sure the flow holes in the plug are downwards.

Fig. 10.12 Pin safety system raising the bottle to fill the vaporiser.

Fig. 10.13 Replacing the pin safety system blank filler plug and securing with the retaining screw before the vaporiser is used.

the gas in the vaporising chamber and so the effect of shaking is eliminated although the vaporiser must be kept upright when charged with halothane (Fluothane).

The liquid capacity of the Fluotec Mark 3 is 135 ml when filled completely, the wicks retain 25 ml. The principle of use can be described as follows.

Figure 10.7 shows diagrammatically the Fluotec Mark 3 in the 'Off' position and Fig. 10.8 in a calibrated 'On' position. In the 'Off' position, gas from the rotameters enters inlet A and as shown by the arrows passes to the channel B in the rotary valve C. The gas continues through the main cover D, thermostat E and along the channel to outlet G and thence to the patient via the corrugated tube and the face mask or endotracheal tube. No vapour is picked up during this journey as the inlets and outlets to the vaporising chamber are closed.

As the control knob K is turned to a calibrated position the 'On' position in Fig. 10.8 is reached. In this position the metered gas in channel B splits into two streams. One stream passes through port H into the vaporising chamber where it comes into very close contact with the wicks, which are soaked with halothane (Fluothane). The gas becomes saturated with halothane vapour and leaves the chamber through port J. From here it enters the channel F and then joins up with the other stream in the main cover D and the mixed streams pass out of the vaporiser at G and thence to the patient.

The concentration of halothane is controlled by the restrictions of the temperature sensitive thermostat E and the control channel F. The restriction of the thermostat E alters according to the operating temperature. Changes in the dial position alter the restriction of control channel F.

A Penthrane thermo-compensated vaporiser is available for the administration of methoxyflurane (Penthrane). The vaporiser (Pentec 2) operates in a similar manner to the Fluotec. Methoxyflurane concentrations between 0·2 and 2 per cent can be delivered in gas flows of about 2 litres per minute.

All these vaporisers are positioned as 'vaporiser out of circuit', i.e., only fresh gases pass through the chamber allowing very accurate percentages to be selected.

Pin safety system. As mentioned previously (page 234), great care must be taken to ensure only the correct anaesthetic agent is added to the vaporiser. Cyprane/Fraser Sweatman Incorporated have introduced a safety pin system for use with thermo-compensated vaporisers. This consists essentially of non-interchangeable bottle units which fit the combined filler and drain of the vaporiser.

The bottle adaptor incorporates a cap which will fit only the correct anaesthetic liquid bottle. Attached to this cap are two flexible tubes. On the delivery end of these tubes is attached a plug which fits into a socket in the filler drain unit. This filler socket is normally sealed by a blank plug N (Fig. 10.9). The plug on the bottle unit is inserted in place of the blank plug (Fig. 10.11). With the holes down, the retaining screw is tightened and the bottle raised to a level higher than the level of the filler (Fig. 10.12). Liquid flows down the outer tube (1) and enters the vaporiser at O. The displaced air passes out of the vaporiser at (2) and up the inner tube P (Fig. 10.9). When the liquid level has risen to the level of the outlet hole P, which corresponds to the full mark on the filler window, the flow will automatically stop because no more air can be displaced.

For draining purposes the adaptor/plug on the bottle unit is fitted into the drain socket U with the holes in the adaptor/plug uppermost. The retaining screw is tightened and drain tap T opened. The anaesthetic liquid flows out of the vaporiser and down the outer tube A. The displaced air in the bottle passes up to inner tube B and is vented to atmosphere via the channel U.

The reservoir bag made of thin anti-static rubber is generally of a 4·5 litre (1 gal) capacity. The anaesthetic gases enter this bag via a drum valve, which is generally a permanently-open 'T' junction.

This bag should be tested regularly for leaks by inflating and submerging in water. There is a tendency for cracks to appear in the folds. The bag should be cleaned and sterilised frequently.

The corrugated tube, made of anti-static rubber and having a wide bore, is joined to the machine at one end and the angle piece at the other by slightly conical metal or hard rubber unions. The union at the angle piece incorporates an expiratory valve.

a. Typical layout of semi-closed system (Magill circuit)

b. Typical layout of to-and-fro absorption system

M = male conical fitting
F = female conical fitting

c. Typical layout of circle absorption system

Fig. 10.14 Typical layouts for breathing attachments of anaesthetic apparatus BSI 3849.

The tube must be checked regularly for punctures as there is a tendency for deterioration to occur in the corrugations. After use it should be stretched and suspended straight for a period, to release condensed moisture which is often lodged in the corrugations and then sterilised at least at the end of a list after each operation.

British Standard 3849 (1965) specifies certain sizes of joint fittings on anaesthetic machines. Basically it requires that the delivery end of the anaesthetic machine shall have a male conical fitting, and the face mask a female conical fitting. The conical fittings on all components of adult size from the male delivery end of the anaesthetic machine shall be in the sequence male-female in the direction of gas flow (Fig. 10.14).

The nominal size of adult cone and socket joints is 22 mm diameter. For paediatric use the size is reduced to a nominal 15 mm diameter except that the female connector to the machine outlet, the male conical fitting leading to the mask and the female conical fitting of the face mask should be of adult size (22 mm).

The expiratory valve on modern apparatus is usually of the Heidbrink type. This is a spring-loaded valve upon which tension may be adjusted to create a slight resistance against the patient's expirations. When closed circuit is used the valve is completely closed and it is necessary to cut the gas flow down to basic oxygen requirements.

Other expiratory valves such as the Coxeter or Magill type may be in use, but basically they are also a spring-loaded valve which acts in a similar manner.

The metal angle piece connects to the face mask, made from anti-static rubber manufactured in a modified funnel shape which, when applied to the patient's face, moulds with the facial contours forming an airtight fit.

The two basic types are (*a*) those having a solid or moulded lip of suitable design and (*b*) those having an inflatable cushion.

Although the cushion type (*b*) must not be over-inflated, even when not in use it should contain a proportion of air to avoid deterioration of the inner surface of the rubber. A small plug blocks the air inlet after inflation, and the mask should be stored on the connecting flange with the cushion upwards or on horizontal pegs as in the Gerrard-Reading dispenser (Fig. 10.3).

The trilene inter-lock unit is mounted in the circuit between the trilene vaporiser and the reservoir bag. This drum valve is so designed that the trilene vaporiser control cannot be moved from the 'Off' position unless the drum is set at open 'circuit'. The danger of using trilene in a circle circuit is that it reacts with heated-up soda lime to form a highly toxic agent di-chloracetylene, which in susceptible patients may cause palsy of various cranial nerves or fatal encephalitis and necrosis of the liver. The interlock device also incorporates an emergency oxygen tap which enables the administration of a plentiful supply of oxygen to the patient if the need arises.

An anti-static rubber harness may be used by the anaesthetist to maintain the face mask in position.

The Clausen and Connell head harness are the two in common use. Both are attached by two or three hooks, either fixed to the face mask or on a ring which fits over it. The Clausen harness has three limbs with several perforations, which may be suitable attached to the three hooks. The Connell has only two specially designed loops which are adjustable and maintain a friction hold on the two limbs.

All rubber items used on anaesthetic apparatus with the exception of endotracheal tubes and some airways have anti-static properties (see chapter 3).

An endotracheal tube and connection may be attached directly to an expiratory valve and the corrugated tube by substituting a Magill catheter connection for the angle piece and the face mask. In this case the corrugated tube and expiratory valve are supported carefully, to avoid pulling on the endotracheal tube after insertion. This is achieved by using adhesive strapping, Sellotape, or a specially designed head harness such as the

Connell, after placing a pad of gauze or sponge rubber between the expiratory valve mount and the patient's face. Under BSI standard the Magill or similar connection must have an internal diameter of not less than 11 mm. This also applies to the machine end of the endotracheal tube connections.

An airway may be used in the patient's mouth to prevent the tongue from falling back (impeding or obstructing respirations), and also prevent teeth clenching an endotracheal tube. There are many varieties, but all are a curved moulded shape which fits comfortably in the pharynx, holding the base of the tongue forward. A metal insert prevents compression of the airway by the teeth if it has been manufactured from a soft material. They may be made from rubber, thermoplastics (Portex vinyl) or less commonly from metal. The most generally used are the Phillips rubber type in six sizes, and the Guedel rubber or plastic in four sizes plus two extra small sizes for infants.

The Heirsch airway is similar to the Phillips, but has an oxygen feed tube fitted to the metal insert, which is of special use in children.

Where the Phillips metal insert has side perforations, it is intended that these perforations remain above the level of the rubber or plastic moulding. This is a safety arrangement whereby the patient's airway would not become obstructed should the main aperture become accidentally blocked, e.g., with the edge of the sheet or blanket.

THE CARBON DIOXIDE ABSORPTION CIRCLE CLOSED CIRCUIT ADDED TO THE BASIC BOYLE'S MACHINE

In the circle apparatus two corrugated tubes are used, one for the delivery of gases to the patient through a one-way inspiration valve, and another through which the expiratory gases are directed into the rebreathing bag via another one-way expiration valve.

Fig. 10.15 A closed or circle circuit (diagrammatic).

Fig. 10.16 The Boyle Mark 4, circle-type absorber. (B.O.C. Medishield.) Key: A Control lever. B Unidirectional valves with 'Visidisks'. C & D Inlet and outlet ports. E Soda lime canister. F Canister seating clamp. G Reservoir bag.

The patient's expirations, from the reservoir bag, pass through the soda lime canister and a selected proportion of carbon dioxide is removed. The expirations then mix with fresh gases from the rotameters which may have been passed through the vaporiser. It is possible also to pass the patient's expirations through a special vaporiser although this is not common practice. (This is then termed vaporiser in circuit.) This gas mixture is directed through the inspiration valve and along the corrugated tube back to the patient, thereby completing the circuit (Fig. 10.15).

The soda lime will only absorb a certain amount of carbon dioxide before it becomes exhausted, but modern methods of manufacture have produced a substance which will allow several hours of use before exhaustion is apparent.

The Boyle circle type absorber, Mark 4. This is designed to use reversible 2 kg capacity re-chargeable canisters or disposable pre-packs of soda lime fitted to a control head by means of a central tube which is screwed into the head with a large plastic hand nut. The canister is made of transparent acrylic material to enable the colour change of indicating soda lime to be seen easily. A condensation trap fitted to the base of the central tube prevents an accumulation of moisture in the soda lime. Unidirectional inspiratory and expiratory valves in the control head incorporate transparent Visidisks, each featuring a coloured 'pip'. These are readily visible, giving immediate confirmation that both discs are in position. The control head of the Mark 4 absorber is of simple one-piece construction. The control lever that allows gases to flow through, or by-pass the canister, has a positive spring-loaded action. A manometer can be fitted which plugs into the control head.

The transparent canister is divided centrally by a perforated metal baffle which effectively reduces 'channelling' of gases (bypassing the soda lime). In use, the gases are routed down through the central tube and up through the soda lime, so that the soda lime in the lower chamber becomes exhausted first. When the colour change in the

Fig. 10.17 Waters' 'to and fro' carbon dioxide absorption canister. (B.O.C. Medishield.)

lower chamber is complete, the soda lime in the chamber may be replaced and the canister refitted with the freshly filled chamber uppermost. When used in conjunction with the Boyle's anaesthetic machine, the absorber can be mounted in four different positions on either side of the table frame, above or below the instrument table. The fresh gas supply tube is plugged into the anaesthetic gas outlet on the manifold panel.

Fresh gases are supplied from the main part of the Boyle's machine and enter the absorber through an inlet at the back.

Soda lime of 4/8 mesh having little or no dust should be used. After refilling the canister, it should be blown through if possible with oxygen, to remove any dust which may have accumulated in the packing.

Modern soda lime preparations such as Calona (B.O.C. Medishield) or Durasorb (M.I.E.) contain a coloured indicator, which retains its colour so long as the soda lime remains active. After four to six hours' use, Durasorb changes from a pink to a cream colour and should be replaced. Calona indicates exhaustion by a change from green to brown. Many machines are now fitted with transparent absorber canisters which permit the colour of the soda lime to be easily observed.

The canister should always be filled to the top with soda lime to utilise the full effect of carbon dioxide absorption.

The Waters' canister 'to and fro' method of carbon dioxide absorption consists of a cylindrical metal or plastic canister containing soda lime, a reservoir bag, conical mount/ expiratory valve with side tube for fresh gases and angled mount for face mask, or Magill mount for endotracheal tube.

The canister is placed as close to the patient as possible. The patient's respirations pass through the canister twice and it is an efficient method of carbon dioxide absorption, although the heavy canister is rather difficult to secure in position.

THE BOYLE INTERNATIONAL MACHINE

This enables the anaesthetist to structure an anaesthetic apparatus to his own requirements. The basic trolley is constructed on a bolt together principle for simple, compact transportation and permits the full range of B.O.C. anaesthetic accessories to be accommodated. Forty different cylinder/pipeline gas supply configurations are available, including cylinder or pipeline models with pin index or overseas yokes. The back bar is designed so that one or two vaporisers can be fitted without the removal of any other components (Fig. 10.18).

ANAESTHETIC MACHINE WITH VENTILATOR

It is possible to utilise almost any type of ventilator with the basic Boyle's apparatus. Figure 10.19 illustrates a Manley Servovent anaesthetic ventilator of the flow generator, volume pre-set type fitted to the Boyle International machine. It provides total, partial and non-rebreathing facilities for use during anaesthesia. The design departs from the 'bag or bellows in pressure chamber' and is able to provide a calibrated tidal volume, together with the facility for spontaneous breathing and manual operation. The unique patient circuit produces inspiration from a calibrated bellows and directs expiration into a bag at atmospheric pressure, from which the bellows fills for the next inspiration. The patient is therefore able to breathe spontaneously throughout the entire expiratory period.

An important feature of the Manley Servovent is that the ventilator drive unit is controlled by a 'fluid logic circuit' whose gas supply is separate from the patient gas circuit. This enables any drive gas to be employed e.g., oxygen or medical compressed air.

In conventional ventilator systems, the drive gas exerts pressure directly on the outside of a bellows or bag enclosed within a pressure chamber, to produce the inspiratory phase. This direct approach gives rise to two main problems; it requires a large volume of drive gas – in excess of the minute volume ventilation of the patient, and the servo system is integrated with the ventilation system which presents difficulties in sterilising the components.

1. Sphygmomanometer. 2. Shelf for accessories such as monitoring apparatus. 3. Bank of four rotameters: oxygen, carbon dioxide, cyclopropane and nitrous oxide. 4. Fluotec halothane vaporiser. 5. Boyle-type ether vaporiser. 6. Gas outlet with flexible corrugated tube for connection to CO_2 absorber unit (16). 7. Suction unit for connection to oxygen supply (15). 8. Oxycaine spray for local topical anaesthesia, operated from oxygen supply (15). 9. Nitrous oxide cylinder supply gauge. 10. Nitrous oxide supply gauge, pipeline. 11. Cyclopropane cylinder supply gauge. 12. Oxygen supply gauge, pipeline. 13. Oxygen cylinder supply gauge. 14. Carbon dioxide cylinder supply gauge. 15. Oxygen supply to operate 7, 8 and 17. 16. Carbon dioxide circle circuit absorption unit. 17. Manley Pulmovent ventilator. 18. Accessories storage drawer.

Fig. 10.18 Anaesthetic machine (Boyle International Anaesthesia Table). (B.O.C. Medishield.)

Fig. 10.19 Manley Servovent anaesthetic ventilator. (B.O.C. Medishield.)

The Manley Servovent operates on a different principle, the driving gas being used to power a piston, which in turn operates the bellows by mechanical linkage. It requires a gas consumption of only a fraction of the minute volume. The inspiratory phase is not determined by the driving gas flow or pressure, but by spring-loaded bellows (set at 68·645 mB,* 70 cm H_2O), which eliminates the possibility of excess pressure being transmitted to the patient. A valve opens if the patient circuit experiences a negative pressure of 9·806 mB (10 cm H_2O) and admits air to prevent ventilation gas deficiency. Noninterchangeable connections ensure that the ventilation system cannot be incorrectly assembled.

Excess gas in the patient circuit is automatically 'dumped' during expiration, through an anti-pollution valve.

As the patient circuit is completely independent of the 'Servo'-drive system it may easily be removed and sterilised in its entirety. An example of an anaesthetic machine which has a permanently fitted ventilator designed as part of the apparatus is the Blease Northwick Park Anaesthetic Trolley (Fig. 10.20).

*Milli Bars.

This machine has the characteristics of a Boyle apparatus but incorporates a variable frequency, variable phase, time cycled pressure or volume limited ventilator of the Manley type. The ventilator is operated entirely by the gas delivered through the anaesthetic unit to the patient. A sensitive manometer, recording both positive and negative pressures, is fitted to the unit. The machine incorporates a closed circle circuit carbon dioxide absorption unit.

A circle or closed circuit has many advantages, including the conservance of expensive anaesthetic vapours or gases such as cyclopropane and halothane (Fluothane); the very accurate control of anaesthetic agents and degree of anaesthesia using minimal anaesthetic (especially useful with the poor risk patient and long operations); the conservance of body moisture and heat.

Figure 10.20 Blease Northwick Park anaesthetic trolley.

1. Bank of four rotameters: oxygen, cyclopropane, carbon dioxide and nitrous oxide.
2. Fluotec halothane vaporiser.
3. Boyle type ether and trilene vaporisers.
4. Oxygen and nitrous oxide cylinder contents gauges; patient circuit pressure gauge.
5. Negative pressure control valve switch.
6. Emergency oxygen lever.
7. Ventilator on/off tap.
8. Tidal volume scale.
9. Manley ventilator.
10. Carbon dioxide circle circuit absorption unit.
11. Accessories storage drawer.

The reader is reminded again that little detail has been given regarding the maintenance of these anaesthetic machines. It is the responsibility of the anaesthetist to ensure that the machines are in good working order, and the degree of simple maintenance by the anaesthetic nurse or technician depends upon his or her experience, mechanical ability and, above all, the anaesthetist's orders in this matter. There should be a routine planned maintenance either by the manufacturer or a specially trained service engineer.

Scavenging systems

Mention was made in Chapter 1 of the need to reduce the level of pollution due to waste anaesthetic gases in the operating theatre atmosphere (page 20). Typical sources of pollution are:
- a. Excess gas from expiratory valves.
- b. Polluted discharge from ventilators, which may or may not include the driving gas.
- c. Expired air from the patient.
- d. Leaks from equipment, poorly fitting face masks, etc.
- e. Spillage e.g. due to filling vaporisers.
- f. Diffusion through tubing (this is thought to be negligible).

An anaesthetic gas disposal (scavenging system) can remove the pollution from sources

Fig. 10.21 Schematic diagram of a scavenging system.

252 Operating Theatre Technique

Use of the Servovent with a conventional anaesthesia circuit

Servovent circuit
1 Tidal volume control
2 Tidal volume scale
3 Pressure gauge
4 Bellows
5 Bellows lock
6 Bacterial filter
7 Plug-in circuit
8 Expiratory valve
9 Hose to anaesthesia circuit
10 Expiratory dump anti-pollution valve
11 Exhaust
12 Air inlet valve
13 Re-breathing bag
14 Springs
15 Piston
16 Non-return valve
17 Pneumatic stop
18 Fluid logic control
19 On-off tap
20 Expiratory time control
21 Inspiratory flow control
22 Driving gas
23 Bleed hole
24 Pressure blow-off
25 Detachable patient circuit

Anaesthesia circuit
26 Fresh gas connected in the normal place
27 Expiratory valves all to be closed
28 Servovent to be connected where re-breathing bag would normally be placed

Fig. 10.22 Use of the Manley Servovent with a conventional anaesthesia circuit. (B.O.C. Medishield.)

a and b, and in principle from c, but has no effect on pollution from sources d, e and f. Pollution from these sources can only be removed by adequate room ventilation. It has been found that pollution can be reduced significantly by:
1. A properly designed and commissioned scavenging system.
2. Adequate room ventilation.
3. Prevention of leaks from equipment, face masks, etc.

There are two types of scavenging systems: passive and active. Passive systems use the patient as the air mover; active systems use a mechanical air mover such as a fan, venturi, vacuum pump or the fan provided for the mechanical extract ventilation. Passive systems are only suitable for a spontaneously breathing patient and cannot remove the high polluted discharge from some ventilators. The performance of a passive system depends on factors such as wind conditions, length of vertical run, etc. and is unpredictable. A passive system is therefore not recommended.

A scavenging system should be capable of removing the polluted discharge from ventilators and an active system is recommended. It should be capable of removing a flow of 100 litres/minute continuous, with peaks of up to 130 litres/minute for up to 0.25 seconds. There are also several systems available commercially which work satisfactorily. The resistance to flow should not exceed 50 Pa at 30 litres/minute, and the maximum resistance should be 1,000 Pa. The maximum suction pressure should not be minus 50 Pa. Safety devices should be provided to ensure patient safety.

A draft British Standard is currently being prepared which covers the design and safety requirements of scavenging systems. Information is also available from DHSS.

Fig. 10.23 Scavenging system using air-break device and mechanical extract as disposal system.

Fig. 10.24 Cape 2000 Ventilator. (Cape Engineering Company Limited.)

The majority of controls and patient monitors are located on the main control panel. Large meters are used to indicate inflation pressure, frequency and tidal/minute volume with phosphorescent pointers for ease of reading in dim light conditions. Additional controls are located on top of the ventilating head.

Frequency – The respiratory rate control on the main control panel allows the frequency to be adjusted between 5 and 50 breaths per minute and this is indicated on the frequency meter.

Preset Volume – The tidal volume is controlled by limiting the travel of the patient bellows in the ventilating head. It is adjusted by the volume INCREASE/DECREASE push buttons on the main control panel to set the lower limit of the patient bellows movement against a scale on the bellows chamber.

Pressure – The upper airway inflation pressure is dependent on the ratio between the patient's vital capacity and the preset tidal volume and also on airway resistance and lung compliance. The pressure is indicated on the pressure meter on the main control panel.

Positive End Expiratory Pressure (PEEP) – The PEEP valve is located on top of the ventilating head.

Inspiratory/Expiratory Ratio – The I/E Ratio may be adjusted to 1:1, 1:2, 1:3 and 1:4 using the relevant control on the main control panel.

Tidal/Minute Volume – The volume meter on the main control panel gives a reading of the tidal volume at the end of each expiratory phase. By depressing the MINUTE VOLUME push button, an instantaneous reading of the minute volume is available.

Intermittent Mandatory Ventilation (IMV) – To activate the IMV system, the IMV control on the main control panel is switched on and set to the desired interval between mandatory breaths (15, 30, 60 or 90 seconds). The ventilator will then automatically deliver one breath of the desired preset volume and inspiratory flow rate at the relevant time intervals. The low pressure alarm is inactivated during IMV but the high pressure alarm still operates.

Inspiratory Flow – The inspiratory flowrate can be adjusted by means of the control located on top of the ventilating head.

DESIGN CONSIDERATIONS

A scavenging system is shown diagrammatically in Figure 10.21. The polluted gases are collected from the patient circuit by the collecting system, which would typically be a modified expiratory valve designed to 'capture' the excess gas. The collecting system should also incorporate a pressure relief valve as shown in Figure 10.23. The polluted gases are then transferred to the receiving system by a transfer tubing. The receiving system is usually part of the fixed installation and may incorporate safety devices, such as a simple air break, to protect the patient, for example in the event of failure of the fan or blockage in the system. The receiving system also often acts as a reservoir. A typical receiving system is the air break device shown in Figure 10.23, originally designed by the North West Thames RHA (NWTRHA, 1980) in the system shown, the mechanical extract ventilation is used to remove and dispose of the gases, but a separate fan could be used instead. The air break device is simple, safe and inexpensive. (Not the hospital medical vacuum system – DHSS, 1976; Spence, 1978; Light, 1979.)

Ventilators

It is now commonplace to use controlled respiration during anaesthesia or following traumatic conditions such as head injuries. This may be accomplished simply by rhythmically squeezing the anaesthetic reservoir bag or by mechanical ventilators.

Many types of ventilators have been developed; some are specifically for use during anaesthesia, whereas others are suitable for mechanically assisted artificial ventilation. There are others which can be used for both purposes, utilising air or a mixture of air and oxygen.

Basically ventilators could be divided into three main groups:

1. *Flow generators.* A *fixed volume* of gases (taken from a constant flow) is delivered into the lungs. A wide *variation in the pressures* reached at the end of inspiration (or inflation) may be observed on the manometer gauge, e.g., when a patient tries to breathe against the machine, irregular patterns result with high and low values at random.

Fibrosed and stiff or congested lungs, airway obstruction including excessive secretion, foreign body, broncho-spasm, etc. (low compliance), all will require high-pressure values. Should this pressure reach a certain level, usually 39·226 mB to 68·645 mB (40 to 70 cm) of water, a safety valve blows off a proportion of the given volume.

Any leak will deprive the patient of the comparable proportion of the original delivered volume and therefore the pressure (manometer) gauge will register a suspiciously low value.

2. *Pressure generators.* With these the ventilator produces a selected pressure within the limits of time imposed by the respiratory rate. The amount of gases required for this pressure depends upon the compliance of the lungs and chest; and will need a variable volume of gases to achieve this. The ventilator will compensate for all but the gross leaks by delivering a larger volume of gases.

3. *Ventilators providing a choice of volume or pressure.* Some ventilators are electrically driven (with a manual control for emergency), others convert a continuous flow of oxygen or compressed air from a cylinder or pipeline, into an intermittent flow to the patient. It would be impossible to mention all the ventilators available and we will therefore confine outselves to a few observations on three, the Cape Bristol Ventilator, the Barnet Ventilator Mark 3 and the Bird Respirator.

THE CAPE 2000

This is basically a volume preset, time cycled flow generator, electrically driven which can be used for long-term ventilation of the lungs post-operatively or in the treatment of respiratory insufficiency.

Fig. 10.25 Cape 200 ventilator – patient system. (Cape Engineering Company Limited.)

(A) The patient system, including the complete ventilating head, the humidifier tank, breathing tubes and connectors are all fully autoclavable in high temperature steam up to 140°C. The only exception is the diaphragm of the pressure operated expiratory (POE) valve which is disposable and is easily removed before autoclaving. A new diaphragm is fitted after sterilisation. The ventilating head is lifted off the ventilator for sterilising and a special stainless steel carrier is provided to hold the head during autoclaving.
(B) If the Positive End Expiratory Pressure control is not required, this is replaced with the glass cover, and plastic diaphragm of the Pressure Operated expiratory valve.
(C) The ventilator head can be removed easily for cleaning and sterilising.
(D) High efficiency pleated membrane filters are fitted to both inspiratory and expiratory sections of the system and are located at the back of the ventilator. The inspiratory filter prevents airborne contamination entering the patient system and the expiratory filter prevents contamina-

Fig. 10.25 (cont'd).

tion from the patient being released into the atmosphere. The expiratory filter is heated to prevent condensation. Thus a high degree of protection is provided for both patient and staff. The inspiratory filter is replaced at approximately 2 monthly intervals. The expiratory filter is replaced at least for every patient.

The tidal volume of gas delivered by the machine can be adjusted between 0–2000 ml, with an infinitely variable frequency of 5–50 respirations per minute and a variable inspiratory/expiratory ratio that can be adjusted to suit patients of all ages. The maximum inflation pressure which can be applied to the patients' lungs is adjustable between 19·61 mB (20 cm H_2O) and 68·64 mB (70 cm H_2O) with the manual positive pressure valve; a positive end expiratory pressure control is also provided which gives accurate adjustment up to a nominal 19·61 mB (20 cm H_2O) pressure.

During long-term ventilation, i.e., via a tracheostomy, a water bath humidifier or ultrasonic nebuliser should be fitted between the machine and the patient on the inspiratory side of the circuit. The water bath humidifier heats the water contained to 55°C which gives an air temperature of approximately 37°C at the patient connection.

A ventilation failure alarm is available which actuates an audible and visual signal if the pressure generated deviates outside the tolerance limits set by the operator. If the pressure falls below a lower pre-set limit, the alarm is immediately actuated after a 14 seconds' delay; this is to avoid false alarms. The alarm is immediately actuated in the event of high pressure. Once the alarm signal is given, it will continue until the fault is corrected. This device can be used with other types of ventilators.

The main feature of this apparatus is the ease with which the patient circuits can be sterilised. The ventilating head and humidifier can be autoclaved and there is a bacteriological filter system on both the inspiratory and expiratory sides (Fig. 10.25).

Fig. 10.26 Humidifier for Cape 2000.

The humidifier operates by surface pick-up from an electronically temperature controlled stainless steel tank which can be sterilised in high temperature steam up to 140°C. The control system is designed to give a tank temperature of 55°C providing a relative humidity of 90–100% at 37°C at the patient 'Y' piece with the standard breathing system. A thermometer indicates the tank temperature and the temperature control system incorporates a safety cut-out to prevent the temperature of the water exceeding 70°C.

Fig. 10.27 Diagrammatic circuitry of the Cape 2000 Ventilator. (Cape Engineering Company Limited.) Key: Dark green – driving gas. Light green – gas to patient. Red – expired gases from patient.

1. Oxygen Inlet
2. Air Inlet
3. Storage Bag
4. Inspiratory Filter
5. Safety Valve (Air)
6. Relief Valve (Excess Pressure)
7. Uni-Directional Valve
8. Bellows
9. Pressure Chamber
10. Volume Scale
11. Uni-Directional Valve (Inspiratory)
12. Flow Control Valve
13. Line Filter (Pressure Monitor)
14. Manual Positive Pressure Valve
15. Humidifier
16. Patient Tubing & Y-Piece
17. Pressure Operated Expiratory Valve
18. Heated Expiratory Filter
19. Bellows Stop
20. Compressor Pre-Filter
21. Compressor
22. Shuttle Valve
23. Spill Valve
24. Solenoid Valve
25. Volume Control Servo Motor
26. I.M.V. Control
27. Frequency Control
28. Frequency Meter
29. I.E. Ratio Control
30. Ventilation Failure Alarm
31. Pressure Meter
32. Tidal/Minute Volume Meter
33. Volume Control
34. Pressure Monitor Sensor

Fig. 10.28 Barnet Mark 3 ventilator.

THE BARNET VENTILATOR MARK 3

This provides electronically controlled time cycling of a volume or pressure generator incorporating either negative phase or patient triggering. The selection of any one cycling system automatically switches the remaining systems out of circuit and therefore the machine can be regarded as three independent ventilators in one unit. Operation of the ventilator is simplified by grouping and colour coding all controls specific to each mode of operation.

Time cycling (colour coded yellow) allows a range of respiratory rates between 6 and 60 per minute with an independent adjustment of inspiratory and expiratory phase times between 0·5 and 5 seconds.

Volume cycling (colour coded orange) is achieved by monitoring the expired tidal volume on the respirometer and adjusting the flow rate control, tidal volume selector and negative pressure control.

Pressure cycling (colour coded green) at required level is selected by setting a calibrated control marked 0–44·13 mB (0–45 cm H_2O).

In operation, volumes between 30 ml and 1,400 ml may be achieved. The positive pressure exerted within the lungs is monitored by a pressure gauge 0–49·032 mB (0–50 cm H_2O); a safety valve limits the maximum positive airway pressure. In expiration, a sub-atmospheric negative phase may be introduced between 0 and minus 12 cm H_2O.

The patient trigger facilities are sensitive to minus 1 cm H_2O, which is equivalent to only 5 ml tidal exchange. If the patient fails to trigger the ventilator, respiration continues automatically at the rate previously selected.

The Barnet ventilator operates electronically through a low voltage battery which is charged by a trickle charger built into the machine. In the event of power failure, the ventilator can be used for periods up to 24 hours away from the mains supply.

Ancillary equipment which can be added includes a humidifier, and CO_2 circle absorption unit. An alarm unit is fitted as standard.

THE BIRD RESPIRATOR

This is a patient-triggered pressure generator operated from an oxygen or compressed air supply.

Basically the respirator consists of a transparent box-like structure divided into two chambers by a diaphragm. As gas flows into one chamber the diaphragm moves valves which allow gas into the second chamber and thence into the patient's lungs, during the inspiratory phase. The expiration is generally passive with the lungs deflating normally by their own elasticity, during this phase fresh gas flows into the respirator ready for the next inspiratory phase.

The sensitivity dial can be adjusted so that either the patient's weakest effort at inspiration will trigger the machine into adequate ventilation, or the patient must make a larger effort in order to do this. The respirator can provide complete controlled ventilation when the sensitivity control is set at zero. A sub-atmospheric pressure can be introduced at the expiratory phase if required.

The Bird respirator is very useful for re-educating the patient to breathe on his own account following conditions which have necessitated prolonged artificial ventilation. In America, where it originates, the machine is much used for inhalation therapy utilising nebulisers for various medicaments.

Terminal disinfection of ventilators presents a number of problems, for with the exception of corrugated tubes, external valves and connections, many of the components cannot be sterilised by heat.

Fig. 10.29 Barnet Ventilator Mark 3 diagrammatic representation of closed circuit (see key). (Reproduced from *Automatic Ventilation of the Lungs* by Mushin et al., by kind permission of the publishers Blackwell Scientific Publications Ltd.)

Key to Figure 10.29.

Gas circuit relevant references

1 Top stroke indicator
2 Weights
3 Microswitch actuating plunger
4 'Inverted top hat'
5 Expiratory bellows
6 Rod with helical spring
7 Centre bellows
8 Centre bellows blow-off valve
9 Closed circuit bellows
10 Beam
11 Cycling selector
12 Time cycling expiratory phase control
13 Time cycling inspiratory phase control
14 Trigger on/off switch
15 Pressure cycling expiratory phase control
16 Upper volume cycling tidal volume control
17 Alarm microswitch contact
18 Volume cycling microswitch contacts
19 Negative pressure control
20 Open connector
21 Negative pressure limiting valve
22 to 24 Non-return valves
25 Open connector
26 Lower volume cycling tidal volume control
27 Volume cycling microswitch contact
28 Alarm microswitch contact
29 Inspiratory solenoid valve
30 Rear closed circuit port
31 Front closed circuit port and exhaust to atmosphere
32 Gas supply to patient port
33 Driving gas, closed circuit port
34 Manual bag port
35 Outlet tube from CO_2 absorber
36 Inlet tube to CO_2 absorber
37 Partitioned soda lime canister
38 Circuit selector control
39 to 46 Poppet valves
47 Gas switch valve
48 Expiratory solenoid valve
49 Wright's respirometer
50 Breathing tubes
51 Diaphragm valve
52 Flow rate control valve
53 Expiratory spill valve
54 Airway pressure gauge
55 Patient Y-piece
56 Pressure relief valve
57 Pressure cycling diaphragm
58 Positive pressure cycling control
59 Trigger pressure diaphragm
60 Trigger pressure control
61 Manual bag
62 Reservoir bag spill valve
63 Closed circuit reservoir bag
64 Air entraining valve
65 Levers exerting spring pressure on beam (10)

Fig. 10.30 The Bird respirator. (Bird Corp. U.S.A.)

For these reasons, no one perfect technique of disinfection has yet been devised. A method has been devised for disinfecting the Cape ventilator and all types of ventilators and this involves the use of formalin (Sykes, 1964 (Lumley)). Liq. Formaldehyde B.P. 100 ml is added to the water in the humidifier (5 per cent solution). A 2-litre reservoir bag and Y-piece is then connected between the expiratory port and inspiratory port. A further 2-litre bag is fitted over the air inlet. The machine is run for four to eight hours to circulate the formalin vapour after which all tubing, traps and the humidifier are washed with tap water. The humidifier is then refilled with a 0·06 per cent solution of ammonia and the machine is allowed to ventilate for eight or more hours until there is no trace of formalin vapour detectable. The humidifier is finally rinsed well with tap water.

Fig. 10.31 Diagrammatic circuitry of the Bird respirator, Mark 8. (By courtesy of the *Nursing Times*, London.)

Another method consists of disinfection of the ventilator circuit by ultrasonic nebulisation (Judd *et al.*, 1969; Stevens, 1969). An ultrasonic nebuliser, such as the DeVilbiss or LKB, NB100, is used to produce a mist of hydrogen peroxide (20 vols) which is circulated through the machine in a similar manner to that described for formalin. This is carried out for a period of 60 minutes followed by ventilation of air for 1–4 hours depending on the type of ventilator. (See Appendix, page 779, for method.)

In the absence of a heat sterilisable or component replaceable ventilator such as the Cape 2000, this method is relatively rapid, bacteriologically effective, technically convenient, safe, and does not interfere with the function of the machine. Any hydrogen peroxide left in the machine will quickly break down into oxygen and water. When using hydrogen peroxide it is wise to protect the hands with rubber gloves to prevent cutaneous desquamation caused by contact with the hydrogen peroxide mist.

The Bird respirator can be stripped down to the actual respirator box and the accessories cleansed in Savlon 10 per cent followed by immersion in two baths of 14 per cent hypochlorite solution for at least 15 minutes each. The respirator itself can be disinfected only in ethylene oxide gas without the use of heat.

Open ether

Even with the advent of the newest and complicated anaesthetic techniques, the administration of open ether is still used occasionally and might well be valuable in the event of a major disaster.

Induction of anaesthesia is accomplished by the patient breathing through a gauze pad on to which is dropped a quantity of ether. Initially, ethyl chloride is commonly used to induce unconsciousness, because it is less unpleasant to breathe than the ether vapour.

Fig. 10.32 Open ether requirements.
1. Airways (Phillip and Guedel).
2. Boxwood wedge.
3. Mouth gag (Mason).
4. Mouth gag (Doyen).
5. Tongue forceps.
6. Pharyngeal swab-holding forceps.
7. Ether bottle with dropper (Bellamy Gardner).
8. Open inhalers, adult and child (Schimmelbusch).
9. Ethyl chloride.

The thickness of gauze should be adequate to prevent the drops of ether from falling on to the patient's face. Twelve to sixteen layers of gauze are usually adequate and these are 'tented' away from the face by a wire frame called a Schimmelbusch mask. As the outer edges of the gauze can become moistened with ether during a long period of anaesthesia, it is preferable to cut this gauze pad to the mask shape (as indicated in Fig. 10.32) to prevent the gauze from actually coming into contact with the skin.

A piece of gamgee measuring about 24 cm by 36 cm (9 in by 14 in), and having a central slit exposing the nose and mouth, is placed to protect the face. A similar piece is placed over the mask and ether dropped through the slit on to the underlying gauze. These pads also prevent the patient from obtaining air round the edges of the mask.

In order to minimise the risk of burns from liquid anaesthetic, the anaesthetist may require petroleum jelly for the lips, and sterile castor oil drops for the eyes after the ether has been administered. These should always be available when open ether is being administered.

Intravenous anaesthesia

A selection of intravenous anaesthetic agents, relaxants, stimulants and antidotes should be clearly labelled and available for the anaesthetist.

The intravenous barbiturates in common use are thiopentone sodium (Pentothal) 2·5 per cent, methohexitone sodium (Brietal) 1 per cent, and the hypnotic propanidid (Epontol) 5 per cent (supplied as a solution) and Ketamine hydrochloride (Ketalar). A 2·5 per cent solution is prepared by dissolving 0·5 g in 20 ml of sterile pyrogen-free distilled water respectively.

Fig. 10.33 Requirements for the intravenous induction of anaesthesia.

1. Succinyl choline (Scoline).
2. Curare (Tubarine).
3. Pethidine (DDA).
4. Atropine.
5. Rubber tubing for tourniquet.
6. File.
7. Spirit-impregnated Mediswabs.
8. Propanidid (Epontol).
9. Water for injection.
10. Thiopentone sodium (Pentothal).
11. Disposable syringes 20 ml, 10 ml and 2 ml.
12. Hypodermic needles Nos. 20, 12 and 1 with needle case.
13. Disposable filling cannula (Kwills).
14. Disposable Gordh needle (Armoven).
15. Mitchell needle.
16. Disposable needle (Plextrocan).

Not illustrated: disposable butterfly needles.

Phenoperidine (Operidine), pethidine and pentazocine (Fortral) are used extensively. Pethidine is often diluted to a 1 per cent solution containing 10 mg per ml.

Relaxants in common use include the 'competitive blocker' muscle relaxants such as curare (Tubarine), gallamine triethiodide (Flaxedil), pancuronium bromide (Pavulon) and alcuronium toxiferine (Alloferin); and depolarising muscle relaxants such as suxamethonium (Scoline).

Stimulants available should include nikethamide (Coramine), aminophylline, methedrine, methoxamine (Vasoxyl, Vasoxine), metaraminol (Aramine), megimide, daptazol, isoprenaline (Insuprel), noradrenaline (Levophed) and adrenaline. Antidotes commonly needed include atropine, prostigmine, nalorphine (Lethidrone) and levallorphan (Lorfan).

It is the anaesthetist's responsibility to prepare these solutions, but if the anaesthetic nurse is permitted to do so, she should check the preparation with a second person and show the anaesthetist the ampoules or bottle from which the injection has been prepared.

A 10 ml or 20 ml disposable sterile syringe is used for barbiturates, and a 2 ml or 5 ml disposable sterile syringe for other drugs, including pethidine, relaxants, antidotes, etc. The integrity of the sterile packet containing the syringe should be checked by trying to squeeze the air from the inside.

The sizes of needles used vary with individual choice but for general purposes a size 12 or 14 hypodermic needle is usual, with perhaps a size 18 for small or delicate veins. The anaesthetist will require a number of 'filling' needles (plastic quills) to aspirate drugs from the ampoules, and larger bore serum needles size 1 for rubber-cap bottles.

For continuous or intermittent intravenous injections, either the syringe and needle are left in position so that small quantities may be injected as required, or a special needle such as the butterfly Gordh or Mitchell is left in the vein and the syringe attached to the needle each time injection is necessary.

Continuous intravenous anaesthesia can be maintained by using a very weak intravenous solution, which is administered via a saline infusion, or small quantities of the drug can be injected into the infusion tube, as required.

Where it is the habit of the anaesthetist to prepare several solutions at the same time, he should label syringes to aid identification.

Medico-legally it is the anaesthetist who is responsible for the right drug being injected. Accidents do occur, and so a nurse should never be offended if the anaesthetist does not appear to trust her spoken word. He must be absolutely certain; where life is concerned, personal considerations are of no account. It is not sufficient to check the name on the outside of the ampoule box. The inscription on the ampoule itself is the *only* proof that the correct drug is being given.

Endotracheal and endobronchial intubation

Apparatus for passing an endotracheal tube must be ready before the commencement of any anaesthetic induction, even if the anaesthetist has not requested its preparation. In resuscitation this procedure will be one of the first performed by the anaesthetist, unless a tube is already in position. Laryngoscopes used when introducing an endotracheal tube include the Magill straight-blade and the anatomical shaped blade Mackintosh types which are illustrated.

There are three basic types of endotracheal tubes, the oral type, both cuffed and non-cuffed and the nasal type. Although each is identical in diameter, the nasal tube is *slightly* softer when pressed between the fingers, and this allows it to comply with the configuration of the nasal space. Some endotracheal tubes are armoured by incorporating a metal or nylon spiral within the tube wall. These tubes have less tendency to become kinked or compressed and are of special use during operations on the skull and chest.

The endotracheal tube is used:

1. When in the opinion of the anaesthetist the airway is liable to be obstructed.
2. For operations in which it is necessary because of surgical technique, e.g., head and chest operations.
3. For upper abdominal operations and artificial ventilation.
4. When the towelling and position of the patient prevents the anaesthetist gaining easy access to the patient's head, and thus guaranteeing a free airway, e.g., craniotomies.
5. To prevent the inhalation of blood or vomit, e.g., emergencies.
6. In the treatment of cardiac arrest.

The anaesthetist generally is likely to use an endotracheal tube which has a terminal cuff which, when inflated with air, impinges upon the tracheal mucosa, thereby sealing the lungs from the upper respiratory passages to prevent the inhalation of blood or vomit. It is important to realise that there is not a fixed volume of air necessary to secure air-tight fitting of the tube within the trachea. The amount may vary between 2 ml and 10 ml of air and this can be tested by the anaesthetist when inflating the lungs (Mackensie et al., 1976).

Fig. 10.34 Requirements for endotracheal intubation.

1. Artery forceps (Spencer Wells).
2. 10-ml syringe.
3. Endotracheal tubes, cuffed (Magill).
4. Endotracheal tubes, nasal (Magill).
5. Endotracheal tubes, oral, plastic (Magill).
6. Endotracheal tubes, oral, rubber (Magill).
7. Endotracheal tube connections (Rowbotham).
8. Endotracheal tube connections (Cobb, plain type).
9. Endotracheal tube connections (Cobb, with suction access).
10. Endotracheal catheter mount (Magill).
11. Laryngoscope (Mackintosh).
12. Laryngoscope (Magill).
13. Endotracheal tube forceps (Magill).
14. Atomiser for topical local anaesthetic.
15. Catheter mount clip.
16. Gauze roll for pharyngeal pack.
17. Anaesthetic swabs.
18. Local anaesthetic for topical application, e.g., 4 per cent lignocaine (Xylocaine).
19. Tube lubricant, e.g., lignocaine (Xylocaine) gel.
20. Endotracheal head harness (Hudson).

Note. Sellotape, or similar, should be available.

A nurse may be asked to clip off the pilot tube when the anaesthetist has inflated the cuff so that it just fits the lumen of the trachea. If a pair of artery forceps is applied, only the tips are used, and as near the syringe as possible; this saves wear and tear of the pilot tube. Endotracheal tubes are now available with pilot tubes which incorporate a self-sealing valve thereby obviating the need to use forceps.

Nasal tube sizes range from 3 mm to 5 mm for a child; 5 mm to 6·5 mm for an adolescent; and 6·5 mm to 9 mm for an adult. Oral tubes range from 3·5 mm to 6·5 mm for a child; 7 mm to 8 mm for an adolescent; and 9 mm to 12 mm for an adult.

The experienced anaesthetic nurse or technician will learn to select the sizes and type of endotracheal tubes required, but where cuffed tubes are to be used, they must always be tested by inflating the cuff before handing to the anaesthetist. All the apparatus should be laid out in the order required, giving special attention to the provision of correct size tube connections, and laryngoscopes in good working order. The electric lamp on the latter must illuminate brightly and if necessary the battery should be changed before use. A second laryngoscope must always be available in case of lamp failure during use. The care of electrical endoscopes has been dealt with in Chapter 2. A tube of lubricant is usually required and this may be combined with a local anaesthetic such as 2 per cent lignocaine (Xylocaine). An example of a non-anaesthetic lubricant is K-Y jelly. A suction machine with long suction catheters is prepared, together with a small bowl of clean water for rinsing the catheters. A surface anaesthetic e.g., 4 per cent lignocaine (Xylocaine) and laryngeal spray may be required. A selection of apparatus is shown in Fig. 10.34.

The endobronchial tube is in effect an extended cuffed endotracheal tube of smaller dimensions, which is passed into the left or right bronchus. Formerly during chest operations, the anaesthetist utilised two tubes, one in the unaffected lung for the purpose of anaesthesia, and one in the other for the purpose of aspiration during operation. Endobronchial tubes have an inflatable cuff to isolate the intubated lung. It is now common practice to use a divided airway or doubled lumen cuffed tube such as the Carlens: this achieves the same purpose. The anaesthetist will require a bronchoscope of suitable type, in addition to the standard laryngoscope, etc., and may also need a long bronchial spray with a surface anaesthetic, e.g., lignocaine (Xylocaine).

All endotracheal and endobronchial tubes must be cleaned thoroughly with a brush and warm antibacterial detergent solution after use. Those having inflatable cuffs are checked before being stored away, care being taken to avoid water entering the cuff or pilot tube. The tubes are always sterilised after use although absolute sterility cannot be guaranteed during intubation.

After use, laryngoscope handles should be cleaned, and the blade dismantled from the handle, cleaned and sterilised. Most modern instruments have nylon insulation and gold-plated electrical contacts which will withstand autoclaving. If they are the older type either subatmospheric steam/formaldehyde or ethylene oxide will have to be resorted to.

Local or regional anaesthesia

This may range from a simple injection for infiltrating a small area, to an extensive nerve block.

Whereas a 10 ml or 20 ml syringe is adequate for a minor procedure, involving the injection of a few millilitres of anaesthetic agent, it is preferable to use a self-filling syringe for larger quantities. The alternative is to leave the needle in position and prepare several syringes filled with anaesthetic agent, using these consecutively.

A fine hypodermic needle of size 18 or 20 will be required for the initial 'weal', followed by a longer one of wider bore. A selection of needles should be available, ranging from 5 cm to 10 cm (2 to 4 in) in length, and 20 to 26 B.W.G. in gauge.

Anaesthetists require exploring needles having long points and others having short points. A short point needle is essential for nerve blocks, especially the brachial plexus block, where a long point needle may increase the risk of pleural puncture or perforation of a blood-vessel.

Amongst the anaesthetic agents most commonly used are lignocaine (Xylocaine), bupivacaine (Marcaine) and procaine (Novocaine).

A 1·5 or 2 per cent lignocaine is used for the initial infiltration or when only a small quantity is required. Where a larger quantity is necessary, the strength of solution is reduced to 1 per cent or 0·5 per cent and the amount injected limited to the maximum dose of the agent (e.g., the maximum dose of plain lignocaine (Xylocaine) in a normal healthy adult is 13 to 15 ml of a 1·5 per cent solution, 23 ml of a 1 per cent solution or 46 ml of a 0·5 per cent solution). Dosage must be reduced in the ill and elderly.

Fig. 10.35 Requirements for local or regional analgesia.

1. 0·5 litre measuring jug.
2. Skin antiseptic.
3. Bonney's blue for marking infiltrated area.
4. Skin pen and nib.
5. Green swabs.
6. Sponge holding forceps, Rampley (2).
7. Sterile towels.
8. Self-filling attachment (Pidkin), for Labet syringe.
9. Locking needles (Labet).
10. Brachial plexus needle (Short point).
11. Filling needle.
12. Hypodermic needles (18, 12 and 1).
13. File.
14. Syringes (Labet).
15. Syringes, 10 ml and 2 ml.
16. Adrenaline 1 in 1000.
17. Lignocaine (Xylocaine) 1·5 per cent.
18. Sterile distilled water.
19. Towel clips.

In order to produce vasoconstriction, and thereby lessen capillary haemorrhage, adrenaline may be added in the proportion of 1 in 400,000 to 1 in 100,000 according to the total amount of solution being injected. A 1 in 400,000 solution may be prepared by adding 1 ml of 1 in 1000 adrenaline to 399 ml of local anaesthetic agent. A 1 in 100,000 solution may be prepared by adding 1 ml of 1 in 1000 adrenaline to 99 ml of anaesthetic agent. A 1 in 100,000 addition of adrenaline also prolongs the action of the local anaesthetic by delaying absorption up to six hours and thereby increases the safety margin for larger doses. In the case of lignocaine the maximum dosage becomes approximately twice that of the plain solution.

An easy way of preparing a small quantity of 1 in 400,000 adrenaline is to add the contents of a 1 ml ampoule of 1 in 1000 adrenaline to a 20 ml ampoule of saline solution from which 1 ml has been withdrawn, leaving 19 ml; 1 ml of this mixture is added to a second 19 ml ampoule containing anaesthetic solution. Should this be done by the anaesthetist, the nurse's watchful eye would make sure that the first ampoule containing the saline is safely discarded after removing 1 ml, so as to avoid accidents.

Fig. 10.36 Epidural or spinal anaesthetic requisites prepared as one packet.

1. Towel clips.
2. Sterile CSF specimen bottle.
3. Aqueous skin antiseptic.
4. Sterile towels.
5. Spinal manometer and connecting tube.
6. Bupivacaine (Marcaine) with 1 in 200,000 adrenaline.
7. Cinchocaine (Heavy Nupercaine).
8. File.
9. Filling needle.
10. Hypodermic needles, size 20, 12 and 1.
11. Three-way tap.
12. Epidural plastic cannula.
13. Green swabs.
14. Sponge holding forceps, Rampley (2).
15. Epidural needles.
16. Spinal needle.
17. Spinal needles.
18. Syringes, 2 ml and 10 ml.
19. Sterile distilled water.
20. Lignocaine (Xylocaine) 1·5 per cent.

It should be pointed out that on occasions the surgeon requires only the effect of the adrenaline and 1 in 100,000 or 1 in 400,000 adrenaline solution is prepared with saline only.

272   Operating Theatre Technique

ESCHMANN BROS. & WALSH LTD.

Frankis Evans Intravenous Needle (Full size)
Sizes available in 45 mm ($1\frac{3}{4}$ in) × 16 B.W.G. cannula.

CHAS. F. THACKRAY LTD.

Hamilton Bailey Intravenous Cannula
Size available: Adult, child and infant.

Mitchell Self-Sealing Intravenous Needle (Full Size)
Sizes available: 38 mm ($1\frac{1}{2}$ in) × B.W.G. 18 and 19 B.W.G.

Gordh Intravenous Needle (Full size)
Size available: 27 mm ($1\frac{1}{16}$ in) × 20 B.W.G.

Tuony Spinal Analgesia Needle (Full size)
Size available: 83 mm ($3\frac{1}{4}$ in) × 16 G.

Howard Jones Spinal Analgesia Needle (Full size)
Size available: 85 mm ($3\frac{1}{8}$ in) × 19 G.

Pannett Spinal Analgesia Needle (Full size)
Size available: 76 mm (3 in) × 21 G.

Fig. 10.37   Intravenous and spinal needles.

The computation of local anaesthetic solutions, with or without adrenaline, is entirely the anaesthetist's responsibility, although selected strengths may be prepared by the pharmacist before they are required. If the anaesthetic nurse is permitted to prepare injections, she should *always* check the preparation with the anaesthetist, retaining all containers for his inspection.

Following operation, when a local anaesthetic has been administered, great care must to taken to avoid injury to areas which may remain analgesic for several hours. This applies especially to the use of hot-water bottles and electric blankets as a post-operative measure.

The topical application of anaesthetic agents such as cocaine to the eyes and lignocaine, etc., to the mucosa of the mouth, pharynx or respiratory tract, requires special after-care. The eyes must always be covered for several hours, as foreign bodies may impinge upon the cornea without the patient feeling their presence. Even with a minor operation, a patient who has had an application of local anaesthetic to the mucosa of the respiratory tract is not permitted to eat or drink for at least four hours following operation and can cough effectively, as the resultant paralysis of the soft palate and epiglottis would allow foreign matter to enter the trachea. Watch also for possible reactions to the local anaesthetic including convulsions. If there is the slightest doubt or history of previous sensitivity a small test dose should be given first.

Spinal and epidural analgesia

Requirements for spinal analgesia should always be autoclaved before use in a special spinal packet.

Spinal analgesia produced by making a spinal intrathecal injection of a heavy or light solution (in relation to the specific gravity of CSF) of anaesthetic agent such as cinchocaine (Nupercaine), lignocaine (Xylocaine) and bupivacaine (Marcaine). In spinal analgesia the drug mixes with the cerebrospinal fluid and bathes a portion of the spinal cord and nerve roots, thereby rendering part of the body analgesic as well as paralysing the muscles. The extent of its desired action is determined by the anaesthetist and depends upon the volume of solution, the specific gravity of the solution and the position of the patient during and immediately after injection.

Epidural analgesia is produced by the slow injection of a larger volume of local anaesthetic agent into the epidural space between the ligamentum flavum and the dura. A special needle or cannula is used to facilitate the introduction of an indwelling nylon catheter through which the anaesthetic agent is injected.

For injection, the patient may either be sitting up with his legs over the side of the operation table, and head and shoulders bent forwards; or lying on the side with his legs drawn up, the head and shoulders being bent towards his knees.

Storage of equipment

Rubber equipment, e.g., endotracheal tubes deteriorate and soften with time, therefore overstocking should be avoided. Rubber should be stored at temperatures below 21°C. No lubricant based on liquid paraffin should be used; it ruins rubber.

Drugs should also be stored at relatively low temperatures. The reserve stock and those particularly sensitive to heat such as scoline and heparin should be kept in a refrigerator.

The patient

So far we have dealt with the apparatus and drugs necessary for the induction of anaesthesia and we must now consider the patient himself.

A patient comes to the theatre with a certain amount of apprehension, even although he may be the last person to admit this. The manner in which he is treated may seriously affect the induction of anaesthesia and his subsequent recovery. He should be made to think that he is the centre of attention, and that all possible skill is being used for his welfare.

In Chapter 1 we stated that the patient should always be accompanied to the theatre by a ward nurse, and if possible this nurse should remain with him until the induction of anaesthesia is complete. The psychological effect of this is very good, for the patient feels reassured by the presence of a ward nurse who is often the person responsible for his nursing after the operation.

Fig. 10.38 Side transfer trolley system which avoids taking a ward trolley into the sterile areas. (A. C. Daniels & Co. Ltd.)

The nursing process

Unfortunately, often due to staffing difficulties, it is not possible for a ward nurse routinely to accompany her patient into the anaesthetic room. In an effort to obviate the disadvantages created by this situation, some operating departments have instituted what is termed the nursing process.

Over the past twenty-five years, with the ever increasing complexities of theatre nursing, the theatre nurse has almost disappeared behind the barriers of the operating theatre.

Furthermore, theatre nurses are gradually being engulfed with an ever increasing load of machinery and equipment, losing some track of the patient (Shaw, 1977).

The nursing process is an attempt to return more to patient-orientated nursing instead of job-orientated nursing. It is an attempt to ensure that each patient is observed and treated as an individual, rather than a 'case to be carried out second on the list'.

The nursing process is not of course confined to the operating theatre; it is a flexible systematic problem-solving approach to planning all forms of nursing care. Published literature includes reference to its application for the surgical patient and it is a concept which is well established in North America (Coates, 1974; Gruendemann, 1973; Rogers, 1975; Saylor, 1975).

In the operating theatre the nursing process consists of three main parts; a pre-operative visit related to a nursing assessment of the patient; care of the patient during surgery; post-operative nursing evaluation of the patient.

Any pre-operative visit must be planned carefully, for if it is carried out either in the wrong way, or by the wrong person irreparable psychological stress may result. The person visiting should be a qualified nurse and one who is to be directly involved in the care of the patient during surgery. A suitable person might be the anaesthetic nurse or theatre sister participating in the theatre operation list the following day. The nurse must be familiar with the techniques of approaching a pre-operative patient, particularly the psychological responses to be expected. The nurse must have a comprehensive knowledge of surgical procedures, although of course it is assumed that the surgeon has already explained the operation planned. The most important aspect of the visit is to be able to answer questions about pre- and post-operative nursing care. But it does give the opportunity for the theatre staff to introduce themselves, and make the patient aware of those who are to be responsible for his nursing care during surgery.

These objectives are summed up in the paper by Hazel Shaw (Shaw, 1977) as:
1. To collect data
2. to lessen the anxieties that the patient may have towards his operation
3. to improve patient care by knowing the patient and his problems before operation and to enable the theatre staff to anticipate equipment that may be needed for his care
4. to help the patient to understand the procedures and equipment that will be used in his care
5. to improve communication between ward staff, theatre staff and surgeons
6. to involve the theatre nurse more with total patient care and to encourage her to keep up-to-date with new procedures and ideas
7. to re-inforce information that the patient has already been given by ward staff and surgeons (the utmost co-operation is needed here to avoid possible confliction of information)

The second part, relating to care of the patient during surgery, does not alter established procedures. However, the first part of the nursing process should enable theatre staff to give a more efficient service, having a sense of security in knowing that patients are receiving the best possible care.

The final post-operative nursing evaluation should be carried out in a similar manner to the pre-operative visit. The main purpose is to enable the theatre nurse to be aware of continuing total patient care. The opportunity should be taken, if appropriate, to ascertain whether the patient may have any comments which could improve care before the anaesthetic induction period. It enables an evaluation of the pre-operative assessment to be made, and widens the nurses' knowledge of the ward situation.

The introduction of the nursing process requires considerable planning and care to become successful. The aspects described refer only to one approach and the reader is directed to other published literature on the subject. For example, another approach is the anaesthetic clinical nurse consultant, which is a staff post aimed at creating a link between the patient and the operating theatre (Millington, 1976).

Assisting the anaesthetist

Some or all of the duties described to assist the anaesthetist may well be performed by the anaesthetic nurse, theatre technician or ward nurse, whichever is most suitable and convenient.

The patient must be accompanied by X-rays, case notes, signed consent for anaesthetic and operation, pathological reports and drug sheet and any other relevant information which will be of use to the surgeon or the anaesthetist. The ward nurse should know the preparation which the patient has had, the time at which food or drink was last taken, the type and amount of pre-operative drugs administered, and the time at which they were given. She is responsible for seeing that any dentures, artificial eyes etc. have been removed, and must know whether the patient has passed urine or has been catheterised, and the time and amount passed, together with any abnormalities detected in routine ward tests.

It is now common practice to transport the patient to the operating department on his bed. The patient is then transferred to a theatre trolley before entering the sterile zone. Alternatively a transfer trolley top system may be utilised (Fig. 10.38). The patient is anaesthetised on the trolley or may be transferred on the underlying canvas stretcher to the operation table in the anaesthetic room.

A patient must *never* be left alone in the anaesthetic room or theatre for he may be confused following the administration of the pre-operative drugs or sedative, and this may lead to accidental personal injury, such as a fall from the trolley or operation table. Identification of the patient, his correct operation and correct site is of paramount importance. This procedure starts in the ward where some identification of the patient's name and case number must be attached to him before he is transferred to theatre. The house surgeon must mark the operation site with an indelible marker indicating the correct side or digit. This is especially important with the unconscious patient, aged or child. The identification can either be in the form of a bracelet (only removable by cutting if off) or details written on the patient by means of a skin pen.

Fig. 10.39 Method of holding upper arm for an intravenous injection, as an alternative to a tourniquet.

Fig. 10.40 Method of holding wrist for an intravenous injection, as an alternative to a tourniquet.

On arrival at the theatre the patient's identification is checked against the case notes and operation list. If conscious, he is further asked his name. The anaesthetic and operation consent form must also be checked (Murray Wilson, 1971).

The surgeon should see the patient before anaesthesia is induced and confirm it is the correct patient, operation and site. This is of vital importance if a limb or digit is to be amputated.

The patient should always be made as comfortable as possible in transit and whilst waiting. Unless the patient is unconscious with the attendant dangers of an obstructed airway, it is a simple matter to remove excess pillows just before induction is commenced. The nurse should see that the patient is kept as quiet as possible, and should not encourage conversation unless it is obvious that the patient feels more relaxed doing so.

During induction the nurse stands by in case the patient becomes restless, but if he does she must not attempt to wrestle with him but must apply gentle restraint, with one arm across the legs just above the knees, using the other arm to prevent any wild flinging about of the patient's arms. She should not hesitate to ask for further assistance in dealing with the obstreperous patient and wild alcoholics.

For intravenous injection, the selected arm is extended towards the anaesthetist and either a quick-release tourniquet applied to the upper arm, or the nurse constricts the venous return by encircling the upper arm with her hands. The patient clenches his fist to make the veins prominent, and after the anaesthetist has aspirated blood into the syringe which probably indicates that the needle is in a vein, the compression of the upper arm veins is released at the anaesthetist's request. The nurse stands at the head of the trolley or operation table to support the patient's jaw when relaxation is complete. The anaesthetist will then apply pressure over the area of injection, which is continued by the nurse when the inhalation anaesthetic is commenced.

Too many nurses regard the maintenance of a good airway in the unconscious patient as just 'holding' up the jaw. Although this *may* suffice in some cases, the nurses must realise the principles behind any method chosen.

Fig. 10.41 Supporting the jaw of an unconscious patient, method one.

Fig. 10.42 Supporting the jaw of an unconscious patient, method two.

When unconscious, the muscles supporting the lower jaw relax, allowing it to sag. The tongue is also paralysed, allowing it to fall backwards, thereby obstructing the patient's airway.

The basis of keeping an airway clear is supporting the jaw and extending the head.

The nurse should place her fingers behind the angle of the jaw on each side, lifting it slightly forwards. This will pull upon the muscle attachments of the tongue, preventing it from falling backwards and thereby maintaining an unobstructed channel between the mouth and larynx. Alternatively the chin can be lifted forwards in a similar manner (Fig. 10.42), but this latter method is not so efficient, especially if the patient has a receding chin.

An unobstructed airway is indicated by quiet respirations, noisy breathing is usually a sign of obstructed breathing. The position of the head or lower jaw may require adjustment to achieve this object – so the nurse should use her hands, sense of hearing and observe the patient's colour and respiration.

As the patient loses consciousness, following the i.v. injection of a barbiturate and relaxant, especially in emergency situations it is possible for regurgitation of stomach contents to occur before the anaesthetist has inserted the endotracheal tube. The nurse or anaesthetic assistant may be required to perform the Sellick manoeuvre as soon as unconsciousness intervenes.

The Sellick manoeuvre (Sellick, 1961) consists of temporary occlusion of the upper end of the oesophagus by backward pressure of the cricoid cartilage against the bodies of cervical vertebrae. This prevents regurgitation of oesophageal or stomach contents during induction of anaesthesia, and also prevents gastric distension from positive pressure ventilation administered by face mask (or mouth to mouth resuscitation).

Before induction, the cricoid is palpated and lightly held between the thumb and second finger. As anaesthesia begins, moderate pressure is exerted on the cricoid cartilage mainly by the index finger. As soon as unconsciousness intervenes, firm pressure can be applied without obstructing the airway and this is maintained until the endotracheal tube has been inserted and the cuff inflated.

Hearing may become very acute as unconsciousness develops and it is the last sense to be depressed. It is therefore unwise for anyone to speak during the initial stages of anaesthesia. Bandages should not be touched, or covers removed until the patient is completely unconscious.

The anaesthetic nurse or technician will hand instruments, etc., to the anaesthetist as required and like the instrument nurse in theatre, will try to anticipate his requirements.

The anaesthetist has many things to watch during the course of anaesthesia, including the colour of the patient, the pulse, respiration, blood pressure, cardiac activity (sometimes by means of an electro-cardiogram), in addition to keeping the general condition of the patient under observation. He *may* assign certain duties to the anaesthetic nurse or technician in this respect, and may require him or her to keep a record of the patient's pulse, and if sufficiently experienced, blood pressure also. He or she will adjust the rate of flow of transfusions, indicated by the anaesthetist, and replace transfusion solutions under his directions.

Guedal describes four stages of anaesthesia which are demonstrable with ether and cyclopropane. However, with the short-acting barbiturates, the patient falls rapidly asleep and excitement is rarely seen.

The first stage is one of analgesia when peripheral sensation is lost, but the nervous system is under control. In the first stage of induction there are frequently swallowing movements, followed by regular respiration and analgesia.

The second stage is one of excitement, with movement of the limbs followed by tonic spasms of the muscles, dilated pupils and roving eyeballs. Quite often this stage is very short and almost absent, especially when anaesthetising the deeply sedated patient.

The third stage is the stage of surgical anaesthesia which may range from moderate to deep according to the type of operation. During this stage, the anaesthetist is on his guard against:
The fourth stage which is respiratory and cardiac arrest.

If the patient collapses on the operation table with acute cardio-circulatory arrest his recovery may well depend upon prompt action by all the theatre staff. Without treatment, irreversible damage may occur in three minutes and a lasting recovery of the brain, and thus the whole body, is impossible after eight minutes.

As the anaesthetist and anaesthetic nurse have a vital part to play, the catastrophe is being dealt with in this chapter.

The following is an outline of the type of scheme most prevalent today.

CARDIOCIRCULATORY ARREST

If this has occurred immediate steps are taken to restore adequate ventilation and circulation. The anaesthetic nurse will be required to keep a record of the time from the first warning, calling out this time, initially, at 15 second intervals with particular emphasis at each minute.

Fig. 10.43 In external cardiac massage, the heart (C) is compressed between the sternum and the spinal column by depressing the sternum with the hands by about 3–4 cm (by kind permission Roche Products Ltd.).

The anaesthetist, having given warning and noted the time, tilts the operation table head downwards, stops the anaesthetic, ensures that the airway is clear, and administers oxygen under pressure. He may later pass an endotracheal tube if one is not already inserted; time is precious.

At the same time the surgeon commences external cardiac massage. (It is now accepted that circulation can generally be maintained in cardiac arrest without thoracotomy and by rhythmic external manual compression of the sternum which in turn compresses the heart between it and the spine, forcing out blood into the aorta. Relaxation of the thoracic cage releases the pressure on the heart and allows it to fill with blood. This must be done on a rigid surface similar to the operation table, boards under a mattress or on the floor.) The compression on the lower half of the sternum must be by the heels of the hands (not the fingers), one on top of the other, aided by the weight of the body. This pressure should not be exerted on the ribs or epigastrium otherwise fracture of the ribs or rupture of the liver or spleen may occur.

Depression of the sternum should be at least 3 to 4 cm with each stroke, with a frequency of between 70 and 90 strokes per minute. This should produce a palpable radial pulse with a blood pressure of 8 to 13 kPa (60 to 100 mmHg). Rhythmic compression of the sternum, whilst giving good temporary artificial circulation, does not produce effective ventilation. This must be accomplished either by manual compression of the anaesthetic machine bag, or attachment of the endotracheal tube to a ventilator.

If the patient responds, the surgeon may instruct his assistant and the scrub nurse to complete any vital stage in the operation. Alternatively he will hand over cardiac massage to the assistant and complete the operation himself

Immediately cardiac massage has been started, the circulating nurse or anaesthetic nurse fetches the cardiac resuscitation set which comprises various drugs, transfusion fluids and equipment, syringes and needles, electrical defibrillator (external or internal) and if possible an electrocardiograph monitor, which should be connected to the patient.

When ventricular asystole is responsible for the arrest of circulation, external massage may re-establish normal rhythm. If there is no response, intracardiac injections may be tried. The most generally used is adrenaline 1 in 10,000 dosage 3 to 5 ml intracardiac or if a very slow ventricular rate has been established, adrenaline 1 in 10,000, 1 ml per minute intravenously. This is for myocardial stimulation.

Calcium chloride, 10 per cent may be given intracardiac or intravenously in a dosage up to 10 ml, this increases tone in a flabby heart.

These measures may provoke ventricular fibrillation which can then be treated with a D.C. counter shock administered by the defibrillator. A D.C. counter shock may also be tried to provoke ventricular fibrillation (if massage is unsuccessful) which can be treated with a second shock. The shock should be given starting (manual control) at 300 J/2 to 4 millisecond.

If a defibrillator is unavailable, ventricular fibrillation can sometimes be treated by intravenous procaine amide (Pronestyl) 1 g or propranolol (Inderal) 5 mg given slowly.

With cardiac arrest of more than the briefest duration, acidosis, both metabolic and respiratory, is likely. If the period of arrest exceeds 2 minutes or if cardiac massage has been carried out for longer than 15 minutes, the patient should have 200/500 ml of 4·2 per cent sodium bicarbonate intravenously.

The blood pressure should be maintained if necessary by the addition of isoprenaline (Aleudrin) or metaraminol (Aramine) to the intravenous fluid.

If pulmonary oedema is suspected or if the volume of intravenous fluid given has exceeded 1500 ml, a diuretic may be given (e.g., frusemide (Lasix) 20 mg or more intravenously).

If normal consciousness does not return fairly quickly, there may be cerebral oedema (which invariably follows a period of anoxia) which may be treated by intravenous 50 per cent sucrose or Urevert.

Two indications for open thoracotomy and direct cardiac massage are (a) inability to restore a radial pulse and satisfactory blood pressure (e.g., in a stout patient when compression of the sternum is difficult or in chest injuries involving the rib cage) and (b) the absence of a D.C. defibrillator when only an A.C. defibrillator is available for direct application to a fibrillating heart.

General outline of procedure for cardiocirculatory arrest:
1. Arrested heart
2. External massage, controlled pulmonary ventilation
3. No beat; adrenaline given or attempt with D.C. shocks, this causes beat or
4. Fibrillation of the heart

Fig. 10.44 The Daniels Cardiac-arrest Trolley was designed in collaboration with the United Cardiff Hospitals. It embraces all the apparatus, instrumentation and drugs required within a minimum of space. The trolley measures 82 cm × 25 cm × 120 cm (33 in × 10 in × 48 in) high and avoids the use of drawers and cupboards in which items can be so easily disarranged and therefore difficult to find at critical times. Each and every item is labelled and made readily accessible in its allotted position. All electrical apparatus is connected to the mains electricity supply via a Mains Control Unit with one mains cable fitted with a universal plug. The upper section contains drugs, endotracheal tubes, laryngoscopes, needles, syringes, etc., in two compartments one of which is hinged to allow closure of this section when not in use. The lower section contains equipment including, defibrillator, ECG, suction machine, Ambu resuscitator and oxygen cylinder. (A. C. Daniels & Co. Ltd.)

Table 10.1 Contents of cardiac resuscitation trolley.

Top of Trolley:
Airways: Sizes 4–00.
Laryngoscopes: Adult Blade.
       Child Blade.
       Pen Torch.
Tongue Depressor.
Mouth Gag.
Magill's Forceps.
Tongue Forceps.
20 ml Syringe (Unsterile).

Elastoplast 75 cm (3 in).
i.v. Cut down set.
i.v. Fluid (Sod. Bic. 8·4%, Glucose 5%, Mannitol 20%).
Disposable Giving Set.
Intracath.
2 i.v. Needles.
Stethoscope.
Receiver with suction catheters.

(*cont'd.*)

Table 10.1 (cont'd.)

Middle Shelf:
Bronchoscopy Tray (Unsterile).
Tracheotomy Tray (with suture material) (Sterile).
Haemorrhage Arrest Tray (Sterile).

Bottom Shelf:
Defibrillator.
Electrode Jelly.
Suction Unit with Yankauers Sucker.
Rubber Gloves.
Battery Unit.
Cyclator Pump.

Left Side of Trolley:
Extension Lead.
Oxygen Cylinder.
Ambu Resuscitator.

Right Side of Trolley:
Drip Stand.
Oxygen Cylinder.
Cyclator Bracket.

Attached to Back of Trolley:
Cardiac Arrest Board.

Lid of Trolley (With Night Light):
Endotracheal Tubes (8).
Sizes from 9·5 to 5·5 (Sterile item) with connections.
Spencer Wells Artery Forceps.
Book for recording used items.
Sphygmomanometer.
3 Files.
Needles: 4 No. 15.
          4 No. 1.
Syringes: 2 × 1 cm³.
          2 × 5 cm³.
          2 × 2 cm³.
Drug Box (with lid).

Connections (3)
  Ambu Bag to Endotracheal.
  Cyclator to Tracheotomy.
  Cyclator to Endotracheal.
Gauze and Lubricant.
Strapping: 12 mm (0·5 in).
Scissors: Small straight Mayo's.
2 Way Resuscitation Tubes (6)
  Sizes from: 00/000 to 3/4.
Labels.
Biro.
Emergency Drugs.
GORD H. Needle (Sterile).
Sterile Intracardiac Needle.

DRUGS ON TROLLEY

Calcium Chloride	10%	10 ml.
Atropine Sulphate		0·6 mgm.
Suxamethonium (Scoline)		100 mgm.
Nikethamide		2 ml.
Aminophylline		250 mgm.
Digoxin		0·5 mgm.
Adrenaline		1/10·000.
Lorfan		1 mgm.
Prostigmine		2·5 mgm.
Methyl Amphetamine		30 mgm.
Methoxamine		20 mgm.
Hydrocortisone		100 mgm Sol.
Noradrenaline		100 mgm.
Procaine Amide		100 mgm. in 1 cm³.
Procaine Hyd.	10%	20 ml.
Lignocaine	1%	10 ml.
Vandid	5% A.	
Propranolol		5 mgm in 5 ml.
Inj. Isoprenaline		5 mgm.
Inj. Aramine		2 mgm.
Lasix		20 mgm in 2 ml.
Sodium Bicarbonate B.P.		8·4% or 4·2%.

5. D.C. defibrillator applied using large moistened, firmly attached electrodes with a surface area of at least 10 cm and supplying in adults 300 to 400 J D.C. over 2 to 4 milliseconds. All staff take hands off patient to avoid a personal electric shock.

6. Beat recommences

7. Intravenous transfusion of 200/500 ml of 4·2 per cent sodium bicarbonate, plus possibly noradrenaline to maintain blood pressure

8. Endotracheal tube passed at earliest opportunity, artificial ventilation continued until normal respirations recommence

9. If external massage unsuccessful, direct massage via a thoracotomy may be considered. If the chest is opened, antibiotics should be given.

Cardiac-respiratory arrest trolley. It is prudent to assemble together the apparatus and drugs required for the treatment of cardiac-respiratory arrest. This may consist of a simple trolley for use within the operating suite or a more complex unit designed to transport the equipment to other parts of the hospital. In the latter case, in addition to laryngoscopes and endotracheal tubes with their connections, Ambu resuscitator, the trolley should contain, a portable suction device, bronchoscope, defibrillator, ECG monitor and equipment for setting up a transfusion.

The drugs most likely to be needed in the treatment of cardiac arrest are:

Cardiac arrest. Adrenaline (epinephrine) 1 in 10,000 10 ml
   Calcium chloride 10 per cent 10 ml
   Lignocaine (Xylocaine) 1 per cent 10 ml
   Sodium bicarbonate 8·4 per cent i.v. (equivalent to 1 mEq/ml) dosage 100 ml initially after 30 seconds arrest or 4·2 per cent dosage 200 ml initially

Supportive cardiac therapy. Isoprenaline 1 mg diluted to 500 ml with a 5 per cent glucose solution i.v.

Fig. 10.45 Rear view of the cardiac arrest trolley with the upper section closed. The top is covered with red Formica to distinguish it from other trolleys. (A. C. Daniels & Co. Ltd.)

Potassium chloride (1·5 g in 10 ml) diluted to 500 ml with a 5 per cent glucose solution i.v. (20 mEq potassium)

Myocardial failure. Digoxin 0·25 mg per ml i.v.
Ouabain (Strophanthin G) 0·5 mg per ml i.v.
Frusemide (Lasix) 20 mg in 2 ml i.v.

Vasopressors. Methoxamine (Vasoxine) 20 mg per ml (dose 4 mg i.v.)
Methylamphetamine 30 mg in 1·5 ml (dose 5 mg i.v.)

Cerebral dehydration and diuresis. Mannitol solution 20 per cent (dose 1 to 200 ml)
Urevert or 50 per cent sucrose

Respiratory complications
Adrenaline 30 ml per ml
Aminophylline 250 mg per 10 ml i.v.
Nikethamide 25 per cent 5 ml i.v.
Nalorphine (Lethidrone) 10 mg per ml i.v.
Levallorphan (Lorfan) 5 mg per 5 ml (dose 1 mg) i.v.
Hydrocortisone 100 mg i.v.

When the operation is completed the anaesthetist will give instructions to the nurse accompanying the patient back to the ward. Under no circumstances must the patient leave the theatre suite until the anaesthetist is satisfied that he is fit to do so.

A good airway must be maintained in the manner described earlier but if there is any doubt regarding this or the possibility that the patient may vomit, he should be placed on his side with the underlying limb flexed, and the shoulders supported.

The patient is transferred carefully to the trolley or bed with minimal movement, and covered with blankets before leaving the theatre suite. After returning him to his bed, if it is necessary to roll him to recover a stretcher, this must be done very gently, not only to avoid injury to the operation area, but a sudden rapid movement of the unconscious patient can cause cardiac arrest.

A tray containing mouth gag, tongue forceps, boxwood wedge, small towel, and vomit bowl or kidney dish should be carried with the patient during transit between the theatre and recovery ward. These instruments must remain by the bed until the patient has recovered consciousness.

An airway or endotracheal tube left in position by the anaesthetist post-operatively should not be removed until the patient attempts to reject it. Attempts at rejection by the patient reveal that his swallowing reflex has returned and that unless there is any clinical contra-indication, the tube may be removed.

If oxygen has to be administered post-operatively to an unconscious patient, it should be given by means of a suitable catheter, mask or oxygen tent. If an endotracheal tube is *in situ*, oxygen may be given via a catheter passed into the lumen of the tube for a few inches. The oxygen flow in this latter case should not be above 3 litres per minute. The recovery of a patient in the recovery ward may be prolonged depending on the anaesthetic used. The awakening from natural sleep is generally quite different to the patient's experience in recovering from anaesthesia (Asbury, 1974). For further information on recovery nursing the reader is referred to a textbook devoted to this subject (Norris and Campbell, 1974, Buxton Hopkin, 1970).

REFERENCES

ASBURY, A. J. (1974) *Nursing Times*, January 24, 106.
BUXTON HOPKIN, D. A. (1970) *Anaesthesia, Recovery and Intensive Care.* London: English University Press.
COATES, L. (1974) *AORN Journal*, **19**, 1091–1104.
DEPARTMENT OF HEALTH AND SOCIAL SECURITY (1976) Pollution of operating departments by anaesthetic gases, HC 76/38.

GRUENDEMANN, B. J. (1973) *The Surgical Patient: Behavioural Concepts for the O.R. Nurse.* St. Louis: Mosby.
HAID, B. AND HOSSLI, G. (1956) *Cardiac and Respiratory Arrest.* Roche Products Ltd.
JUDD, P. A., TOMLIN, P. J., WHITBY, J. L., INGLIS, T. C. M. AND ROBINSON, J. S. (1968) *Lancet,* **ii**, 1019.
LIGHT, S. (1979) *Nursing Mirror,* January 11, 20.
LUMLEY, J. (1976) *British Journal of Anaesthesia,* **48**, 3.
MACKENSIE, C. F., KLOSE, S. AND BROWNE, D. R. G. (1976) *British Journal of Anaesthesia,* **48**, 105.
MILLINGTON, C. (1976) *Natnews,* **13**, 18–22.
MURRAY WILSON, A. (1971) *Nursing Times,* November 11, 1406.
NORRIS, W. AND CAMPBELL, D. (1974) *Anaesthetics, Resuscitation and Intensive Care.* Edinburgh: Churchill Livingstone.
NORTH-WEST THAMES REGIONAL HEALTH AUTHORITY (1980) Personal communication.
ROGERS, P. M. (1975) *AORN Journal,* **21**, 1278–1288.
SAYLOR, D. R. (1975) *AORN Journal,* **22**, 624–636.
SELLICK, B. A. (1961) *Lancet,* **ii**, 494–496.
SHAW, H. (1977) The Nursing Process, the Operating Theatre and Patient. Unpublished paper; Theatre Nursing Education and Research Fellowship Fund.
SPENCE, A. A. AND KNILL-JONES, R. P. (1978) *British Journal of Anaesthesia,* **50**, 713.
STEVENS, H. R. (1969) *Lancet,* **i**, 732.
SYKES, M. K. (1946) *British Medical Journal,* **i**, 561.

11
GLOSSARY OF TECHNICAL TERMS AND WORDS COMMONLY USED IN THE THEATRE

Some of the technical terms used in the theatre often appear very complicated, and may be rather difficult to understand at first. It is for this reason that the glossary has been placed before the chapters dealing with specific operations.

Definitions of some of the more common suffixes and roots may help the nurse to understand the descriptions of various operation instrument sets.

SUFFIXES

—desis: a fusion operation, e.g., arthrodesis or fusion of a joint.
—ectomy: describes the removal or excision of a structure, e.g., gastrectomy, or excision of the stomach.
—graphy: representing, recording or describing, e.g., ventriculography.
—otomy: refers to incising or dividing a structure, e.g., laparotomy, making an opening into the abdomen; or tenotomy, dividing a tendon.
—ostomy: making an artificial opening between one organ and another, or one organ and the surface of the body, e.g., gastroenterostomy, an opening between the stomach and small intestine; gastrostomy, an opening between the stomach and the surface of the abdomen, usually for the purpose of feeding.
—orrhaphy: a repair operation, e.g., herniorrhaphy, repair of a hernia; perineorrhaphy, repair of the perineum.
—oscopy: inspection of the interior of a duct, cavity or organ by means of an endoscopic instrument. These instruments usually incorporate their own illumination in the form of a minute electric lamp (or bundle of optic fibres which transmit light to the area being examined) and often having magnifying viewing attachments, e.g., the cystoscope, for examining the bladder; the sigmoidoscope, for examining the sigmoid flexure of the colon.
—pexy: suturing or fixing in place, e.g., nephropexy, suturing a 'wandering' kidney to the posterior abdominal wall.
—plasty: is used to describe a plastic operation for the repair of tissues or organs which have been damaged by injury or disease, e.g., rhinoplasty, the rotation of a skin flap from the forehead and scalp, to cover a defect of the nose; arthroplasty, an operation on a joint to increase mobility.

ROOTS

Adeno:	gland, e.g., Adenoma
Angio:	vessel, e.g., Angiography
Arthro:	joint, e.g., Arthroplasty
Broncho:	bronchus, e.g., Bronchoscopy

Cardio:	heart, e.g., Cardiotomy
Cholecyst:	gall bladder, e.g., Cholecystectomy
Col:	colon, e.g., Colectomy
Colpo:	vagina, e.g., Colporrhaphy
Cranio:	skull, e.g., Cranioplasty
Cysto:	sac containing fluid, e.g., Cystectomy
Gastro:	stomach, e.g., Gastrectomy
Herni:	abnormal aperture, e.g., Herniorrhaphy
Hyster:	uterus, e.g. Hysterectomy
Laryn:	larynx, e.g., Laryngoscopy
Mast:	breast, e.g., Mastectomy
Nephr:	kidney, e.g., Nephrectomy
Oöphor:	ovary, e.g., Oöphorectomy
Orchid:	testis, e.g., Orchidectomy
Osteo:	bone, e.g., Osteotomy
Pharyng:	throat, e.g., Pharyngotomy
Pneum:	lung, e.g., Pneumonectomy
Prostate:	prostate, e.g., Prostatectomy
Pyel:	kidney or pelvis, e.g., Pyelolithotomy
Rhino:	nose, e.g., Rhinoplasty
Thoraco:	chest, e.g., Thoracotomy
Ureter:	ureter, e.g., Ureterolithotomy
Vulv:	vulva, e.g., Vulvectomy

Adenoidectomy: Removal of adenoid tissue from the naso-pharynx.

Adrenalectomy: Excision of an adrenal gland for tumour, treatment of hypertension or relief of pain in malignant conditions e.g., carcinoma of breast.

Advancement: An operation to correct squint, also known as strabismus operation.

Albee's operation: *Hip* – arthrodesis effected by removing the upper surface of the femur and corresponding edge of acetabulum; *Spine* – arthrodesis effected by splitting spinous processes and inserting a bone graft obtained from the tibia.

Anastomosis: The establishment of an intercommunication between two hollow organs, blood vessels or nerves.

Angiography: Serial X-ray examination of the cerebral vascular tree following injection of radio-opaque medium into a neck artery.

Antrostomy: Making an opening into the maxillary antrum to provide external drainage. The Caldwell Luc operation is an extensive form of antrostomy.

Appendectomy: Removal of the appendix.

Arteriectomy: Excision of an artery or part of an artery.

Arteriorrhaphy: Suturing an artery.

Arteriotomy: Incision of an artery.

Arthrectomy: Excision of a joint.

Arthrodesis: An operation to permanently stiffen a joint and performed to prevent movement by obliterating the joint.

Arthrography: X-ray examination of a joint, often after the injection of a radio-opaque substance.

Arthroplasty: An operation to effect increased movement of a joint. The operation usually consists of replacing the joint surface or surfaces with a metallic or plastic prosthesis.

Arthroscopy: Examination of the interior of a joint by means of an arthroscope.

Arthrotomy: Incising a joint for the purpose of examination or subsequent drainage.

Bankhart's operation: For recurrent dislocation of the shoulder – repair of the glenoid rim defect supplemented by plication of the joint capsule and subscapularis muscle.

Bilroth's operation: A partial gastrectomy with either 1. anastomosis of the remaining section of the stomach to the duodenum or 2. closure of the lines of section followed by gastrojejunostomy.

Biopsy: Excision of small piece of tissue for examination.

Blalock's operation: Performed usually for Fallot's tetralogy – anastomosis of the pulmonary artery (distal to a pulmonary stenosis) to a branch of the aorta.

Bronchoscopy: Examination of the interior of the bronchial tree by means of a bronchoscope. Certain operative manipulations are possible through the instrument, including removal of a foreign body or section of a growth for pathological investigation.

Caesarean section: Removal of a foetus at or near term through an abdominal incision.

Capsulectomy: Excision of a capsule – generally a joint, lens or kidney.

Capsulotomy: Incision of a capsule e.g., that surrounding the lens of the eye.

Caudal block: see epidural.

Cervicectomy: Amputation of the uterine cervix.

Cholecystectomy: Excision of the gall-bladder.

Cholecystenterostomy: Constructing an opening between the gall-bladder and the small intestine for the drainage of bile. This is performed when there is an obstruction of the common bile duct as may occur by pressure due to a growth, e.g., carcinoma of the head of pancreas.

Cholecystotomy: Making an opening into the gall-bladder, generally for the removal of gall-stones.

Choledochotomy: Making an opening into the common bile duct generally for the removal of stones.

Chordotomy: The division of nerve tracts within the spinal cord.

Circumcision: Excision of the prepuce or foreskin.

Coccygectomy: Excision of the coccyx.

Colpotomy: Incision of the vaginal wall, usually performed to drain an abscess in the pouch of Douglas through the vagina.

Colectomy: Excision of a portion of whole of the colon.

Colostomy and Caecostomy: These are terms used when making a fistula or an opening between the colon or caecum and the surface of the abdomen, to act as a temporary or permanent anus for the discharge of faeces. The most common sites for a colostomy are at the level of the transverse or pelvic colon.

Colporrhaphy: A repair operation of the vaginal wall in the treatment of pelvic prolapse. Prolapse of the uterus and stretching of the anterior vaginal wall may cause the bladder and urethra to bulge into the vaginal canal, creating the condition known as cystocele. Similarly, a posterior prolapse, with stretching of the posterior vaginal wall, allows prolapse of the rectum, forming a rectocele. A cystocele is treated by the operation of anterior colporrhaphy, and a rectocele by posterior colporrhaphy. Both these operations are often combined with perineorrhaphy.

Commissurotomy: Splitting a stenosed valve, e.g., mitral or aortic.

Corneoplasty: Excision of opaque corneal tissue and replacement with a healthy, transparent, human donor cornea (Keratoplasty).

Craniectomy denotes removal of bone from skull vault, e.g., osteoplastic flap.

Cranioplasty: A plastic operation on the skull.

Craniotomy: This is a term used when opening the cavity of the skull, e.g., in the treatment of cranial injuries such as depressed fractures: for the removal of an intracranial tumour; for the drainage of an abscess.

Cryosurgery: Using the effect of freezing on tissue in surgery.
Culdoscopy: Examining the uterus by passing a culdoscope through the posterior vaginal fornix behind the uterus to enter the peritoneal cavity.
Curettage: The removal of tissue by means of a curette, or spoon, using a scraping action. The most frequent curettage is that of the interior of the uterus and the removal of overgrown lymphatic tissue in the nasopharynx (adenoids).
Cyclotomy: An incision through the ciliary body as a drainage operation for the relief of glaucoma.
Cystectomy: Excision of the urinary bladder, most commonly for a malignant tumour.
Cystodiathermy: The application of a diathermy current to the walls of the urinary bladder via a cystoscope or by open operation.
Cystoscopy: Inspection of the interior of the bladder by means of an examining cystoscope. An operating cystoscope may be used for catheterising the ureters, cauterising papillomata, and obtaining a biopsy of bladder or tumour tissue. A resectoscope is used for resecting part of the prostate via the urethra.
Cystostomy: Temporary or permanent suprapubic drainage of the bladder.
Dacryocystectomy: Excision of part or all of the lacrymal sac.
Dacryocystorhinostomy: Performed for obstruction of the naso-lacrymal duct to establish drainage from the lacrymal sac to the nose.
Debridement: Thorough cleansing of a wound, removal of foreign matter, and damaged or infected tissue.
Decortication: Excision of the cortex or outer layer of an organ e.g., visceral pleura of the lung.
Diathermy: A high-frequency electric current in the form of electromagnetic waves. These waves are concentrated at the point of the surgeon's electrode, producing great heat which is utilised to coagulate the tissues (e.g., sealing blood-vessels). When the frequency of the current is increased, the diathermy electrode may be used like a knife to divide the tissues, giving minimal coagulation.
Disobliteration: Endarterectomy – removal of intimal plaques which are blocking an artery – rebore.
Dissect: To cut or separate tissues.
Ectopic Gestation: The implantation and development of a fertilised ovum outside the uterus, most frequently in a Fallopian tube. Rupture of the ectopic gestation causes severe bleeding and shock, requiring urgent surgical intervention.
Embolectomy: An operation for the removal of an embolus, usually a blood-clot, from an artery.
Encephalography: X-ray examination of the ventricular system and subarachnoid spaces surrounding the brain by fractional replacement of cerebrospinal fluid with filtered air. (See also ventriculography.)
Endarterectomy: See disobliteration.
Endoscopy: Inspection of any body cavity by means of a scope.
Enterostomy: The establishment of an intestinal fistula.
Enucleation: Removal of the eye is described under this heading. The term means also the removal of a tumour as a whole, compared to its removal in sections (eviscerate or gut).
Epididymectomy: Excision of the epididymis, which is a series of tubules lying behind the testis, and continuous with the vas deferens.
Epidural block: Injection of local anaesthetic, usually into the lumbar or caudal region before surgery or for prolonged analgesia.
Episiotomy: Involves the incision of the perineum during labour, to prevent excessive laceration.

Excision: Cutting away or taking out.

Fasciotomy: Incision of fascia.

Fenestration: Establishment of a fenestra or window in the horizontal semicircular canal to re-establish sound conduction to the inner ear of a suitable patient suffering from otosclerosis.

Fothergill's operation: Colpoperinorrhaphy including amputation of the cervix – i.e. repair of a cystocele and rectocele – see also Manchester repair.

Fulguration: Destruction of tissue by diathermy.

Gallie's operation: Radical repair of a hernia using fascia lata strips taken from the lateral aspect of the thigh.

Ganglionectomy: Excision of a ganglion.

Gastrectomy: Excision of the stomach. The most usual operation is partial gastrectomy in the surgical treatment of gastric or duodenal ulcers. Total gastrectomy, although nowadays a relatively rare operation, is generally reserved for malignant conditions.

Gastroenterostomy: Making an opening between the stomach and small intestine, usually the jujunum, for the purpose of short circuiting the stomach contents, which normally pass through the pylorus into the duodenum.

Gastroscopy: Inspection of the stomach cavity via the oesophagus, or via a gastrostomy, using a gastroscope.

Gastrostomy: Making an artificial opening between the stomach and the abdominal surface for the purpose of feeding. This is generally done for the patient having an oesophageal stricture which cannot be relieved by dilation with bougies.

Gastrotomy: Opening the stomach for the purpose of exploration, or the removal of a foreign body.

Gilliam's operation: Shortening of the round ligament to correct retroversion of the uterus. See also hysteropexy, ventrosuspension.

Girdlestones operation: The original procedure is described as removal of part of the acetabulum and the femoral head and neck with a muscle mass stitched between the bone ends. Nowadays removal of part of the femoral head and neck only is often called Girdlestones.

Glossectomy: Excision of the tongue.

Haemorrhoidectomy: The ligation and excision of internal piles.

Harris' operation: A transvesical, suprapubic prostatectomy.

Hemicolectomy: Excision of approximately half of the colon.

Hepatectomy: Excision of part of the liver.

Herniorrhaphy: The repair of an abnormal aperture in the walls of a cavity which has allowed the protrusion of a viscus. An example of this is the direct inguinal herniorrhaphy in which a sac containing viscera protruding from the abdomen through Hesselbach's triangle is obliterated.

Herniotomy: A simple operation for hernia, with return of hernia contents to their normal position and ligation of the sac.

Hymenectomy: Excision or trimming of an imperforate or rigid hymen.

Hypophysectomy: Excision of the pituitary gland.

Hysterectomy: Removal of the uterus via the abdomen or vagina. A subtotal hysterectomy means the removal of the body of the uterus, but leaving the cervix: total hysterectomy implies excision of the entire uterus: pan-hysterectomy generally means the excision of the uterus, Fallopian tubes and ovaries also: radical hysterectomy describes removal of the uterus, appendages, upper part of the vagina and adjacent connective tissue. This latter operation is known also as Wertheim's operation.

Hysteropexy: A plastic operation on the uterus performed in the treatment of a retroverted uterus. See also ventrosuspension.

Hysterotomy: Opening into the uterus usually for the removal of a foetus a good period before term.

Iridectomy: Removal of a section of the iris of the eye, thus forming an artificial pupil. This is performed as a preliminary to cataract extraction and in the relief of tension in glaucoma.

Ileocolostomy: A fistula or opening made between the ileum and colon to by-pass an obstruction or inflammation.

Ileocystoplasty: A plastic operation, utilising a section of isolated ileum to increase the urinary bladder.

Ileostomy: A fistula or opening made between the ileum and the surface of the abdomen.

Ileoureterostomy: Transplantation of the lower ends of the ureters into an artificial bladder formed from an isolated loop of ileum which is made to open on to the surface of the abdomen.

Jejunostomy: Making an opening into the jejunum.

Keller's operation: For hallux valgus or rigidus – excision of the proximal half of the proximal phalanx, also exostosis of the metatarsal head.

Keratectomy: Excision of a portion of the cornea.

Keratoplasty: see corneoplasty.

Laminectomy: Cutting through and removal of the spinal laminae as a preliminary of approach to the spinal cord or intervertebral discs.

Laparotomy: Opening the abdominal cavity for the purpose of inspection of, or operation upon the organs within. An emergency laparotomy is performed for many conditions which come under the heading 'acute abdomen'. When an accurate diagnosis is uncertain this may reveal acute appendicitis, perforated ulcers of the stomach or bowel, intestinal obstruction, e.g., malignant growth, strangulated hernia, etc.

Laryngectomy: Excision of the larynx.

Laryngofissure: Splitting the thyroid cartilage of the larynx to expose the vocal cords.

Laryngoscopy: Inspection of the interior of the larynx, either by means of an illuminated laryngoscope (direct laryngoscopy), or by a mirror and reflected light (indirect laryngoscopy). The anaesthetist uses a laryngoscope to inspect the entrance to the larynx and to assist in the insertion of an endotracheal tube into the trachea by direct vision.

Laryngotomy: Opening the larynx to introduce a tube for the purpose of aiding respiration. This operation should more correctly be termed laryngostomy, meaning a temporary or permanent opening into the larynx. Like tracheostomy, this operation is often performed in cases of extreme urgency when the glottis is blocked.

Leucotomy: An operation in the frontal area of the brain for division of some white nerve fibres. Performed for relief of certain mental conditions associated with extreme anxiety or emotional stress.

Lithotomy: Incision for removal of a stone or calculus.

Lithotrity or **Litholapaxy:** The crushing and removal of a calculus or stone lying in the bladder by using a lithotrite passed per urethra.

Lobectomy: Excision of one lobe of the lung.

Lymphadenectomy: Excision of a lymph node or nodes.

Manchester repair: Colpoperinorrhaphy including amputation and reconstruction of the cervix. See also Fothergill's operation.

Mastectomy: Removal of the breast. This operation is performed for carcinoma of the breast and is generally combined with some form of radiotherapy. A more extensive operation called radical mastectomy involves excision of the breast, together with the underlying pectoral muscles and adjacent lymph glands.

Mastoidectomy: The removal of diseased mastoid air cells as a result of mastoiditis.
Meniscectomy: Removal of a torn semilunar cartilage usually from the knee joint.
Myomectomy: Removal of a fibroid from the uterus.
Myringotomy: Incision of the tympanic membrane of the ear to allow drainage of the middle ear.
Nephrectomy: Removal of a kidney.
Nephropexy: A plastic operation to secure a 'wandering kidney' to the posterior abdominal wall.
Nephrostomy: Making an opening between the pelvis of the kidney and the abdominal surface for the purpose of drainage. It is usual to employ a self-retaining catheter, such as the De Pezzer type, which may be connected to a suitable receptacle.
Nephrotomy: Incising the kidney, usually for the removal of a renal calculus. The operation is then called nephrolithotomy.
Neurectomy: Excision of a part of a nerve.
Neuroplasty: Surgical repair of nerves.
Neurorrhaphy: Anastomosis of the two ends of a divided nerve.
Neurotomy: Incision into a nerve.
Oesophagectomy: Excision of the oesophagus, generally for a malignant condition.
Oesophagoscopy: Inspection of the interior of the oesophagus by means of an illuminated oesophagoscope. Biopsy of a tumour or the removal of an impacted foreign body may also be carried out.
Oöphorectomy: Excision of one or both ovaries.
Oöphorosalpingectomy: Excision of an ovary and its associated Fallopian tube.
Orchidectomy: Removal of the testis.
Osteoplasty: Any plastic operation on a bone.
Osteotomy: Division of a bone. Normally an osteotome is used for this purpose and the instrument has two bevelled edges as opposed to a chisel which has only one bevelled edge, the other being straight. The operation is generally performed to correct bone deformity, or as a part of an arthroplastic procedure.
Pallidotomy: Division of nerve fibres from the cerebral cortex to the corpus striatum to relieve Parkinson tremor.
Pancreatectomy: or radical excision of the pancreatic head: Excision of the head of pancreas, duodenum, part of the jejunum, stomach, lower half of the common bile duct and part of the pancreatic duct.
Paul-Mikulicz operation: After excising a section of the colon, the two cut ends of the bowel are kept exposed outside the peritoneal cavity on the abdominal surface. After a period these cut ends are anastomosed without the peritoneal cavity being opened.
Pericardectomy: Excision of a thickened pericardium of the heart.
Parathyroidectomy: Excision of one or more parathyroid glands.
Parotidectomy: Excision of the parotid salivary gland.
Patellectomy: Excision of the patella.
Perineorrhaphy: This is the repair carried out when the pelvic floor has become weakened, allowing the uterus to prolapse.
Pharyngolaryngectomy: Excision of the pharynx and larynx.
Pharyngotomy: Opening the pharynx as a preliminary to removing a malignant growth of the upper part of the oesophagus.
Phlebectomy: Excision of a vein or part of.
Phlebotomy: Incision into a vein.
Phrenic Avulsion: In order to produce paralysis of one dome of the diaphragm and collapse of the lower part of the lung on that side, the fibres of the phrenic nerve are torn

from their attachment. Another operation is crushing of the phrenic nerve to produce a temporary effect.

Pneumonectomy: Excision of one lung in the treatment of malignant conditions and tuberculosis, etc.

Pneumothorax (Artificial): Air in the pleural space. The air is introduced into the pleura via a hollow needle and using the pneumothorax apparatus.

Proctoscopy: Examination of the rectum and anal canal, using a proctoscope.

Prostatectomy: Removal of the prostate gland either suprapubically, retropubically, transurethrally or by the perineal route.

Pyelography (Retrograde): The injection of a radio-opaque substance into the pelvis of the kidney via the ureteric catheter. Subsequent radiological examination reveals the outline of the renal pelvis on the X-ray plate.

Pyelolithotomy: Removal of a stone from the kidney pelvis.

Pyloro-myotomy: In the treatment of congenital pyloric stenosis in infants, the muscular coat of the pyloric section of the stomach is incised down to the level of the mucosa to provide relief. This is known as Ramstedt's operation.

Pyloroplasty: A plastic operation on the pylorus to widen the orifice.

Radium or Radiotherapy:

Atomic or Nuclear Reactor: A machine for producing radioactive isotopes, such as radioactive iodine and cobalt.

Cobalt: A radioactive isotope, which has a half-life of 5·3 years and decays eventually into nickel.

Disintegration or Decay: This is a spontaneous process in which the radioactive material emits an alpha, beta or gamma ray.

Half-Life: Radioactive material is made up of a large number of radioactive nuclei. As these disintegrate during the decay of the material and give off alpha, beta or gamma rays, the total number of nuclei in the material diminishes, and consequently the activity of the isotope gradually becomes weaker. The half-life is defined as 'the amount of time which is required for one half of a large number of identical nuclei (making up the isotope) to disintegrate'. For example, in the case of radium which has a half-life of roughly 1,700 years; in 1,700 years the radium contains half as many radioactive nuclei than when it was formed, and in 3,400 years this figure will be approximately one quarter of the original number of nuclei.

Radiation: The diffusion of rays from a point (in this case gamma rays which cause biological damage to the tissues). Malignant tumours are often more susceptible to radiation than normal tissue but over-exposure to these rays may cause normal tissue to become damaged and produce diseases such as leukaemia (where the white cells of the body are over-produced).

Radium: A radioactive isotope, with a half-life of about 1,700 years.

X-ray: A penetrating electromagnetic radiation which is generated by bombarding a metal target (in the X-ray tube) with energetic electrons. X-rays and gamma rays for practical purposes may really be regarded as the same thing.

Ramstedt's Operation: See pyloro-myotomy.

Rectosigmoidectomy: Excision of the rectum and sigmoid colon.

Rhinoplasty: A plastic operation on the nose for reformation due to injury or cosmetic reasons.

Salpingectomy: Excision of a Fallopian tube.

Salpingo-oöphorectomy: Excision of a Fallopian tube and ovary.

Shelf operation: Open reduction of congenital dislocation of hip.

Sigmoidoscopy: Inspection of the rectum or sigmoid flexure of the colon, using an illuminated endoscope passed per anum.

Skeletal Traction: The insertion of a pin or wire through a bone for the purpose of traction. A Steinmann pin and Kirschner wire are the two most commonly used, and these may be inserted into the fractured bone itself, or a bone below the fracture forming part of an appendage to it. The most usual sites are the tibial tubercle for fractures of the femoral shaft and the lower tibia for fractures of the tibial shaft.

Splenectomy: Removal of the spleen. The most common condition requiring its removal is traumatic rupture, although certain diseases involving enlargement of the organ may require surgery also.

Stapedectomy: Excision of stapes for otosclerosis and insertion of Teflon piston, vein graft or plug of fat.

Stereotactic Surgery: Deep ablative surgery of the white matter, basal ganglia or brain stem projection fibres by electro-coagulation or cryo-probe.

Sympathectomy: Partial excision of sympathetic nerve.

Synovectomy: Excision of a joint synovial membrane often in rheumatoid conditions.

Tarsorrhaphy: Suturing the eyelids together as a temporary measure in certain conditions, e.g., fifth cranial nerve damage.

Tenoplasty: A plastic operation on a tendon.

Tenorrhaphy: Anastomosis of the two ends of a cut tendon.

Tenotomy: Division of a tendon.

Thoracoplasty: Removal of several ribs on one side to produce collapse of the underlying lung.

Thoracotomy: Opening the chest cavity, e.g., as a preliminary to heart surgery.

Thoracoscopy: Inspection of the pleural space, using a thoracoscope passed through a small incision in the chest wall.

Thromboendarterectomy: Removal or a thrombus from an artery followed by re-boring.

Thymectomy: Excision of the thymus.

Thyroidectomy: Removal of approximately seven-eighths of each lobe of the thyroid gland leaving the parathyroid glands intact.

Tonsillectomy: Excision of the tonsils.

Trachelorrhaphy: Repair of a lacerated uterine cervix.

Tracheostomy: Often incorrectly termed tracheotomy, is an operation for the insertion of a tube into the trachea as an aid to respiration. Generally, the trachea is opened at the level of the thyroid isthmus, but in emergency the opening may be made through the upper rings of the trachea. This latter operation is called a 'high tracheostomy', and may be performed rapidly, as the tracheal rings are close to the skin.

Trendelenburg's Operation: Usually refers to ligation of internal saphenous vein in varicosed leg veins, also an operation describing pulmonary embolectomy.

Trephine Operation: This term is applied to the removal of a disc of tissue. Trephining of the skull, in the true sense of the word, involves the removal of a disc of bone, although today craniotomies are usually performed by drilling a hole with suitable perforators and burrs. The resultant pulverised bone may be returned to the hole after operation but this is not always considered necessary.

Removal of a small disc of the sclerotic coat of the eye in the treatment of chronic glaucoma is also called trephining.

Turbinectomy: Removal of the turbinate bones.

Ureterectomy: Excision of a ureter.

Ureterocolostomy: Transplantation of the ureters into the colon.

Ureteroileostomy: See ileoureterostomy.

Ureterolithotomy: This describes the operation for opening the ureter to remove a calculus.

Urethrotomy: A rather uncommon operation now for incising the urethra in the treatment of strictures. Internal urethrotomy is performed with a guarded knife passed into the urethra. External urethrotomy involves opening the urethra through an incision made in the perineum.

Vagotomy: Division of the vagus nerves often in conjunction with gastro-enterostomy in the treatment of peptic ulcer or pyloroplasty.

Valvotomy: Incision of a valve generally in the heart or major blood vessels.

Vasectomy: Excision of a section of the vas deferens.

Ventriculo-atrial or **ventriculo-peritoneal shunt:** The establishment of artificial CSF drainage to heart or peritoneal cavity in cases of primary or secondary hydrocephalus (Pudenz or Spitzholter valve).

Ventriculo-cysternostomy: The establishment of artificial drainage between the ventricles and cysterna magna. (Torkildsen operation.)

Ventriculography: This is radiography of the cerebral ventricles accomplished by removing cerebrospinal fluid and replacing it with a small quantity of air, using hollow ventricular needles. Trephine holes are made in the skull and the ventricular needles passed into the ventricles (see also encephalography).

Ventro-suspension: A plastic operation on the uterus for shortening the round ligaments which run forward to the inguinal canal, thereby suspending the uterus in the anteverted position. This operation is known also as hysteropexy.

Vulvectomy: Excision of the vulva.

Wertheim's hysterectomy: For carcinoma of the cervix – extensive excision involving the uterus, upper vagina, Fallopian tubes, ovaries and regional lymph glands.

INSTRUMENTS FOR PARTICULAR OPERATIONS

There are two methods of instrument selection: (*a*) enough instruments are prepared for a particular operation; (*b*) basic instrument sets are used and specialised instruments are added to these as required.

In this book method (*a*) is used only for highly specialised or very minor procedures. Method (*b*) is used extensively, for it ensures that the instruments to which the surgeon is accustomed are always at hand and is a method which is suited to the pre-set tray system of sterilisation. Also, by arranging the instruments in groups, the teaching of nurses and technicians is simplified.

Except in minor procedures, the general set, or when only a few instruments are needed, the more common instruments are not illustrated. This is to allow greater prominence to the special instruments described.

12
OPERATING MICROSCOPES

During the last 15 years or so, binocular operating microscopes have become indispensable equipment for many surgeons. A great number of new surgical interventions that were previously impracticable have evolved from the continued application of microsurgical techniques.

Microsurgery in its present form, is thought to have started with Dr. Karl Nylen of the University of Stockholm in 1922, when he used for the first time a low power monocular operating microscope for ear surgery. He then took a Zeiss Slit Lamp, added a light source and suitable support for its stereoscopic microscope, and thereby created the first true operating microscope.

In spite of this success, binocular loupes and loupes mounted to spectacle frames predominated over the use of compound microscopes for three decades until in 1953, when the first complete operating microscope designed primarily for ear surgery was introduced by Carl Zeiss in West Germany.

The introduction of this new microscope led the way for microsurgery to extend into other disciplines such as ophthalmology, neurosurgery and plastic reconstructive surgery, until the present day when the operating microscope has been adopted by the majority of surgical disciplines.

Basic principles

The operating microscope achieves two purposes. The first is to provide a magnified image of small objects, and the second is to provide a magnified view of larger areas on which more precise surgery can be performed (Fig. 12.1).

The operating microscope consists of a stereo microscope, which in principle is two monocular instruments placed side by side. Each of the monocular systems provides a slightly different angular view of the object, thereby providing a three-dimensional image. This three-dimensional image is essential for providing depth perception, so that the surgeon may place his instruments and sutures accurately on the required spot.

The microscope body most commonly used for microsurgery consists of four basic components. These are (1) binocular tube, which contains the eyepieces, attached to (2) the main body of the instrument which incorporates (3) optics for varying the magnification, and screwed in to this on the lower part, (4) is an objective or lens, which can be interchanged to give various distances between it and the operative area. In addition to this viewing unit, an illuminaton system is attached. This allows light from a suitable source to be fed via the microscope body through the objective and on to the operating area.

The whole of this viewing and illumination system is attached to a fine focusing slide, and then fitted to a stand by means of couplings which may vary according to the type of surgery being performed. The stand is commonly a column of 2 m height fixed to a tripod base, to which are attached castors for manoeuvrability. Although this floor stand is

Fig. 12.1 Diagrammatic representation of an operating microscope head. (Zeiss, W. Germany.)

in common use, the most convenient and modern form of supporting the microscope is on a ceiling suspension unit.

In addition to the basic microscope set-up, it is usual to attach accessories for enabling assistants and theatre staff to observe through the microscope. It is also possible to attach still, ciné and television cameras to enable the proceedings to be recorded, and in the case of closed circuit television, relayed to a remote position for teaching purposes.

The use of microscopes

The wide range of operating microscope parts and accessories available for use in microsurgery, may be used in a large number of permutations and combinations. It is not feasible to attempt a description of their use and function in detail within the limited confines of this chapter. It is therefore recommended that full use is made of available material such as manufacturer's instruction and assembly booklets. In addition, information is generally readily available from the specialist technical representatives from the various companies.

Although some surgical specialities, particularly ENT, have been using operating microscopes for many years, it is useful to consider the relatively new microsurgical techniques in neurosurgery and plastic/hand surgery.

Neuro-microsurgery – Although pioneer work was done in microneurosurgical techniques during the late 1940s it is only in the last decade or so that the microscope has been accepted as routine equipment. The microscope itself has certainly been responsible for the development of new techniques in neurosurgery, particularly microvascular anastomosis, which is probably responsible for the acceptance of microsurgery as an essential part of neurosurgical procedures.

Fig. 12.2 Suitable for ENT and neurosurgery the OPM16H microscope has a binocular from 0° to 60° from the vertical. The microscope will give magnifications from 4× to 20× and the light source is tungsten halogen. (Zeiss, W. Germany.)

Fig. 12.3 Accessories for microscopes: a. camera; b. photoadaptor with iris; c. short observer tube; d. beam splitter; e. long observer tube; f. binocular stereo assistant's tube. (Zeiss, W. Germany.)

At the present time the microscope is routinely used for intracranial procedures, spinal and peripheral nerve surgery (Fig. 12.2). The procedures undertaken include the clipping of aneurysms, excision of arterial venous malformations, vessel anastomosis and the resection of brain tumours, intradural tumours, excision of arterial venous malformations, and the repair of congenital anomalies. It has been reported that even lumbar disc removal can involve the use of the microscope.

As an example, the microscope set-up for the clipping of an aneurysm would require an objective of 250 or 300 mm focal length and an inclined binocular, eyepieces $12.5 \times$ to $16 \times$, in order to provide a variable magnification range of about 4 to 20 times. The microscope body would be mounted via a geared coupling to the stand (the geared coupling is a most important part of the equipment, as it allows very fine angular adjustment of the microscope, enabling the optical axis to be aligned perfectly with the pathology). A camera, if to be used, would be attached to the left of the beam splitter, and the assistant's observation system to the right, the microscope stand being positioned to the left of the surgeon.

It is essential to note that as the microscope support arm for neurosurgery may well be fully extended, the base of the microscope stand must be orientated correctly; that is with the long tripod foot positioned under the microscope arm and pointing in the same direction. Failure to observe this precaution could result in the microscope being out of balance, with the inevitable consequences.

Modern microscope techniques require the use of many accessories fitted to the microscope (Fig. 12.3), and because of the extra weight added new stands have been appropriately designed, indeed in many cases older equipment may be fitted with additional weights and/or extension feet to give the required stability. However, the ceiling mounted microscope must be recommended for its inherent safety, ease of use and the freeing of valuable theatre floor space for the vast array of support equipment commonplace today (Figs. 12.4 and 12.5).

Fig. 12.4 This OPM16 microscope is suitable for ophthalmic surgery is combined with a slit illuminator. The radius of the curved arm enables the slit illuminator to be moved from a centre position in both directions either by motor or manually. Adjustment by motor is possible at a speed of 5 degrees per second. This illustration shows the microscope suspended on an electro hydraulic ceiling mount with $x-y$ coupling. (Zeiss, W. Germany.)

Plastic and hand surgery – Like so many modern techniques this has developed with the availability of good quality microscopes and ultrafine sutures, many of which despite their small size still have to be made by hand.

Plastic and hand surgery for the most part require two pairs of hands, and for this reason, the two surgeons require an identical field of view at the same magnification and through the same optical system. For this purpose, microscopes have been developed such as that as shown in Figure 12.6, giving surgeons exactly the view they require, with ample illumination from the tungsten halogen powered fibre optic light source. The microscope set-up here requires a 200 mm objective, two straight binocular tubes, a stereo beam splitter, $12.5\times$ eyepieces, a tilting coupling allowing a small degree of movement away from the vertical, and a stand with a motor head to allow fine focus movement in the vertical plane. In this case the light source is contained in a fan-ventilated housing mounted on to the microscope stand, and the light is transmitted through a fibre optic bundle along the microscope arm to an outlet on the microscope body.

Fig. 12.5 Electromotive ceiling mount with microscope.
1. outlet for microphone; 2. outlet for electronic flash; 3 & 4. outlets for foot or hand control panels; 5. switch for halogen lamps; 6. outlet for foot switch (8·5 V overload and film advance); 7. switch for two modes of operation: motorized stand and freely moveable counterweight stand; 8. fuses for 12 V halogen lamps, for 7 V and 24 V AC jacks; 9. signal lamps: white = in operation, green = stand in upper position of rest; 10. power socket (on request)
Top inset shows OPM18F microscope with still and ciné cameras. (Zeiss, W. Germany.)

Microsurgical procedures inevitably involve a number of surgeons and assistants all grouped round a relatively small operative area, and this can make life difficult for the scrubbed nurse who must know precisely what is happening. If equipment and space permit, the ideal solution is to provide the scrubbed nurse with an additional observer tube, so that a direct view of the microsurgical area may be obtained. Alternatively, a method which gives more freedom is to attach a small closed circuit colour or monochrome television camera to the microscope, and position the viewing monitor in the most convenient position.

Fig. 12.6 OPM17 Microscope used for plastic and reconstructive surgery. Enables surgeon and assistant to work in a face to face position, observing the operative field through the same optical system and under the same angle with the aid of a stereo beam splitter. Illumination is provided by a fibre light generator fitted to the upper part of the stand. The floor stand is easily moveable and can be fixed in position by a foot control. The swivel arms are fully adjustable, and the microscope head carriage slides easily up or down the column, being counter balanced with weights so that it remains in position at any desired height without clamps. The stand base houses the power supply units and controls apparatus. Alternatively this microscope could be ceiling-mounted (see Fig. 12.4). (Zeiss, W. Germany.)

Fig. 12.7 Colposcope. This has a motorised zoom system 1:5 and the motorised axial fine focusing are controlled with a hand or foot control. Magnification is continuously variable from 1·6 × to 50 × with a field of view diameter between 125 mm and 4 mm. (Zeiss, W. Germany.)

Care and maintenance

Care and maintenance of operating microscope as far as theatre staff is concerned is a relatively simple matter provided that:
1. At least two members of staff are given total responsibility for checking, setting-up and storing the instrument.
2. Appropriate instruction books have been read from cover to cover.
3. The responsible staff know precisely which adjustments and maintenance may be carried out by themselves and when it is necessary to call in a specialist service engineer.

4. Ample supplies of spare parts such as bulbs, fuses and sterilizeable caps or disposable drapes are always kept in stock.

Consideration should be given to arrangements for a regular servicing contract with the manufacturers or agents, and if doubt, or problems arise, they should be contacted for advice. The operating microscope is a piece of precision equipment which, if it is to function properly, must be treated with the same care accorded to other delicate instruments.

Fig. 12.8 Simple microscope OPM19. This is an 'economy version' microscope which can be stand, wall or ceiling mounted. By selecting a wide range of optical and mechanical accessories the instrument can be adapted to a particular task. There is a choice of interchangeable objectives with a working distance from 100 to 400 mm in steps of 25 mm. The magnification ranges from 2 × to 50 × with field of view diameters of 100 mm to 4 mm. (Zeiss, W. Germany.)

Assembly of microscope

To set up the microscope for an operation, there are several aspects to consider.
1. Positioning of the microscope for the specific operation and also for the comfort of the surgeon.
2. Each operation requires a different working distance and magnification. Also the position of the microscope body has to be perpendicular in relation to the pathology.
3. The optical parts of the microscope, i.e., objective, binocular (straight or inclined) stereo observation tubes etc.
4. Photographic accessories including connection of a camera and possibly a television monitor and recorder.

For example, the microscope set up for a corneal graft would require a 175 mm objective, an inclined binocular tube and a variable magnification range of approx. 4 to 20 times. The assistant's observation tube will be on one side of the beam splitter, and perhaps a camera on the other. The microscope stand is positioned to the left or right of the surgeon, according to which eye is being operated on.

However, familiarisation with specific parts of the operating microscope will help to understand various microscope assemblies, and also the terminology commonly used.

Objective – this is a lens which is interchangeable and screwed to the underside of the microscope. Various focal lengths are available to allow for different working distances.

Beam splitter – this is an optical attachment fitted between the binocular and microscope body, which divides the light rays between the operator and the camera or observation tubes.

Binocular tube – this is obtainable in a straight, inclined or inclinable version. The inclinable version enables the binocular to have the angle varied between straight and 60° to the vertical. Eyepieces or oculars are fitted into the tubes of the binocular; available in various magnifications according to the application. Reticules or graticules (grid lines or measuring scales) may be fitted into eyepieces to help visualize the portion of the field suitable for photography, or that which will appear on a television screen. The graticule or reticule also serves to assist focusing when taking the photograph.

Magnification changer or zoom system – these are the optical systems built into the body of the microscope, which allow the magnification to be varied to suit the conditions prevailing. A magnification changer has usually five steps of magnification available; whereas the zoom system provides a continuous change of magnification without losing the view of the subject. Zoom systems are generally operated by foot or other controls leaving the hands free to continue with the operation.

306   Operating Theatre Technique

Fig. 12.9   Fig. 12.10
Neurosurgery
FIG. 12.9 Acoustic neuroma – later excised preserving the facial nerve. Fig. 12.10 Aneurysm of the left posterior communicating artery which later had its neck toughened by bi-polar coagulation followed by a clip. (Figs. 12.9 and 12.10 taken through Zeiss (W.G.) Operating Microscope by Mr A. E. Booth, FRCS, Walsgrave Hospital, Coventry.)

Fig. 12.11   Fig. 12.12

Fig. 12.13

ENT surgery
Fig. 12.11 Tympanoplasty following previous operation. Replacement of the stapes. (Taken through Zeiss (W.G.) Operating Microscope by Dr H. Schobel, St Polten.) Fig. 12.12 Exposure of the roof of the middle ear. Fig. 12.13 Chronic inflammation of the papilla extension. (Figs. 12.12 and 12.13 taken through Zeiss (W.G.) Operating Microscope by Dr I. Bejar, Mexico.)

Operating Microscopes   307

Fig. 12.14   Fig. 12.15

Peripheral vascular surgery
Fig. 12.14   A completed micro-arterial anastomosis (about 1·2 mm diameter). Fig. 12.15 Two strands of nerve graft attached to the same digital nerve. (Figs. 12.14 and 12.15 from Dept. of Medical Illustration, Queen Victoria Hospital, East Grinstead.)

Fig. 12.16   Fig. 12.17   Fig. 12.18

Ophthalmic surgery
Fig. 12.16   Exposure of the ciliary body for examination. Fig. 12.17   After opening the conjunctiva and sewing on a fleringa ring, a corneo-scleral cut and radial cuts in the sclera are fashioned. Fig. 12.18   Closing the incision following removal of a malignant melanoma. (Figs. 12.16, 12.17 and 12.18 taken through Zeiss (W.G.) Operating Microscope by Prof. G. Mackensen, U.A.K. Freiburg.)

13
FIBRE OPTIC ENDOSCOPY

Fibre optics

Fibre optics have replaced, to a great extent, the conventional optic and light systems in endoscopes. Fibre optic instruments are available for many applications; the use of specific instruments such as cystoscopes and arthroscopes is included in the appropriate chapters. However, it is opportune here to describe the basic principles of fibreoscopy, relevant to the field of gastroenterology where the most significant advances have been made in endoscope design.

Fibre optics is a term applied to a system for transmitting light and images through thin fibres of optical glass by the phenomenon of total internal reflection (Hollanders, 1979). Remarkable efficiency has been achieved in optics with present instruments, but there are limitations to the degree of perfection obtainable, and these include:

1. Limitation of light transmission by fibres, amounting to 70 per cent of the core diameter of each.
2. Up to 10 per cent loss of light intensity for each 30 cm length of fibre bundle from the light source.
3. Good transmission of red and green light through the fibres, but poor transmission of blue light, an important consideration when selecting materials for colour photography.
4. Resolution depends on diameter of fibre and packing density.
5. Some fibres will inevitably break during use, and users have to adapt to the effect of a few 'black' spots in the image formed.

The fibre optic system consists of three basic parts: the light source or generator unit, the insertion tube and optical image guide bundle, and the instrument or endoscope control section.

The light source. The light is supplied by a high-intensity lamp which has an in-built parabolic reflector. This reflector, which although focussing the visible light rays into the optical bundle, allows the long (or hot) infra red rays to pass through. This ensures cold light is passed to the instrument or endoscope. Special lamps such as quartz iodine, metal halide and xenon have been developed to give a high intensity of light up to 500 watts, which overcomes some of the optical limitations described previously.

The light guide or fibre light bundle. This is connected at one end to the light source and at the other to the endoscope; it contains about 20,000 flexible optical fibres, which are incoherent (not capable of carrying an image). The bundles transmit a pre-focused light of high intensity and even density to the endoscope; they are sheathed in metal and PVC, and are extremely flexible (Carr-Locke, 1, 1977; Hollanders, 1979).

The intensity of light output at the patient end of the optical bundle varies with the working distance from the object. This may be as high as 5,000 ft candles at 25 mm (1 in) distance, but generally averages 1,600 to 2,800 ft candles intensity. The degree of intensity can be adjusted.

The instrument or endoscope. This is optically continuous with the fibre cable for the purpose of illumination. In addition, a separate set of optical fibres terminating proximally at an eyepiece, and distally at an appropriate lens, carry an image through the scope. Both these sets of optical glass fibres are contained in a protective sheath, which generally incorporates additional channels for suction, gas inflation/irrigation, and the passage of flexible biopsy or operative forceps and electrodes. (Fig. 13.13.)

Care of fibre optic endoscopes. The principles for the care of endoscopes have already been described in Chapter 5, but it is important to emphasise the special care required for

Fig. 13.1 Endoscope storage cupboard. (Courtesy, Dr Carr-Locke.)

fibre optic instruments after use. It can be said that 'the useful life of endoscopic instruments is inversely proportional to the number of people using them'.

Fibrescopes are exceptionally expensive, comparable with their complexity; in 1977 a gastroscope cost in the region of £5,000. It is therefore essential to adhere to the manufacturer's instructions regarding cleaning and maintenance (NATN, 1979).

Debris and mucus must be removed from the instrument immediately, after use using a mild detergent such as Savlon 1 per cent, followed by copious rinsing in warm water. Great emphasis is placed on cleaning rather than sterilising which is virtually impossible. After thorough cleaning, the insertion tube only of the endoscope can be terminally disinfected by immersion in a chemical fluid such as gluteraldehyde (Cidex). If the instrument has been used on a patient known or suspected to have a viral disease such

Fig. 13.2 Olympus Gastrointestinal Fibrescope type GIF P2, forward viewing. (Keymed.)

Fig. 13.3 Lower portion of oesophagus, oesophageal varices. (Courtesy, Dr D. L. Carr-Locke and *Nursing Times*.)

Fig. 13.4 Lesser curve gastric cancer. (Courtesy, Dr D. L. Carr-Locke and *Nursing Times*.)

Fig. 13.5 Olympus Gastrointestinal Fibrescope, type TGF 2S, side viewing. (Keymed.)

Fig. 13.6 Gastric ulcer on posterior wall of the gastric antrum. (Courtesy, Dr D. L. Carr-Locke.)

Fig. 13.7 Gastric ulcer on posterior wall of stomach being biopsied. (Courtesy, Dr D. L. Carr-Locke.)

Fig. 13.8 Endoscope trolley. (Keymed.)

Biopsy forceps (Alligator type)	Biopsy forceps (with needle)	Forceps (Suture cutting)	Endoscopic injector	Grasping forceps (Alligator jaws)
Grasping forceps (Basket)	Grasping forceps (W-shape)	Grasping forceps (Rubber tips)	Clip fixing device	Surgical scissors
Grasping forceps (Rat tooth)	Grasping forceps (Pelican type)	Grasping forceps (Tripod)	Cytology brush	Cytology brush (with sheath)

Fig. 13.9 Biopsy forceps and brush. (Keymed.)

as hepatitis, it will have to be subjected to ethylene oxide (Chapter 6). After cleaning and disinfection, flexible fibrescopes should be stored as shown in Figure 13.7. Care must be taken not to drop or damage the optical bundle as this will cause individual fibres to shatter.

Endoscopes penetrating tissue i.e., laparoscopes, arthroscopes, thorascopes, etc., must be used in a sterile condition. Although some instruments may be compatible with steam sterilisation, the others will have to be processed by the ethylene oxide method described in Chapter 6, page 150.

Gastrointestinal fibrescopes (including gastroscopes and duodenoscopes)

Before the advent of fibreoptics, the rigid instruments available had many limitations. Fibre optics enabled the development of endoscopes which not only have a flexible shaft, but give an operator the ability to manoeuvre the tip of the instrument by changing its configuration.

There are three basic types of instruments:
1. Forward or oblique viewing for examination/biopsy.
2. Side or lateral viewing for examination/biopsy/operative procedures.
3. Forward/oblique/side viewing with channel for complex operative procedures.

The first type of instrument is suitable for examining the oesophagus, most of the stomach and the upper part of the duodenum, and serves 90 per cent of situations.

The second type, side or lateral viewing instrument is needed in 10 per cent of cases, when full examination of oesophagus, stomach and duodenum is required. This includes the fundus of the stomach and fornices of the duodenal bulb.

The third type of instrument is generally larger in diameter than the previous two (although there are exceptions), which enables suitable dimension of channels to be incorporated for operating instruments. A wide range of procedures can be undertaken, including the removal of polyps and diathermising various lesions.

All three types of instruments can be obtained from several manufacturers, although for the purpose of this only two will be mentioned: American Cystoscope Manufacturing Inc. and Olympus Optical Co. Ltd. (marketed by Keymed in the United Kingdom).

Examples of type 1 are the ACM F-8 or F7 and the Olympus GIF-K (diameter 13·3 mm, forward/oblique viewing, suitable for examination/biopsy); type 2 includes ACM F-5b, Olympus GIF-P2 (small diameter, 8·6 mm, forward viewing, suitable for examination/biopsy/removal of foreign bodies), GIF-D3 and JF-B3; (a gastro/duodenofibrescope suitable for carrying out retro grade cholangio-pancreatography by cannulation of the papilla of Vater); an example of type 3 would be the Olympus TGF-2S (diameter 14·5 mm, side viewing suitable for removal of polyps from the stomach).

Fig. 13.13 (Keymed).
The air feeding, lens cleaning and suction capabilities are essential to ensure clear visualization and good photographs. The ingenious arrangement of air/water and suction pipes contributes much to the famous single-handed control of Olympus fibrescopes (Fig. A).
Air feeding and lens cleaning:
Air, driven by the air-pump built into the light source, flows constantly out of the air/water button hole. When the hole is closed with a fingertip, the air flow is diverted toward the distal end (Figs B and F). When the occluded button is depressed all the way, the air flow is led into the water bottle and forces the water to flow through the air/water pipe to the distal port (Figs C and E).
Suction:
An external aspirator attached to the suction connector constantly draws air through the suction button hole. When the occluded button is depressed all the way, fluid is drawn through the biopsy/suction channel outlet at the distal end (Figs D and G).

Fig. 13.10 Olympus Duodeno fibrescope, type JFB3, side viewing. (Keymed.)

Fig. 13.11 ERCP catheter partially inserted into the ampula of Vater. (Courtesy, Dr D. L. Carr-Locke.)

Fig. 13.12 Diagrammatic view of ampullary cannulation. (Courtesy, Dr D. L. Carr-Locke and *Nursing Times*.)

Fig. 13.13 Olympus one-touch insufflation and suction mechanism (legend opposite).

Upper Gastrointestinal endoscopy

DEFINITION

The examination of the interior of the oesophagus, stomach or duodenum, using a fibrescope.

POSITION

Left lateral or sitting.

INSTRUMENTS

Suitable fibrescope (e.g., forward, side or multiangle viewing depending on whether oesophagus/stomach/duodenum are to be examined)
Fibreoptic light source/diathermy power supply
Plastic mouth guard
Biopsy forceps (these include those suitable for cutting, grasping, taking cytology specimens etc., Fig. 13.9)
Accessories for endoscopic diathermy (e.g. snares, cutter, electrodes Fig. 13.14)
Angled tongue depressor
Pharyngeal spray
Topical anaesthetic, e.g., 1 per cent lignocaine (Xylocaine)
Lubricant e.g., Lignocaine (Xylocaine) gel
Oesophageal bougies and tubes sizes 16 and 18 Charriere gauge may be required
Water container/irrigator
Medical vacuum
Camera.

OUTLINE OF PROCEDURE

The patient is usually sedated with intravenous diazepam; a calm atmosphere and gentle technique can do much to reduce anxiety, complications and the need for heavy sedation. In addition, a topical anaesthetic is applied to the pharynx (1 per cent lignocaine spray). An assistant stands behind the patient (who is sitting or lying on his left side), supporting his head, and encouraging him to bend his neck forward to relax his neck muscles and to avoid moving his head from side to side (Hollanders, 1979).

A plastic mouth-guard is then placed between the gums and teeth, the lubricated fibrescope is passed through the guard and over the tongue, and the patient is asked to swallow. This usually opens the upper oesophageal sphincter (cricopharyngeus) so that the instrument can be advanced into the oesophagus. If, because of severe retching, the instrument cannot be passed, an attempt may be made to pass it under direct vision. If this fails a small oesophageal dilator may be passed in order to relax the cricopharyngeus sufficiently to permit passage of the instrument. No force should ever be employed in this procedure as perforation of the oesophagus can occur. If the patient is in a sitting position, when the instrument is well past the cricopharyngeus, the patient is placed on his left side for completion of the examination.

Examination of the oesophagus. The patient's head is elevated 10–15°, and a partial examination is carried out as the instrument is advanced towards the stomach. Complete examination is usually left until the end of the endoscopy procedure, unless obvious pathology is found in the oesophagus.

The examination is started by inflating the oesophagus with air until a view of the lumen is obtained. Successful examination requires nearly continuous use of air, water and suction to keep the lens clean and the oesophagus distended. The operator keeps the fibrescope in the centre of the lumen by coordinated use of the angle control knob and flexible tube rotation.

Special care is exercised to avoid mucosal trauma when passing the instrument through the hiatus and into the stomach. In case of strictures, when the hiatal opening is visualised, a biopsy forceps is passed through the suction channel into the stomach and the scope is gently passed over the forceps safely into the stomach. The forceps are then withdrawn.

Fig. 13.14 (Keymed). Accessories for endoscopic diathermy.

At the end of the procedure, a more complete inspection of the oesophagus is carried out as the instrument is withdrawn. This would include relation of the gastro-oesophageal mucosal junction to the diaphragmatic hiatus (possible hiatus hernia); state of oesophageal mucosa (possible eosophagitis, varices and tumours). If necessary biopsy forceps are introduced into the suction channel and specimens taken for histology; brush cytology specimens may also be taken.

Examination of the stomach. The patient's head may be tilted downwards 10–15°, and the instrument is then passed through the hiatus 2–3 cm into the stomach. Sufficient air is inflated to open up the body of the stomach, the objective lens is rinsed and the scope is positioned in the centre of the gastric lumen. Combined with intermittent suction to remove secretions and the air inflation the instrument is manoeuvred along the greater curvature of the stomach to the pylorus. It may be necessary to place the patient on his back in order to pass the instrument through the pylorus into the duodenum and if difficulty is experienced a similar procedure to that described for entry to the stomach may be carried out, utilising a biopsy forceps as a guide.

When examination of the duodenum is completed, a detailed examination of the stomach is carried out as the instrument is withdrawn. The objective is to achieve complete examination of the stomach paying special attention to areas which can easily become 'blind' spots in the examination e.g., the lesser curvature, severe cascade deformaties of the stomach wall, the cardia and fundus. Operative procedures may include biopsy with forceps and brush cytology, removal of foreign bodies; diathermy excision of polyps. The biopsy forceps is a delicate precision instrument which must be used with great care. Biopsies are torn off as opposed to cutting with the forceps to avoid using force to close the jaws when the biopsy is taken, which may separate the attachment of the pull wire from the forceps tip. The endoscopist will manoeuvre the forceps in and out, operating the controls of the fibrescope, whilst an assistant opens or closes the forceps jaws as required.

Examination of the duodenum. As with the oesophagus and stomach the duodenum is best examined as the fibrescope is withdrawn. The organ is inflated with air and the scope manoeuvred into the second part of the duodenum. During a slow withdrawal of the instrument, a careful examination is carried out and if necessary biopsies or brush cytology specimens are taken. Duodenal ulcers are generally shallow and small and tend to be found in the folds of the duodenal cap. Retrograde cholangiopancreatography can be undertaken by cannulation of the papilla of Vater (Schiller and Peachey, 1978).

Withdrawal of instrument. When examination of the oesophagus has been completed the angle free control is released and the instrument gently withdrawn. The operator may inspect the larynx, possibly the trachea, and the pharynx before the instrument is completely removed.

Lower Gastrointestinal endoscopy

DEFINITION

The examination of the interior of the colon using a fibrescope.

POSITION

Usually left lateral

INSTRUMENTS

Colonofibrescope
Fibreoptic light source/diathermy power supply
Biopsy forceps (these include those suitable for cutting, grasping, taking cytology specimens etc. (Fig. 13.9)
Accessories for endoscopic diathermy (e.g., snares, cutter, electrodes (Fig. 13.14)
Colon stiffening tube
Lubricant e.g., ligocaine (Xylocaine) gel
Water container/irrigator
Carbon dioxide gas source
Medical vacuum
Camera.

OUTLINE OF PROCEDURE

Good colonoscopy is a procedure which requires good pre-operative radiology with adequate double contrast barium enema pictures of the whole colon. The most common indication for colonoscopy examination is to clarify an abnormality revealed radiologically by barium enema; colonoscopy may also be carried out for persistent symptoms such as rectal bleeding, passage of mucus or colonic pain despite negative investigations such as sigmoidoscopy and barium enema.

Thorough preparation of the bowel is essential if the operator is to achieve a complete examination. Although such preparation is not a part of this operative description it is useful to note that this preparation may consist of a low residue diet for two days before examination and the administration of purgative enemas. (Carr-Locke, 2, 1977.) Therapeutic colonoscopy often includes the removal of polyps (polypectomy). The colonoscope has the facility for blowing in carbon dioxide so that explosive gas mixtures do not form in the bowel whilst polyps are being removed by diathermy. Complete colonoscopy requires X-ray screening facilities, although left-sided examinations can be done without.

Fig. 13.15 Olympus Colono fibrescope. (Keymed.)

Fig. 13.16 Snare loop approaching colonic polyp. (Courtesy, Dr D. L. Carr-Locke.)

Fig. 13.17 Just after colonic polyp has been removed by diathermy. (Courtesy, Dr D. L. Carr-Locke.)

The patient may be sedated with diazepam; if discomfort or pain is felt during the procedure this may be supplemented by intravenous pethidine or inhaled nitrous oxide 50 per cent with oxygen 50 per cent (Entonox). The patient at first lies on his left side but may find it more comfortable to turn prone as the examination proceeds.

A well-lubricated colonoscope is introduced into the rectum and gently advanced along the centre of the bowel under direct vision. Great skill is required to manoeuvre the scope along the sigmoid colon and through the various bends into the ascending colon. However, it is safe to progress if the bowel mucosa is seen to slip past the instrument tip. Examination of the whole colon can take up to two hours.

As with upper gastrointestinal endoscopy, the best views of the interior of the colon are usually obtained on withdrawal of the instrument. It is at this stage that biopsies or cytology specimens are taken and polypectomy performed. For polypectomy the bowel gas is replaced with carbon dioxide and a diathermy snare loop (Fig. 13.16) passed through the suction/biopsy channel. With a special diathermy power source and appropriate precautions (Chapter 2, page 60), a diathermy current is applied to the snare which has been tightened around the base of the polyp which is cut away without bleeding. The cut polyp can be removed with biopsy holding forceps and sent for histology. The angle controls are returned to normal and the instrument gently withdrawn.

Fig. 13.18 Proctoscopy and sigmoidoscopy.

1. Sigmoidoscope light lead and light attachment.
2 and 3. Large and small proctoscope (Kelly).
4 and 5. Large and small sigmoidoscopes (Norton Morgan).
6. Eyepiece for sigmoidoscope.
7. Biopsy forceps, cutting jaws (e.g., Brunings cup, Yeaman, etc.).
8. Telescope attachment.
9. Dissecting forceps, non-toothed.
10. Soft paraffin lubricant.
11. Gallipot containing Savlon 1 per cent.
12. Wool and gauze swabs.
13. Towel clips.
14. gloves and dressing towels.

Not illustrated:
Double inflation bellows, and battery or transformer.

Proctoscopy and sigmoidoscopy

DEFINITION

An examination of the rectum or sigmoid flexure of the colon, using an illuminated endoscope passed per anum. (The fibre optic aspect would consist only of the illumination device.)

POSITION

Left lateral, lithotomy or kneeling.

INSTRUMENTS. As Figure 13.18.

OUTLINE OF PROCEDURE

The lubricated endoscope is passed via the anus. When the surgeon uses a sigmoidoscope, the walls of the colon are kept separate by inflating with air. Small pledglets of cotton-wool are held with the long forceps to swab the area in view, and the biopsy forceps may be used to obtain a specimen of tissue for histology. Sometimes a rectal or colonic polyp may be diathermised and in this case the indifferent electrode is applied to the patient's leg, observing the precautions listed in Chapter 2. The active electrode is inserted through a special attachment at the proximal end of the endoscope.

REFERENCES AND FURTHER READING

CARR-LOCKE, D. L. (1977) Gastrointestinal endoscopy – 1. *Nursing Times*, 73, 1348.
CARR-LOCKE, D. L. (1977) Gastrointestinal endoscopy – 2. *Nursing Times*, 73, 1403.
NATIONAL ASSOCIATION OF THEATRE NURSES (1979) *A Report on the Care and Sterilisation of Fibre Optic Endoscopes. Staffing and Training Sub-Committee*, September.
SCHILLER, K. F. R. AND PEACHEY, J. (1978) Gastrointestinal fibre-endoscopy. *Nursing Mirror*, November, 30.
HOLLANDERS, D. (1979) *Gastrointestinal Endoscopy*. London: Baillière-Tindall.

14
GENERAL INSTRUMENTS

The general set. (Figs. 14.1 to 14.28)

The general set of instruments is arranged according to the kind of operation, and preference of the surgeon; but this set must include sufficient basic instruments for any of the operations performed in that particular theatre. However, the instruments listed, indeed any of the operation sets described in the following chapters, are intended to act only as a guide and must, of course, be adjusted in type, size or number to suit a surgeon's individual requirements.

A basic general set of instruments could consist of the following:
Scalpel handles Nos. 3 and 4, with Nos. 10 and 20 blades (Bard Parker), 2.
Dissecting forceps, toothed, small (Lane), 2.
Dissecting forceps, toothed, large (Bonney), 2.
Dissecting forceps, non-toothed, small and large, 2.
Scissors, curved on flat, small and large (Mayo), 2.
Scissors, straight (Mayo).
Scissors, straight, stitch.
Artery forceps, curved on flat (Kelly Fraser/Dunhill/Halstead), 10.
Artery forceps, straight (Moynihan), 10.
Artery forceps, straight 20 cm (8 in) (Spencer Wells), 5.
Dissector (MacDonald/Durham/Watson-Cheyne).
Aneurysm needle.
Photoclips for anchoring soiled dressing bag, diathermy leads or suction tubing etc., 3.
Curetting spoons, medium and large (Volkmann), 2.
Probe, malleable silver.
Sinus forceps.
Sponge-holding forceps (Rampley), 5.
Needle holder, large (Mayo), 2.
Needle holder, small (Kilner), 2.
Towel clips (Backaus), 5.
Tissue forceps (Lane), 5.
Tissue forceps (Allis), 5.
Retractors, single hook, sharp and blunt, 2.
Retractors, double hook, blunt, 2.
Retractors, medium (Langenbeck), 2.
Retractors, large (Morris), 2.

General Instruments 323

Fig. 14.1 Duray Scalpel Handles Sizes 3, 4 and 5.

Fig. 14.2 Disposable Scalpel Blades Sizes 10–25.

Fig. 14.3 Stitch Scissors.

Fig. 14.4 Mayo Scissors (Straight).

Fig. 14.5 Mayo Scissors (Curved).

(Chas. F. Thackray Ltd.)

Fig. 14.6   Lane Toothed Dissecting Forceps.

Fig. 14.7   Treves Toothed Dissecting Forceps.

Fig. 14.8   Non-Toothed Dissecting Forceps.

Fig. 14.9   Bonney Toothed Dissecting Forceps.

Fig. 14.10   Crile Artery Forceps.

Fig. 14.11   Dunhill Artery Forceps.

Fig. 14.12   Halstead Mosquito Artery Forceps.

Fig. 14.13   Spencer Wells Artery Forceps.

(Chas. F. Thackray Ltd.)

General Instruments

Fig. 14.14 Macdonald Dissector.

Fig. 14.15 Durham Dissector-Raspatory.

Fig. 14.16 Watson-Cheyne Dissector.

Fig. 14.17 Syme Aneurysm Needle.

Fig. 14.18 Volkmann Curetting Spoon. (Double end. Four sizes A, B, C and D. Zimmer Orthopaedic Ltd.)

Fig. 14.19 Rampley Sponge-Holding Forceps.

Fig. 14.20. Mayo Needle Holder.

Fig. 14.21 Kilner Needle Holder, Simple Pattern.

Fig. 14.22 Mayo Backhaus Towel Forceps.

(Chas. F. Thackray Ltd.)

326   Operating Theatre Technique

Fig. 14.23   Lane Tissue Forceps.

Fig. 14.24   Allis Tissue Forceps.

Fig. 14.25   Single Hook Retractor.

Fig. 14.26   Double Hook Retractor.

Fig. 14.27   Morris Retractor.

Fig. 14.28   Langenbeck Retractor.

15
GENERAL OPERATIONS ON THE ABDOMEN

The laparotomy set. (Figs. 15.1–15.7)

Combined with the general set, this is the basis for all major operations on the abdomen and is suitable for a midline, paramedian, transverse or elliptical incision. Bowel clamps and special instruments are added as required.

Gall-bladder forceps, curved on flat (Moynihan), 6.
Long tissue forceps (Lane), 6.
Artery forceps, curved on flat (Kelly Fraser), 25.
Long scissors, curved on flat (McIndoe).
Hernia director (Key).
Hernia bistoury, curved.
Aneurysm needle, large (Moynihan).
Artery forceps, straight 20 cm (8 in) (Spencer Wells), 25.
Deep retractors, curved narrow blade (Deaver), set of 4.
Retractor, self-retaining abdominal (Gosset/Denis Browne).
Deep retractor, right-angled narrow blade (Kelly).

Not illustrated:
2·5 and 3 (2/0 and 0) Chromic catgut or Dexon for ligatures.*
2·5, 3, 4, and 5 (2/0, 0, 1 and 2) Silk or thread for ligatures.
4 or 5 (1 or 2) Chromic catgut, Dexon or silk on large half-circle, round-bodied needles for peritoneum, and large half-circle cutting needles for rectus or linea alba. (Proportionally smaller for children.)
5 (2) Nylon (strong) on curved cutting needles for tension sutures (optional).
2·5 (2/0) Nylon or silk on curved or straight cutting needles for skin.
Fine rubber tubing or buttons for tension sutures.
Michel or Kifa skin clips (optional).

Types of central abdominal incisions

HIGH MIDLINE INCISIONS

These are used for operations on the stomach, liver, gall-bladder, spleen, etc. A vertical midline incision is made through the skin, extending from just below the xyphisternum to the umbilicus where it curves outwards to avoid this landmark. The incision is continued through the linea alba to expose the peritoneum, which is picked up with forceps and incised.

---

*In all the following chapters, suture sizes are described in metric sizes followed by the original BPC sizes in parentheses.

328 Operating Theatre Technique

Fig. 15.1 Moynihan Cholecystectomy Forceps.

Fig. 15.2 Moynihan Aneurysm Needle.

Fig. 15.3 Metzenbaum Dissecting Scissors (Curved).

Fig. 15.4 Kelly Retractor.

Fig. 15.5 Deaver Retractor With Shaped Handle.

Fig. 15.6 Gosset Self-Retaining Retractor With Panting Adjustable Centre Blade.

Fig. 15.7 Denis-Browne Retractor Set.

LOW MIDLINE INCISIONS

These are used for operations on the lower bowel, bladder, uterus and rectum, etc. A vertical midline incision is made through the skin, extending from the pubis to the umbilicus where it curves outwards. The anterior rectus sheath is split following the line of the linea alba, and the peritoneum is picked up with forceps and incised.

PARAMEDIAN INCISIONS

These are used primarily to gain access to one side of the abdomen and are placed accordingly. A vertical skin incision is made 2 cm from the midline. The extent of the incision depends upon the operative procedure; e.g., for caecal or lower colon operations the incision would extend from just above the level of the umbilicus to the pubis, for gastric or gall-bladder operations the incision would extend from just below the costal margin to the umbilicus. For extensive procedures the incision would be a combination of both types just given.

The anterior rectus sheath is incised 2 cm from the midline and the rectus muscle retracted laterally or split between its fibres. The posterior rectus sheath and peritoneum together are picked up with forceps and incised.

Transverse (Kocher's type) incisions are not often used as there is danger of damage to the nerves supplying the rectus muscle. An oblique skin incision is made below the costal margin. The rectus muscle, external oblique and underlying internal oblique and transversus muscles are divided across in line with the skin incision, and the peritoneum is opened in the usual manner.

PFANNENSTIEL TRANSVERSE ELLIPTICAL INCISION

This is favoured by the gynaecologists. The skin is incised elliptically just above the pubis. The anterior rectus sheath is incised transversely in line with the skin incision, and is retracted to expose the rectus muscles which are freed from the sheath. The rectus muscles are separated from the midline and the peritoneum is picked up with forceps and incised vertically.

Closure of central abdominal incisions

The peritoneum and posterior rectus sheath are sutured with a continuous chromic catgut or Dexon on a round-bodied needle. Non-absorbable tension sutures on curved cutting needles may be inserted in midline and paramedian incisions. These tension sutures pass from one side of the incision through the skin, figure-of-eight manner through the muscle, and out through the skin again on the opposite side of the incision. The sutures are tied over a button or thin rubber tubing after the muscles have been approximated. Alternatively, several interrupted sutures of silk, nylon or polyester material may be inserted to approximate the muscles before using chromic catgut.

For midline and paramedian incisions, the anterior rectus sheath or linea alba is sutured with interrupted or continuous chromic catgut, Dexon or monofilament nylon on a cutting or lance point needle.

Kocher's incision is closed by approximating the muscles with interrupted mattress sutures of chromic catgut or Dexon, which are left long and tied when all have been placed.

The skin is closed with interrupted or continuous silk or nylon on a curved or straight cutting needle, sometimes used in conjunction with Michel or Kifa skin clips (lower midline incisions especially).

Fig. 15.8 An outline drawing of the anterior abdominal wall in which the course of the nerves are shown by interrupted lines and the position of some of the commoner incisions are indicated by continuous lines

(A) Mayo-Robson's modified paramedian incision for biliary tract operations.
(B) Right supra-umbilical paramedian incision (for stomach and duodenum).
(C) Kocher's paracostal incision for stomach and spleen, and on the right side for biliary tract.
(D) Left pararectal incision for colon.
(E) Battle's incision for appendectomy.
(F) Right iliac gridiron incision for appendectomy.
(G) Lanz incision for appendectomy.
(H) Transverse incision for subrapubic cystotomy.
(I.H.) Iliohypogastric nerve.
(I.ING.) Ilio-inguinal nerve.
(Bruce. Walmsley and Ross.)

Appendectomy

DEFINITION

Removal of the appendix.

POSITION

Supine.

Fig. 15.9 (above left) Paramedian incision. The rectus mucle has been retracted laterally to expose the posterior sheath, which is then incised together with the peritoneum.

Fig. 15.10 (above right) Closure of paramedian incision. The rectus muscle covers the suture line in the posterior sheath. Tension sutures have been inserted. The anterior sheath is being repaired by a continuous suture. (Farquharson and Rintoul.)

Fig. 15.11 Lower abdominal transverse incision with vertical seaparation of the recti. The incision is curved so as to lie in the skin creases. After the anterior sheaths have been incised, and the superior flap elevated upwards, the recti are separated and held apart by retractors. Transversalis fascia and peritoneum are then incised in a vertical direction. (Farquharson and Rintoul.)

Figs. 15.12 (left) and 15.13 (right) Gridiron incision, in which the muscles are not divided, but are split in the line of their fibres—external oblique in the line of the skin incision, internal oblique and transversus in a more or less transverse direction. The muscles are held apart by retractors, to expose transversalis fascia and peritoneum, which are then incised as one layer. The method of closing the incision is shown. (Farquharson and Rintoul)

INSTRUMENTS

General set (Figs. 14.1–14.28)
Bowel-holding forceps (Hamilton Bailey)
Long artery forceps, curved on flat (Moynihan gall-bladder or Gordon Craig artery forceps), 5
Suction tubing, nozzles and tube anchoring forceps
2·5 and 3 (2/0 and 0) Chromic catgut, Dexon or silk for ligatures
2·5 (2/0) Chromic catgut or Dexon on a non-traumatic curved or straight intestinal needle for purse-string suture
3 or 4 (0 or 1) Chromic catgut or Dexon on a small half-circle round-bodied needle for peritoneum and first muscle layer
3 or 4 (0 or 1) Chromic catgut or Dexon on a small half-circle cutting needle for muscle aponeurosis
2·5 (2/0) Silk or nylon on a medium-curved or straight-cutting needle for skin sutures (Michel or Kifa skin clips may be required)
(Medium-sized tube drain or corrugated drain may be required).

OUTLINE OF PROCEDURE

Incisions used for this operation include the McBurney 'grid iron', the Battle type and the right lower paramedian. (If a paramedian approach is used, the instruments for laparotomy are selected.)

The centre of a McBurney incision lies in the right iliac region, situated over a point which is at the junction of the outer with the inner two-thirds of an imaginary line joining the umbilicus with the anterior superior iliac spine. It is about five or seven cm in length, and is approximately parallel with the inguinal ligament. The aponeurosis of the external oblique is incised in line with the skin incision. The underlying fibres of the internal oblique and transversus muscles are separated at right angles to the external oblique to expose the peritoneum. The peritoneum is picked up with forceps and incised.

A Battle incision is made more towards the midline, and the rectus muscle is retracted medially to expose the peritoneum which is picked up with forceps and incised.

The caecum is identified and the appendix grasped with a pair of tissue forceps. The meso-appendix is ligated with chromic catgut, Dexon or silk, and the base of the appendix is crushed and ligated with chromic catgut or Dexon. A purse-string suture is placed around the appendix base, the appendix is removed and the stump invaginated before tying the purse-string suture. All instruments which have come in contact with the transected stump are discarded before the operation proceeds.

When the appendix is adherent in a retrocaecal position, the surgeon may divide it and invaginate the stump before ligating the meso-appendix.

The wound is closed by suturing the peritoneum with continuous chromic catgut or Dexon on a round-bodied needle, the internal oblique and transversus muscles with similar (but interrupted) sutures and the external oblique with a continuous chromic catgut or Dexon suture on a cutting needle. Finally the skin is closed with interrupted silk or nylon sutures on a cutting needle or by inserting skin clips.

Fig. 15.14 Technique of appendicectomy

(A) Meso-appendix clamped and divided; base of appendix crushed with forceps.
(B) Meso-appendix tied off; appendix ligatured at base; purse-string suture inserted.
(C) Appendix clamped distal to ligature and about to be divided against swab.
(D) Appendix stump about to be invaginated before tightening of purse-string suture.
(Farquharson and Rintoul.)

If the appendix has perforated, the surgeon may insert a drainage tube through a separate stab incision before closing the wound.

Drainage of an intrapelvic abscess (1)

DEFINITION

The establishment of a temporary drainage tract for an intraperitoneal pelvic abscess.

Fig. 15.15 Schematic drawing to show the relations of the gall bladder and bile ducts to the duodenum and head of pancreas. (Farquharson and Rintoul.)

POSITION.

Supine.

INSTRUMENTS

General set (Figs. 14.1–14.28)
Artery forceps, straight, 20 cm (8 in) (Spencer Wells), 5
Deep retractors, narrow blade (Deaver), 2
Suction tubing, nozzles and tube anchoring forceps

Long plastic drainage tubing and wound suction apparatus (Redivac, Portovac)
Ligatures and sutures as for appendectomy (or laparotomy).

OUTLINE OF PROCEDURE

A long plastic drainage tube is inserted into the pelvis through a McBurney or lower paramedian incision and connected to a wound suction apparatus. The wound is closed in the usual manner for that particular incision.

OPERATIONS ON THE GALL-BLADDER AND COMMON BILE DUCT

Cholecystostomy

DEFINITION

An opening made into the gall bladder to establish drainage of bile.

POSITION

Supine, with liver bridge elevated (optional)

INSTRUMENTS

General set (Figs. 14.1–14.28)
Laparotomy set (Figs. 15.1–15.7)
Liver retractor (Nuttall)
Gall-stone forceps (Desjardin)
Common bile duct probes (Bake)
Intestinal occlusion clamp, curved (Doyen)
Gall-stone probe (Desjardin), 3 sizes.
Malleable scoop and probe (Moynihan)
Catheters, self-retaining (De Pezzer and Malecot, sizes 16 and 18 Charrière gauge), page 651
Catheter introducer, page 651
Gall-bladder trocar and cannula
Long plastic drainage tube
'T' drainage tubes (Kehr), assorted sizes
Haemostatic agent (gelatine sponge)
10 ml syringe and exploration needle
Suction tubing, nozzles and tube anchoring forceps
Laparotomy ligatures and sutures
2·5 (2/0) Chromic catgut or Dexon on a small curved non-traumatic intestinal needle for purse-string suture.

OUTLINE OF PROCEDURE

Through a right paramedian or transverse incision, a purse-string suture is placed in the tip of the gall-bladder. A trocar and cannula is inserted at a point in the centre of this purse-string suture and the bile evacuated. Desjardin's forceps may be used through

Fig. 15.16
Desjardin Gall-Stone Probe.

Fig. 15.17
Moynihan Gall-Stone Probe and Scoop.

Fig. 15.18
Bakes Common Bile Duct Dilators.

3, 4, 5, 6, 7, 8, 9, 10, 11 mm

Fig. 15.19 Kehr 'T' Tube. Sizes available: 12, 15, 18, 21, 24 and 27 Charrière gauge. Rubber or plastic.

Fig. 15.20 Ochsner Gall-Bladder Trocar.

Fig. 15.21 Desjardin Gall-Stone Forceps.

Fig. 15.22 Moynihan Gall-Stone Scoop.

the stab opening to extract any gall-stones. A long drainage tube is inserted and secured by tying the purse-string suture.

The wound is closed in the usual manner and the drainage tube connected to a sealed bottle or disposable plastic bag.

Cholecystectomy

DEFINITION

Removal of the gall-bladder.

POSITION

Supine, with the liver bridge elevated (optional)

INSTRUMENTS

(As above).

Fig. 15.23 Cholecystectomy by the retrograde method—exposure of the cystic duct at its junction with the common hepatic duct, in the right free border of the lesser omentum. The inset diagram shows cystic duct divided between ligature and clamp, and cystic artery displayed. (Farquharson and Rintoul.)

OUTLINE OF PROCEDURE

The incision is as above; the cystic duct and artery are identified, clamped, ligated with chromic catgut, Dexon or silk, clamped distally, and divided. The gall-bladder is freed from the liver and removed. The raw surface of the liver may either be sutured over with 2·5 (2/0) chromic catgut or Dexon on a small curved non-traumatic intestinal needle, or a haemostatic agent (e.g., gelatine sponge or Surgicel) applied.

A long drainage tube is inserted and the wound closed in the usual manner.

Fig. 15.24 (above left)   Method of opening the supra-duodenal part of the common bile duct by an incision made directly over the calculus. Note index finger in epiploic foramen.

Fig. 15.25 (above right)   Removal of a calculus in the lower part of the common bile duct by means of long slender forceps introduced through an incision in the supra-duodenal part of the common bile duct.

Fig. 15.26 (left)   T-tube drainage of the common bile duct. The incision in the duct is sutured *above* the emerging limb of the tube in order to avoid any drag on the suture line when the tube is withdrawn. (Farquharson and Rintoul.)

Choledochotomy

DEFINITION

An incision into the common bile duct, usually for the extraction of gall-stones.

POSITION

Supine, with the kidney bridge elevated (optional).

INSTRUMENTS

As above, plus malleable probes, bougies, irrigation syringe, catheter and warm saline.

OUTLINE OF PROCEDURE

The incision is as above; the common bile duct is identified and two long 'stay' sutures of 2·5 (2/0) chromic catgut or Dexon on a small (20 mm) non-traumatic intestinal needle are inserted. The duct is opened between these sutures, suctioned and explored with probes and Desjardin's forceps. The duct may be irrigated with saline before inserting a Kehr's T-tube; and the incision in the duct is sutured with further 2·5 (2/0) chromic catgut or Dexon sutures, *above* the emerging limb of the tube in order to avoid any drag on the suture line when the tube is withdrawn.

An additional long drainage tube is placed in the vicinity of the duct and the wound is closed in the usual manner.

Cholecystogastrostomy

DEFINITION

Anastomosis between the gall-bladder and the stomach.

POSITION

Supine.

INSTRUMENTS

(As above)

OUTLINE OF PROCEDURE

The incision is as above; the gall-bladder is drained with a trocar and cannula and then approximated to the stomach. Curved occlusion clamps are applied and an anastomosis made with two layers of 2·5 (2/0) chromic catgut or Dexon sutures on a small or medium cuved non-traumatic intestinal needle. A long drainage tube is inserted in the vicinity of the anastomosis and the wound closed in the usual manner.

Cholecystoenterostomy

DEFINITION

The procedure is as above but the anastomosis is made between the gall-bladder and the jejunum, often with jejuno-jejunostomy.

Choledochoduodenostomy

DEFINITION

Anastomosis between the common bile duct and the duodenum.

POSITION.

Supine.

INSTRUMENTS

As above, plus 2 (3/0) chromic catgut or Dexon on a small curved non-traumatic intestinal needle.

OUTLINE OF PROCEDURE

The incision is as above; the common bile duct is mobilised and anastomosed to the duodenum with two layers of 2 (3/0) chromic catgut or Dexon. A long drainage tube is inserted in the vicinity of the anastomosis and the wound is closed in the usual manner.

Radical resection of the head of the pancreas

DEFINITION

The head of pancreas, duodenum, part of the jejunum and stomach are resected, together with the lower half of the common bile duct and part of the pancreatic duct.

POSITION

Supine.

INSTRUMENTS

General set (Figs. 14.1–14.28)
Laparotomy set (Figs. 15.1–15.7)
Gall-bladder set (Figs. 15.16–15.22)
Gastrectomy set (Fig. 15.30)
Suction tubing, nozzles and tube anchoring forceps
Diathermy leads, electrodes and lead anchoring forceps
Laparotomy ligatures and sutures.
2, 2·5 and 3 (3/0, 2/0 and 0) Chromic catgut or Dexon on small and medium half-circle
 and curved non-traumatic intestinal needles for anastomoses
2·5 (2/0) Silk on small curved non-traumatic intestinal needles.

OUTLINE OF PROCEDURE

Through a midline incision a partial gastrectomy, duodenectomy, partial jejunectomy, pancreatectomy and choledochectomy is performed. The stump of the pancreas is joined to the remaining portion of the jejunum (pancreaticojejunostomy) as an end to end anastomosis. The end of the common bile duct is anastomosed to the jejunum (choledochojejunostomy), using interrupted silk sutures in both cases. The stomach is anastomosed to the jejunum (gastrojejunostomy) in the usual manner and the wound is closed.

Ramstedt's operation

DEFINITION

An operation performed for the relief of congenital pyloric stenosis and which consists of division of the circular muscle fibres of the pylorus.

POSITION

The patient is placed in the supine position or immobilised on a padded crucifix if local anaesthesia is being used.

Fig. 15.27 Rammstedt's operation for congenital pyloric stenosis. An incision 2 to 3 cm in length is made in the long axis of the pylorus, and should divide all except the deepest of the circular muscle fibres. The remaining fibres are then gently teased apart with a blunt dissector. Arrow indicates the point where special care must be taken to avoid penetration of the mucosa. (Farquharson and Rintoul.)

INSTRUMENTS

Sponge-holding forceps (Rampley), 5
Towel clips, 5
Scalpel handles No. 3, with Nos. 10 and 15 blades (Bard Parker), 2
Fine dissecting forceps, toothed (Gillies), 2
Fine dissecting forceps, non-toothed (McIndoe), 2
Scissors, straight, 13 cm (5 in) (Mayo)
Scissors, curved on flat, 18 cm (7 in) (Mayo)
Long scissors, curved on flat (McIndoe)
Sinus forceps
Blunt dissector (Watson Cheyne)
Blunt dissector (MacDonald)
Fine artery forceps, curved on flat (mosquito), 5
Fire artery forceps, straight (mosquito), 5
Small retractors, double hook, 2
Medium retractors (Czerny), 2
Fine tissue forceps (McIndoe), 5
Skin or tetra towel forceps (Moynihan), 4 for the sides of the wound and 2 for the ends of the wound (Optional)
2 and 2·5 (3/0 and 2/0) Chromic catgut or Dexon for ligatures
2·5 and 3 (2/0 and 0) Chromic catgut or Dexon on small half-circle round-bodied needles for peritoneum and muscles
2 (3/0) Silk or nylon on a small curved or straight cutting needle for skin sutures.

OUTLINE OF PROCEDURE

Through a small midline or paramedian incision, the pylorus is delivered into the wound and an incision made through the tumour wall into the circular muscle fibres, care being taken to avoid incising the mucosa. These fibres are stretched with artery or sinus forceps until the mucosa herniates into the muscle incision. The wound is closed in the usual manner.

Gastroenterostomy

DEFINITION

The establishment of an opening between the stomach and the jejunum.

Fig. 15.28 Posterior gastro-jejunostomy. The jejunum is brought through an opening in the transverse mesocolon, and is anastomosed to the posterior wall of the stomach. (Farquharson and Rintoul.)

Fig. 15.29 Anterior gastro-jejunostomy. The jejunum is brought round as a long loop below the transverse colon, and is anastomosed to the anterior wall of the stomach.

POSITION

Supine.

INSTRUMENTS

General set (Figs. 14.1–14.28)
Laparotomy set (Figs. 15.1–15.7)
Intestinal occlusion clamps, straight (Doyen), 2
Intestinal occlusion clamps, curved (Doyen), 2
Twin occlusion clamps (Lane), optional
Fine tissue forceps (McIndoe), 5
Fine artery forceps, straight (mosquito), 5
Suction tubing, nozzles and tube anchoring forceps
Laparotomy ligatures and sutures
2·5 and 3 (2/0 and 0) Chromic catgut or Dexon on medium or small curved non-traumatic intestinal needles for anastomsosis
2·5 (2/0) Silk on small curved non-traumatic intestinal needles for anastomosis.

OUTLINE OF PROCEDURE

Through a left paramedian or midline incision an opening is made in the avascular space of the transverse mesocolon. The posterior wall of the stomach is grasped with tissue forceps on the lesser and greater curvatures at each end of the proposed line of anastomosis. The jejunum is grasped with tissue forceps also, and occlusion clamps applied to the stomach and jejunum. A continuous 2·5 (2/0) chromic catgut or Dexon suture or interrupted silk sutures are used for the posterior seromuscular layer joining the stomach and bowel. The stomach and jejunum are then opened and gastric contents evacuated with the suction tube. The second posterior row of sutures consists of a continuous 2·5 or 3 (2/0 or 0) chromic catgut or Dexon through and through all layers of the stomach and bowel, and this is continued around the stoma to form the first anterior layer. If continuous chromic catgut has been used for the first posterior layer, this suture is continued to form the second seromuscular layer of the anastomosis; alternatively, interrupted silk sutures are used. The opening in the mesocolon is sutured to the stomach before wound closure. This operation is often combined with vagotomy.

Partial gastrectomy

DEFINITION

Resection of a portion of the stomach with anastomosis between the remaining portion of the stomach and the duodenum or jejunum.

POSITION

Supine.

INSTRUMENTS

General set (Figs. 14.1–14.28)
Laparotomy set (Figs. 15.1–15.7)
Gastrectomy set (Fig. 15.30)
Fine artery forceps, straight (McIndoe), 5

Suction tubing, nozzles and tube anchoring forceps
Laparotomy ligatures and sutures
2·5 and 3 (2/0 and 0) Chromic catgut or Dexon on small and medium curved and half-circle non-traumatic intestinal needles for anastomosis
2·5 (2/0) Silk on a small curved or half-circle non-traumatic needle for anastomosis.

OUTLINE OF PROCEDURE

There are several variations in the technique of gastric resection but basically the initial dissection is the same. The incision may be right paramedian or midline and possibly transverse.

The Billroth I or Schoemaker Operation. The omentum on the greater curvature of the stomach is dissected free down to the duodenum, clamping, dividing and ligating the blood vessels in the process. The right gastric vessels on the lesser curvature of the stomach are identified and divided between stout ligatures of chromic catgut or silk. A

Fig. 15.30 Gastrectomy and resection of bowel.

1. Twin occlusion clamp for stomach or intestine (Lane).
2. Intestinal crushing clamps (Joll), 2.
3. Intestinal occlusion clamps, curved (Doyen), 2.
4. Intestinal occlusion clamps, straight (Doyen), 2.
5 and 6. Intestinal crushing clamps, double action, small and large (Payr), 2 of each size.
7. Fine tissue forceps (McIndoe), 4.

crushing clamp is placed across the duodenum at its junction with the stomach, and then alongside this but just distally an occlusion clamp is also applied. The duodenum is divided with a scalpel, which is then discarded. The left gastric or coronary vessels and the vessels in the omentum on the upper left side of the stomach are ligated with stout chromic catgut or silk and then divided. An occlusion clamp is applied across the stomach at the desired level and the organ resected.

The cut end of the stomach is funnelled with two layers of sutures towards the greater curvature and the anastomosis made to the duodenum. The first posterior and second anterior seromuscular layers of the anastomosis consist of continuous 2·5 (2/0) chromic catgut or Dexon suture or interrupted silk sutures. The second posterior and first anterior layers consist of a continuous 3 (0) chromic catgut or Dexon suture placed through and through all layers of the stomach and bowel. Instruments used for the anastomosis are discarded before wound closure.

Billroth II Operation. In all the following variations of this operation, the duodenum is divided between crushing clamps and closed with a continuous chromic catgut suture followed by a second layer of catgut or interrupted silk sutures. The stomach is resected and anastomosed to a loop of jejunum. With the original Billroth II operation, now rarely performed, the cut end of the stomach is closed and the jejunum joined to a fresh opening in the stomach. The Polya operation is perhaps the most common and consists of an end to side anastomosis between the entire cut end of the stomach and the jejunum, posterior to the transverse colon. An anterior Polya resection consists of an end to side anatomosis made in a similar manner but anterior to the transverse colon. The Hoffmeister resection consists of closing the cut end of the stomach, leaving a 51 mm (2 in)

BILROTH 1

POLYA TYPE

Fig. 15.31 The main types of partial gastrectomy. (MacFarlane and Thomas)

Fig. 15.32 Polya type of gastrectomy

Mobilisation of stomach; division and closure of duodenum

(A) The stomach and first part of duodenum are mobilised, and the latter is divided between clamps.
(B) The duodenal stump is closed with an invaginating sero-muscular suture passed from side to side above the clamp.
(C) Closure of the duodenal stump is reinforced with a second invaginating suture. If this is impracticable the first suture line is covered with omentum or is buried by being sutured against the pancreas.
(D) The left gastric vessels are identified and divided between ligatures about 2 cm (1 inch) below the oesophageal orifice.

Fig. 15.32 (cont'd.) Polya type of gastrectomy

Retro-colic anastomosis of valvular (small-stoma) type

- (E) The proximal loop of jejunum is brought through an opening in the transverse mesocolon, and, with the aid of twin clamps, is anastomosed to the stomach at the selected level. The first layer of suture is shown.
- (F) The stomach has been divided and the distal segment removed; the upper part of the cut end is then closed, and the lower part only is used for the anastomosis.
- (G) Diagram to show the reputed effect of the valvular stoma in directing gastric contents into the efferent loop of jejunum.
- (H) The margins of the opening in the mesocolon are sutured to the stomach wall immediately above the anastomosis. (Farquharson and Rintoul.)

stoma on the greater curvature to which the jejunum is anastomosed. Alternatively, a central 51 mm (2 in) stoma may be formed by partially closing the cut end of the stomach from each side. The loop of jejunum is then anastomosed to the opening.

Vagotomy (Adominal approach)

DEFINITION

Division of the vagus nerves often in conjunction with gastro-jejunostomy in the treatment of peptic ulcer or pyloroplasty.

POSITION

Supine.

Fig. 15.33 Total gastrectomy by the abdominal approach. (A) The duodenum is divided and the completely mobilised stomach is turned upwards to expose the posterior surface of the oesophagus. (B) The method of anastomosing oesophagus to a loop of jejunum is shown. (C) Finally an entero-anastomosis is performed, and a tube is led down into the efferent loop of jejunum. (Farquharson and Rintoul.)

INSTRUMENTS

General set (Figs. 14.1–14.28)
Laparotomy set (Figs. 15.1–15.7)
Gastro-enterostomy set (page 343) if gastro-jejunostomy is to be carried out.
Laparotomy ligatures and sutures.

Fig. 15.34 Trans-abdominal vagotomy. Exposure of the lower 2 inches of the oesophagus, with the left (anterior) vagus nerve on its surface. (Farquharson and Rintoul.)

Fig. 15.35 Trans-abdominal vagotomy. Resection of a portion of both vagus nerves—(A) the left (anterior), and (B) the right (posterior). (Farquharson and Rintoul.)

OUTLINE OF PROCEDURE

The incision may be midline or paramedian. The left triangular ligament is divided to mobilize the left lobe of the liver, which is displaced to the right with a pack.

The transverse colon and small intestine are displaced downwards with a pack. Utilising deep retractors and traction, the stomach is drawn downwards to expose the gastro-oesophageal junction. After incising the covering peritoneum, a finger is passed upwards to gently mobilize the oesophagus within the posterior peritoneum.

The lower 5 to 8 cm (2 to 3 inches) of the oesophagus is drawn into the abdomen and immoblised with a tape or tubing sling. The anterior (left) vagus nerve, which may have two divisions is identified and sectioned between forceps. The upper end is ligated with non-absorbable ligatures, and the lower end withdrawn to expose other branches of the nerve. These are excised for a length of 3 to 5 cm (1½ to 2 inches).

The posterior (right) vagus nerve lies behind the oesophagus. This is identified and excised in a similar manner to the anterior nerve. If a gastro-jejunostomy is to be carried out, this follows the vagotomy. The abdomen is closed as for laparotomy.

Total gastrectomy

This is occasionally performed for malignancy and the dissection approximates to that for partial gastrectomy but is more extensive. Although the procedure may be carried out by the abdominal route as illustrated, in most instances a thoraco-abdominal approach is employed. A Billroth I type of anastomosis may be used, joining the oesophagus to the duodenum, but more commonly an oesophagojejunostomy is established.

Intussusception

DEFINITION

Obstruction from invaginated bowel.

POSITION

Supine with Trendelenburg for colonic invagination.

INSTRUMENTS

As for gastrectomy (p. 343) (resection of bowel may be necessary).

OUTLINE OF PROCEDURE

Through a paramedian or midline incision, the deformity is reduced by gentle pessure exerted on the head of the invaginated portion of the bowel. Warm packs are applied and if the bowel is non-viable, it is resected in the usual manner and the wound closed.

Resection of small bowel

DEFINITION

Resection of a portion of the small intestine.

POSITION

Supine.

INSTRUMENTS

As for gastrectomy (p. 343).

OUTLINE OF PROCEDURE

The incision may be paramedian or midline (an exception being when treating a strangulated hernia and in this case the bowel may be delivered via the hernial orifice).

Fig. 15.36 Technique of resection in small bowel. (Farquharson and Rintoul.)

The mesenteric vessels supplying the loop of bowel are identified and ligated with chromic catgut or silk. Crushing and occlusion clamps are applied at each side of the affected section of bowel which is then resected. The occlusion clamps are retained until an end to end or side to side anastomosis has been made, using two layers of continuous chromic catgut or Dexon. Anastomosis instruments are discarded before wound closure in the usual manner.

Right hemicolectomy

DEFINITION

Resection of the right half of the colon.

POSITION

Supine.

INSTRUMENTS

As for gastrectomy (p. 343).

OUTLINE OF PROCEDURE

Through a right paramedian or midline incision, the ascending colon and distal part of the ileum are mobilised from the lateral peritoneal fold. The ureter and duodenum are identified, the mesentery incised, and the mesenteric vessels ligated with chromic catgut or silk before division. If the anastomosis is to be made side to side, crushing clamps are applied across the transverse colon and the ileum. The bowel is then resected and the stumps closed with a layer of continuous 3 (0) chromic catgut or Dexon through

Fig. 15.37 Resection of small bowel with side-to-side anastomosis.

(A, B and C) Division of bowel and closure of cut-end with inverting suture.
(D) Method of anastomosis. The first layer of sutures has been inserted, and the seromuscular coat has been incised. (Farquharson and Rintoul.)

Fig. 15.38 Right-sided hemicolectomy.

(A) Terminal ileum and mobilised right side of colon about to be divided between clamps. A ligature is shown applied to right colic and ileo-colic arteries.
(B and C) Closure of cut ends of bowel.
(D) Side-to-side anastomosis completed. (Farquharson and Rintoul.)

and through sutures and a seromuscular layer of interrupted silk sutures. Curved occlusion clamps are applied and a side to side anastomosis made in the usual mnner. If the anastomosis is to be end to end, crushing and occlusion clamps are applied transversely across the colon and obliquely across the ileum. The bowel is resected and the occlusion clamps retained until the anastomosis is completed in the usual manner. The instruments used for the anastomosis are discarded, the defect in the posterior peritoneum and mesentery sutured and the wound closed.

Total colectomy

DEFINITION

Resection of the ascending, transverse and descending colon.

POSITION

Supine with some degree of Trendelenburg.

INSTRUMENTS

As for gastrectomy (p. 343).
Intestinal occlusion clamps, right-angled (Finch), 2.

OUTLINE OF PROCEDURE

The incision may be midline or paramedian. The colon is mobilised from the distal end of the ileum to the sigmoid flexure, ligating and dividing the mesenteric and superior haemorrhoidal vessels with stout chromic catgut, Dexon or silk. Resection of the colon between two sets of crushing and occlusion clamps is performed and anastomosis made between the ileum and the rectum (ileorectostomy) in the usual manner, or the rectum is closed with interrupted silk sutures and an ileostomy performed. If the resection is low, the rectal anastomosis may be made with a series of interrupted mattress sutures of 3 (0) chromic catgut, Dexon or silk which are left long and not tied until all have been placed in position.

Abdominoperineal resection of the rectum and part of the colon

DEFINITION

Mobilisation of the diseased portion of the colon which is pushed into the hollow of the pelvis for removal via the perineal route, and the establishment of a terminal colostomy.

POSITION

Lithotomy and Trendelenburg with a sandbag or similar support under the buttocks.

INSTRUMENTS

Anterior Part of the Operation
  General set (Figs. 14.1–14.28)
  Laparotomy set (Figs. 15.1–15.7)
  Long scalpel handle No. 4L with No. 20 blade (Bard Parker)
  Long dissecting forceps, toothed, 25 cm (10 in)
  Long dissecting forceps, non-toothed, 25 cm (10 in)
  Long scissors, curved on flat, 23 cm (9 in) (Nelson)
  Scissors, straight, 20 cm (8 in) (Mayo)
  Intestinal occlusion clamps, straight (Doyen), 2
  Intestinal occlusion clamps, curved (Doyen), 2
  Intestinal crushing clamps (Payr or Joll), 2
  Intestinal crushing clamps (de Martel or Zachary Cope), set of 3
  Suprapubic retractor (Doyen)

Suction tubing, nozzles and tube anchoring forceps
Diathermy leads, electrodes and lead anchoring forceps
Ligatures and sutures as for laparotomy
Long tissue forceps, 20 cm (8 in) (Lane's or Fagge's), 5

Posterior Part of Operation
General set (Figs. 14.1–14.28)
Extra towel clips, 5
Long scalpel handle No. 4L with No. 20 blade (Bard Parker)
Long tissue forceps, 20 cm (8 in) (Lane's or Fagge's), 5

Fig. 15.39 Parker-Kerr Intestinal Clamp (Crushing).

Fig. 15.40 De Martel Intestinal Clamps (Crushing).

Fig. 15.41 Mikulicz Enterotome (Crushing).

Fig. 15.42 Lloyd Davies Rectal Excision Clamp.

Deep retractors, narrow blade (Paton), 2
Rugines curved and straight (Faraboeuf)
Bone nibbling or gouge forceps (single action)
Bone nibbling or gouge forceps (compound action)
Bone cutting forceps, curved (Liston)
Long scissors, straight, 20 cm (8 in) (Mayo)
Long scissors, curved on flat, 20 cm (8 in) (Mayo)
Urethral catheter, 18 to 20 Charrière gauge (Jacques, Nélaton, or Foley self-retaining)
(If Foley catheter is used, a syringe containing 5 to 30 ml of sterile water to inflate the catheter cuff, and a ligature for the pilot tube will be required, unless this is self-sealing.)
Spigot

Fig. 15.43 Abdomino-perineal excision of rectum—abdominal dissection.

The pelvic colon has been mobilised by incision of the peritoneum along its lateral side. Note the position of the left ureter crossing the bifurcation of the left common iliac artery, and how it may be endangered by the dissection. The inferior mesenteric artery is elevated on the forceps and is about to be divided just below the origin of its upper left colic branch. (Farquharson and Rintoul.)

Fig. 15.44 Abdomino-perineal excision of rectum—abdominal dissection.

(A) A Payr's clamp has been introduced through a *circular* incision in the left iliac fossa, and applied to the bowel at the level for division; a second clamp has been applied immediately below. The bowel is about to be divided between the clamps, when the proximal cut end can be brought out to form the colostomy.
(B) Method of closing the peritoneal gutter lateral to the bowel. (Farquharson and Rintoul.)

Extra-peritoneal colostomy.

(C) Cut end of pelvic colon drawn to exterior through the extra-peritoneal tissues.
(D) Re-peritonisation completed. (Golligher, by kind permission.)

Large rubber or plastic drainage tube
3 and 4 (0 and 1) Chromic catgut or Dexon for ligatures
4 or 5 (1 or 2) Chromic catgut or Dexon on a large half-circle cutting needle for deep sutures
5 (2) Silk on a large half-circle cutting needle for anal purse-string sutures
2·5 (2/0) Silk or nylon in large curved cutting needles for skin sutures.

OUTLINE OF PROCEDURE

Generally this operation is performed as a synchronous-combined procedure by two operation teams. In this case the instrument sets must be available on two trolleys for simultaneous use and it is very important that the swab count of each team is kept separate. To assist this, the instrument nurse assisting the surgeon performing the anterior part of the operation will ensure that only 'taped' swabs or packs are used in the vicinity of the pelvis and that instruments are not interchanged between the teams.

The Anterior Part of the Operation. Through a lower midline incision the bowel is mobilised from the point of transection to the coccyx, ligating and dividing the inferior mesenteric vessels. Slender crushing clamps such as the de Martel's are applied across the colon, above the diseased portion. The bowel is divided and the proximal end brought out through an incision at the selected site for the permanent colostomy. A rubber glove is secured over the distal clamp to prevent soiling of the peritoneum, and the diseased

Fig. 15.45 Perineal dissection for excision of the rectum—patient in the lithotomy position. The coccyx has been disarticulated, and the levator ani on the right side is about to be divided between two fingers which have been passed forwards above it. *Inset* shows incision. (Farquharson and Rintoul.)

portion of the bowel and rectum is pushed into the hollow of the pelvis for removal by the surgeon performing the perineal part of the operation. The pelvic peritoneum is sutured with a continuous 2·5 (2/0) or 3 (0) chromic catgut or Dexon before general wound closure.

The Posterior Part of the Operation. A urethal catheter is inserted and the bladder emptied. The rectum is sealed by placing two purse-string sutures around the anus, and an elliptical incision made round the rectum exposing the levator ani muscles, which are divided. The urethra is identified and in co-operation with the surgeon performing the anterior part of the operation, the rectum is freed with scissors. The diseased bowel and rectum is removed through the posterior incision and the muscles approximated with chromic catgut. A long drainage tube (which will be attached to a suitable sterile bottle) is used to drain the pelvic space before skin closure with silk or nylon.

Anterior resection of the rectum and part of the Colon

DEFINITION

A sphincter-saving resection of the rectum and part of the colon with re-establishment of continuity by anastomosis.

POSITION

As for abdominoperineal resection.

Fig. 15.46 Anterior (trans-abdominal) resection of the rectum—division of the bowel between clamps below the tumour. (Best, by kind permission.) (Farquharson and Rintoul.)

Fig. 15.47 Anterior (trans-abdominal) resection of the rectum—anastomosis of pelvic colon to stump of rectum—using AutoSuture® stapling technique. (Auto-Suture Ltd.)

INSTRUMENTS

As for abdominoperineal resection
Minus de Martel clamps
Plus Intestinal occlusion clamps, right-angled (Finch), 2
Plus Proctoscope (Fig. 13.18).

OUTLINE OF PROCEDURE

Through a lower midline incision, the colon is mobilised from the point of transection to the ano-rectal junction, ligating and dividing the inferior mesenteric vessels. It is then divided between clamps, one a right-angled clamp (Finch) placed proximally to the two.

The mesorectum is separated from the back of the rectum at the level selected for division below the growth (not less than 6 cm from its inferior edge). The mesorectum is

Fig. 15.48 Technique of transverse colostomy.

(A) Loop of colon mobilised.
(B) Colostomy rod in position.
(C and D) Double barrel defunctioning type of colostomy.
(E) Method of suturing colostomy to skin. Stitches are placed to pick up the mucosal edge, the bowel wall about 2 cm below (not penetrating the lumen), and finally the skin margin.
(A, B, C and E: Farquharson and Rintoul, D: Macfarlane and Thomas.)

then clamped with two large artery forceps, divided and ligated leaving the rectum bared all round over a segment about 4 cm long.

The bowel is then clamped at the upper end of this bared segment with right-angled clamps, the rectum is transected, and the colon clamp brought into proximity to the open stump of the rectum. A row of seromuscular mattress Lembert sutures are inserted both laterally and medially and left untied. A further row of through and through mattress sutures are inserted and when all are placed the sutures are tied. This slides the colon down to the cut edge of the rectum, invaginates the suture line and completes the anastomosis. Finally the clamp is removed and the pelvic peritoneum sutured over the anastomosis to extraperitonealise the suture line. Stapling instruments are available which complete the anastomosis in one action, and enable resection to within about 2 cm ($\frac{3}{4}$ inch) segment of the rectal margin (Heald, 1980).

A drainage tube is inserted and the wound closed in layers in the normal manner.

Colostomy

DEFINITION

The establishment of a temporary or permanent opening in the colon.

POSITION

Supine.

INSTRUMENTS

General set (Figs. 14.1–14.28)
Laparotomy set (Figs. 15.1–15.7)
Long scissors, curved on flat (McIndoe)
Fine artery forceps, straight (mosquito)
Fine tissue forceps (McIndoe), 6
Glass or plastic colostomy rod and tubing
Diathermy cable and electrodes
Paraffin gauze dressing or colostomy bag (i.e. colostomy is to be opened immediately)
Ligatures and sutures as for laparotomy.

OUTLINE OF PROCEDURE

The incision can be paramedian, midline or in the iliac region as described for apendicectomy. The colon is mobilised and a loop brought either through the original incision or through a separate stab wound (inguinal colostomy). An opening is made in the mesentery of this loop of bowel, and a glass or nylon rod (attached at one end to a short piece of tubing) is passed between the skin and bowel. The tubing is then attached to the other end of the rod, forming a D-shaped loop which retains it in position. The wound is closed and petroleum jelly gauze placed around the exteriorised bowel. The colostomy is usually opened with a diathermy knife or cautery, but the apparatus should be available in case the surgeon decides to open the bowel in theatre. If the colostomy is opened immediately after operation, a self-adhesive colostomy bag may be applied, in this instance the cut edge of the bowel is sutured as shown in Figure 15.48E.

Closure of colostomy

DEFINITION

Re-establishment of intestinal continuity.

POSITION

Supine.

INSTRUMENTS

General set (Figs. 14.1–14.28)
Deep retractors, narrow blade (Paton), 2
Intestinal occlusion clamps, straight (Doyen), 2
Fine tissue forceps (McIndoe), 5
Fine artery forceps, curved on flat (mosquito), 10
2·5 (2/0) Chromic catgut, Dexon or silk for ligatures
2·5 (2/0) Chromic catgut or Dexon and silk on a small curved non-traumatic intestinal needle for closure of bowel
3 or 4 (0 or 1) Chromic catgut or Dexon on a medium half-circle round-bodied or Mayo needle for peritoneum and muscle
2·5 (2/0) Silk or nylon on a large curved or straight cutting needle for skin sutures.

OUTLINE OF PROCEDURE

An extraperitoneal or intraperitoneal closure may be performed. If an extraperitoneal closure is contemplated, the spur between the upper and lower portion of the colostomy will have been crushed previously by an enterotribe (see Fig. 15.41).

For extraperitoneal closure an elliptical incision is made around the colostomy and the skin and bowel freed down to the peritoneum. The segment of skin attached to the colostomy is excised and the opening in the colon closed with one layer of continuous chromic catgut or Dexon and one layer of interrupted silk sutures. The peritoneum and muscle are plicated over the sutured colon and the wound is closed.

For intraperitoneal closure the dissection is the same except that the peritoneum is opened at each side of the exteriorised colon. The bowel is sutured in the manner already described or is divided at each side of the colostomy, and an end to end anastomosis made. The wound is closed.

Ileostomy

DEFINITION

The establishment of an opening into the ileum (generally permanent).

POSITION

Supine.

INSTRUMENTS

As for colostomy
Intestinal occlusion clamps, straight (Doyen), 2
2·5 (2/0) Chromic catgut or Dexon on a small curved non-traumatic intestinal needle for ileum closure. Ileostomy bag.

OUTLINE OF PROCEDURE

This operation is usually done for ulcerative colitis. Through a low paramedian or midline incision, the ileum is mobilised and two occlusion clamps applied at the selected

Fig. 15.49 The types of operation performed for ulcerative colitis. (A) Ileostomy. (B) Ileostomy with resection of the colon and rectum. (C) Resection of colon with ileorectal anastomosis. (Macfarlane and Thomas.)

Fig. 15.50 Splenectomy (left). The spleen is lifted forwards and is mobilised by incision of the peritoneum passing from its lateral surface on to the posterior abdominal wall, *i.e.* the posterior layer of the lieno-renal ligament. (right) The gastro-splenic ligament is divided between clamps and ligatured. The thin anterior layer of the lieno-renal ligament is then incised to expose the splenic vessels and the tail of the pancreas. (Farquharson and Rintoul.)

point for ileostomy. The ileum is transected and the proximal end brought out through a small circular wound made in the right side of the abdomen. The distal end of the ileum is closed with 2·5 (2/0) chromic catgut or Dexon and the wound is closed. The base of the exteriorised ileum is sutured to the abdominal wall and the mucosa is then everted. The cut edge of the mucosa is sutured to the skin with 2·5 (2/0) chromic catgut or Dexon. An ileostomy bag is usually applied immediately at the end of the operation.

Splenectomy

DEFINITION

Removal of the spleen.

POSITION

Supine.

INSTRUMENTS

As for laparotomy, including ligatures and sutures (p. 329).

OUTLINE OF PROCEDURE

A midline, left paramedian or transverse incision is made. The spleen is palpated, and if there are any adhesions these are clamped with forceps before dividing. The gastrosplenic ligament is first divided and then the lateral peritoneal fold of the lienorenal ligament is incised, allowing the spleen to be brought forward into the wound. The major splenic vessels are either clamped with sets of two strong artery forceps and divided, or are individually ligatured with double strong silk or thread and cut after the ligatures have been tied. The spleen is then free and may be removed. The wound is closed in layers.

Inguinal or scrotal herniorrhaphy

DEFINITION

The obliteration of a sac containing viscera, which have protruded from the abdomen, either as a direct hernia through Hesselbach's triangle, or as an indirect hernia through the internal ring.

POSITION

Supine.

INSTRUMENTS

General set (Figs. 14.1–14.28)
2·5 and 3 (2/0 and 0) Chromic catgut or Dexon for ligatures
3 or 4 (0 or1) Chromic catgut or Dexon on a small or medium half-circle round-bodied needle for the hernial sac, and on a half-circle cutting needle for the muscle tendon
Repair material of choice, e.g., monofilament, braided nylon; braided silk; polyethylene; polyester; linen thread; stainless steel wire; and mesh made from nylon,

Fig. 15.51 Diagrammatic sections of the long axis of the inguinal canal.

In all three diagrams the external spermatic fascia is shown to be continuous with the aponeurosis of the external oblique muscle.

(1) The upper diagram shows the normal spermatic cord and its coverings.
(2) The middle diagram shows an oblique inguinal hernia. Note the relationship of the hernial sac to the inferior epigastric artery. In an oblique hernia the sac descends within the coverings of the spermatic cord.
(3) The lowest diagram shows a direct inguinal hernia. Note the relationship of the neck of the hernial sac to the inferior epigastric artery. In a direct inguinal hernia the external spermatic fascia is the only covering which the hernia shares with the spermatic cord. (Bruce, Walmsley and Ross.)

braided silk or wire (Chapter 7); small or medium stout half-circle needles, such as Mayo needles, or special types such as fish-hook shape may be used to facilitate the suturing with the chosen material

2·5 (2/0) Silk or nylon on medium or large curved or straight cutting needles for skin sutures

(Alternatively, Michel or Kifa clips may be used.)

Fig. 15.52 Simple herniotomy for oblique inguinal hernia; incision in external oblique aponeurosis, separation of sac by gauze dissection, transfixion ligature of the sac at its neck, and repair of external oblique aponeurosis. (Farquharson and Rintoul.)

Fig. 15.53 The Bassini method of repair in inguinal hernia—approximation of the conjoined muscles and tendon to the inguinal ligament, behind the spermatic cord; this is held out of the way, under cover of the lower flap of external oblique. (Farquharson and Rintoul.)

Gallie's Repair, Extra Instruments
   Fascia forceps, right and left, 2
   Fasciatome or fascia stripper
   Gallie's living suture needles—small, medium and large
   2·5 and 3 (2/0 and 0) Silk on small half-circle round-bodied needles for securing graft.

OUTLINE OF PROCEDURE

Through an incision overlying the inguinal canal, the spermatic cord is mobilised and retracted with a piece of ribbon gauze or tubing. By separating the coverings of the cord, the hernial sac is found and isolated. It is opened to make quite sure that it is empty, transfixed, ligated with 3 or 4 (0 or 1) chromic catgut or Dexon at the internal ring, and is cut off. This is all that is necessary in infants who require no repair of the muscles at this stage.

There are many repair procedures, including the *Bassini operation* which consists of interrupted silk sutures from the border of the internal oblique and transversus abdominus muscles to the inguinal ligament deep to the spermatic cord. In *Gallie's repair* a strip of fascia lata is removed from the lateral aspect of the thigh either with a fasciatome or via a long incision extending from just above the knee to the great trochanter. This fascia is then sutured 'zigzag' fashion across the posterior inguinal wall to strengthen it. A *nylon darn* consists of a continuous monofilament or braided nylon suture, introduced forwards and backwards across the posterior inguinal wall, extending from the internal oblique and transversus abdominus muscles to the inguinal ligament without actually drawing them into approximation.

Stainless steel wire or braided nylon/silk mesh may be used to strengthen the posterior wall. A piece of suitable shape and size is sutured around its periphery to the muscles described above.

The hernia repair may be further strengthened by overlapping the external oblique, suturing the upper margin to the inguinal ligament and using the part below the incision for an overlap. This means that the anterior wall of the inguinal canal has a double instead of a single layer of external oblique. The wound is closed.

Femoral herniorrhaphy

DEFINITION

This is similar to an inguinal hernia but the sac protrudes through the femoral ring into the femoral canal.

POSITION

As for inguinal hernia.

INSTRUMENTS

As for inguinal hernia (p. 364).

OUTLINE OF PROCEDURE

The hernial sac is exposed below the inguinal ligament, freed, ligated and excised as previously described. The femoral canal is then usually closed from above by opening the inguinal canal and suturing the conjoined tendon to the pectineal ligament with interrupted silk or thread sutures. The operation then proceeds as for inguinal hernia.

Umbilical hernia

DEFINITION

A protrusion of intestine through the umbilicus or muscle surrounding the umbilicus. (In congenital form, the loop of intestine can easily be seen through a thin transparent membrane and is not strictly speaking a true hernia, for the bowel has never been inside the abdomen. The aquired hernia in children is due to the scar of the umbilicus giving way because of some strain (e.g., coughing). In adults usually the obese patient, the hernia occurs above or below the umbilical scar itself.)

POSITION

Supine.

INSTRUMENTS

As for inguinal hernia (p. 364).

OUTLINE OF PROCEDURE

A transverse elliptical incision is made above or below the umbilicus. The sac is isolated, opened, and the omentum contained either dissected free or clamped and resected. The redundant sac is excised, and the peritoneal opening closed with 4 or 5 (1 or 2) chromic catgut or Dexon. Repair is accomplished by overlapping the aponeurosis transversely with interrupted silk or thread mattress sutures (Mayo procedure). The skin wound is closed.

Ventral hernia

DEFINITION

A protusion of abdominal viscera through an opening in the linea semilunaris, linea alba or through the scar of an abdominal incision.

POSITION

Supine.

INSTRUMENTS

As for inguinal hernia (p. 364).

OUTLINE OF PROCEDURE

Through the selected incision the sac is identified and obliterated. The abdominal wall is repaired either with a fascial strip or a non-absorbable suture material (see inguinal hernia) and the wound is then closed.

Fig. 15.54 Mayo's operation for umbilical hernia—repair by overlapping or fascial sutures.

(A) Clearance of the aponeurosis centrally towards the neck of the sac.
(B) Circular division of the neck of the sac and its fibrous covering.
(C) Mattress sutures inserted to draw one flap under cover of the other.
(D) Overlapping completed by suturing down free edge of superficial flap.

Fig. 15.55 (*Left*) Repair of scar hernia (median sub-umbilical) by overlapping of the anterior rectus sheaths, relaxation incisions being made on each side.

Fig. 15.56 (*Right*) Repair of scar hernia (median sub-umbilical) by a double layer of fascial sutures, without any attempt to dissect out the individual muscle layers. (Farquharson and Rintoul.)

Strangulated hernia

DEFINITION

Gangrene of an intestinal loop contained within a hernial sac, due to compression of its mesentery and blood-vessels.

POSITION

Supine.

INSTRUMENTS

As for inguinal hernia (p. 364)
Fine tissue forceps (McIndoe), 5
Fine artery forceps, straight (mosquito), 5
Intestinal occlusion clamps, straight (Doyen), 2
Intestinal occlusion clamps, curved (Doyen), 2
Intestinal crushing clamps (Payr, Joll or Schoemaker), 2
Artery forceps, straight, 20 cm (8 in) (Spencer Wells), 10
Long artery forceps, curved on flat (Moynihan gall-bladder), 5
Hernia director and bistoury
2·5 and 3 (2/0 and 0) Chromic catgut or Dexon on small or medium non-traumatic intestinal needles for resection anastomosis
Ligatures and sutures as for inguinal hernia.

OUTLINE OF PROCEDURE

The approach and dissection follows that for inguinal hernia or umbilical hernia, etc. The sac is opened and the gangrenous contents prevented from slipping into the abdomen whilst the constricting area is divided, perhaps with a director and bistoury under direct vision. Warm, moist packs are applied to the bowel and if it does not appear viable after five minutes, a resection of the affected part is carried out in the usual manner. Repair is carried out in the usual manner.

Haemorrhoidectomy

DEFINITION

The excision of internal piles.

POSITION

Lithotomy or jack-knife.

INSTRUMENTS

Sponge-holding forceps (Rampley), 5
Towel clips, 5
Rectal speculum (Kelly, Gabrial, etc.)
Scalpel handle No. 3 with No. 10 blade (Bard Parker)
Dissecting forceps, toothed, 2
Scissors, straight, 15 cm (6 in) (Mayo)

Scissors, curved on flat, 15 cm (6 in) (Mayo)
Artery forceps, straight (Moynihan), 10
Dissectors (MacDonald and Durham), 2
Pile clamps (Kocher, curved), 6
Aneurysm needle
2·5 (2/0) Chromic catgut or Dexon for fine ligatures
6 (3) Chromic catgut, Dexon or silk on a medium curved round-bodied needle for pile transfixion and ligation
Stout rubber or plastic drainage tube and safety-pin
(Three small packs made from petroleum jelly gauze, or ribbon gauze soaked in antiseptic, may be required to pack around the tube to control oozing from pile areas after operation.)

Fig. 15.57 Haemorrhoidectomy by the dissection-ligature technique. (Farquharson and Rintoul.)

OUTLINE OF PROCEDURE

The three piles are each clamped with forceps and individually dissected upwards off the muscular coat of the anal canal until a pedicle is formed. This pedicle is transfixed at the base, ligated and two-thirds of the pile cut off together with the tag of skin corresponding to the pile. A drainage tube may be inserted.

Anal fissure

DEFINITION

A small vertical ulcer at the anal margin.

POSITION

Lithotomy or jack-knife.

INSTRUMENTS

As for haemorrhoidectomy
Malleable probe
Small retractors, double hook, 2
Sinus forceps
Curetting spoon, double end (Volkmann)
Petroleum jelly gauze roll.

Fig. 15.58 Excision of an anal fissure. (Farquharson and Rintoul.)

OUTLINE OF PROCEDURE

The anal margins are retracted and a knife directed against the floor of the ulcer dividing the internal sphincter fibres. There is usually a small tag of skin (the so-called 'sentinel pile') in the region of the fissure, and this is cut away to provide free drainage. The wound is plugged with petroleum jelly gauze.

Fistula in ano

DEFINITION

A sinus or sinuses between the anal canal and the skin in the region of the anus.

POSITION

Lithotomy or jack-knife.

INSTRUMENTS

As for anal fissure.

OUTLINE OF PROCEDURE

The sinuses are opened to provide free drainage, care being taken to divide only the subcutaneous sphincter muscle, otherwise, incontinence may result. The surgeon may require a sterile dye to assist identification of the sinuses and indigo carmine or methylene blue together with a syringe and cannula should be available.

REFERENCES AND FURTHER READING

FARQUHARSON, E. L. AND RINTOUL, R. F. (1972) *Textbook of Operative Surgery*. Edinburgh: Churchill Livingstone.
HEALD, R. (1980) *Nursing Mirror*, **150**, No. 1, 30.
MACFARLANE, D. A. AND THOMAS, L. P. (1972) *Textbook of Surgery*. Edinburgh: Churchill Livingstone.

16
OPERATIONS ON THE BREAST

Incision of breast abscess
DEFINITION

The incision and drainage of an abscess due to acute mastitis.

POSITION

Supine.

INSTRUMENTS

    Sponge-holding forceps (Rampley), 2
    Towel clips, 5
    Scalpel handle No. 3 with No. 10 blade (Bard Parker)
    Dissecting forceps, toothed, 2
    Dissecting forceps, non-toothed, 2
    Scissors, curved on flat, 13 cm (5 in) (Mayo)
    Sinus forceps, 18 cm (7 in)
    Probe, malleable silver
    Artery forceps, straight (Moynihan), 5
    20 ml syringe with wide-bore exploration needles
    Sterile culture tube
    2·5 (2/0) plastic drainage tubing and safety-pin
    Latex rubber or plastic drainage tubing and safety-pin
    2·5 (2/0) Silk or nylon on a large curved cutting needle for securing drainage tubing.

OUTLINE OF PROCEDURE

An incision or incisions are made radiating from the nipple. If the abscess is loculated, care is taken to drain each compartment. A split drainage tube is inserted and secured to the skin with a suture. A firm dressing is applied.

Excision of simple adenoma or amputation of the breast (simple mastectomy)
DEFINITION

The removal or a simple adenoma; or amputation of the mammary gland, most commonly for chronic mastitis.

POSITION

Supine, with arms extended on narrow arm boards (Fig. 4.12).

INSTRUMENTS

    Genral set (Figs. 14.1–14.28)
    Local infiltration set (Fig. 10.35) with adrenaline 1:400,000 (optional)
    Artery forceps, curved on flat (Kelly Fraser, Dunhill, etc.), 25
    Large tissue forceps (Lane or Fagge), 5
    Diathermy leads, electrodes and lead anchoring forceps
    Short rubber or plastic drainage tube and safety-pin for adenoma; or long drainage tube and Redi-vac or Portovac for mastectomy
    2·5 and 3 (2/0 and 0) Chromic catgut or Dexon for ligatures
    2·5 (2/0) Silk or nylon on a large curved or straight cutting needle for skin sutures.

OUTLINE OF PROCEDURE

A simple adenoma is removed through an incision placed over the swelling, but extending radially from the nipple to conserve the secreting ducts. The wound is closed with or without drainage.

For simple mastectomy, the skin and subcutaneous tissues over the incision line may be infiltrated with 100 to 300 ml of a 1:400,000 adrenaline solution to minimise bleeding. An elliptical, vertical incision is then made extending from the axilla to the sternum, enclosing the nipple in the centre of the ellipse. The skin is dissected from the breast until the surgeon has reached the limits of the gland in all directions. The breast is peeled off the deep fascia (without cutting into it) towards the axilla, using light strokes of the knife, until the axillary tail of the gland is reached. The blood vessels at this point are ligated before freeing the breast, which is then removed. A drain is placed in the lower end of the wound which is closed in the usual manner. A negative pressure may be applied to this drainage tube in the manner described on page 378.

Radial mastectomy

DEFINITION

Removal of the mammary gland, together with the pectoralis minor and major muscles, and the axillary glands. The operation is performed for malignant tumours of the breast.

POSITION

Supine with arms extended on narrow arm boards, or only one secured and the other (operation side) held by a seated assistant. The arm is more easily supported in a flexed position, holding the elbow in one hand and the wrist in the other. The elbow must not be allowed to drop below the plane of the operation table or abducted more than a right angle to the body, for the nerves may be stretched over the humeral head and cause paralysis.

INSTRUMENTS

    General set (Figs. 14.1–14.28)
    Local infiltration set (Fig. 10.35) with adrenaline 1:400,000 (optional)
    Artery forceps, curved on flat (Kelly Fraser, two-thirds serrated jaws), 25
    Artery forceps, curved on flat (Dunhill, fully serrated jaws), 25
    Large tissue forceps (Lane or Fagge), 6
    Diathermy leads, electrodes and lead anchoring forceps

Fig. 16.1 Extent of dissection required in the operation of radial mastectomy. (Farquharson and Rintoul.)

Long plastic drainage tube and Redi-vac
2·5 and 3 (2/0 and 0) Chromic catgut or Dexon and silk or thread for ligatures
3 (0) Chromic catgut or Dexon on a medium half-circle round-bodied needle for axillary sutures
2·5 (2/0) Silk or nylon on a large cuved or straight cutting needle for skin sutures
(Skin graft instruments may be required, page 621).

OUTLINE OF PROCEDURE

The skin and subcutaneous tissues over the incision line may be infiltrated with 100 to 300 ml of 1:400,000 adrenaline solution to minimise bleeding. An elliptical, vertical incision is then made, keeping at least 50 mm (2 in) from the growth all round, which is in the centre of the ellipse. The skin flaps over the axilla are reflected to expose the pectoralis major and minor muscles which are severed from their insertions. The fat and glands contained in the axilla are cleared by dissection, carefully avoiding damage to the major blood vessels, subscapularis nerve and the nerve of Bell. The skin flaps overlying the breast are reflected and the breast removed together with the pectoralis muscles underneath, extending from the sternum medially to the border of the latissimus dorsi muscle.

Fig. 16.2 Perforated suction catheter in position prior to wound closure (inset shows catheter protruding from separate stab incision). Operation depicted is that on a limb although a similar technique is used for draining a mastectomy wound. (Zimmer Orthopaedic Ltd.)

Fig. 16.3 The Redi-vac suction device showing vacuum bottle, suction catheter and insertion trocar. (Zimmer Orthopaedic Ltd.)

Fig. 16.4 Portovac portable wound suction unit. (Howmedica (U.K.) Ltd.)

A long drainage tube is inserted into the axilla through a separate stab incision, the skin flaps are approximated with tissue forceps and the wound is closed.

The long drainage tube is either coupled to an under-water collection bottle (Chapter 25), or preferably a slight negative pressure is applied by connecting a Redi-vac bottle to the open end of the tube.

FURTHER READING

FARQUHARSON, E. L. and RINTOUL, R. F. (1972) *Textbook of Operative Surgery*. Edinburgh: Churchill Livingstone.

17
DENTAL OPERATIONS

Dental extraction

DEFINITION

The removal of a tooth or root either under local or general anaesthesia.

POSITION

Supine, or sitting with the head and neck extended slightly.

INSTRUMENTS

Mouth gag (Mason or Doyen)
Dental props, set
Tongue forceps
Angled tongue depressor
Dental conveying forceps, stout and fine, 2
Dental extraction forceps, set
Dental elevators and probes, set
Mouth mirror
Local anaesthetic, e.g., 2 per cent lignocaine (Xylocaine) and dental syringe may be required
Mouth wash.

Fig. 17.1 Examples of upper and lower dental extration forceps. (Birmingham Dental Hospital.)

OUTLINE OF PROCEDURE

If general anaesthesia is to be administered, mouth props are inserted to prevent the patient from closing his jaw. Following the administration of a local anaesthetic, five minutes are allowed to elapse before the operation is commenced. The teeth are extracted and the patient is allowed a gentle mouth wash before leaving the dental chair.

Fig. 17.2 Removal of impacted wisdom tooth.

1. Dental mirror.
2. Dental conveying forceps, fine and stout, 2.
3. (A) Root elevator straight.
   (B) Probe.
   (C) Probe and scaler.
   (D) Specula and spoon.
4. Spatula.
5. Curette (Volkmann).
6. Apical elevators, left and right, 2.
7. Apical elevators, left and right, 2.
9. Small gouges (Jenkins), 3 mm, 4 mm, 6 mm, and 8 mm, 4.
10. Small mallet (Rowland).
11. Dental cavity syringe.
12. Dental extraction forceps, appropriate shape.
13. Root elevators (Winter), 4.
14. Root elevators (Hospital), right and left, 4.
15. Root elevator (Read).
16. Retractors, cheek, 2.
17. Retractors, cheek, 2.
18. Dental drill handpieces, straight and angled, 2.
19. Dental burrs, fissure and rose-end type.
20. Bone-nibbling or gouge forceps, 2 sizes.
21. Gag (Brunton).
22. Mouth prop (Hewitt).

Not illustrated:
Suction tubing, fine nozzles and tube anchoring forceps.

Dental Operations

Removal of impacted wisdom tooth

DEFINITION

The removal of the third molar tooth, the eruption of which is partially or completely prevented by its contact against the second molar tooth.

Fig. 17.3 Wiring of mandible, utilising teeth.

1. Towel clips, 4.
2. Right-angled tongue depressor.
3. Mouth gag (Mason).
4. Tongue forceps (Mayo).
5. (A) Collar pliers.
   (B) Collar pliers.
   (C) Collar pliers.
   (D) Snipe nose pliers.
   (E) Contouring pliers.
6. Cheek retractors, 2.
7. Root elevators (Winter), right and left, 2.
8. (A) Wire-cutting forceps, straight.
   Wire-cutting forceps, angled on flat.
9. Scissors, curved on flat, 13 cm (5 in) (Mayo).
10. Silk or thread, stout.
11. Stainless-steel wire.

POSITION

Supine, with some reverse Trendelenburg.

INSTRUMENTS

As Figure 17.2.

OUTLINE OF PROCEDURE

An incision is made in the gum overlying the impacted tooth. The cortex of the bone which covers the tooth is drilled or gouged away. The tooth is removed and the incision closed either with 2 (3/0) chromic catgut, Dexon or Silk.

METHODS OF IMMOBILISING FRACTURES OF THE MANDIBLE

Fig. 17.4 When there are teeth in both fragments, a fracture may be immobilised by interdental or arch wiring, or by cap splints. When the jaw is edentulous, a Gunning splint (or preferably the patient's dentures), circumferential wiring or the two-pin splint is used. (J. N. Wilson and Watson Jones.)

Treatment of a fractured mandible

DEFINITION

Reduction of a fractured mandible, followed by immobilisation, in this case by wiring the upper and lower teeth together.

POSITION

Supine, with some reverse Trendelenburg.

Fig. 17.5 Interdental eyelet wiring. (Photo, courtesy Mr N. L. Rowe, F.D.S.R.C.S., M.R.C.S., L.R.C.P. Consultant in Oral Surgery, Queen Mary's Hospital, Roehampton.)

Figs. 17.6 and 17.7 Double fracture of the mandible immobilised by two-pin splints, one on each side of the jaw. Fracture of an edentulous mandible immobilised by a Gunning Splint with circumferential wiring. (Courtesy R. Watson-Jones.)

INSTRUMENTS

As Figure 17.3.

OUTLINE OF PROCEDURE

With a pharyngeal pack in position; wires with loops are wound around the necks of two adjacent teeth on one side of the lower jaw. The wires are twisted together so that the loops or eyelets protrude at gum level from the space between the two teeth.

This procedure is repeated on the other side of the lower jaw and at correspondingly opposite positions around the teeth in the upper jaw. This results in protruding eyelets spaced evenly around the jaw.

The wires are now passed through eyelets on opposing jaws. The pharyngeal pack is removed, the tie wires tightened and the lower teeth secured in normal occluion with the upper teeth; this immobilises the fracture.

Alternative methods of jaw immobilisation are shown in Figs. 17.4, 17.6 and 17.7.

FURTHER READING

WILSON, J. N. (1976) *Watson Jones: Fractures and Joint Injuries.* Edinburgh: Churchill Livingstone.

18
EAR, NOSE AND THROAT OPERATIONS

SURGICAL APPROACHES TO THE MIDDLE EAR AND MASTOID

There are four methods of approach to the middle ear space and mastoid; permeatal, endaural, postaural and posterior tympanotomy. Each of these approaches are suited to specific surgical procedures, although the selection of any particular one will depend on clinical assessment of the possible range and extent of the proposed procedure.

Fig. 18.1 Anatomical cross section of the ear. (Down's Surgical Ltd.)

Permeatal approach

This approach is often used for stapedectomy, ossicular chain reconstruction or examination, destruction of the membranous labyrinth in uncontrolled unilateral Ménière's disease associated with severe sensorineural deafness, tympanic neurectomy and removal of some glomus—jugulare tumours. A curved incision is made in the posterior canal skin which is then reflected forwards from the bone beneath by blunt dissection to expose the posterior part of the mesotympanum (Fig. 18.2A).

Fig. 18.2 Permeatal surgical approach. (A) The incision. (B) Reflection of the tympanomeatal flap. (C) Exposure of the middle ear cavity. (Ballantyne.)

Exposure of the posterior half of the middle ear cavity reveals the chorda tympani, and nerve situated just behind the tympanic membrane (Fig. 18.2C). Gentle reflection of the nerve reveals the long process of incus, incudostapedial joint and the oval window region.

The posterosuperior part of the middle ear cavity is exposed fully by curetting the bony meatal wall and this reveals the stapedius tendon, pyramidal process, stapes and oval window. The tympanic meatal flap is replaced at the conclusion of the operation.

Endaural approach

The endaural approach is used mainly for removal of cholesteatoma in the epitympanum, correction of acquired mental stenosis and occasionally modified radical mastoidectomy or fenestration.

The incision is commenced in the cartilage-free gap between the anterior end of the helix posteriorly and the tragus anteriorly, and continued in a circular fashion between the cartilaginous and bony meatus (Fig. 18.3A). The periosteum in the lower meatal part of the incision is reflected off the bone to expose the supramental spine (of Henle), the supramental triangle (of Macewen) and the bony cortex of the mastoid process (Fig. 18.3B).

The temporalis muscle is reflected upwards, the meatal skin mobilised from the bone down to the tympanic ring to expose the epitympanum (Fig. 18.3C). The mastoid antrum and air cells are exposed with a power driven cutting burr, the attic is visualised by drilling forwards from the antrum (Fig. 18.3D). The short process of the incus and malleo–incudal joint are identified. The horizontal semi-circular canal is exposed by removal of the incus.

Postaural approach

This approach is often used as it provides good visualisation of the entire mastoid bowl, the epitympanum and the anterior recess of the deep meatus. The operations most frequently carried out via this approach include: simple, modified radical and radical

Fig. 18.3 *Endaural approach.* (A) Incision. (B) Exposure of the mastoid and temporalis fascia. (C) Reflection of meatal skin. (D) Exposure of mastoid antrum.

Fig. 18.4 *Postaural approach.* (A) Incision. (B) Reflection of periosteum. (C) Reflection of meatal flap.

Fig. 18.5 *Posterior tympanotomy.* (A) Reflection of meatal flap. (B) Posterior tympanotomy. (Ballantyne.)

mastoidectomy, combined approach tympanoplasty, in Menière's disease, facial nerve surgery, tumours in the middle ear cavity, extensive glomus-jugulare tumours and some cases of congenital atresia.

A curved incision is made behind the ear and division of subcutaneous tissues and muscle carried out by diathermy. The overlying periosteum is divided, the flaps separated to expose the mastoid cortex, suprameatal triangle and bony posterior meatal margin (Figs. 18.5A and B).

The temporalis muscle is displaced upwards exposing the zygoma root. The posterior canal skin is reflected from the bone as far as the tympanic margin (Fig. 18.5B). The mastoid antrum is exposed as in the endaural approach (Figs. 18.3C and D).

Posterior tympanotomy

This is an extension of the postaural approach used for patients with cholesteatoma of the mastoid bowl, attic and mestotympanum and is often combined with tympanoplasty (p. 397). It may also be used for patients with generalised and irreversible active mucosal disease of the mastoid bowl and tympanic cleft.

The incision and reflection of periosteum are as for the postaural approach (Figs. 18.4A and B). The posterior canal skin is reflected forwards from the bone, and the tympanic membrane reflected from the sulcus to determine the extent of the middle ear disease. The meatal flap may be reflected forwards after mobilisation if attic or posterior marginal perforation is present. The mastoid antrum is exposed as for the endaural approach.

A simple mastoidectomy is carried out, exentering the entire mastoid bowl. The bony dissection is continued into the root of the zygoma to expose the epitympanum, short process of the incus and malleo-incudal joint (Fig. 18.4C).

A posterio tympanotomy is performed, by gradually thinning down the posterior meatal bony wall, thereby connecting the mastoid cavity and the posterior mesotympanum. The slot is lateral to the facial nerve and medial to the tympanic annulus.

OPERATIONS ON THE EAR

Myringotomy

DEFINITION

Incision of the tympanic membrane.

POSITION

Supine, with the head inclined away from the affected ear.

INSTRUMENTS

Sponge holding forceps, small (Ramply)
Aural speculae (Yearsley or Pritchard) 3 sizes
Jobson Horne probe
Myringotome (Agnew)
Dressing forceps (Heath)
Suction tubing, fine nozzles and tube anchoring forceps
Operating microscope.

OUTLINE OF PROCEDURE

The operation is almost always carried out with the aid of an operating microscope. A speculum is placed into the outer ear and a myringotome used to make an incision in the tympanic membrane. The discharge which wells forth is gently aspirated by suction.

In secretory otitis media (blue drum, or 'glue' ear) a Shephard's teflon grommet drain tube may be inserted in the ear drum to ventilate the middle ear. This is usually left in position until it comes away by itself (Fig. 18.24).

Fig. 18.6   Heath Aural Forceps.

Fig. 18.7   Agnew Myringotome.

Fig. 18.8   Jobson Horne Probe.

Fig. 18.9   Yearsley Aural Specula.

Figs. 18.7 to 18.9   Instruments for myringotomy. (Down's Surgical Ltd.)

Fig. 18.10   Tilley Aural Forceps, extra fine, with box-joint.

Fig. 18.11   Hartmann Aural Forceps, dressing and polypi, with screw-joint.

Fig. 18.12   Henckel Aural Forceps, fine, with fenestrated scoop blades.

Fig. 18.13   Pritchard Aural Forceps, with box-joint.

Fig. 18.14   Hartmann Crocodile Action Forceps, with serrated jaws, stainless steel.

Fig. 18.15   Wishart Guillotine Forceps, for head of malleus, right.

Figs. 18.10 to 18.15   Aural instruments. (Down's Surgical Ltd.)

Ear, Nose and Throat Operations

Fig. 18.16 Kerrison Ronqeurs, upward cutting, four widths.

Fig. 18.17 Lempert Nibbling Forceps, angular, 3 mm jaws, compound action.

Fig. 18.18 Lempert rugines, broad and narrow

Fig. 18.19 Lempert Scoops, oval, 6 sizes, 3·5 to 6 mm.

Fig. 18.20 Freer separator and elevator, fine.

Fig. 18.21 Dundas Grant Seeker, stainless steel.

Fig. 18.22 Lempert Suction and Irrigation Tube, with Tucker Valve Plate, with Stilette to clean out after use, 6 F.G., 2 mm diam., electro-plated.

Figs. 18.16 to 18.22 Aural instruments. (Down's Surgical Ltd.)

Fig. 18.23 Myringotomy. In acute suppurative otitis media the incision is as shown. For a diagnostic paracentesis a small stab is usually made anteriorly in a radial direction. (Hall and Coleman.)

Figs 18.24 and 18.25 Shepard Grommet Drain tube, Teflon. (Down's Surgical Ltd.)

Mastoidectomy

DEFINITION

The removal of diseased mastoid air cells.

POSITION

Supine, with some reversed Trendelenburg and the head inclined away from the affected side.

INSTRUMENTS

Sponge-holding forceps (Ramply), 5
Towel clips, 5
Scalpel handles No. 3 with No. 10 and No. 15 blades (Bard Parker), 2
Dissecting forceps fine toothed (Lane and Gillies), 2
Dissecting forceps fine non-toothed (McIndoe), 2
Artery forceps, curved on flat (Kilner), 10
Aural forceps (Hartmann)
Aural forceps (Heath)
Dressing forceps (Pritchard)
Hook aural (Hartmann)
Probe aural (Jobson Horne)
Needle holder (Kilner multiple joint or Gillies)
Raspatory (Lempert)
Raspatory (Freer)

Fig. 18.26 Mastoidectomy. A post auricular incision is made, the periosteum and meatal flap reflected and the mastoid antrum exposed (Fig. 18.4A to C). (A) Antrum exposed. (B) Air cells removed, extenteration complete, bony cavity formed with antrum as its deepest point, bounded above by the dural plate, posteriorly by the sinus plate, and anteriorly by the bony meatal wall and aditus. (C) Wound closed with drainage. (Ballantyne.)

Medium retractors (Czerny), 2
Retractors, self-retaining (Mayo angled, and West straight), 2
Fine scissors, curved, 10 cm (4 in) (Kilner)
Stitch scissors, 13 cm (5 in)
Power drill, range of cutting burrs, connecting tubing or drive cable
Cartridge syringe for 2 ml adrenaline cartridges (1 : 250,000)
Fine exploring needles, sizes 18 and 14
Gelatine sponge, ribbon gauze, adrenaline, bone wax, B.I.P.P. paste in gallipot
2 (3/0) Plain catgut or Dexon for ligatures
2 (3/0) Plain catgut or Dexon on a small half-circle cutting needle for subcutaneous sutures
2 (3/0) Silk or nylon on a small curved cutting needle for skin sutures
Operating microscope.

OUTLINE OF PROCEDURE

If the operation is for acute mastoiditis, a conservative mastoidectomy is performed. The skin over the incision line is infiltrated with a 1 in 250,000 adrenaline solution to minimise bleeding. A curved incision is made behind the junction of the auricle with the scalp, and a periosteal elevator used to reflect this skin flap and ear to expose the underlying bone above and behind the external auditory meatus.

The bone over the mastoid antrum is drilled away till the antrum is opened, the diseased cells removed, but the middle ear is not opened. Either the mastoid cavity is packed with ribbon gauze impregnated with B.I.P.P., etc., and a portion of the gauze left protruding from the wound, or a post-auricular drain consisting of rubber or plastic drainage tubing is inserted. The wound is closed with catgut or Dexon, and silk or nylon skin sutures. The surgeon may also pack the external auditory canal with suitably impregnated ribbon gauze.

Modified radical mastoidectomy

In a radical mastoidectomy the middle ear and mastoid are turned into one cavity, drained permanently to the outside through an enlarged external auditory meatus. It is now customary to complete the operation with the creation of a new ear drum with a graft of temporal fascia.

The bone of the posterior wall of the external auditory meatus is removed and any middle ear pathology dealt with. Care is taken to avoid damage to the facial nerve which runs along the inner wall of the middle ear. The mastoid cavity and the middle ear are packed as previously described and the wound closed.

Mastoidectomy may also be performed through an endaural incision. This is known as Lempert's approach.

Microtia and meatal atresia of the external auditory canal

DEFINITION

Correction of maldevelopment of the external auditory meatus which is often associated with maldevelopment of the middle ear. Depending on the degree of congenital abnormality the operation usually consists of repositioning the pinna and refashioning of the middle ear.

POSITION

As for mastoidectomy.

INSTRUMENTS

As for mastoidectomy (p. 392).
Skin grafting set.

OUTLINE OF PROCEDURE

Microtia. This abnormality may be due to maternal rubella or the taking of thalidomide during pregnancy. The new pinna may have to be reconstructed in stages with a skin tube pedicle (Chapter 24). Cartilage taken from the patient's rib, from the mother, or from another person may be used. A new ear drum is constructed, often from cialit-preserved homologous dura mater, or temporal fascia. The newly constructed external auditory canal is skin grafted. The operation may be carried out in several stages.

Meatal atresia. There are various degrees of abnormality but the pinna is always situated away from its normal position forwards and downwards towards the angle of the jaw. A 'Z' plasty is carried out behind the ear to eventually move the external auditory meatus to a normal position (Fig. 18.27A).

The mastoid process is generally exposed via a postaural incision (Figs. 18.4A and B, p. 387), and exenteration of the autrum completed. The ossicles are exposed and where the meatus is present, the meatal skin is elevated, followed by enlargement of the underlying bony meatus with a cutting burr (Figs. 18.27B and C). The meatal skin tube is then refashioned and packed into position with a B.I.P.P. pack; the 'Z' plasty is closed (Fig. 18.27F) and a week later the defect in front of the pinna is skin grafted. Where the meatus is not present there are often abnormalities of the ossicles. This necessitates refashioning of the ossicles and tympanoplasty; the combined approach may be used (p. 399).

Fig. 18.27 Surgery of meatal atresia. (A) Z plasty incision, the more normal the pinna the shorter the distances a–b and b–c are made. (B and C) Exposure of the ossicles. (D and E) Elevation of the meatal skin and enlargement of the underlying bony meatus. (F) Closure of the Z plasty leaving a bare area in front of the pinna which is skin grafted in a second stage operation. (Ballantyne.)

Otoplasty (See Chapter 24)

Osteoma of the external auditory canal

DEFINITION

Removal of a simple bony tumour of the external auditory canal.

POSITION

As for mastoidectomy.

INSTRUMENTS

As for mastoidectomy, p. 392.

OUTLINE OF PROCEDURE

The exposure is similar to that for mastoidectomy. The skin is elevated off the tumour which is drilled away, often using diamond paste burrs.

Operations to improve Aural Function

Stapedectomy

DEFINITION

Removal of stapes in cases of conductive or mixed deafness due to otosclerosis in which there is a good bone-air gap, and insertion of a prosthesis in order to re-establish sound conduction to the inner ear.

POSITION

As for mastoidectomy.

INSTRUMENTS

As for mastoidectomy (p. 392).
Stapedectomy set etc. (Fig. 18.30).
Saline irrigation set.

Fig. 18.28 (A and B). Shea Teflon piston attached to tip of the incus with the lenticular process seated in a cup at the prosthesis head. By fitting on to the tip of the incus where the stapes was formerly attached, the prosthesis closely approximates the original angle to the oval window and provides a more normal reconstruction. (C and D) Shea slotted prosthesis. (E) Prefabricated wire loop with gelatine sponge. (Down's Surgical Ltd.)

OUTLINE OF PROCEDURE

Previously mobilisation of stapes was carried out but this seldom gave permanent results as the stapes usually became fixed again. Stapedectomy is carried out via a permeatal approach (Fig 18.29); the favoured procedure being to remove the stapes, seal off the oval window with a piece of temporal fascia, vein or gelatin sponge and to replace the stapes with a prosthesis such as a specially shaped polyethylene tube of suitable length, or a teflon piston, or a piece of stainless steel hooked over the incus. This is to connect the incus to the oval window, thereby restoring the function of the ossicular chain.

Fig. 18.29 Stapedectomy, approach by permeatal incision (Fig. 18.2). (A) The stapedius tendon is cut with a curved sickle knife. (B) Fracture of the stapedial cura. (C) Removal of the stapes superstructure. (D) Removal of the footplate to accommodate the prosthesis (in Ménière's disease, the whole of the stapes footplate would be removed if the labyrinth is to be destroyed). (E) Insertion of stainless steel piston. (F) Sealing the gap between the piston and oval window with gelatin sponge. (Ballantyne.)

Tympanoplasty

DEFINITION

Repair of the ear drum by myringoplasty (a graft of temporal fascia, vein or Cialit-preserved homograft (duramater) and if necessary reconstruction of the ossicular chain with polyethylene, teflon, or stainless steel, or grafts of cartilage taken from the nasal septum, or bone chips, or sterile preserved ossicles taken from cadavers or other patients and preserved in the deep freeze, or patients own refashioned ossicles.

POSITION

As for stapedectomy.

Fig. 18.30 Zoellner's Tympanoplasty Instruments. As used at the Royal National Throat, Nose and Ear Hospital, London. (Down's Surgical Ltd.)

INSTRUMENTS

As for stapedectomy.
Tympanoplasty instruments (Fig. 18.30).

OUTLINE OF PROCEDURE

Tympanoplasty is a delicate procedure to reconstruct the sound conducting mechanism in cases of chronic otitis media or other types of disease or trauma, which have resulted in disruption of the mechanism thereby producing hearing loss. It is often combined with procedures for erradication of chronic disease – such as generalised cholesteatosis and intractable catarrahal otitis media. The operation of choice is 'combined approach tympanoplasty' which enables eradication of disease from the middle ear and mastoid air cell system, with minimal disturbance of the external meatus and the sulcus tympanicus. This enables ossicular chain reconstruction to be carried out if necessary, in a middle ear of normal dimensions. The extent of the procedure depends on the complexity of the disease encountered, and therefore this account will be confined to the basic operative stages.

A postaural approach is carried out (Fig. 18.4) and a mastoidectomy performed within the area bounded by the dotted lines in Figure 18.31A. The mastoid antrum is identified and the mastoid air cells removed, this reveals the head of the malleus, the body of incus and the lateral semi-circular canal (Fig. 18.31B). A superior tympanotomy is carried out (Fig. 18.31C) followed by a posterior tympanotomy (Fig. 18.31D).

Removal of the posterior wall of the facial recess and the chordal ridge reveals the stapes superstructure, and stapedectomy can be undertaken as described in Figure 18.29A–D. Examples of ossicular reconstruction are shown in Figures 18.29E and F. The wound is closed as for mastoidectomy.

◀ Key:
- A. Zoellner's scissors, bayonet shaped, tubular model, with upward cut, lateral action.
- B. Zoellner's scissors, angular, with upward cut, lateral action, screw joint.
- C. Zoellner's fine raspatory, curved to right, with thumb grip, matt finish.
- D. Ditto, curved to left, with thumb grip, matt finish.
- E. Zoellner's fine spear-pointed needle, curved to right, with thumb grip, matt finish.
- F. Ditto, curved to left, with thumb grip, matt finish.
- G. Zoellner's knife, upward cutting, with thumb grip, matt finish.
- H. Ditto, downward cutting, with thumb grip, matt finish.
- I. Zoellner's small hook, with thumb grip, matt finish.
- J. Zoellner's rack to hold instruments above, figs. C to I with three space clips for additional similar instruments; arranged to protect the knives, etc. during sterilisation and afterwards to make the different instruments easily discernible.
- K. Zoellner's suction tube, nickle plated with fine detachable end, 5 sizes 18, 20, 22, 24 and 26 s.w.g. × 19 mm ($\frac{3}{4}$ in) long.
- M. Zoellner's raspatory, curved on flat, narrow bladed on metal handle.
- N. Ormerod's aural scissors, extra fine, curved upwards crocodile action, black finished.
- O. Ormerod's aural forceps with extra fine circular cup crocodile action jaws, black finished.
- P. Ormerod's aural forceps with extra fine elongated cup crocodile jaws, black finished.
- Q. Hartmann's aural forceps with extra fine serrated crocodile action jaws, black finished.
- R. Aural forceps extra fine, double cup oval jaws 1·75 mm × 0·75 mm crocodile action, black finished.
- S. Scissors, extra fine, crocodile action jaws, black finished.
- T. Zoellner's Skin Graft Plate, 152 × 76 mm (6 × 3 in) with three holes 22, 28, 32 mm ($\frac{7}{8}$, $1\frac{1}{8}$ and $1\frac{1}{4}$ in) diameter.

Fig. 18.31 Combined approach tympanoplasty (A) Mastoidectomy. (B and C) Superior tympanotomy. (D) Posterior tympanoplasty – extent. (E) Facial recess and chordal ridge removed, stapes superstructure visualised. (F and G) Dissection of tympanic membrane. (Ballantyne.)

Repair of the ear drum (myringoplasty) is best carried out using the patient's own tissue. Various incisions may be employed via the transmeatal route. The scar tissue is first removed around the whole circumference of the perforation. Starting at the edge of the perforation the outer epithelial layer is dissected from the fibrous layer (Figs. 18.31F and G). The aim is then to apply the graft as an overlay, underlay or sandwiched in between the layers of the ear drum, bridging the perforation.

Other Operations on the Middle and Inner Ear

Ménière's disease

DEFINITION

Surgical relief of Ménière's disease (attacks of rotational vertigo, tinnitus and deafness) after failure of conservative treatment. There are many specialised operations for this condition including labyrinthectomy in which the membranous labyrinth is removed either after opening a semi-circular canal, or by suction through the oval window in a procedure similar to stapedectomy. This operation abolishes further attacks of vertigo, but produce total deafness in the operated ear.

Other operative procedures include, division of the vestibular nerves without injuring the facial nerve or cochlear nerve, and less frequently now the application of ultrasound to the membranous labyrinth.

Acoustic neuroma

DEFINITION

Removal of tumour of the eighth cranial (acoustic and vestibular) nerve through the mastoid and labyrinth.

INSTRUMENTS

As for mastoidectomy and also stapedectomy type microscopic instruments; microscope; dental drill with diamond paste burrs, general surgery set to take fat from abdomen or thigh to seal cerebrospinal fluid leak.

OPERATIONS ON THE NOSE AND ACCESSORY SINUSES

Pre-operative nasal packing

DEFINITION

Packing of the nasal cavity before operation either to effect local anaesthesia (e.g., lignocaine (Xylocaine) 4 per cent) or to provide vasoconstriction and haemostasis for the surgeon (e.g., 5 to 10 per cent cocaine solution with 1 in 10,000 adrenaline added. Too much adrenaline may cause ventricular fibrilation if halothane or trilene general anaesthesia is used).

POSITION

Supine.

INSTRUMENTS

Speculae Nasal (Thudichum), set
Dressing forceps, nasal (Tilley or Wilde)
Roll of 25 mm (1 in) ribbon gauze
Lignocaine 4 per cent
Adrenaline 1 in 10,000
Graduated measure, 15 ml ($\frac{1}{2}$ oz)

Head light, or head mirror and lamp
Towel or swab to protect the patient's lips.

OUTLINE OF PROCEDURE

The ribbon gauze is impregnated with solution, and one or both nasal cavities are packed using a nasal speculum and dressing forceps. The ribbon gauze is first passed into the posterior part of the cavity, and successive layers are applied until it is filled. The pack is left in place for at least 15 minutes before operation, and is removed gently to avoid trauma of the nasal mucosa. Spraying the nose with 5 per cent cocaine first makes packing with ribbon gauze less unpleasant if the patient is conscious.

Reduction of a nasal fracture

DEFINITION

Anatomical re-alignment of a fractured nasal bone.

Fig. 18.32 Anatomical cross-section of nose. (Down's Surgical Ltd.)

Ear, Nose and Throat Operations

POSITION

Supine.

INSTRUMENTS

Dressing forceps nasal (Tilley)
Re-dressing or re-fracture nasal forceps (Walsham)
Mallet small (Rowland), optional
Specula nasal (Thudichum)
25 mm (1 in) ribbon gauze which may be impregnated with petroleum jelly
Scissors, dressing
Suction tubing, fine nozzles and tube anchoring forceps
Plaster of Paris strips 50 mm (2 in) × 150 mm (6 in) or Stent material, and hot water in a small bowl
Adhesive strapping and a few small swabs

Fig. 18.33 Walsham Nasal Re-Dressing Forceps.

Fig. 18.34 Tilley Dressing Forceps.

Fig. 18.35 Thudichum Nasal Speculum.

Fig. 18.36 Grunwald Nasal Turbinate Forceps, with narrow punch jaws, 3 patterns.

Figs. 18.33 to 18.36 Nasal Instruments. (Down's Surgical Ltd.)

404 Operating Theatre Technique

Fig. 18.37 Ballenger Swivel Knife.

Fig. 18.38 Luc Punch Forceps.

Fig. 18.39 Nasal Gouge.

Fig. 18.40 St Clair Thompson Nasal Speculum.

Fig. 18.41 Killian Nasal Speculum.

Fig. 18.42 Howarth Nasal Raspatory.

Fig. 18.43 Hill Nasal Raspatory.

Figs. 18.37 to 18.43 Nasal Instruments. (Down's Surgical Ltd.)

Heymann Angled Nasal Scissors

Henckel-Tilleys Punch Forceps

Jansen Middleton Nasal Septum Forceps

Figs. 18.44 to 18.46   Nasal Instruments (cont'd.). (Down's Surgical Ltd.)

OUTLINE OF PROCEDURE

If the injury is old the nasal bone may be re-fractured with a small mallet, utilising a swab to protect the skin.

One jaw of the Walsham's forceps is introduced into the nose and pressed against the nasal bone on the selected side. The other jaw provides counter-pressure against a swab placed on the outside of the nose.

The fragments of the nasal bone are manipulated into anatomical position and the nose packed with ribbon gauze. If the fracture fragments are stable no further procedure is carried out. If unstable, the fracture is immobilised either with three strips of plaster of Paris (two diagonally across the bridge of the nose extending from forehead to cheek, one across the forehead) or Stent. A Stent splint is fashioned by softening the material in hot water and moulding it into shape. The splints are retained in position with adhesive plaster.

Nasal polypectomy

DEFINITION

Removal of nasal polypi, either under general or local anaesthesia.

POSITION

Supine.

Fig. 18.47 Submucous resection of the nasal septum. (A) Incision on one side of nasal septum. (B) and (C) Plane of cleavage between cartilage and perichondrium opened by blunt dissection. (D) to (G) Cartilage incised, opening second plane of cleavage between cartilage and perichondrium on other side. (H) Removal of cartilage with Ballenger's swivel knife. (I and J) Groove of perichondrium lying on crest of maxilla and vomer. The crest of the bone is freed from soft tissue, fractured in the mid-line, and then removed with a hammer and gouge or bone forceps. (Ballantyne.)

INSTRUMENTS

Nasal speculae (Thudichum) set
Nasal speculae (St Clair Thompson), set
Nasal dressing forceps (Henckel-Tilley)
Nasal snare, wire
Punch forceps, small and large (Weil), 2
25 mm (1 in) ribbon impregnated with petroleum jelly
Suction tubing and fine nozzles and tube anchoring forceps.

OUTLINE OF PROCEDURE

Using a nasal speculum, the wire loop of the snare is manoeuvred around each polyp in turn and withdrawn, bringing the excised polyp with it; the Weil's forceps are used to grasp and remove tags, avulsing them with a twisting action. Packing the nasal cavity or cavities completes the operation.

Turbinotomy or turbinectomy

DEFINITION

The removal part of hypertrophied nasal turbinate.

INSTRUMENTS

Nasal specula (Thudichum), set
Nasal specula (St Clair Thompson), set
Nasal dressing forceps (Tilley or Wilde)
Nasal snare, wire
Punch forceps, small and medium (Weil or Luc), 2
Nasal scissors, angled (Heymann)
25 mm (1 in) ribbon gauze impregnated with petroleum jelly
Suction tubing, fine nozzles and Robin tube anchoring forceps.

OUTLINE OF PROCEDURE

Using a nasal speculum, the surgeon inserts the angled scissors and divides the turbinate bone along its base for a short distance. The wire snare is inserted and the loop passed over the turbinal with the barrel of the snare lying along the cut made. The snare is withdrawn and the enlarged portion of the turbinal removed with forceps.

The nasal cavity or cavities are packed with ribbon gauze in the usual manner.

Submucous resection of the nasal septum

DEFINITION

The removal of the deflected bony and cartilaginous parts of a nasal septum to rectify an obstructed airway.

POSITION

Supine.

INSTRUMENTS

Sponge-holding forceps (Rampley), 5
Scalpel handles No. 3 with No. 10 and No. 15 blades (Bard Parker), 2
Towel clips, 5
Fine dissecting forceps, toothed (Gillies)
Dressing forceps, angled (Tilley)
Dressing forceps, angled (Wilde)
Gauges nasal, angled (Tilley and Killian)
Knife nasal (Dundas Grant)
Knife swivel (Ballenger)
Mallet (Heath)
Mouth gag (Mason)
Probe, malleable silver
Punch forceps (Luc) medium and small
Punch forceps (Weil)
Raspatory, nasal (Hill)
Raspatory, nasal (Howarth)
Retractors, small single hook, 3
Scissors, nasal angled (Heymann)
Septum forceps, nasal (Jansen Middleton)
Speculum, nasal, self-retaining (Killian)
Speculae, nasal, long (St Clair Thompson) set of 3
Speculae, nasal, short (Thudichum) set of 4
Tongue depressor, angled
Tongue forceps (Mayo)
Suction tubing, fine nozzles and tube anchoring forceps
Needle holder (Kilner multiple joint)
2 (3/0) Chromic catgut or Dexon on a small half-circle cutting needle for mucosa sutures
B.I.P.P. (optional)
Lubricant in galli-pot e.g., liquid paraffin
Rubber glove fingers for nasal pack (distended with ribbon gauze) optional
Plaster of Paris strips or Stent impression material for nasal splint (optional).

OUTLINE OF PROCEDURE

A small incision is made behind the junction of the skin and mucous membrane on one side of the nasal septum. A Thudichum's nasal speculum is inserted, and using a long raspatory through this incision, the mucoperichondrium is dissected free from the septum along one side.

An incision is then made through the cartilage along the line of the original incision and the raspatory introduced to strip off the mucoperichondrium on the other side of the septum. Care is taken not to puncture the mucosa on this side. The small nasal speculum is changed for a longer one (St Clair Thompson's), which is inserted so that the blades pass between the nasal septum and mucosa on each side. This separates the mucosa away from the septum and the cut edge of the septal cartilage lies in the centre of the speculum.

As much as necessary of the cartilage is removed with a Ballenger's swivel knife, which is first passed backwards and then downwards, and finally forwards. Pieces of the vomer and vertical plate of the ethmoid are removed with punch forceps and the irregular spur which is usually present along the lower edge of the septum is removed with an angled gouge.

The long speculum is removed and the tubinates are examined using a Thudichum's speculum. If these are hypertrophied, a turbinotomy or turbinectomy may be performed.

Some surgeons suture the mucosal incision before inserting two rubber glove fingers (one in each nostril) which have been packed with petroleum jelly gauze.

Fig. 18.48   Tilley Antrum Trocar.

Fig. 18.49.   Tilley Lichwitz Antrum Trocar and Cannula.

Fig. 18.50   Luer Jansen Gouge or Punch Forceps.

Fig. 18.51   Kerrison's Rongeur, Upward Cutting.

Fig. 18.52   Citelli Gouge or Punch Forceps.

Figs. 18.48 to 18.52   Antrum Instruments. (Down's Surgical Ltd.)

Antrostomy (intransal operation)

DEFINITION

An intransal opening into the maxillary antrum usually performed for chronic suppuration.

POSITION

Supine.

INSTRUMENTS

Sponge-holding forceps (Rampley), 5
Scalpel handle No. 3 with No. 15 blade (Bard Parker)
Towel clips, 5
Curetting spoon (Volkmann)
Dissector (Hill)
Dressing forceps nasal (Tilley or Wilde)
Small gouges 4 mm, 6 mm, 8 mm, (Jenkins)
Harpoon antrum (Tilley)
Irrigation syringe and warm saline
Power drill, cutting burrs, connecting tubing or drive cable
Punch forceps (Citelli)
Punch forceps, small and medium (Luc)
Punch forceps, small and medium (Weil)
Probe, malleable silver
Scissors, nasal, angled (Heymann)
Snare nasal wire
Speculae nasal (Thudichum) set
Speculae nasal (St Clair Thompson) set
Trocar antrum and cannula
Suction tubing, nozzles and tube anchoring forceps
(Two rubber glove fingers distended with petroleum jelly ribbon gauze may be required).

OUTLINE OF PROCEDURE

An intra nasal antrostomy consists of performing a turbinectomy or turbinotomy (removing the anterior end of the inferior turbinate) followed by the insertion of an antrum harpoon, or using burrs to make an opening through the lateral nasal wall into the antrum. This opening is then enlarged with a burr or punch forceps, followed by irrigation of the antrum with warm water. The nasal cavity may be packed using two rubber glove fingers as previously described.

Radical antrostomy or Caldwell Luc operation

DEFINITION

An opening into the antrum approached via the mouth through the anterior wall of the maxilla, leaving a large antrostomy into the nose.

POSITION

Semi-sitting head and neck flexed
or Supine.

INSTRUMENTS

Sponge-holding forceps (Rampley), 5
Scalpel handle No. 3 with Nos. 10 and 15 blades (Bard Parker)
Towel clips, 5
Curetting spoon (Volkmann)
Dissecting forceps, toothed (Lane), 2
Dissecting forceps, non-toothed, 13 cm (5 in), 2
Dressing forceps, angled (Tilley)
Dressing forceps, angled (Wilde)
Gouge forceps (Jansen)
Gouge or punch forceps (Citelli)
Harpoon antrum (Tilley)
Irrigation syringe and warm water
Mouth gag (Mason)
Needle holder (Kilner multiple joint)
Punch forceps nasal (Grunwald)
Punch forceps (Luc) large and medium
Punch forceps (Weil)
Raspatory nasal (Hill)

Fig. 18.53 Caldwell – Luc operation. (A) Incision. (B) Soft tissue elevated from bone, antrum opened, enlargement of bony opening with punch forceps. (C) Removal of antral lining. (D) Site of antrostomy opening into nose. (Ballantyne.)

Raspatory nasal (Howarth)
Power drill, burrs, connecting tubing or drive cable
Retractors, malleable, medium
Rugine (Faraboeuf)
Scissors, curved on flat, 13 cm (5 in) (Mayo)
Scissors, stitch, 13 cm (5 in)
Scissors, nasal angled (Heymann)
Speculum nasal self-retaining (Killian)
Speculae, nasal, long (St Clair Thompson), set of 3
Speculae, nasal small (Thudichum), set of 4
Tongue depressor, angled
Tongue forceps (Mayo)
Trocar, antrum and cannula
Cartridge syringe for 2 ml adrenaline cartridge 1 : 250,000
Fine exploring needles, sizes 18 and 14
Suction tubing and tube anchoring forceps
3 or 2·5 (0 or 2/0) Chromic catgut, Dexon or silk on a small half-circle round-bodied needle for mucosa suture
Lubricant in galli-pot e.g., Liquid paraffin
2 Rubber glove fingers for nasal pack (distended with ribbon gauze).

OUTLINE OF PROCEDURE

The upper lip on the affected side is retracted upwards and the tissues just above the gingivolabial reflection infiltrated with adrenaline 1:250,000 solution. An incision is made in the mucosa lying over the anterior wall of the maxilla. The mucous membrane is reflected from the surface of the bone, and an opening fashioned in the wall of the antrum, using a power driven burr followed by punch forceps.

Any diseased mucosa in the antrum is scraped away, and the cavity is irrigated with warm saline. An opening is made into the nasal cavity through the lateral bulge at the interior meatus using a burr. The opening is enlarged with punch forceps to about 1·5 cm long by 1 cm wide, and an incision made through the mucosa which is then incised to create an opening which matches the bony opening. The cavity may then be packed with B.I.P.P. ribbon gauze, the end of which is brought out via the antrostomy opening and taped to the cheek. The gum is then closed with catgut or dexon sutures.

Ethmoidectomy (intranasal operation)

DEFINITION

Removal of the anterior wall of the ethmoidal labyrinth and ethmoidal cells for chronic allergic inflammatory conditions.

POSITION

Supine.

INSTRUMENTS

As for submucous resection (p. 408)
Frontal sinus probe
Frontal sinus curette

Fig. 18.54 Exposure of the frontal, ethmoidal and sphenoidal sinuses. (A) The incision. (B) Ligation of the ethmoidal vessels either with ligatures or clips. (C) Exposure of the ethmoidal sinuses. (D) Exposure of the frontal sinus. (E) Maintenance of frontal sinus drainage. (Ballantyne.)

OUTLINE OF PROCEDURE

A submucous resection of the nasal septum may be performed to provide better access to the ethmoidal labyrinth.

Basically, the operation consists of removing the ethmoid cells which lie around the passage leading from the frontal sinus to the nasal cavity. The operation is performed almost entirely with a long nasal speculum, frontal sinus probe, punch forceps, such as Luc's and the frontal sinus curette.

Fronto-ethmoidectomy

DEFINITION

Removal of diseased ethmoid cells and the creation of a drainage channel through that area from the frontal sinus.

POSITION

Supine.

INSTRUMENTS

Sponge-holding forceps (Rampley), 5
Towel clips, 5
Scalpel handles No. 3 with Nos. 10 and 15 blades (Bard Parker), 2
Bone nibbling forceps, curved on flat
Artery forceps fine curved on flat, mosquito, 10
Dressing nasal forceps (Tilley)
Curette frontal sinus
Dissecting forceps, toothed (Gillies and Lane), 2
Dissecting forceps non-toothed 13 cm (5 in), 2
Needle holder (Kilner multiple joint, or Gillies)
Power drill, burrs, connecting tubing or drive cable
Punch forceps frontal sinus (Citelli)
Punch forceps, small and medium (Luc)
Rasps frontal sinus (Watson-Jones), set of 3
Retractors small double hook
Retractors, self-retaining (Mayo hinged and West straight or Ferris Smith), 2
Rugines, small, curved and straight (Farabacue), 2
Scissors, curved on flat 13 cm (5 in) (Mayo)
Scissors, fine curved, 10 cm (4 in) (Kilner)
Scissors, stitch, 13 cm (5 in)
Skin hooks (Gillies), 2
Speculae, nasal (St Clair Thompson), set of 2
Tissue forceps, fine (McIndoe), 5
Suction tubing, fine nozzles and tube anchoring forceps
2 (3/0) Plain cutgut or Dexon for ligatures
2 and 2·5 (3/0 and 2/0) Chromic catgut or Dexon on small half-circle round-bodied needles for subcutaneous sutures
1·5 (4/0) Silk or nylon on a small curved cutting needle for skin sutures.

OUTLINE OF PROCEDURE

A curved incision is made medial to the medial canthus of the eye. The periosteum is reflected off the maxilla, and frontal bone and medial orbital wall. The lacrymal sac is displaced laterally and the ethmoidal vessels exposed, and ligated.

The thin ethmoidal bone medial to the orbit is penetrated and ethmoid cells exenterated to expose the anterior wall of the ethmoid sinus which is then removed. Exenteration of the anterior ethmoid cells, working in an upwards direction exposes the frontal sinus. The bony wall of the frontal sinus floor is removed and the diseased contents evacuated.

A plastic or rubber tube may be inserted between the cavity and the nose, being left to protrude at one end of the nostril, where it is secured with a suture. Haemostasis is secured and the subcutaneous tissues approximated before closing the skin with fine silk or nylon sutures.

OPERATIONS ON THE THROAT AND MOUTH

Direct laryngoscopy

DEFINITION

Direct examination of the larynx with an endoscope which places the mouth, pharynx and larynx in a straight line (the Boyce position).

POSITION

Supine.

INSTRUMENTS

Laryngoscope with appropriate size of blade (Mackintosh Magill or Chevalier Jackson, etc.) (Chapter 10, p. 268)
Tongue forceps (Mayo)
Angled tongue depressor
Laryngeal swab holders and small mops
Laryngeal biopsy forceps
Adrenaline 1 in 1,000
Graduated measure
Suction tubing, nozzles and tube anchoring forceps
Diathermy leads, electrodes and lead anchoring forceps.

OUTLINE OF PROCEDURE

The patient is anaesthetised and with his neck flexed and head extended the laryngoscope is inserted. A biopsy may be taken with the biopsy forceps and the area swabbed with small mops soaked in adrenaline solution, or diathermised.

For bronchoscopy and oesophagoscopy, see Chapter on Thoracic Operations.

Peritonsillar abscess or quinsy

DEFINITION

An abscess between the surgical capsule of the tonsil and the superior constrictor muscle and fascia of the adjacent lateral pharyngeal wall.

POSITION

Sitting, facing the surgeon, or lateral position with the table in slight Trendelenburg.

INSTRUMENTS

Scalpel handle No. 3 with No. 15 blade (Bard Parker) wrapped with adhesive plaster, tip only exposed.
Sponge-holding forceps (Rampley) and small sponges or swabs, 5
Mouth gag (Mason or Doyen)
Tongue forceps (Mayo)
Angled tongue depressor
Scissors, straight with sharp outer edges.
Sinus forceps
Pharyngeal spray and 4 per cent lignocaine
Sterile throat swab
Mouth washes (used with great caution and with patient bending forwards).

OUTLINE OF PROCEDURE

A little topical anaesthesia is generally employed. An incision is made with the guarded knife through the maximum bulge in the soft palate, parallel with the posterior margin and extending approximately about 2 cm inwards from the anterior pillar of the fauces. Sinus forceps are introduced quickly into the incision and separated.

Tonsillectomy and adenoidectomy

DEFINITION

Enucleation of the tonsils either by dissection or guillotine, and curetting of the adenoids.

POSITION

Dissection. Supine, with the head and neck in extension. A 'jack' may be used to support the mouth gag during operation. One of the best gag supporters is two Draffin poles, one on each side, resting on the operating table, thus leaving the patient's chest unobstructed. Adenoidectomy as below.

Guillotine: First supine with the head to one side, and then lateral for adenoidectomy.

INSTRUMENTS

Sponge holding forceps (Rampley), 5
Towel clips, 5
Dissector (Hill)
Dissector tonsil and pillar retractor (Beavis)
Artery forceps, tonsil, curved and straight (Negus, Birkett)
Compression clamps, tonsil (Beneys)
Curette, adenoid (St Clair Thompson)
Dissecting forceps, long fine, toothed and non-toothed (Waugh)
Guillotine, tonsil, haemostatic
Holding forceps, tonsil (Denis Browne)

Ear, Nose and Throat Operations

Fig. 18.55 Negus Tonsil Artery Forceps (curved).

Fig. 18.56 Birkett Tonsil Artery Forceps (straight).

Fig. 18.57 Gwynne Evans Tonsil Dissector.

Fig. 18.58 Irwin Moores Tonsil Needle

Fig. 18.59 Mollinson Tonsil Dissector and Pillar Retractor.

Fig. 18.60 Eves Tonsil Snare.

Fig. 18.61 Beneys Tonsil Compressor.

Figs. 18.55 to 18.61 Tonsil Instruments. (Down's Surgical Ltd.)

418 Operating Theatre Technique

Fig. 18.62 Barnhills Adenoid Curette.

Fig. 18.63 Denis Browne Tonsil Holding Forceps.

Small spare blade.

Fig. 18.64 St Clair Thompson Adenoid Curette.

Fig. 18.65 Woods Curved Tonsil Scissors.

Fig. 18.66 Poppers Haemostatic Tonsil Guillotine (Enculeator).

Figs. 18.62 to 18.66 Tonsil and Adenoidal Instruments. (Down's Surgical Ltd.)

Ligature needle, tonsil (Irwin Moores)
Mouth gag and blades (Boyle-Davis)
Mouth gag (Mason)
Scissors, tonsil, curved and straight (Wilson)
Snare, tonsil (Eve)
Tongue forceps (Mayo)
Angled tongue depressor
Suction tubing, nozzles and tube anchoring forceps
2 (3/0) Silk, linen thread, catgut or Dexon for ligatures
Adrenaline 1 in 1,000 (optional)
Graduated measure
Iced water.

OUTLINE OF PROCEDURE

Dissection Operation: A Boyle-Davis mouth gag is inserted, and if an endotracheal tube has not been placed in position, the anaesthetic gases are conveyed to the back of the pharynx through a tube attached to the side of the tongue blade.

Fig. 18.67 (A) Shows incision of anterior pillar. Tonsil is drawn out with forceps putting pillar on the stretch to define the attachment to tonsil. (B) Blunt dissection of tonsil by scissors inserted through incision in anterior pillar. Dissection is done by forceps, dissector or scissors. (C) Shows tonsil dissected out of its bed, leaving pedicle below the lower pole. (D) Snare placed round the pedicle. (Hall and Colman.)

The tonsil is grasped with holding forceps and drawn inwards, exposing the anterior pillar of the fauces. Using curved scissors, or a dissector, an incision is made through the mucous membrane at the junction between the tonsil and the anterior pillar. The tonsil is freed by blunt dissection, first at the upper part and then the lower. After the tonsil has been removed, bleeding vessels are clamped and tied, or under-run and tied with silk or linen thread. The other tonsil is removed in a similar manner and both tonsil beds are inspected for complete haemostasis before gag is removed.

Guillotine Operation: A mouth gag is inserted and the tongue grasped with tongue forceps. The guillotine is passed into the mouth and the right tonsil positioned in the ring. With the haemostatic type instrument (tonsil enucleator), the clamp mechanism is closed to crush the tonsil 'pedicle' for about 20 seconds before depressing the knife blade to separate the tonsil from its bed. With the simple type instrument, when the tonsil has been pressed well into the ring, the knife blade is depressed and the tonsil removed by a slight twist of the guillotine. The second tonsil is removed, and compression clamps applied to a taped swab in each tonsil fossa. The child is immediately turned on its side for the removal of the adenoids. The guillotine operation is now less common than dissection.

Adenoidectomy. The adenoids are removed with a curette which is passed behind the soft palate, pressed hard against the posterior pharyngeal wall, and moved in a downwards sweeping action. Care is taken to avoid damage to the mucosa of the posterior pharyngeal space.

The patient's face and neck are bathed with ice-cold water, and if haemorrhage persists a Boyle-Davis gag may be inserted for further inspection of the tonsil fossae.

Tracheostomy

DEFINITION

The establishment of an opening into the trachea below the larynx, and the insertion of a tube for the purpose of supplying an airway.

POSITION

Supine, with a sandbag under the shoulder blades, neck extended, with the head thrown well back and the chin in the midline. (Fig. 4.13, p. 80).

INSTRUMENTS

As for tracheostomy (Fig. 18.69)
Sponge-holding forceps (Rampley), 5
Towel clips, 5
Needle holder (Kilner)
Suction tubing, nozzles and tube anchoring forceps
2·5 and 3 (2/0 and 0) Chromic catgut or Dexon for ligatures
3 (0) Chromic catgut or Dexon on a small half-circle round-bodied needle for muscle sutures.
2 (3/0) Silk or nylon on a small curved cutting needle for skin sutures
(Local anaesthetic requisites (Fig. 10.35) may be required).

OUTLINE OF PROCEDURE

Emergency tracheostomy is carried out less frequently nowadays. Endotracheal intubation is usually carried out first for respiratory obstruction. Where this is impracticable, or

Ear, Nose and Throat Operations

for prolonged pulmonary mechanical ventilation, effective tracheostomy may be undertaken and an appropriate plastic or rubber cuffed tube inserted. Silver tracheostomy tubes are still used for maintaining an airway either before or after operations on the larynx.

A tracheostomy set of tubes and instruments arranged in the correct order of use should be kept sterile and ready in all operating theatres. It is important that the tapes are already attached to the outer tubes, as many valuable minutes may be lost placing these in position during operation.

Fig. 18.68 Elective tracheostomy (transverse incision). (A) Incision. (B) Separation of sternothyroid and hyoid muscles. (C) Identification of thyroid isthmus, incision through pretracheal fascia, separation of thyroid isthmus. (D) Division of thyroid isthmus between haemostats. (E) Incision of trachea, creation of circular opening. (F) Tracheostomy tube inserted, retained by tapes passed around the neck and secured with a reef knot. (Ballantyne.)

It is important that the head and neck are maintained perfectly in the midline during the whole operation. A transverse or vertical midline incision is made over the upper part of the trachea just below the cricoid cartilage. The incision is extended through the deep fascia, and the sternothyroid and hyoid muscles retracted laterally.

The isthmus of the thyroid gland is either clamped across, divided and ligated, or displaced. Another layer of the fascia is incised, the cricoid cartilage steadied with a single sharp hook, and the trachea is opened through a vertical stab wound which divides about two rings of cartilage. The trachea dilators are inserted into this incision, separated, and a tracheal tube inserted. Some surgeons cut a small flap of cartilage when making their

Fig. 18.69 Tracheostomy or laryngostomy.

1. Scalpel handle No. 3 with No. 10 blade (Bard Parker).
2. Scalpel handle No. 9 with No. 15 blade (Bard Parker).
3. Fine dissecting forceps, toothed (Gillies), 2.
4. Fine dissecting forceps, non-toothed (McIndoe), 1.
5. Scissors, curved on flat, 13 cm (5 in) (Mayo).
6. Scissors, stitch.
7. Fine artery forceps, straight, mosquito, 6.
8. Fine artery forceps, curved on flat, mosquito, 6.
9. Artery forceps, straight, 18 cm (7 in) (Spencer Wells), 2.
10. Small retractors, sharp and blunt, single hook, 2.
11. Small retractors, double hook, 2.
12. Medium retractors, malleable copper.
13. Retractor, self-retaining (West).
14. Tracheal dilating forceps (Bowlby or Trouseau).
15. Long tracheostomy tubes (Chevalier Jackson), assorted sizes. A, outer tube; B, inner tube; C, pilot or introducer.
16. Medium tracheostomy tubes (Parker), assorted sizes. A, outer tube; B, inner tube; C, pilot or introducer.
17. Laryngotomy tube (Butlin), 3 sizes. A, tube; B, pilot or introducer.

Ear, Nose and Throat Operations

Fig. 18.71 Trouseau Tracheal Dilating Forceps. Sizes available 16–34 Charrière gauge.

Fig. 18.70 Chevalier Jackson Tracheostomy Tubes. (Down Bros Ltd.)

(Medishield)

(Portex)

A. Morrant Baker Plastic Tracheostomy Cannula, with fixed plastic flange slotted for retaining tape.
B. Morrant Baker Rubber Tracheostomy Cannula, with fixed rubber flange slotted for retaining tape and detachable inflatable rubber cuff.
C. James Rubber Tracheostomy Cannula, with detachable rubber flange slotted for retaining tape and fixed inflatable rubber cuff.
D. Portex Cuffed Plastic Tracheostomy Tube.

Fig. 18.72 Tracheostomy Cannulae or Tubes. Sizes available: A, B and C, 27, 30, 33, 36, 39 and 42 Charrière gauge or 3 to 12 Magill tube scale.

incision in order to accommodate the circumference of the tube better, especially the cuffed, rubber variety (which may be used as an alternative to those illustrated, see Figs. 18.69–18.71). This cartilage flap is sutured to the skin to prevent it slipping back accidentally into the trachea should the tube become displaced, and to help in changing the tube.

The skin is closed in the usual manner. The tapes secured round the neck and a dressing of tulle gras applied under the tube flange.

Laryngofissure

DEFINITION

An opening through the thyroid cartilage into the larynx to remove a tumour or tumours.

POSITION

As for tracheostomy.

INSTRUMENTS

General set (Figs. 14.1–14.28)
Laryngofissure and laryngectomy set (Fig. 18.73)
Tongue forceps (Mayo)
Angled tongue depressor
Mouth gag (Mason)
Suction tubing, nozzles and tube anchoring forceps
Diathermy leads, electrodes and lead anchoring forceps
Connection and tubing for anaesthetic machine
Corrugated rubber or plastic drainage tubing
2·5, 3 and 4 (2/0, 0 and 1) Chromic catgut or Dexon for ligatures
2·5 and 4 (2/0 and 1) Chromic catgut or Dexon (or stainless-steel wire) on medium half-circle cutting and round-bodied needles for larynx and muscle sutures.
2·5 or 2 (2/0 or 3/0) Silk or nylon on a medium curved cutting needle for skin sutures.

OUTLINE OF PROCEDURE

A preliminary tracheostomy may have been performed. A midline incision is made from the hyoid bone to the cricoid cartilage. Soft tissues are retracted and the thyroid cartilage divided with shears or a cartilage saw, care being taken to divide the mucous membrane of the larynx in the midline. (This is to avoid damage to the vocal cords.) The cut edges of the cartilage are retracted to expose the interior of the larynx. The tumour is excised, haemostasis secured with diathermy, and the wound closed in layers, with drainage. Stainless-steel wire or chromic catgut is used to close the larynx.

Laryngectomy

DEFINITION

Removal of the entire larynx, and establishment of a permanent tracheostomy.

POSITION

As for laryngofissure.

INSTRUMENTS

As for laryngofissure.
Silk may be used in preference to catgut sutures for the deep closure.

Fig. 18.73 Laryngofissure or laryngectomy.

1. Scissors, straight 20 cm (8 in) (Mayo).
2. McIndoe bone cutting forceps.
3. Retractor, self-retaining (West).
4. Retractor, self-retaining (Mayo, angled).
5. Tracheal dilators (Bowlby or Trouseau).
6. Cartilage saw.
7. Small retractor, sharp single hook.
8. Long tracheostomy tube (Cheválier Jackson, large size).

OUTLINE OF PROCEDURE

A midline incision is made from the hyoid bone to the cricoid cartilage. The body of the hyoid bone may be divided in the midline and the ends retracted.

The muscle attachments at the sides of the larynx are freed and the trachea is severed. The endotracheal tube is withdrawn, and a wide tracheostomy tube (wrapped with tulle gras) is inserted into the severed end and connected to the anaesthetic machine.

The larynx is elevated and freed, clamping the vessels as dissection proceeds. The pharynx is then opened and the larynx removed. When haemostasis is complete, the pharynx is closed with interrupted chromic catgut, Dexon or silk sutures.

The incision is closed, with drainage, and the skin margins in the lower part of the wound are sutured around the tracheal opening.

There are a variety of post-laryngectomy tubes (e.g., Lombard's which is metallic), but a very satisfactory tube can be fashioned from the lower 6 cm (2·5 in) or so of a size 10 Magill endotracheal tube with a safety pin put across it. If the rubber produces skin irritation, a plastic tube can be used. In laryngectomy and pharyngo-laryngectomy a feeding tube is passed either beforehand in the ward, or towards the end of the operation in the theatre.

Partial amputation of the tongue

DEFINITION

Removal of varying amounts of the tongue for carcinoma, but usually not less than half when the growth is limited to one side. Radical dissection of the cervical glands (Chapter 22) may also be performed, either before, during, or after this operation.

POSITION

Supine.

INSTRUMENTS

As for tracheostomy
General set (Figs. 14.1–14.28)
Mouth gag (Doyen or Mason)
Tongue forceps (Mayo)
Angled tongue depressor
Fine artery forceps, curved on flat mosquito, 10
Fine artery forceps, straight, mosquito, 10
Fine tissue forceps (McIndoe), 5
Suction tubing, nozzles and tube anchoring forceps
Diathermy leads, electrodes and lead anchoring forceps.
2 and 2·5 (3/0 and 2/9) Chromic catgut or Dexon for ligatures
2·5 and 3 (2/0 and 0) Chromic catgut or Dexon on small half-circle round-bodied needles for sutures
3 (0) Silk on a medium half-circle round-bodies needle for stay sutures.

OUTLINE OF PROCEDURE

A preliminary tracheostomy is performed and the pharynx packed with ribbon gauze. Three stay sutures are inserted into the tongue and left long. One of the sutures is placed behind the growth and the other two at each side of the tip of the tongue.

The mucous membrane on the floor of the mouth is freed and the tongue split longitudinally down the centre. The tongue is freed from the hyoid bone and the posterior position divided across well behind growth. Any blood-vessels seen during dissection are picked up with artery forceps and ligated or under-run, if possible before they are divided. Haemostasis may be achieved also with diathermy.

The cut edge of the tongue is sutured and the mucous membrane approximated also if possible.

Partial excision of the jaw

DEFINITION

Partial removal of the mandible for malignancy. This operation is usually combined with radical dissection of the cervical glands (Chapter 22).

POSITION

Supine, with sandbag under the shoulder blades, neck extended and head thrown well back, with the chin central and in the midline.

INSTRUMENTS

    As for partial amputation of the tongue
    Wire saw and handles (Gigli or Olivercrona)
    Saw guide (de Martel)
    Jaw saw (Wood)
    Bone awls, set
    Bone-nibbling forceps, small and medium, 2
    Bone-cutting forceps (Liston)
    Bone-cutting forceps (Horsley compound action)
    Small rugines, curved and straight (Faraboeuf), 2
    Bone-holding forceps (St Thomas)
    Ligatures as for partial amputation of the tongue, plus 2/0 and 0 Silk.

OUTLINE OF PROCEDURE

An L-shaped or T-shaped incision is made over the neck and lower mandible. Radical dissection of the cervical glands is carried out and the muscles attached to the mandible are freed. The tongue and the parotid gland are retracted and the portion of the jaw to be removed is divided with a saw. The bone is disarticulated from the joint and resected.

The wound is closed in layers with drainage in the usual manner. If the mucosa cannot be approximated, the wound will be partially packed and an intra-oral or buccal skin graft will be performed at a later date by the plastic surgeon. In order to restore the facial contours after such an extensive excision, the dental surgeon may co-operate with the otolaryngologist and plastic surgeon to provide a prosthesis, which will also help to maintain the graft in position during healing.

REFERENCES AND FURTHER READING

BALLANTYNE, J. (1976) *Operative Surgery: The Ear*. London: Butterworth.
BALLANTYNE, J. (1976) *Operative Surgery: Nose and Throat*. London: Butterworth.
HALL, I. S. AND COLMAN, B. H. (1976) *Diseases of the Nose, Throat and Ear*. Edinburgh: Churchill Livingstone.

19
OPERATIONS ON THE FACE

Excision of superficial ulcer of the face

DEFINITION

The removal of a superficial dermal ulcer.

POSITION. Supine.

INSTRUMENTS

Sponge-holding forceps (Rampley), 2
Towel clips, 4
Scalpel handles Nos. 3 and 9 with Nos. 10 and 15 blades (Bard Parker)
Fine dissecting forceps, toothed (Gillies), 2
Fine dissecting forceps, non-toothed (McIndoe), 2
Scissors, curved 10 cm (4 in) (Kilner or strabismus)
Fine pointed scissors, curved (iris)
Fine double-hook retractors, 2
Skin hooks (Gillies or Kilner), 2
Fine tissue forceps (McIndoe), 4
Artery forceps, straight, mosquito, 5 to 10
Artery forceps, curved on flat, mosquito, 5 to 10
Fine needle holder (Gillies, Kilner, etc.)
2 and 1·5 (3/0 and 4/0) Plain catgut or Dexon for ligatures
2 (3/0) Plain catgut or Dexon on a small curved round-bodied needle for fat sutures
1·5 or 1 (4/0 or 5/0) Silk or nylon on a small curved non-traumatic cutting needle for skin sutures
(Skin graft instruments may be required (Fig. 24.15).)

OUTLINE OF PROCEDURE

An elliptical incision is made following the facial lines and with the ulcer in the centre of the ellipse. The ulcerated skin is dissected free and the surrounding skin flaps undermined. If the skin can be approximated, it is closed with fine interrupted sutures; if it cannot, a skin flap is rotated or a split-skin graft performed, using a soft textured graft such as that which can be obtained from the inner aspect of the upper arm.

Removal of sebaceous or dermoid cysts, naevi, etc.

This is similar to the operation above but with the addition of the following instruments:
Dissector (MacDonald or Durham)
Double-end curetting spoon (Volkmann)
Medium retractors, double hook, 2.

20
GYNAECOLOGICAL AND OBSTETRIC OPERATIONS

Excision of Bartholinian cyst

DEFINITION

The removal of a cyst due to blockage of the duct of the Bartholin gland which is in the labium majora on either side.

POSITION

Lithotomy, Figure 4.11.

INSTRUMENTS

Sponge-holding forceps (Rampley), 5
Towel clips, 5
Scalpel handle No. 3 with No. 10 blade (Bard Parker)
Dissecting forceps, toothed (Lane), 2
Dissecting forceps, non-toothed, 15 cm (6 in)
Scissors, curved on flat, 13 cm (5 in) (Mayo)
Tissue forceps (Allis), 5
Dissector (MacDonald or Durham)
Fine artery forceps, straight, mosquito, 10
Needle holder (Mayo)
2·5 (2/0) Chromic catgut or Dexon for ligatures
3 (0) Chromic catgut or Dexon on a small half-circle round-bodied needle for deep sutures.

OUTLINE OF PROCEDURE

An incision is made over the swelling in the long axis of the labium majora, and deepened down to the cyst wall. The cyst is removed by blunt dissection and any blood-vessels encountered are picked up and ligated. The incision is closed with chromic catgut, drawing the walls of the cyst cavity together.

Excision of the vulva (vulvectomy)

DEFINITION

Removal of the vulva.

POSITION

Lithotomy.

INSTRUMENTS

General set (Figs. 14.1 to 14.28).
Urethral catheter, self-retaining (Foley size 18 Charrière gauge)
20 ml syringe and sterile water for inflating catheter balloon
Proflavine emulsion or similar gauze pack
2·5 and 3 (2/0 and 0) Chromic catgut or Dexon for ligatures
4 or 5 (1 or 2) Chromic catgut or Dexon on a medium half-circle Mayo's needle with a trocar point for sutures.

OUTLINE OF PROCEDURE

An outer, oval incision is made, surrounding both labia majora if necessary. An inner, oval incision is also made and this lies just within the mucocutaneous junction, to include the urethral orifice, passing around the vaginal orifice. The incisions are extended down to the urethra. Just above the urethra the cut edges are united together, but the cut edge of the vagina below is approximated to the cut edge of the skin all around. A self-retaining catheter is inserted and the vagina packed with a length of gauze to control bleeding.

Perineorrhaphy

DEFINITION

Repair of a complete or incomplete rupture of the perineum.

POSITION

Lithotomy.

INSTRUMENTS

As vulvectomy
Ligatures and sutures as vulvectomy
3 (0) Chromic catgut or Dexon on a small half-circle round-bodied needle for plication of rectum
3 (0) Chromic catgut or Dexon on a curved non-traumatic intestinal needle for rectal closure (complete rupture only).

OUTLINE OF PROCEDURE

Incomplete Rupture, where a Segment of Perineum Remains. Tissue forceps are applied to the estimated edge of the original vaginal opening. Traction on these forceps stretches the torn edge of the perineum which is cut away between the forceps to expose an edge of mucosa and skin. The edge of the mucosa is dissected up and the posterior vaginal wall freed from the rectum. A triangular-shaped piece of vaginal wall (with its base at the perineum) is excised, and the levator ani muscles identified and drawn together with mattress sutures of chromic catgut or Dexon. The triangular gap is approximated longitudinally with a continuous chromic catgut or Dexon suture, and the vagina is packed in the usual manner. The procedure is completed by inserting a self-retaining catheter into the bladder.

Complete Rupture. This operation is similar to that just described, but in addition it is necessary to reconstruct the rectum and the anal sphincter.

The septum separating the rectum and vagina is cut away, so exposing the mucous membrane of both. The rectum is freed and the torn ends of the sphincter identified. The rectum is sutured and the sphincter brought together with strong chromic catgut or Dexon. The operation then resembles incomplete rupture with repair of the levator ani muscles and closing the triangular gap formed by partial excision of the posterior vaginal wall. Finally, a catheter and vaginal pack are inserted.

Anterior colporrhaphy, amputation of cervix and posterior colpoperineorrhaphy (Manchester or Fothergill repair)

DEFINITION

Repair of a cystocele (prolapse of the bladder into the vagina) and repair of a rectocele (prolapse of the rectum into the vagina).

POSITION

Lithotomy.

INSTRUMENTS

General set (Figs. 14.1 to 14.28)
Dilation and curettage set (Fig. 20.2)
Artery forceps, straight (Moynihan), 24
Urethral catheter, self-retaining (Foley size 18 Charrière gauge)
20 ml syringe and sterile water for inflating catheter balloon
2·5 and 3 (2/0 and 0) Chromic catgut or Dexon for ligatures
3 (0) Chromic catgut or Dexon on a small half-circle round-bodied needle for plication of the bladder
4 or 5 (1 or 2) Chromic catgut or Dexon on a small half-circle Mayo needle with a trocar point for sutures
Proflavine emulsion or similar gauze pack for the vagina.

OUTLINE OF PROCEDURE

Anterior Colporrhaphy. An Auvard's speculum is inserted and the cervix grasped with vulsellum forceps. The surgeon may then perform a dilation and curettage of the uterus if the patient is post menopausal and has cervical bleeding.

Traction is placed on the vulsellum forceps, pulling the cervix down and thereby stretching the anterior vaginal wall. An incision is made just above the junction of the cervix with the vaginal wall and blunt pointed scissors are inserted to separate the bladder from the vagina. A bladder sound is inserted, and the dissection continued up to a point just below the urethra, and the vaginal wall is then split up the midline along the extent of the separated portion. These skin flaps are retracted laterally and the bladder mobilised from the cervix and up and away from view. The cystocele is repaired by plicating the pubocervical fascia with 3 (0) chromic catgut or Dexon, thereby making a buttress between the bladder and vagina.

Amputation of the Cervix. If there is a vault prolapse, then a partial amputation of the cervix is performed. This is done after dissecting up two flaps of mucous membrane from the cervix, one in front and one behind. The partial amputation of the cervix is per-

Fig. 20.1 Anterior colporrhapy, amputation of cervix and posterior colpoperineorrhaphy. (A) Opening up the anterior vaginal wall. (B) Mobilising cystocele from cervix. (C) Placing the tightening suture as far laterally as possible. (D) Obliteration of the cystocele completed. (E) Removing redundant vaginal wall. This is followed by closure with a continuous catgut suture. (F) The cystocele has been repaired. The cervix is being stripped of vaginal wall. (G) Posterior vaginal wall being stripped back. Elongated transverse cervical and uterosacral ligaments have been sutured and divided. (H) Amputation of cervical stump. (I) Covering the posterior stump with vaginal wall.

formed and the two flaps of mucous membrane sutured so that the mucosa is invaginated towards the lining of the cervix to form a reconstructed cervical os.

The anterior incision is closed with several mattress sutures which are placed lateral to the cut edge of the vaginal wall on each side. These sutures are tied and the redundant vaginal wall excised, so narrowing the vagina. The procedure is completed with a row of interrupted chromic catgut or Dexon sutures.

Posterior Colpoperineorrhaphy. The Auvard's speculum is removed and an elliptical transverse section of skin excised with scissors. The rectum is freed with dissecting scissors and the posterior vaginal wall is slit up the midline. The rectocele is repaired by approximating the levator ani muscles with mattress sutures of chromic catgut or Dexon. The redundant vaginal mucosa is excised and the edges brought together with continuous chromic catgut sutures.

Fig. 20.1 (*cont'd.*)

(J) Tying the transverse cervical ligaments in front of the cervix and so shortening them and raising the uterus. (This is the so-called Fothergill suture: sometimes two are put in). (K) Covering cervical stump and closing the vaginal wall. On release of the cervical stump the uterus returns to the pelvis. (L) Mobilisation of the posterior vaginal wall. (M) Separating rectocele from posterior vaginal wall. (N) Obliterating the rectocele by tightening the fascial layer. (O) Excess vaginal skin is removed. The perineal muscles are sutured over the obliterated rectocele. The skin and vagina are closed as in perineorrhaphy. (Garrey, Govan, Hodge and Callander.)

The transverse incision in the posterior vaginal wall is sutured longitudinally, which again tightens the vagina. The operation is completed by inserting a self-retaining catheter into the bladder and packing the vagina with a proflavine emulsion gauze or similar pack.

Dilation of the cervix and curettage of the uterus

DEFINITION

Dilation of the cervix and scraping away the uterine mucosa.

POSITION

Lithotomy.

INSTRUMENTS

As Figure 20.2.

Fig. 20.2 Dilatation of the cervix and uterine curettage.

1. Sponge-holding forceps (Rampley), 2.
2. Vaginal speculum (Auvard).
3. Vulsellum forceps (Teale), 2.
4. Uterine sound (Horrock).
5. Uterine dilators (Hegar), set of various sizes.
6. Uterine curette (Sim), double end.
7. Flushing curette (Rheinstadter).
8. Ovum forceps (Greenhalgh).
9. Towel clips, 4.
10. Vaginal speculum (Sim).
11. Spiked-end probe (Playfair).
12. Bladder sound.
13. Female catheter, metal.
14. Uterine dressing forceps (Jessop Hospital pattern).

OUTLINE OF PROCEDURE

An Auvard's speculum is inserted and the cervix drawn down and steadied with one or two vulsellum forceps. The position and length of the uterus are gauged with a uterine sound and progressively larger sizes of uterine dilators are inserted until the os is large enough to introduce the curette. The surgeon always holds each dilator between his thumb and forefinger, with the other fingers extended at the side, so that should the dilator slip, these extended fingers will come into contact with the buttocks and prevent the dilator penetrating too deeply. A uterine curette is inserted and the mucosa scraped gently and systematically. The curetted mucosa is sent for histological examination.

If the procedure is being carried out for retained products of conception, the initial stages follow that described above, but in this case the retained products are removed preferably with ovum or sponge-holding forceps instead of a curette, and the uterine sound is not used. A gauze pack may then be inserted into the vagina.

Fallopian insufflation and salpingography

DEFINITION

Insufflation of the Fallopian tubes with CO_2 to test their patency; and injection of a radio-opaque medium for X-ray examination of the interior of the uterus and Fallopian tubes.

POSITION

Lithotomy.

INSTRUMENTS

Salpingography (Fig. 20.3).

OUTLINE OF PROCEDURE

A bi-valve speculum is inserted and the cervix drawn down and steadied with one or two pairs of vulsellum forceps. The position and length of the uterus are gauged with a uterine sound and progressively larger sizes of uterine dilators are inserted up to the outside diameter of the insufflation nozzle. The insufflation nozzle is inserted into the cervical canal and CO_2 under pressure is injected into the uterus up to 180 mmHg. Patency of the Fallopian tubes is determined either by applying a stethoscope to the abdominal wall and listening to the gas escaping into the peritoneal cavity from each tube as the pressure is applied, or observing a direct reading Kymograph which records pressure variations as the CO_2 is injected. (The dilation may then be continued followed by endometrial biopsy.)

For salpingography, a Sim's speculum is inserted and the radio-opaque medium (Urografin 76 per cent) injected into the uterine cavity with a special syringe. An X-ray is taken immediately.

Cervical and uterine polypus, biopsy and cauterisation of the cervix

DEFINITION

Removal of a polypus from the cervix or interior of the uterus; biopsy of the cervix for histological examination; cauterisation for cervical erosion and chronic cervicitis.

POSITION

Lithotomy.

INSTRUMENTS

Dilation and curettage (Fig. 20.2)
Scalpel handle No. 3 with No. 10 blade (Bard Parker)
Dissecting forceps, toothed (Lane), 2
Dissecting forceps, non-toothed, 18 cm (7 in), 2
Scissors, curved on flat, 18 cm (7 in) (Mayo)
Needle holder (Mayo)
Diathermy or cautery apparatus, leads and electrodes for cervical cauterisation
3 or 4 (0 or 1) Chromic catgut or Dexon on a small half-circle Mayo needle with a trocar point for sutures.

OUTLINE OF PROCEDURE

Cervical Polypus. A Sim's speculum is inserted and the polyp grasped with ring forceps or artery forceps. The polypus is twisted until it comes away, and the cervical canal is gently scraped with a small curette.

Uterine Polypus. A Sim's speculum is inserted and the cervical os dilated until the opening is large enough to graps the polyp with forceps and twisted as described above. If bleeding is persistent and cannot be stopped with hot irrigations, the surgeon will pack the uterine cavity with a length of gauze.

Fig. 20.3 Apparatus for Testing and Recording Tubal Patency and Functional Activity. (From *Textbook for Midwives* by Margaret Myles, by kind permission.)

Instruments for endometrial biopsy:
2 sponge-holding forceps.
1 Sim's speculum.
1 teneculum forceps.
1 uterine sound.
2 endometrial biopsy curettes.
1 dissecting forceps.

Instruments for tubal insufflation:
2 cannulae.
1 uterine sound.
1 teneculum forceps.
1 Sim's speculum.
2 sponge-holding forceps.

Cervical Biopsy. This operation is generally performed in conjunction with dilatation and curettage of the uterus, sometimes following a Papanicolaou cervical smear in which suspicious cells have been found. A small wedge or cone of cervix is excised and sent for histological examination, and the incision is approximated with chromic catgut or Dexon. The vagina may be packed with a proflavine emulsion or similar gauze pack.

Fig. 20.4 Extensive cone biopsy of the cervix. (A) The method of covering the raw area, the blood vessels which lie laterally have been underpinned and ligatured. (B) A long catgut suture is introduced as shown in the vaginal wall posteriorly. (C) The needle has then been passed through the whole thickness of the cervix to emerge through the vaginal wall. The needle is then threaded through the other end of the suture and passed as shown. When the suture is tied the posterior part of the raw area is covered. A similar suture is introduced anteriorly, and finally lateral sutures are passed to cover the raw area completely. (Hawkins and Bowne.)

Cervical Cauterisation. A bi-valve or Sim's speculum is inserted and heat applied to the ulcerated area by means of a cautery or diathermy electrode. If diathermy is being used, the indifferent electrode is applied to the patient's thigh with the usual precautions (Chapter 2). The vagina will be packed with a proflavine emulsion or similar gauze pack. Spiritous antiseptics must not be used for skin preparation due to the danger of explosion with diathermy or cautery. (Cauterisation using a laser beam is a fast developing technique.)

Laparoscopy (peritoneoscopy)

DEFINITION

Inspection of the peritoneal cavity by means of a laparoscope introduced through the abdominal wall.

POSITION

Either supine or slight Trendelenburg with legs in lithotomy.

INSTRUMENTS

Laparoscopy
Sponge-holding forceps (Rampley), 2
Towel clips, 5

Scalpel handle No. 3 with No. 10 blade (Bard Parker)
Dissecting forceps, toothed (Lane), 2
Dissecting forceps, non-toothed, 15 cm (6 in)
Scissors, curved on flat, 13 cm (5 in) (Mayo), 1.
Needle holder (Mayo), 1
Laparoscope, such as the Frangeheim (as Fig. 20.5)
Palmer biopsy drill forceps (Fig. 20.6)
Verres trocar and cannula
Diathermy leads and electrodes
Fibre light projector
2·5 or 3 (2/0 or 0) chromic catgut or Dexon for ligatures and on small half-circle cutting needle for subcutaneous sutures if required
2·5 (2/0) silk or nylon on straight or curved cutting needle for skin sutures.
Vaginal examination
Instruments as for D and C may be required
Gentian violet solution and 10 ml syringe with cannula.

OUTLINE OF PROCEDURE

The Verres needle is inserted through a small 2 cm skin incision made transversely just below the umbilicus. The same incision is used later for inserting the laparoscope trocar and cannula. (The point of the Verres needle is first covered with K-Y or similar jelly.)

The needle is manipulated until the point is felt to pass through the outer layer of the rectus sheath then impinging upon the posterior layer and with a little more pressure enter the abdominal cavity. The sudden dropping of the inner core into the needle (Fig. 20.7) is a further indication that the point has entered the abdominal cavity.

Fig. 20.5 Frangenheim laparoscope. (Down's Surgical Ltd.)

Fig. 20.6 Palmer Biopsy forceps.

Fig. 20.7 (A) Needle at skin surface, inner core fully extended. (B) Needle in abdominal wall, inner core fully retracted at point, air intake raised above shoulder. (C) Needle point through abdominal wall, inner core descends rounded end now prevents point of outer sheath from damaging bowel, etc. Air intake sits down on shoulder as point enters peritoneal cavity.

The needle is then connected to a carbon dioxide supply controlled through an apparatus such as the Semm's automatic insufflator and some three litres of gas are allowed to pass into the abdominal cavity. This takes three to four minutes and care is taken not to raise the intra-abdominal pressure by more than 20 mmHg as this could seriously interfere with the return of blood to the heart by stopping the flow in the inferior vena cava which could lead to acute hypotension.

The lubricated laparoscope trocar and cannula are now inserted slightly diagonally (alongside the Verres needle) through the rectus sheath and into the abdominal cavity. The trocar is removed and the telescope with its accompanying light carrier is passed through the cannula into the abdominal cavity.

PROCEDURES CARRIED OUT WITH THE LAPAROSCOPE (FISHER, 1970)

1. *Infertility*. Tubal patency can be demonstrated by dye installation through a cervical cannula by a second operator. A solution of gentian violet, is instilled into the uterus; with the laparoscope the surgeon by visualising dye transit can confirm tubal patency. Similarly the restriction of dye dispersal by fine adhesions is easily demonstrated. At the same time ovarian biopsy can be taken to establish the presence of primordial follicles or functioning corpora lutea or graffian follicles.

2. *Ectopic Pregnancy*. When there are doubts in cases of early tubal abortion laparoscopy can reveal the presence of the tubal gestation and the surgeon can then proceed to laparotomy and definitive surgery. Conversely, a ruptured retention cyst which is settling can be left alone and thus laparotomy avoided.

3. *Acute Infection*. In the presence of abdominal pain where the differential diagnosis

includes acute salpingitis, ectopic pregnancy and ruptured retention cysts, laparoscopy has been used to identify the engorged and distended Fallopian tubes in cases of acute salpingitis, thus permitting conservative treatment and avoiding laparotomy.

4. *Amenorrhoea.* The investigation of amenorrhoea today will include a laparoscopy, visualising the ovaries and enabling a biopsy to be taken. This step can be most useful in establishing the likelihood of the ovaries responding to treatment. In the absence of primordial follicles there is little evidence that stimulation by gonadotrophins will be of value. Similarly, the presence of multiple micro-cysts in the ovary indicate the need for extreme caution in the management of gonadotrophin stimulation therapy.

5. *Sterilisation.* It is possible by introducing suitably insulated forceps through a second small incision to divide the Fallopian tubes by diathermy coagulation in one or more places and thus effect sterilisation by interrupting tubal continuity.

6. *Unexplained Abdominal Pain.* Much of the gynaecologist's practice concerns pain in the pelvis. In these instances laparoscopy provides a means of obtaining a correct diagnosis in cases of unsuspected endometriosis and other causes of pelvic inflammatory response. Thus definitive treatment is possible and the patient's pain relieved.

At the close of the operation the carbon dioxide is first expelled from the abdominal cavity via the cannula which is then removed. The skin incision is closed with silk or nylon, alternatively subcutaneous sutures of catgut or Dexon may be used.

Abdominal hysterectomy

DEFINITION

Partial or entire removal of the uterus through an abdominal incision.

POSITION

Trendelenburg, Figure 4.7.

INSTRUMENTS

General set (Figs. 14.1 to 14.28)
Laparotomy set (Figs. 15.1 to 15.7)
Hysterectomy set (Fig. 20.8)
2·5 and 3 (2/0 and 0) Chromic catgut or Dexon for ligatures, fine and medium
5 (2) Chromic catgut or Dexon on large half-circle Mayo needles with trocar points for transfixion sutures and uterine, vaginal vault, peritoneum and muscle sutures
3 (0) Chromic catgut or Dexon on a medium half-circle round-bodied needle for reconstruction of pelvic floor
2·5 (2/0) Silk or nylon on a large straight or curved cutting needle for skin sutures
(Kifa and Michel clips may be required.)

OUTLINE OF PROCEDURE

The vagina is swabbed with antiseptic solution and plugged with a length of antiseptic gauze, which is left protruding for subsequent removal during operation. Removal and safety ensuring removal will be easier if a pair of sponge-holding forceps is attached to this pack and left lying between the patient's legs.

The abdomen is opened through a subumbilical midline incision which passes through the skin, linea alba and peritoneum. The bowel which may protrude is displaced towards the diaphragm with two or three large gauze packs. The uterus is drawn out of the pelvis and two pairs of Kocher's or Mayo-Oschner forceps are applied across the broad ligament either inside or outside the ovaries, depending on whether they are to be removed or not. It is usual to try to leave at least one ovary for endocrine function. The broad ligament is opened on each side between these forceps and a flap of peritoneum is cut from the front

Fig. 20.8 Abdominal hysterectomy, etc.

1. Suprapubic retractor (Doyen).
2. Long, heavy scissors, curved on flat 25 cm (10 in).
3. Artery forceps, curved on flat (Mayo-Oschner), 6.
4. Vulsellum forceps (Teale), 2.
5. Needle holder and needles (Bonney-Reverdin), 3 sharp point and 1 blunt point.
6. Uterine dressing forceps (Jessop Hospital pattern).
7. Sponge-holding forceps (Rampley), 2.
8. Vaginal retractor (Collins).
9. Vaginal speculum (Sim).

of the uterus. The bladder is separated from the front of the cervix by blunt dissection and is pushed well below the point of transection. Pairs of clamps are placed across the cardinal ligaments and uterine arteries on each side, carefully avoiding the ureters, and the vessels are divided between the clamps.

For subtotal hysterectomy, the uterus is removed by cutting across the cervix; for part or total hysterectomy the pack is removed from the vagina, the fornix of the vagina is cut into, the cervix seized with a pair of vulsellum forceps and drawn upwards, and the uterus is removed by dividing the vagina from the cervix all round.

Transfixion sutures are placed and tied around the clamped stumps of the ovarian

Fig. 20.9 Subtotal hysterectomy. (A) Broad ligaments clamped and divided between forceps, anterior peritoneal flap being reflected. (B) Clamping the uterine artery. (C) Amputation of cervix. (D) Transfixion sutures being secured around clamped stumps of ovarian vessels. (E) Burying left ovarian pedicle. (F) Burying right ovarian pedicle. (Bonney.)

vessels, round ligament and uterine arteries. For subtotal hysterectomy, the stump of the cervix is closed over with a few interrupted chromic catgut or Dexon sutures, and for total hysterectomy the cut edge of the vagina is closed with interrupted or continuous chromic catgut or Dexon sutures. The flap of peritoneum is sutured over the cut edge of the posterior peritoneum, covering the cervical or vaginal stump and the transfixed round ligaments. The surgeon may suture the round ligaments to the vault of the vagina before reconstructing the pelvic floor with 4 (0) chromic catgut or Dexon sutures. The abdominal wound is closed in layers.

Wertheim's hysterectomy

DEFINITION

Total hysterectomy, bilateral salpingo-oöphorectomy, with removal of the upper part of the vagina and lymphatic glands which drain the pelvis.

POSITION

Tredelenburg, Figure 4.7.

INSTRUMENTS

As for abdominal hysterectomy
Hysterectomy clamps, right-angled (Wertheim), 2
Diathermy leads, electrodes and lead anchoring forceps
Urethral catheter, self-retaining (Foley size 18 Charrière gauge)
20 ml syringe, and sterile water to inflate catheter balloon
Ligatures and sutures as for hysterectomy.

OUTLINE OF PROCEDURE

This follows the procedure of total hysterectomy but with the following additions.

The rectum is freed from the vagina which is divided across well beyond the cervix, after applying strong right-angled clamps (Wertheim's). In this way, when the uterus is removed, the growth on the cervix is covered by a section of the vagina clamped over it, thereby preventing soiling of the peritoneal cavity. After the vagina has been closed and the vessels ligatured, the connective tissue on the side walls of the pelvis and around the vessels is carefully dissected free, together with the iliac and obturator glands.

The pelvic floor is reconstructed as before and the wound closed in layers. As the bladder has been extensively separated, it is usual to leve a catheter *in situ* for a few days post-operatively.

Vaginal hysterectomy

DEFINITION

Removal of the uterus through the vagina.

POSITION

Lithotomy.

444   Operating Theatre Technique

A
- Medial stump of the round ligament
- Lateral stump of the round ligament
- Lateral stump of the infundibulopelvic ligament
- Medial stump of the infundibulopelvic ligament

B

C

D
- Lateral stump of the uterine vessels
- Lateral stump of the Cardinal ligament
- Uterosacral ligament separated from its rectal attachment

E

F
- Horizontal connective tissue ground bundle
- Ureter
- Medial stump of the Cardinal ligament
- Medial stump of the uterine vessels

INSTRUMENTS

General set (Figs. 14.1 to 14.28)
Artery forceps, straight, 20 cm (8 in) (Spencer Wells), 10
Deep retractors, narrow blade (Deaver or Paton), 2
Artery forceps, heavy curved on flat (Mayo-Oschner or Kocher), 6
Vulsellum forceps (Teale), 2
Scissors, heavy curved on flat, 20 cm (8 in) (Mayo)
Vaginal speculum (Auvard)
Urethral catheter, self-retaining (Foley size 18 Charrière gauge)
20 ml syringe, and sterile water to inflate catheter balloon
4 and 5 (1 and 2) Chromic catgut or Dexon for all ligatures, transfixion sutures and closure sutures on large half-circle Mayo needles with trocar points
Proflavine emulsion or similar gauze pack may be required for vagina.

OUTLINE OF PROCEDURE

An Auvard's speculum is inserted, and the cervix grasped with vulsellum forceps, pulled down and steadied. An incision is made below the urinary orifice and round the cervix. The bladder is freed from the uterus in front, and the rectum from the uterus posteriorly. The anterior and posterior peritoneum is opened and traction applied to the cervix so that clamps can be applied to the cardinal ligament and uterine arteries. The fundus of the uterus is delivered from the abdomen and clamps applied to each round ligament. The round ligament is severed between the clamps and the uterus is removed. The vessels and ligaments are transfixed and ligated with chromic catgut or Dexon. The anterior and posterior peritoneum are sutured together, exteriorising the round ligaments and uterine vessels which are sutured over by closing the vaginal wall.

A catheter is inserted and the vagina plugged with a proflavine emulsion gauze or similar pack.

◀ Fig. 20.10 Wertheim's hysterectomy for carcinoma of cervix – extent of excision.
(A) The abdomen has been opened and the round ligaments have been divided. The infundibulopelvic ligament has also been divided between ligatures. The ligatures are left long and act as retractors. The peritoneum in front of the uterus has been cut through so that the broad ligament has been opened up.
(B) The right external iliac vessels and their lymph nodes have been exposed by the division of the peritoneum between the right ovariopelvic ligament and the right round ligament. A taped swab has been placed in the right paravesical fossa to arrest bleeding. The glands and cellular tissue are being cleared from the left external iliac vessels. The uterus is drawn well over to the opposite side so that the obturator fossa is exposed. The obturator nerve, artery and vein are well seen and the left ureter can be seen passing under the uterine artery.
(C) The uterine artery has been divided between ligatures and the roof of the ureteric canal cut through. The cardinal ligament can be seen in the diagram with the aneurysm needle placed below it. In front of the cardinal ligament lies the paravesical space while behind the ligament lies the pararectal space.
(D) The cardinal ligament has been divided on each side. The uterus has been drawn forwards, the peritoneum of the pouch of Douglas has been cut through transversely and the bowel has been separated from the posterior vaginal wall.
(E) The uterosacral ligament on the left side has been clamped and divided. A clamp has been placed across the left cardinal ligament, and the tissues distal to the clamp have been cut through.
(F) The uterus and appendages have been separated from their attachments, the cardinal ligaments and the uterosacral ligaments having been divided. A large Wertheim clamp has been placed over the vagina. On each side of the vagina below this level the paravaginal tissues which form the horizontal part of the ground bundle have been clamped and divided.

Oöphorectomy, salpingectomy, myomectomy

DEFINITION

Removal of an ovary; Fallopian tube; or one or more uterine fibroids.

POSITION

Trendelenburg. (Supine for ectopic gestation.)

INSTRUMENTS

As for abdominal hysterectomy (p. 440).
Suction tubing, nozzles and tube anchoring forceps for ectopic gestation.

OUTLINE OF PROCEDURE

The uterus is exposed through a subumbilical midline incision. For *oöphorectomy* and removal of ovarian cyst, the pedicle of the ovary or tumour is transfixed with strong chromic catgut or Dexon, clamping with Mayo-Oschner forceps before division. The tumour is removed and the raw edges of the tied pedicle are covered with peritoneum secured with fine chromic catgut sutures.

In *salpingectomy*, the inflamed tubes are usually adherent behind the uterus. They are carefully freed by blunt dissection and clamped across with double clamps before dividing. A catgut or Dexon transfixion ligature is now passed around the cut tube and vessels at each side of the division. This operation is performed also for ruptured ectopic gestation and in this case suction is used to remove blood from the peritoneal cavity.

For sterilisation the Fallopian tube is drawn up with dissecting forceps in a position where the broad ligament is relatively bloodless and curved clamps are placed in position on each side. The tissue enclosed by the two clamps is then excised with a scalpel.

Fig. 20.11 Removal of the Fallopian tube for ectopic gestation. Further clamps are placed across the broad ligament so that no part escapes ligation.

Subsequently the tissues enclosed in the clamps are ligatured. No effort is made to bury the cut ends of the Fallopian tube. Although the operation is simple, it gives excellent results and subsequent adhesions have been shown to cause no trouble.

In *myomectomy*, the uterus is incised and the fibroids shelled out. The uterine incision is closed with two layers of chromic catgut or Dexon and the abdominal incision closed in the usual manner. The common complications are haemorrhage and sepsis.

Fig. 20.12 Operation for sterilisation. The method of the Viennese school.

Fig. 20.13 Myomectomy (A) Enucleation of the tumour from the uterus. The myoma is drawn out with a vulsellum forceps, and adhesions separated with the help of Mayo's scissors. (B) In this case the cavity of the uterus has been opened and the mucous membrane is being closed with interrupted catgut sutures. The peritoneal flap is then sutured back in position. (Howkins and Bourne.)

Fig. 20.14 Ventrosuspension of the uterus (Gilliam's operation) (A) Forceps, preferably curved, being introduced between the anterior rectus sheath and the rectus muscle. (B) The surgeon has passed the forceps round the outer border of the rectus and manoeuvred the points inwards to the internal abdominal ring. The peritoneum has been nicked over the points which are slightly opened to receive the ends of the suture used to plicate the round ligament. (C) The round ligament suture is now withdrawn along the track of the forceps and its ends are secured by threading them on a needle which anchors them to the anterior rectus sheath. (D) When tied this suture firmly draws the uterine cornu against the peritoneal surface of the posterior aspect of the rectus muscle and holds the uterus in a position of anterversion. (Howkins and Bourne.)

Hysteropexy

DEFINITION

A plastic operation on the uterus, performed for retroversion.

POSITION

Trendelenburg.

INSTRUMENTS

As for laparotomy (Figs. 14.1 to 14.28 and 15.1 to 15.7)
Artery forceps, curved (Mayo-Oschner or Kocher), 2.

OUTLINE OF PROCEDURE

There are several operations for this condition, but only one, that of ventrosuspension or shortening of the round ligaments (Gilliam's operation), will be described here.

A transverse, curved incision is made just above the pubis. This incision is carried down to the rectus sheath only, which is then incised in a vertical direction and the peritoneum is opened. The uterus is raised and a transfixion ligature placed on each round ligament about 1 cm (half an inch) from where it joins the uterus. The two ends of this ligature are left about 25 cm (10 in) long.

The skin is separated from the anterior rectus sheath for a small area on each side of the incision. Using scissors, the anterior rectus sheath is separated from the rectus muscle in a downward and outward direction towards the inernal abdominal ring. Curved artery forceps are manoeuvred along this so-formed track on each side of the incision to the internal ring. They pass through the internal abdominal ring and are manoeuvred along the round ligament to the point of ligature, where they are pushed through a stab incision in the peritoneum. The ligature is grasped and the forceps withdrawn, pulling the round ligament through the internal abdominal ring to appear between the anterior rectus sheath and muscle. The round ligaments are secured to the anterior rectus sheath with sutures of strong silk and the ligatures are used as an additional suture to make fixation doubly sure.

This procedure shortens the round ligaments by doubling them over and the suspension of the uterus is tightened, thereby correcting retroversion. The wound is closed in layers.

Caesarean section

DEFINITION

Removal of the foetus through an incision in the abdominal wall and the uterus.

POSITION

Supine, followed by Trendelenburg. 10°–20°.

INSTRUMENTS

As for hysterectomy
Uterine forceps (Green-Armytage), 5
Obstetric forceps
Suction tubing, nozzles and tube anchoring forceps
2 ml syringe and needles with ergometrine 0·5 mg
Mucus extractors and general apparatus for resuscitation of the child (cord clamps, scissors, etc.).

OUTLINE OF PROCEDURE

The patient comes to theatre with a catheter *in situ* which is released but not removed during the operation. A midline incision is made extending from the umbilicus to the pubis. The bowel is displaced towards the diaphragm with packs and a 10 cm (4 in)

Fig. 20.15 Lower segment Caesarean section. (A) The peritoneum has been divided transversely just above the dome of the bladder. Using finger and gauge dissection, the peritoneal flaps are separated from the bladder and uterus. (B) The incision through the lower segment has been completed with scissors and the baby's head is presenting. (C) Delivery of the deeply engaged head using obstetric forceps, the retractor is usually removed during delivery. (D) Repair of the uterine wall, the second suture layer is being inserted. (Farquharson and Rintoul; Movair, 1972.)

incision made in the uterus. For lower segment operations (the majority of procedures), the incision is made horizontally in the uterus (after separating the bladder from the uterus) just where the peritoneum is reflected off the bladder, and for upper segment operations, the incision is in the midline vertically. This requires a clean scalpel. The incision is completed with scissors and by manual stretching. The foetus is delivered and the umbilical cord clamped with forceps and divided. Whilst the midwife or paediatrician resuscitates the child, the placenta is delivered and the cut edges of the uterus grasped with Green-Armytage forceps. Suction is used to remove amniotic fluid.

Ergometrine is injected intravenously to cause contraction of the uterine muscles and thereby arrest haemorrhage. The incision in the uterus is closed with two layers of chromic catgut or Dexon sutures, the first layer passing through the muscle coat but not the mucosa, and the second layer is inserted to invert the first layer. The uterovesical peritoneum is sutured and the wound closed in the usual manner.

Clots are expressed from the vagina by pressure on the abdomen and a pad applied to the vulva.

REFERENCES AND FURTHER READING

GARREY, M. M., GOVAN, A. D. T., HODGE, C. H. AND CALLANDER, R. (1972) *Gynaecology Illustrated*. Edinburgh: Churchill Livingstone.
HOWKINS, J. AND BOURNE, G. (1971) *Shaw's Textbook of Gynaecology*. Edinburgh: Churchill Livingstone.
MACLEOD, D. AND HOWKINS, J. (1966) *Bonney's Gynaecological Surgery*. London: Baillière Tindall.
MOVAIR, T. J. (1972) *Hamilton Bailey's Emergency Surgery*. Bristol: Wright.

21
NEUROSURGICAL OPERATIONS

Angiography

DEFINITION

Serial X-ray examination of the cerebral vascular tree following the injection of a radio-opaque medium into a main artery in the neck, (the needle being introduced percutaneously) or via a femoral catheter.

POSITION

Supine, with the head extended, preferably on a Lysholm skull table.

INSTRUMENTS

Sponge-holding forceps, (Rampley), 5
Towel clips, 5
Scalpel handle (Bard Parker) with No. 11 blade
20 ml syringes, 3
Sterile normal saline, pyrogen-free, 60 ml
Arterial puncture needles, i.e., Lindgren arterial needles; carotid or vertebral type needles, adult and child size; or femoral arterial catheters, trocar and cannula
Adaptors and silicone tubing, 15 cm in length
Local anaesthetic requisites (Fig. 10.35)
Contrast medium, e.g., Hypaque 35 per cent or Conray 420.

OUTLINE OF PROCEDURE

After cleansing the skin and draping, a bleb of local anaesthetic is raised anterior to the sternomastoid, and then the carotid sheath or region of the vertebral artery is infiltrated. The needle is mounted on a syringe filled with saline and is inserted into the appropriate artery through a nick in the skin. After ensuring that there is a good backflow of blood from the selected vessel, the assembly is kept patent by slow injection of saline.

After positioning the patient for radiography, the saline-filled syringe is exchanged for a syringe containing contrast medium which is then rapidly injected intra-arterially whilst X-rays are taken. Normally these consist of three views, antero-posterior, lateral and oblique, taken serially. Each time, 8 to 10 ml of contrast medium is injected. Alternatively, if vertebral or multiple aneurysms are suspected, 4-vessel angiography is carried out via a femoral catheter. The groin is cleansed and draped in the usual manner, and the trocar and cannula inserted through the palpated external iliac artery. The trocar is withdrawn, and the cannula is pulled back until its presence within the vessel is indicated by a flow of arterial blood. The catheter guide wire is threaded through the cannula until it reaches the selected level in the aorta. The catheter is then passed over the guide wire for the

Fig. 21.1 Cross section of skull showing brain. (Down's Surgical Ltd.)

Fig. 21.2 Vertical section of brain. (Down's Surgical Ltd.)

predetermined distance, and after confirmatory radiographs to check its position, the guide and cannula are withdrawn, leaving the catheter in place. The injection of radio-opaque medium follows in a similar manner to that for carotid angiography.

Air encephalography

DEFINITION

X-ray examination of the ventricular system and subarachnoid spaces surrounding the brain by fractional replacement of cerebrospinal fluid with filtered air.

POSITION

Sitting, with head flexed 20°, usually in an encephalography chair.

INSTRUMENTS

Spinal set (Fig. 10.36).

OUTLINE OF PROCEDURE

Local anaesthesia and lumbar puncture is performed, omitting manometry. Using 5 ml quantities, 30 to 40 ml of c.s.f. is gradually replaced with air (filtered through a swab whilst being sucked into the syringe), an X-ray being taken after 10 ml replacement to check that air is entering the brain ventricles. After adequate air replacement the lumbar puncture needle is removed, the patient placed supine and further X-rays are taken. A sample of the aspirated c.s.f. is sent for analysis.

Myelography

DEFINITION

X-ray examination of the spinal canal after the injection of a radio-opaque medium into the subdural space.

POSITION

Lateral with knees and neck moderately flexed, or sitting.

INSTRUMENTS

Spinal set (Fig. 10.36)
Myodil or Metrizamide contrast medium.

OUTLINE OF PROCEDURE

Local anaesthesia and lumbar puncture is performed in the third or fourth lumbar interspace. Pressure readings without, and then with jugular compression are taken and 5 to 6 ml of c.s.f. withdrawn for analysis. The contrast medium is then injected and the patient X-rayed supine and prone on a tilting table. The contrast medium is left *in situ.*

Cysternal puncture

DEFINITION

The subarachnoid injection of Myodil or Metrizamide for myelography in cases of 'failed lumbar puncture' due to 'dry tap' secondary to total spinal block. The contrast medium is injected into the cysterna magna.

POSITION

Sitting with the neck flexed.

INSTRUMENTS

Spinal set (Fig. 10.36)
Cysternal puncture (short bevel) needle
Needle guard
Steel rule, 15 cm (6 in).

OUTLINE OF PROCEDURE

A skin bleb of local anaesthetic is raised in the mid-line of the neck, halfway between the external occipital protuberance and the sixth cervical spinous process. After infiltration of the neck musculature, the cysternal puncture needle (with the guard set at 55 mm) is then slowly inserted in the mid-line to traverse the posterior atlanto-occipital membrane and enter the cysterna magna at the base of the brain. After withdrawing 5 to 6 ml of c.s.f. for analysis, contrast medium is injected, the needle withdrawn and X-rays taken as in myelography.

Ventriculography

DEFINITION

An X-ray examination of the ventricular system of the brain after partial replacement of the ventricular c.s.f. with air, or occasionally Myodil or Metrizamide.

POSITION

Supine or sitting in the neurosurgical chair.

INSTRUMENTS

Sponge-holding forceps (Rampley), 5
Scalpel handle No. 4 with No. 22 blade (Bard Parker)
Scalpel handle No. 5 with No. 15 or 11 blade (Bard Parker)
Fine dissecting forceps, non-toothed (McIndoe)
Fine dissecting forceps, toothed (Gillies)
Medium dissecting forceps, non-toothed
Medium dissecting forceps, toothed (Lane's)
Artery forceps, straight (Moynihan), 5
Scissors, stitch
Scissors curved (Metzenbaum)
Scissors curved (strabismus)

Scissors straight (Iris)
Dura hooks, sharp and blunt
Periosteal elevator (Adson)
Dissector (McDonald)
Trephine seeker/small aneurysm needle
Dura separator (Sergeant's)
Dressing forceps (Tilley or Olivecrona)
Bone nibblers, curved on flat and angled on side 2
Skull perforators and burrs (Hudson)
Skull brace (Hudson)
Retractors, self-retaining (Shnitkers)
Fine needle holder (West)
Diathermy leads, electrodes, scabbard and lead anchoring forceps
Spinal manometer
CSF specimen bottles
10 ml syringe
Bonney's Blue
Steel rule and skin pen
Ventricular cannula
Towel clips 5
Irrigation syringe
Pint measure with warm saline
Local anaesthetic requisites (Fig. 10.35)
Suction tubing, fine nozzles and tube anchoring forceps
Fine Nélaton catheters, polyvinyl or latex rubber with spigots, 5
250 ml conical flask fitted with a two-holed rubber stopper, glass air-vent and 100 cm of silicone tubing and fine metal concentric connector
Horsley's bone wax gelatine sponge, patties
2 or 1·5 (3/0 or 4/0) Silk on small curved round-bodied needles for dura
2 (3/0) Silk on small curved cutting or straight cutting needles for skin.

OUTLINE OF PROCEDURE

Local anaesthetic is infiltrated into the areas selected for ventricular puncture. A 5 cm straight incision is made 3·5 cm from the midline, either on the frontal or parietal eminences. Two artery forceps are clipped on to the deepest galeal layer as retractors and after clearing back the periosteum, the artery forceps are replaced with a self-retaining retractor which by virtue of pressure from the blades creates haemostasis.

The hole is drilled first by using the perforator and then the appropriate matching burr. The dura is elevated with a dural hook, incised in a cruciate fashion and the lifted edges diathermised. The underlying brain is diathermised and incised at the entry point for insertion of the cannula. The lateral ventricles are cannulated on either side and c.s.f. pressure measured if required. Samples of c.s.f. are taken separately from each side for analysis.

The cannulae may be exchanged for fine catheters through which c.s.f. is fractionally replaced with filtered air in 5 to 10 ml increments to give a total replacement of 30 to 40 ml with normal size ventricles. If Myodil is used only 5 to 6 ml is injected.

The catheters are spigoted and the scalp closed in two layers after haemostasis has been secured. Following radiography, the catheters (which project through the suture line) are either removed, or in cases of chronic raised intracranial pressure, one is left coupled to the drainage flask for 24 to 48 hours to minimise the risk of brain compression or 'coning'.

Neurosurgical Operations 457

Fig. 21.3 Hudson Brace Perforator Spherical and Cylindrical Burrs.

Fig. 21.4 Schnitker Scalp Retractor, curved, self-retaining with blunt swivel blades.

Fig. 21.5 Sergeant-Horsley Dura Mater Separator.

Fig. 21.6 Adson Fraser Brain Suction Tube.

Fig. 21.7 Adson Curved Periosteal Elevator.

Figs. 21.3 to 21.7 Neurosurgical instruments – craniotomy/burr hole. (Down's Surgical Ltd.)

Fig. 21.8 Cairns Dural Hook, fine, sharp.

Fig. 21.9 Jefferson Ventricular Cannula and Tubing Connection.

Fig. 21.10 Dandys Ventricular Drainage Cannula. (Full size approx.)

Fig. 21.11 Luer-Jansen Rongeur, double action, slightly curved on flat.

Fig. 21.12 Gigli Wire Saw and Handle. (Used in pairs.)

Fig. 21.13 Cairn-De Martel Wire Saw Guide.

Fig. 21.14 Cairns Rongeur with fine angled on flat jaws, curved handles.

Figs. 21.8 to 21.14 Neurosurgical instruments – craniotomy/burr hole (*cont'd.*) (Down's Surgical Ltd.)

Burr hole and biopsy abscess drainage

DEFINITION

Diagnostic needle biopsy of pathological intracerebra tissue or cyst drainage via a burr hole.

POSITION

Supine, lateral or prone depending on selected site for biopsy.

INSTRUMENTS

As for ventriculography
Glass microscope slides, 7·6 cm × 2·5 cm (3 in × 1 in)
In cases of brain abscess a selection of short rubber tubing of medium bore, 5 cm long will be required. Also antibiotic solution.

OUTLINE OF PROCEDURE

Up to and including the dural incision the procedure approximates that for ventriculography. The burr hole is sited so that on 'needling' the brain a relatively 'silent' area is traversed.

The brain substance is explored with a fine brain needle passed in radiate fashion, to discover pathological tissue or cysts. When a possibly pathological area of brain is entered, a gentle aspiration biopsy is taken through the needle and pressure-smeared between two microscope slides which are placed in formol saline and sent for pathological examination.

Cysts and abscess cavities are drained through medium-bore tube drains. Antibiotics are instilled and abscess cavities are assessed thereafter by EMI brain scanner. The scalp is closed in two layers.

Craniotomy and craniectomy

DEFINITION

Craniotomy is incision through the scalp and underlying muscle, with fashioning of a muscle-hinged osteoplastic flap of the skull in order to gain access to the brain. *Craniectomy* denotes removal of a bone from the skull vault, either by enlargement of burr holes or removal of osteoplastic bone flap, again to afford access to the brain. Included under this heading is reduction of a depressed fracture of the skull vault.

POSITION

Supine for frontal, temporal or parietal exposures; prone for occipital and posterior fossa exposures; sitting for posterior fossa exposures or lateral for temporo-parietal flaps.

INSTRUMENTS

General set (Figs. 14.1 to 14.28), except large retractors
As for ventriculography (p. 455)
Artery forceps, curved on side, 24
Dissector, double end (Durham)

460 Operating Theatre Technique

Fig. 21.15 Raney scalp clip and applying/removing forceps.

Fig. 21.16 Olivecrona Angled Neuro Dressing Forceps.

Fig. 21.17 Cairns Artery Forceps, curved-to-side, box-joint.

Fig. 21.18 Adson Dressing Forceps, serrated points.

Fig. 21.19 Schmeiden (or Taylor) Dural Scissors, angular with probe-pointed under blade, screw-joint.

Fig. 21.20 Selverstone Micro Alligator Forceps, light smooth jaws.

Figs. 21.15 to 21.20 Neurosurgical instruments – craniotomy/burr hole (*cont'd.*). (Down's Surgical Ltd.)

Neurosurgical Operations 461

Fig. 21.21 Air powered driver.

Fig. 21.23 Sweet Angular Crocodile Forceps with fine jaws, from shoulder to tip.

Fig. 21.22 Craniotome handpiece.

Fig. 21.24 Cairns Malleable Strip Retractors.

Fig. 21.25 Cushing Rongeur. For Pituitary Body. Maybe straight (not illustrated), angled forwards (A) or angled backwards (B).

Figs. 21.21 to 21.25 Neurosurgical instruments – craniotomy/burr hole (*cont'd.*). (Down's Surgical Ltd.)

462   Operating Theatre Technique

Fig. 21.26   Dissecting Forceps, straight.

Fig. 21.27   Micro Forceps, taper jaws, with smooth Tungsten Carbide inserts.

Fig. 21.28   Micro Needleholder, Straight, spring handles, Tungsten Carbide faced smooth jaws.

Fig. 21.29   Jacobson Micro Scissors, Straight, spring handle.

Fig. 21.30   Yasargil Micro Forceps.

Fig. 21.31   Micro Instruments, squeeze action, angled shaft.

Figs. 21.26 to 21.31   Neurosurgical micro instruments. (Down's Surgical Ltd.)

Aneurysm needles small and medium
Scissors, dura mater (Schmeiden)
Micro instruments, various
Brain retractors, malleable, various sizes
Punch forceps (Hajecks, DeVilbiss)
Wire saw and handles (Gigli or Olivecronas)
Saw guard (Cairn-de-Martel)
Haemostasis clips and insertion/removal forceps (Raney)
Dissecting forceps (Adson)
Rongeur, pituitary, straight and angled (Cushing).

Craniotomy

INSTRUMENTS

Retractors, self-retaining (West, Mayo hinged, etc.), 2
Fine needle holders (West or Kilner), 2
20 ml syringe
Elastic rubber bands for securing forceps in groups
Plastic drainage tubing and Redivac wound suction apparatus
Diathermy leads, electrodes, scabbard and lead anchoring forceps
(Bone awl or micro hand drill with twist drills and drill guard may be needed, plus stainless steel wire)
2 or 1·5 (3/0 or 4/0) Silk on small curved round-bodied needles for dura
2 (3/0) Silk on small curved cutting or straight cutting needles for skin.

OUTLINE OF PROCEDURE

Depending on the site and extent of brain exposure required, either a solitary burr hole will be made which is enlarged as necessary to form a limited craniectomy (e.g., for access to the Gasserian ganglion, certain temporal haematoma, subtemporal decompressions or emergency intracranial vascular surgery); or alternatively several burr holes are made in rhombic form and linked with a wire saw to form a bony 'trapdoor' hinged on the temporal muscle. This is the classical osteoplastic flap.

Elevation of a depressed fracture of the skull vault. To gain access to the fracture margins, a skin incision is made which possibly will include existing scalp wounds if the fracture be compound. The galeal bleeding is arrested with artery forceps which are grouped conveniently with rubber bands and clipped to the drapes.

The periosteum is reflected from the fracture lines for 5 to 10 mm each side and a burr hole made on sound bone to one side of the depression in order to afford access to the extradural space. Alternatively small comminuted fragments of bone often found impacting the fracture in the depressed position are nibbled away, any extradural haematoma being removed by suction. The dura is freed from the skull and an Adson elevator or bone spike inserted into the burr hole or bony defect. Using intact bone as the fulcrum, the depressed fragments are gently elevated into anatomical position and haemostasis is secured.

If the dura is penetrated resulting in a c.s.f. leak, the rent must be exposed and explored. Minimal pulped brain is gently irrigated, removed with suction and finally haemostasis secured with diathermy or Cushing clips. The dural rent is closed with fine silk interrupted sutures or a fascial patch, the donor site being conveniently temporal fascia or even fascia lata.

The scalp is closed (after inserting a drain) as for venticulography.

Evacuation of extradural haematoma. (This may only require instruments as for ventriculography providing the additional cranial instrument set is kept sterile for immediate use.)

A limited temporal craniectomy is made as previously described. The bleeding point is exposed – usually where the middle meningeal vessels emerge from the bony tunnel in the temporal bone to cross to the dura. Bleeding is arrested by coagulation or by under-

Fig. 21.32 Cutting a burrhole utilising skull perforator and spherical burr. (Gillingham.)

Fig. 21.33 Method of elevating a depressed fracture of the skull through an opening made with burr or trephine in *undamaged* bone adjoining the defect. In compound fractures all bone fragments should be removed. (Farquharson and Rintoul.)

running the vessel with a fine suture. The dura is then secured with dural 'hitch' stitches to the pericranium thereby occluding dead space and preventing extradural ooze under the bone edges, which can predispose towards extradural clot reaccumulation. After haemostasis is secured and a suction drain inserted the scalp is closed routinely with two layers of silk sutures to both muscles and scalp.

Subdural haematoma. (This may only require instruments as for ventriculography as above.) These are removed normally by making two burr holes at suitable sites and then after dural incision the fluid or clot is aspirated by suction. Any remaining clot is flushed out by gentle irrigation utilising a fine catheter, the saline being introduced at one burr hole and the clot expelled via the other. If the clot be solid and too firm to evacuate, an osteoplastic flap must be turned and the clot removed under direct vision.

In chronic subdural haematoma the brain shrinks and there is often some difficulty in expanding it to refill the space left by the evacuated haematoma. In this case saline is injected either via a lumbar puncture, or the lateral ventricle is cannulated and filled directly with saline via a Cushing brain needle.

Fig. 21.34 Operation for extra-dural haemorrhage. The initial opening in the skull is made with a burr or trephine, and is then enlarged with Rongeur forceps to allow adequate access to the clot. *Inset* shows area to be infiltrated with local anaesthetic and the incision employed. (Farquharson and Rintoul.)

Raising an osteoplastic flap. This is a preliminary procedure for all extensive intracranial procedures. The initial stages follow those previously described but a larger planned scalp incision is made. After scalp reflexion to the base of the planned incision, bleeding points are diathermised and the scalp flap covered with a saline soaked pack.

Two radial diathermy incisions are made down to bone in the temporal muscle, so that a fan-shaped section over the site of the osteoplastic bone flap will remain attached to temple and also to the reflected bone. This soft-tissue bridge is responsible for revascularisation of the bone flap after replacement when the operation is completed.

Five or six trephine holes are made at intervals on the circumference of the proposed bone flap. After deflecting the underlying dura from beneath the margins of the burr holes, first the bone base of the flap beneath the temporalis muscle is divided or narrowed enough to fracture through when the flap is reflected. The remaining burr holes are then linked one after the other with a de Martel saw guide and wire saw, or craniotome chamfering the bone edges to prevent the replaced bone flap from sinking inward.

The bone is then rapidly prised up and reflected, followed by removal of any bone spikes at the base. It is then wrapped with a saline soaked pack, which is secured to the drapes with rubber bands and towel clips. Occasionally the bone flap may be totally removed at this stage when a large decompression is needed rapidly. Bone haemostasis is secured with diathermy or bone wax and the edges are then covered with moist lintine strips followed by a fresh towel to cover all instruments *in situ* to that moment.

The dura is always reflected toward the vertex of the skull. A point near to the bone margins toward the base of the skull and free from blood vessels is selected and picked up with a sharp hook. It is then nicked with a scalpel and the nick enlarged with a director and scalpel sufficiently to introduce a small patty. The brain being protected by the patty, the dura is opened with dural scissors. Vessels to be traversed are coagulated, or under-run. The dural flap is reflected and covered with a moist patty or guttapercha strip. The dura is kept moist throughout the operation.

Tumours are gently separated out with brain retractors, scissors, diathermy and suction tube, or removed 'piecemeal' with a diathermy loop as in the case of large meningiomata. The cavity left by infiltrative tumours is gently irrigated until haemostasis is complete. Oozing is controlled with gelatin sponge, Oxycel or Surgicel covered with a moist cotton-wool pack which is sucked dry. This pack is later removed with the aid of irrigation.

For closure the dura is first 'hitch stitched' to the pericranium as described previously, then closed with interrupted silk sutures. The bone flap is replaced *in situ* and sutured in place with periosteal silk sutures. In some cases the flap is fixed with twisted loops of

Fig. 21.35 Method of turning down an osteoplastic flap based on the temporalis muscle. A wire saw is shown in position between two burr holes. (It is now the custom to open the dura by means of a U-shaped flap, rather than by a cruciate incision.) (Farquharson and Rintoul.)

stainless steel wire inserted in holes drilled in the flap and surrounding intact vault bones. Whilst drilling, the brain is guarded to avoid accidental deep penetration. The scalp may be drained using a subgaleal suction drain.

Posterior fossa exploration. A midline, 'crossbow' or lateral linear incision is made through previously infiltrated neck musculature. Artery forceps on each side of the incision are grouped together with rubber bands. The neck musculature is incised with diathermy down to bone and the occipital bone bared widely, stripping the muscles back with a periosteal elevator and large self-retaining retractors.

Fig. 21.36 Sub-occipital approach to the cerebellum and brain stem. The occipital sinus is shown about to be divided between ligatures. (Farquharson and Rintoul.)

Two burr holes are made one on either side of the midline over the cerebellum. Using nibblers, a large craniectomy is made bilaterally and the crest of midline bone between these removed. The posterior aspect of the foramen magnum rim is removed, as is usually the posterior arch of the atlas and even the axis together with the axis' spinous process.

The dura is opened widely in stellate fashion and held back with 'hitch stitches'. The brain is explored by 'needling' and retraction, pathological tissue being dealt with as previously described. The dura is left open and the muscles closed in layers to effect a watertight closure. Skin is then closed in two layers.

Cranioplasty

DEFINITION

Repair of skull defects with bone, acrylic resin or Vitallium prostheses.

POSITION

As for the appropriate craniotomy. If iliac bone or rib is to be used for a bony cranioplasty, the patient is placed in the lateral or half-lateral position.

INSTRUMENTS

As for craniotomy
Bone graft set (Fig. 23.91)
Pistol grip hand drill, twist drills and drill guard
Stainless steel wire
Prosthesis; acrylic polymer and monomer, acrylic plate or Vitallium plate.

OUTLINE OF PROCEDURE

The cranial defect is exposed by reflexion of the scalp flap and careful sharp dissection to leave freshened bone margins and intact dura underlying the defect. The bone edges are 'stepped or chamfered' until the prepared prosthesis sits snugly in position. Holes are drilled in the surrounding bone at suitable intervals and the prosthesis is firmly wired into place with stainless steel wire. After twisting the wire ends these are cut and buried in the drill holes. The scalp is closed in two layers often with a suction drain in place for 24 hours post-operatively.

If an autogenous bone graft is used to repair the defect the bone is removed from the appropriate donor site. A plate of cortical and cancellous bone can be removed *en bloc* from the inner aspect of the ileum, alternatively two or three sections of rib of sufficient length to bridge the skull defect may be used. A rib is split lengthwise and wired *in situ* in parallel strips to roof over the defect. Any cancellous chippings are lightly packed in the interspaces and the scalp closed routinely.

Prefrontal leucotomy

DEFINITION

Severing of the fronto-thalamic association fibres in both frontal lobes of the brain.

POSITION

Sitting or supine, with head flexed forward.

INSTRUMENTS

As for ventriculography (p. 455)
Narrow brain retractors, 4
Leucotome.

OUTLINE OF PROCEDURE

There are many individual variations of the operation, the usual procedure is a modified Freeman and Watts operation. The coronal suture is localised by skin markings 13 cm along the midline from the nasion toward the vertex. A small vertical incision is made bilaterally along the coronal suture centred 3 cm behind the zygomatico-frontal suture and 6 cm above the superior margin of the zygoma. A burr hole is made and enlarged to 2 by 3 cm. The dura is incised in cruciate fashion, haemostasis being secured with diathermy.

A brain needle is inserted horizontally just in front of the anterior horn of the lateral ventricle and the depth to the falx determined which is usually 55 mm or thereabouts. If the ventricle is opened, section is made anterior to the needle track to avoid the former.

A leucotome is inserted with the blade held horizontally and a cut made parallel to the zygoma, 10 mm less in depth to that of the falx in order to avoid the pial vessels on the medial orbital gyrus. The section is carried forward as far as possible using a sweeping action, with the brain surface as the axis. The leucotome is then withdrawn and a vertical section made of similar depth in the coronal plane. After finally withdrawing the leucotome the wound is irrigated until bleeding stops and then closed routinely.

Stereotactic surgery

DEFINITION

Deep ablative surgery of the white matter, basal ganglia or brain stem projection fibres by means of a special probe utilising electro-coagulation or extreme cold (cryoprobe) as the destructive agent. Accuracy of siting is accomplished by means of a stereotactic frame applied to the skull coupled with contrast radiography demonstrating fixed intracerebral landmarks as points of reference.

POSITION

Sitting (Leksell and cryoprobe); or prone (Guiot) depending on which stereotactic frame is used.

INSTRUMENTS

As for ventriculography (p. 455)
Micro hand drill, twist drills and drill guard
Lead shot
Cryoprobe or electro-coagulation unit
Stereotactic frame (Leksell, Cooper, Guiot Gillingham, etc.).

OUTLINE OF PROCEDURE

One stage procedure. The ventricles are outlined by contrast radiography and the stereotactic frame applied to the skull. By reference to a standard sterotactic atlas, the probe is inserted and localised into the required position and a lesion performed in increments until the desired effect is obtained in the conscious patient.

Two stage procedure. The preliminary stage is performed followed two days later by the main operation. An example is stereotactic thalamopallidotomy, designed to relieve the tremor and rigidity of Parkinsonism.

Stage one consists of inserting lead shot landmarks on the surface of the skull. Using the stereotactic frame bar as a guide, three incisions are made through the scalp one traverse frontally as low as possible towards the nasion; another longitudinally over the coronal suture and a third longitudinal or transverse incision low on the occipital bone towards the external occipital protuberance. All the incisions are placed in the midline. Using a guarded drill, several holes are drilled in the outer table of the skull so that five or six lead shot can be inserted and secured with bone wax, arranged in a W fashion to give a 'spread' of shot across the skull midline at the three sites.

The scalp is closed routinely and an air encephalogram taken with several radiographic views to include the lines of shot and the septum pellucidum as well as the third ventricle. By computation by consideration of the position of lead shot and various other intracranial landmarks, accurate co-ordinates of the globus pallidus and ventro-lateral nucleus of the thalamus are worked out. From this, the position of the parietal burr hole required in a direct line behind these targets is also worked out.

Stage two, the patient is conscious, placed in the prone position, with the head resting in a neurosurgical horseshoe and the limbs exposed. The original incisions are re-opened and the lines of lead shot exposed. The shot selected for siting an anchor point for the Guiot frame is removed and after enlarging the socket left behind, a special screw is driven home into the outer skull table. The procedure is repeated at the other incisions and after removing all surplus lead shot markers, the bar of the Guiot frame is secured to the anchor points and the wounds closed around the screws.

Two burr holes are then made and the dura incised to expose brain. The first is sited over the frontal horn of the lateral ventricle which is then catheterised. The second burr hole is made over the parietal eminence on the side for the lesion, a pre-determined site, usually about 3 to 3·5 cm above the external occipital protuberance and centred 16 mm from the midline.

Fig. 21.37 Guiot Gillingham stereotactic frame. (Eschmann Bros and Walsh Ltd.)

The Guiot frame is secured to the central bar with the depth electrode touching the brain surface. Myodil or Metrizamide contrast medium 3 ml is instilled into the ventricle and by manipulating the head is manoeuvred into the third ventricle to outline the anterior and posterior commissure. The sights of the Guiot frame are then aligned on the globus pallidus by using these points of reference and an image intensifier.

The contrast medium is aspirated and the frontal burr hole closed. The electrode is slowly inserted into the brain 16 mm from the midline until the ventro-lateral nucleus of the thalamus is entered, this usually results in a dramatic cessation or diminuation of tremor. A radiofrequency current of known strength and duration is then passed through the electrode to make a small spherical lesion in the thalamus. Alternatively the cryoprobe tip is cooled to -30 to $-100°C$ and after a predetermined time, warmed up again (Chapter 22).

After an acceptable result is achieved, the electrode is pushed further anteriorly, traversing the internal capsule to enter the globus pallidus. A second lesion is then made, which usually dramatically improves dexterity and alleviates the increased rigidity. The apparatus is then removed and the incisions closed.

By similar techniques, electrodes and probes can produce lesions in the frontal association to cause a controlled, more exact leucotomy; suprafellar cysts can be approached and ascending pain fibres in cases of intractable pain can be destroyed in the brain stem, with minimal interference to brain function.

Torkildsen operation (Ventriculo-cysternostomy)

DEFINITION

The establishment of artificial drainage between the lateral ventricles and cysterna magna.

POSITION

Prone with the neck flexed.

INSTRUMENTS

As for craniotomy
Silicone tubing 8 to 10 Charrière gauge.

OUTLINE OF PROCEDURE

A vertical midline incision is made in the occipital region, haemostasis secured and self-retaining retractors placed to retract the muscles. Two parietal burr holes are made followed by a limited posterior fossa craniectomy, the dura not being opened initially. Silicone drainage tubes are introduced into both lateral ventricles via supratentorial dural incisions. These tubes are laid in channels cut in the outer skull table between the burr holes and the craniectomy.

The cerebellar dura is opened for 1 cm, and the silicone tubes, after trimming for length, are inserted through the arachnoid into the cysterna magna. The dura is then closed around the tubes and the scalp sutured in layers.

Insertion of ventriculo-atrial or ventriculo-petritoneal shunt

DEFINITION

The establishment of artificial c.s.f. drainage to heart or peritoneal cavity in cases of primary or secondary hydrocephalus.

POSITION

Supine, with head rotated to the left, sandbag under the shoulders and an X-ray film cassette beneath the patient's chest.

INSTRUMENTS

As for ventriculography (p. 455)
Fine arterial bulldog clamps, 3
Small gauges, 3 mm, 4 mm, 6 mm (Hahn or Jenkins), 3
Suitable valve (Pudenz of Spitz-Holter)
Fine bore silicone tubing assorted sizes
Eynard connectors, 2.

Fig. 21.38 Pudenz valve for ventriculo-atrial shunt.

Fig. 21.39 Spitz-Holter valve for ventriculo-atrial shunt.

OUTLINE OF PROCEDURE

Ventriculo-atrial shunt, (Pudenz valve insertion). A preliminary chest radiograph confirms the level of the right atrium. A right sub-mandibular incision is made and the posterior branch of the common facial vein or the right internal jugular vein is exposed and freed from surrounding tissues.

A supramastoid occipital scalp incision 5 cm (2 in) long is made well above the line of the lateral sinus, and using a small gouge a hole is drilled in the attenuated skull. The dura is incised and the enlarged occipital horn of the lateral ventricle is catheterised with the top-half of the Pudenz catheter. This is then occluded with the bulldog clip to prevent leakage of c.s.f.

(*It is not normally necessary to insert the patent flushing disc in the shunt circuit. If this is required, the gouge-hole must be enlarged to fit the rim of the disc snugly and bone haemostatis secured with bone wax. A 5 cm length of top catheter is then cut off and tied to the centre of the outlet of the flushing disc with fine silk. The disc is then inserted and sutured to the periosteum margins of the bone defect. This step is omitted if no flusher is required.*)

Two silk ligatures are passed around the right internal jugular vein, or the posterior branch of the common facial vein if the latter is of sufficiently large calibre to admit the Pudenz tube valve. The top ligature is tied to occlude the vessel. The Pudenz atrial catheter is checked for correct functioning of the four slit valves at the atrial end. The vessel is nicked and the catheter inserted toward the superior vena cava until it is estimated to be within the right atrium.

A few millilitres of Hypaque 35 per cent is injected via an Eynard connector whilst a radiograph of the chest is taken to verify correct positioning of the valve. Alternatively the catheter can be inserted under ECG control using hypertonic saline instilled. After any necessary adjustment, so that the valve tip is well within the right atrium, the Pudenz tube is secured in the neck with the lower ligature. The tubing of the lower end of the valve is then tracked from the neck incision to the scalp incision, using large artery forceps forced along the subcutaneous tissues. After trimming to a suitable length, the top and bottom tubes are linked over a fine connector supplied with the valve (or to the flushing disc) with silk ties. After checking fontanelle tension and the flusher if fitted, for correct function, both wounds are closed in two layers.

Ventriculo-peritoneal shunt. Ventricular catheterisation is performed as above with a single length of fine silicone tubing with several side holes cut near the top end. The tubing is then tunnelled subcutaneously, if necessary with supplementary small incisions down the neck and across the right anterior chest wall to a secondary incision sited just below the right costal margin.

The peritoneal cavity is opened at this site and after trimming to length and cutting several side holes in the silicone tubing, the latter is inserted into the suprahepatic space and sutured to peritoneum with watertight closure. The wounds are closed in layers.

Trans-sphenoidal Hypophysectomy

DEFINITION

Surgical excision of the normal pituitary or pituitary tumours with only limited intra cranial extension, via a transethmoidal – sphenoidal approach.

POSITION

Supine, in reversed Trendelenberg.

474 Operating Theatre Technique

Fig. 21.40 Love Kerrison Rongeurs, extra small, upward and downward cutting.

Fig. 21.41 Bateman pituitary forceps.

Fig. 21.42 Hardy modified Cushing Bi-valve speculum.

Fig. 21.43 Angell James dissectors.

Fig. 21.44 Bateman curved suction tube (insulated).

Fig. 21.45 Angell James diathermy needle.

Figs. 21.40 to 21.45 Instruments for Trans-sphenoidal Hypophysectomy. (Down's Surgical Ltd.)

INSTRUMENTS

As for fronto-ethmoidectomy (p. 414)
Bi-valve speculum (Hardy modified Cushing)
Dissector (Angell James) set
Rongeurs, upward and downward cutting (Love Kerrison)
Pituitary forceps (Bateman)
Nasal septum instruments may be required (p. 408)
Diathermy needle, leads and lead anchoring forceps
Curved suction tube (insulated)
Ligatures and sutures as for Fronto-ethmoidectomy (p. 414)
B.I.P.P. and ribbon gauze
Operating microscope.

OUTLINE OF PROCEDURE

This approach is used more frequently now as an alternative to transcranial removal of the pituitary. The normal pituitary gland may be removed for the hormonally-dependent tumour, as in metastatic spread of carcinoma of the breast or prostate, and cases of uncontrolled complications of diabetis such as retinopathy. Tumours of the pituitary requiring excision are usually associated either with Cushings disease, acromegaly, or pressure on the optic chiasma which may cause blindness.

Ethmoidosphenoidal exenteration is carried out either by the Patterson approach (infra-orbital – Fig. 21.46A), or by the Howarth approach – Fig. 21.46B. The intersphenoidal septum is perforated and removed after exposure of the right sphenoidal sinus, and the operating microscope is brought into use.

A long-handled power driven burr is used to remove the central section of the anterior wall of the pituitary fossa. The burr hole is enlarged with punch forceps.

The pituitary gland is exposed through a cruciate incision in both layers of the dura, the extent being dependent on the size of the extent of the intercavernous venous system. Pituitary dissectors are used to separate the gland which is removed from the fossa with forceps, care being taken to excise all remnants.

Fig. 21.46 Trans-sphenoidal hypophysectomy. (A) i-Patterson approach, ii-Howarth approach. (B) Perforation of the intersphenoidal septum. (C) Anterior wall of pituitary fossa perforated with burr and aperture enlarged with punch; cruciate incision in dura. (D) Removal of pituitary. (Gillingham.)

The fossa is plugged with a graft of muscle, usually excised from the lateral aspect of the patient's thigh; this is to control oozing of blood or cerebro-spinal fluid. The nose is packed with B.I.P.P. gauze and the incision sutured as for fronto-ethmoidectomy.

Repair of spina bifida and meningocoele

DEFINITION

The repair of a congenital defect in the vertebral column which allows herniation of the malformed meninges and the spinal cord or caudu equina.

POSITION

Prone.

INSTRUMENTS

General set (Figs. 14.1 to 14.28)
Fine artery forceps, curved on flat, mosquito, 25
Fine dissecting forceps, toothed (Gillies), 2
Fine dissecting forceps, non-toothed (McIndoe), 2
Fine tissue forceps (McIndoe), 12
Fine scissors, curved on flat, iris, 2
Long scissors, curved on flat (McIndoe)
Suction tubing, fine nozzles and tube anchoring forceps
Diathermy leads, electrodes, scabbard and lead anchoring forceps
2 (3/0) Plain catgut or Dexon on small curved round-bodied needles
2 (3/0) Silk on small curved cutting needles.

OUTLINE OF PROCEDURE

The margins of the herniated sac or exposed neural disc are freed from the overlying skin which is then retracted gently. The underlying neural tissue is gradually freed from the surrounding fascia on the margins of the lamina defect with preservation of all possible neural tissue. Haemostasis must be meticulous. The edges of the neural disc are then sunk beneath a flap of reflected fascia tailored from the paravertebral tissues. This layer is closed with fine silk, plain catgut or Dexon to secure a watertight closure.

In the case of meningocoele when no neural disc is exposed, after freeing adherent nerve roots from the sac of the meningocoele, the sac is excised, the roots returned to the spinal canal and the sac edges resutured together.

The skin is closed, if necessary with the formation of rotation flaps and extensive undermining, in two layers to give a tensionless three layer closure in all.

Laminectomy

DEFINITION

Removal of laminae, usually to provide access to a prolapsed intervertebral disc which may be pressing on a nerve root.

POSITION

Knee/elbow, as Fig. 4.17, or lateral, or prone position of flexion.

INSTRUMENTS

General set (Figs. 14.1 to 14.28)
Laminectomy set (Fig. 21.47)
Diathermy leads, electrodes and lead anchoring forceps
Suction tubing, nozzles and tube anchoring forceps

Fig. 21.47 Laminectomy – removal of prolapsed intravertebral disc.

1. Scalpel handle No.5 with No. 15; blade (Bard Parker).
2. Long fine dissecting forceps, toothed and non-toothed (Waugh), 2 of each.
3. Dissector (Macdonald).
4. Nerve hook, medium (Adson), 2.
5. Nerve hook, large (Love).
6. Nerve hook, small (Adson).
7. Seeker (Horsley).
8. Dura mater separator (Sergeant-Horsley).
9. Rugines, large (Mitchell), straight and round end.
10. Rugine, small (Faraboeuf).
11. Gouge or bone-nibbling forceps, angled on side.
12. Gouge or bone-nibbling forceps, angled on flat.
13. Gouge forceps, angled on side, compound action.
14. Irrigation syringe.
15. Pituitary forceps (Cairn Cushing).
    A. Straight, small.
    B. Straight, medium.
    C. Straight, large.
16. Pituitary forceps (Cairn Cushing).
    A. Angled, small.
    B. Angled, medium.
17. Retractor, self-retaining (Little).
18. Retractor, self-retaining (Adson).
19. Broad osteotomes, 38 mm (1½ in) and 25 mm (1 in).
20. Mallet (Heath).
21. Punch forceps (Duggan), forward and backward cutting.
22. Retractors, laminectomy (Charnley), 2.
23. Retractors, laminectomy (Hibb), 2.
24. Retractors, laminectomy (Penrose), 2.
25. Ribbon gauze 25 mm (1 in) and 50 mm (2 in).
26. Bone wax (Horsley).
27. Patties made from cottonoid, large and small.
28. Rubber or plastic corrugated drain.

Corrugated drainage tubing
2·5 (2/0) Plain catgut or Dexon for ligatures
1 (5/0) Silk on a small curved round-bodied non-traumatic needle for dural tears
4 or 5 (1 or 2) Chromic catgut or Dexon or silk, etc., on a large half-circle cutting needle for muscle sutures
3 (0) Silk or nylon on a large curved cutting needle for skin sutures.

OUTLINE OF PROCEDURE

A midline incision is made over the spines of the vertebrae from which the laminae are to be removed. This incision is deepened and the erector spinae muscles are reflected from the vertebrae with a rugine of broad osteotome (Fig. 21.50A).

The dura is exposed by excising the ligamentum flavum with a scalpel and the overlying lamina with bone-nibbling forceps. Retraction on the nerve root exposes the intervertebral disc which, if bulging, is incised with a fine scalpel and extracted with pituitary forceps. It may be necessary to expose a disc space above or below that selected if the findings are inconclusive in the first instance.

The wound is closed with or without drainage.

Excision of spinal cord tumour

DEFINITION

The removal of a spinal cord tumour following cervical, dorsal or lumbar laminectomy.

POSITION

Prone neurosurgical position (Fig. 4.15) with some flexion of the spine; lateral flexed position or laminectomy position (Fig. 4.17).

Fig. 21.48 (*Left*) Laminectomy for intervertebral disc protrusion. Stripping of soft tissues from the spinous processes and laminae.

Fig. 21.49 (*Right*) The ligamentum flavum and the contiguous margins of two laminae have been removed on the affected side. The nerve root and the main theca have been retracted to expose the protrusion of the disc.

INSTRUMENTS

As for laminectomy
Dura scissors (Schmeiden)
Micro instruments (p. 462)
Ligatures and sutures as for laminectomy.

OUTLINE OF PROCEDURE

A midline incision is made over the spines of the vertebrae. This incision is deepened and the erector spinae muscles reflected from the vertebrae with a rugine or broad osteotome (Fig. 21.50A). Self-retaining retractors are inserted. Sufficient spinous processes and interspinous ligaments, are removed to expose the area of exploration. The laminae are removed initially without disturbing ligamentum flavum.

Further operative stages will depend upon the type and extent of the tumour, but generally the exposed ligamentum and extra dural fat is excised for intra dural tumours by incision of the dura with scalpel and scissors. Stay sutures are placed in the edges of the cut dura to act as retractors and these lie over moist lintine strips arranged along each side of the wound.

The tumour is freed by sharp and blunt dissection together with adherent meninges, and haemostasis is secured with diathermy, gelatine sponge, Oxycel or Surgical. The dura is closed with interrupted silk sutures, and if excision of the tumour has left a defect this is covered with gelatine sponge or film. The wound is closed as for laminectomy, with or without drainage.

Fig. 21.50. (A) Reflection of the erector spinae muscles from vertebrae. (B) Self-retaining retractors inserted. (Gillingham.) (C) Removal of spinous processes. (Farquharson and Rintoul.)

Fig. 21.51 Spinal cord tumours. (A) Extra-dural neoplasm. (B and C) Ependymoma. (D and E) Neurofibroma, the tumour may be submerged under portions of the cauda equina. (Gillingham.)

Lumbar sympathectomy

DEFINITION

Removal of the lower three lumbar sympathetic ganglia and intervening trunk for vasospastic disturbances.

POSITION

Supine.

INSTRUMENTS

As for laparotomy (Figs. 15.1 to 15.7)
Illuminated retractor (Coldlight)
Long dissecting forceps, non-toothed, 25 cm (10 in), 2
Long dissecting forceps, toothed, 25 cm (10 in)
Long scissors, curved on flat, 23 cm (9 in) (Nelson)
Silver clips and galley (McKenzie)
Insertion forceps for silver clips
Ligatures and sutures as for laparotomy (p. 327).

OUTLINE OF PROCEDURE

The chain of ganglia may be approached by either of two incisions. If the sympathectomy is unilateral, an incision, rather like a kidney incision is made, but rather further forward. This incision extends from the margin of the twelfth rib towards the umbilicus, splitting the external oblique and transversus muscles in line with their fibres in the manner described for appendectomy in Chapter 13. The ganglia are approached by retracting the peritoneum which is not opened.

If the sympathectomy is bilateral, the approach *may* be midline or paramedian, opening the peritoneum anteriorly, retracting the viscera and opening the posterior peritoneum to expose the ganglia situated on each side of the abdominal aorta.

The second, third and fourth lumbar ganglia and the intervening trunk are dissected free and removed after ligating the proximal and distal points with silver clips. The wound is closed in the usual manner for laparotomy.

Division of the sensory root of the trigeminal nerve (Dandy's operation)

DEFINITION

Intracranial fractional division of the sensory root of the trigeminal nerve for the relief of intractable trigeminal neuralgia.

POSITION

Sitting with the head in a frontal horse-shoe to afford access to the temporal region and face on affected side.

INSTRUMENTS

As for ventriculography (p. 455)
Trigeminal retractor, large self-retaining (Dandy's)
Brain retractors, malleable

Headlight
Blunt meningeal hooks, 2
Silver clips and galley (Cushing's)
Insertion forceps for silver clips
Bone-cutting forceps (de Vilbiss)
Dural scissors (Dott)
Ligatures and sutures as for ventriculography (p. 455).

OUTLINE OF PROCEDURE

A moderate sized temporal craniectomy is made extending well downward to the floor of the middle cranial fossa. The middle meningeal vessels are clipped or diathermised and divided. An extradural subtemporal dissection is made toward the midline until the dural fold overlying the trigeminal ganglion is exposed.

The dura is incised and by blunt dissection with meningeal hooks the sensory root of the trigeminal nerve is isolated and the motor root identified. The appropriate sensory division of the trigeminal nerve is then divided and the temporalis muscle is sutured in two layers after haemostasis has been secured. The scalp is sutured routinely in two layers without drainage.

Peripheral nerve anastomosis

DEFINITION

Repair of an injured peripheral nerve by anastomosis.

POSITION

Musculospiral (radial), ulnar or medium nerves; supine, with the arm extended on an arm table. Sciatic or popliteal; prone.

INSTRUMENTS

General set
Fine dissecting forceps, toothed (Gillies), 2
Fine dissecting forceps, non-toothed (McIndoe), 2
Micro dissecting forceps (Figs. 21.26, 21.27 and 21.56)
Micro scissors (Figs. 21.29 and 21.53)
Micro artery forceps (Fig. 21.56)
Fine artery forceps, curved on flat (Mosquito), 6
Fine artery forceps, straight (Mosquito), 6
Iris scissors, straight, sharp points
Iris scissors, curved on flat, sharp points
Razor blade breaker and holder (Fig. 21.52)
Razor blades
Plastic tubing or tape for nerve traction
Retractor, self-retaining (Mayo)
Plaster of Paris back slab, or similar splint

Nerve Sutures for both Operation Areas
   1 or 0·75 (5/0 or 6/0) Silk or Dacron on a small curved round-bodied non-traumatic needle
   19 Micron metallised nylon suture

Fig. 21.52 Razor Blade Breaker and Holder.

Fig. 21.53 Jacobson Micro Scissors, Straight, spring handle.

Fig. 21.54 Yasargil Artery Forceps, serrated jaws, spring handles with catch.

Fig. 21.55 Micro Needleholder, Straight, spring handles, Tungsten Carbide faced smooth jaws.

Fig. 21.56 Jacobson Dissecting Forceps, fine, smooth, straight jaws.

Figs. 21.52 to 21.56   Micro nerve instruments. (Down's Surgical Ltd.)

Ligatures and Sutures for an Arm Operation
   2 and 2·5 (3/0 and 2/0) Plain catgut or Dexon for ligatures
   3 (0) Chromic catgut or Dexon on a medium half-circle cutting needle for muscle sutures
   2·5 (2/0) Silk or nylon on a medium curved cutting needle for skin sutures.

Fig. 21.57 Classical method of nerve suture. Note how, in order to avoid rotation of the two segments of nerve, guide sutures are inserted into the sheath at corresponding points on the circumference, and are held on dissimilar pairs of forceps. Very fine silk stitches are used for the repair; these should pick up the sheath alone without traumatising the nerve fibres. (Farquharson and Rintoul.)

Ligatures and Sutures for a Leg Operation
   2·5 and 3 (2/0 and 0) Plain catgut or Dexon for ligatures
   4 or 5 (1 or 2) Chromic catgut or Dexon on a medium or large half-circle cutting needle for muscle sutures
   2·5 or 0 (2/0 or 0) Silk or nylon on a large or medium curved cutting needle for skin sutures.

OUTLINE OF PROCEDURE

The incision is made and the muscles split or retracted to expose the nerve. The proximal and distal portions of the divided nerve are mobilised so that they can be brought together without tension. This usually means that the skin incision must be extended and the nerve mobilised for a considerable distance proximal to the division.

Fig. 21.58 Funicular repair of a digital nerve inserting a metallized nylon microsuture through the nerve sheath (see also Fig. 12.14, p. 306).

Fig. 21.59 Secondary repair of a digital nerve with the metallized 19 micron nylon suture. (O'Brien.)

The bulbous fibrous neuroma is excised with the razor blade, and 'stay' sutures are placed in the nerve sheath. These 'stay' sutures are used as temporary retractors and to approximate the nerve ends, which are anastomosed with interrupted silk or metalised nylon sutures placed through the nerve sheath only. Care is taken to complete the anastomosis without rotation of the nerve ends. A piece of Millipore or Dacron silastic material may be wrapped around the anastomosis to form a protective tunnel.

The muscle is sutured over the nerve and the skin is closed. The limb is immobilised with a splint and bandages in a position which affords the least tension on the nerve suture line.

Fig. 21.60 Exposure and transposition of the ulnar nerve at the elbow. (Farquharson and Rintoul.)

Transposition of ulnar nerve

DEFINITION

Anterior translocation of the ulnar nerve from its normal position behind the medial epicondyle to a soft tissue channel made medially in the flexor carpi ulnaris, thereby alleviating recurrence of symptoms due to stretching of the nerve.

POSITION

Supine, with the arm extended on an arm table and small sandbag.

INSTRUMENTS

As for peripheral nerve suture.

OUTLINE OF PROCEDURE

A curved incision is made, extending above and below the elbow, with its centre lying over the medial epicondyle. The skin flaps are reflected and the nerve dissected free from behind the epicondyle. Loops of rubber tubing or tape are placed around the nerve which is retracted medially. The flexor carpi ulnaris is partially detached from the epicondyle, and reflected to form a channel into which the nerve is laid.

The muscle can be sutured over the nerve with interrupted chromic catgut, Dexon or left unsutured and the skin closed with interrupted silk or nylon.

FURTHER READING

FARQUHARSON, E. L. AND RINTOUL, R. F. (1972) *Textbook of Operative Surgery*. Edinburgh: Churchill Livingstone.
GILLINGHAM, F. J. (1970) *Neurosurgery*. London: Butterworth.
O'BRIEN, B. McC. (1977) *Microvascular Reconstructive Surgery*. Edinburgh: Churchill Livingstone.

22
OPHTHALMIC OPERATIONS

A very large proportion of ophthalmic operations are performed under local anaesthesia if the patient is co-operative. In small children, restless adults and also major procedures such as retinal detachment general anaesthesia is usually administered. The operating microscope is used extensively (see Chapter 12).

Local anaesthesia consists of installation of cocaine 4 per cent at intervals before operation. In addition, for operations on the eyelids a 1 or 2 per cent lignocaine (Xylocaine), amethocaine or ophthaine is injected subcutaneously. For operations on the eyeball itself and ocular muscles, a retrobulbar injection of lignocaine (Xylocaine), amethocaine or

Fig. 22.1 Anatomical cross-section of eye.

ophthaine is made. The lignocaine (Xylocaine) solution may be combined with 1 in 100,000 adrenaline which acts as a haemostic agent. Local anaesthesia is often used in conjunction with sedatives such as pethidine and phenergan or basal anaesthetics.

Excision of chalazion

DEFINITION

The removal of a cystic degenerated Meibomian gland in the eyelid.

POSITION

Sitting or supine with head elevated.

INSTRUMENTS

Sponge holding forceps (Rampley), 2
Scalpel handles, No 3 with Nos 15 and 11 blades (Bard Parker)
Fine dissecting forceps, toothed and non-toothed, fixation
Fine scissors, curved on flat, blunt points (Strabismus)
Iris scissors, curved on flat, sharp points
Iris scissors, straight, sharp points
Eyelid retractors (Desmare), 2
Eyelid guard (Stallard)
Tarsal cyst forceps (Greene)
Meibomian cyst curettes, 3 sizes
Fine needle holder (Barraquer)
Towel clips (Backhaus), 4
Hand cautery and points
Cartridge syringe with fine hypodermic needle
0·7 (6/0) Black silk on small cutting needle for skin closure.

OUTLINE OF PROCEDURE

The cyst is usually removed via the conjunctiva but occasionally through the skin. In either case, the skin overlying the lesion is infiltrated with local anaesthetic, and if the cyst is to be removed through the conjunctiva, this may be ballooned out with local anaesthetic injected into the inferior or superior cul-de-sac.

A chalazion clamp is applied with the cyst projecting into the ring of the forceps. Approach to the cyst through the conjunctiva is made through an incision vertical to the lid margin, for this type of wound closes readily without sutures. The cyst is curetted unless it is large, or has recurred in which case it is dissected out with sharp scissors or a scalpel.

If the cyst is approached through the skin, the incision is made parallel with the lid margin and is closed afterwards with a few interrupted silk sutures.

Ectropion correction

DEFINITION

The correction of an eyelid deformity (usually the lower lid), where relaxation of the skin and muscles of the eyelid cause permanent exposure of the conjunctiva.

Fig. 22.2   Fixation Forceps (Non-toothed).

Fig. 22.3   Fixation Forceps (Toothed).

Fig. 22.4   Lang Eye Speculum (Full size).

Fig. 22.5   Clark Eye Speculum (Full size).

Fig. 22.6   Snellen Entropion Forceps.

Fig. 22.7   Greene Tarsal Cyst Forceps.

Fig. 22.8   Desmarres Retractors (Sizes A, B and C).

Fig. 22.9   Iris scissors, curved on flat.

Fig. 22.10   Barraquer needle holder.

Fig. 22.11   McHardy meibomian curette.

Figs. 22.2 to 22.11   Instruments for eyelid operations. (Chas. F. Thackray Ltd and Down's Surgical Ltd.)

POSITION

Supine.

INSTRUMENTS

As above, plus
Eyelid retractors, left and right (Clark or Lang), 2
Fine skin hooks (Kilner), 2
Mapping pen and gentian violet
1 (6/0) Chromic catgut or Dexon on small cutting needle for orbicularis.

Fig. 22.12 Ectropion and entropion correction, (A and B) V-Y operation for ectropion excision of arrow-headed area of skin which is sutured as a Y. (C) Fox's operation for entropion of lower lid, resection of tarsus, skin and muscle. (Stallard.)

OUTLINE OF PROCEDURE

There are several operations for this condition, including skin grafting procedures. Basically the operation consists of tightening the lower lid to correct the abnormal position. One such operation is the V-Y procedure.

Kilners hooks are used to bring together the eyelid skin to a point where the ectropion is corrected. A mapping pen, dipped in gentian violet may be used to mark the redundant fold. An incision is made along the marked line and an arrow headed area excised (Fig. 22.12A).

Entropion correction

DEFINITION

The correction of an eyelid deformity where inward rotation or inversion of the eyelid may cause trauma by the rubbing of the lashes on the cornea.

POSITION

Supine.

INSTRUMENTS

As Ectropion.

OUTLINE OF PROCEDURE

There are several plastic operations for atonic (senile) entropion. The objective is to space the atrophic tarsus and atonic orbicularis muscle which have allowed the lid to become too long from side to side. A lid clamp is used to evert the lower lid and a triangular segment of conjunctiva and tarsus excised with its open at the lid margin, and just lateral to the centre of the eyelid.

Fox's operation is an additional procedure in which a triangle of skin, base up and just temporal to the lateral canthus is excised and also an ellipse of orbicularis muscle is resected.

Chromic catgut or Dexon sutures are used to unite the resected tarsus and conjunctiva. The orbicularis muscle is also sutured with catgut or Dexon and the skin incision is closed with interrupted sutures of 0·7 (6/0) black silk.

Dacrocystorhinostomy

DEFINITION

The establishment of a permanent opening between the lacrimal sac and the nasal cavity.

POSITION

Supine (Head clamp may be used).

INSTRUMENTS

Sponge holding forceps (Rampley), 2
Scalpel handles No. 3 with Nos. 10 and 15 blades (Bard Parker), 2
Fine dissecting forceps, toothed, fixation, 2
Fine dissecting forceps, toothed (Gillies), 2
Fine dissecting forceps, non-toothed (McIndoe), 2
Fine scissors, curved dissecting points (Kilner)
Spring scissors (Wescott)
Fine artery forceps, curved on flat, mosquito, 10
Fine tissue forceps (McIndoe), 5
Dissectors (Howarth and Stallard)
Elevator, muco-periosteal (Traquair)
Hooks (Kilner), 2
Nasal forceps, angled (Wilde)
Nasal speculum (St Clair Thompson)
Retractors, claw (Lane), 2
Retractor, self retaining (Bishop Hartmann)
Dilator, canaliculus (Nettleship)
Lacrimal probes, set
Punch forceps (Citellis and Duggan or Ferris-Smith), 3
Power driven diamond burrs, connecting tubing or cable
 or
Small gouges, 4 mm, 6 mm, 10 mm
Small chisels or osteotomes, 4 mm, 6 mm, 10 mm
Small mallet (Rowland)
Needle holders (Castroviejo and Barraquer), 2
Syringe and lacrimal cannula

Fig. 22.13 Dacrocystorhinostomy. (A) Using a diamond burr to remove bone from lacrimal fossa. (Hall.) (B) Left lacrimal sac cut transversely at entrance to naso-lacrimal duct. (C) T incisions in nasal muscosa. (D) Suture of posterior panels of lacrimal sac. (E) Suture of anterior panels. (F) Suture of posterior panels of nasal mucosa. (Stallard.)

Fine suction nozzles, tubing and tube anchoring forceps
Diathermy electrodes, cable and cable forceps or hand cautery and points
Irrigation syringe and cannula
Towel clips (Backhaus), 4
1 (6/0) Chromic catgut or Dexon on ½ circle spatulated needle for lacrimal sac and deep sutures
2 (4/0) Silk on small ½ circle cutting needle for traction sutures
1 (6/0) Silk on small curved cutting needle for skin sutures.

OUTLINE OF PROCEDURE

A curved incision is made to expose the whole of the anterior lacrimal crest. Claw retractors are inserted to facilitate reflection of the orbicularis muscle, with an elevator, from the frontal process of the maxilla medial to the lacrimal crest. After haemostasis by diathermy or cautery, a self-retaining claw retractor is inserted.

The lacrimal fascia is incised and the lacrimal sac separated by blunt dissection from the lacrimal fossa down to the opening of the naso-lacrimal duct. The sac is retracted and 2 to 3 mm of bone removed from the anterior lacrimal crest and lower part of the lacrimal fossa using a power driven diamond burr, punch forceps or gouges. The thin parchment – like bone of the posterior part of the lacrimal fossa is fractured with a blunt dissector, and using punch forceps or a power burr the opening is enlarged, care being taken to avoid damage to the underlying mucosa.

Scissors are used to make a transverse cut across the end of the sac where it enters the naso-lacrimal duct. After checking the patency of the sac lumen, the medial wall is opened vertically with one blade of the spring scissors almost down to the fundus where a T-cut is made (Fig. 22.13B). The nasal mucosa is incised to match the opening in the lacrimal sac (Fig. 22.13C) and the patency and position of each canaliculus checked with a lacrimal probe.

The anastomosis between the sac and nasal mucosa is carried out as illustrated in Figures 22.13D to 22.13F. The orbicularis incision is closed with interrupted catgut or Dexon sutures and the skin sutured with silk.

Strabismus operations

DEFINITION

Advancement or recession of the ocular muscles in the treatment of squint.

POSITION

Supine.

Fig. 22.14 Graefe Strabismus Hooks.
(A) Large; (B) Medium; (C) Small.

Fig. 22.15 Prince Strabismus Forceps.

Fig. 22.16 Recession operation for squint. (A) Recession of left medial rectus, edges of Tenons capsule retracted, muscle elevated with strabismus hook, traction sutures being inserted. (B) Division of muscle at its insertion. (C) Marking position of recession with calipers. (D) Suturing muscle to new scleral insertion. (E) Closure of Tenons capsule. (F) Closure of conjunctiva. (Stallard.)

A   B

Fig. 22.17   Resection of left lateral rectus. (A) Muscle for resection held with two pairs of forceps, resection completed with sutures. (B) Suturing of rectus to new scleral insertion. (Stallard.)

INSTRUMENTS

    Eye speculum, guarded (Lang)
    Eyelid retractors (Desmarre), 2
    Strabismus hooks (Graefe or Chavasse), 2
    Fine artery forceps, curved on flat (Mosquito), 4
    Fine dissecting forceps, toothed (Jayles or Fixation)
    Fine dissecting forceps, non-toothed (Fixation)
    Strabismus scissors, curved on flat, blunt points
    Scissors, spring (Wescott)
    Muscle forceps (Prince)
    Needle holder (Barraquer)
    Screw callipers
    Rule, stainless steel 15 cm (6 in)
    Hand cautery and points
    Towel clips (Backhaus), 4
    2 (4/0) Silk on small curved cutting needle for traction
    1·5 (5/0) Plain catgut or Dexon
        or
    0·5 (8/0) Virgin silk on small curved cutting needle for conjunctiva.

OUTLINE OF PROCEDURE

These operations are usually performed under general anaesthesia. Eye muscle action is weakened by recession and strengthened by resection.

An eye speculum is inserted, traction sutures are placed just into the sclera, and a crescentic incision made in the conjunctiva, parallel with, or at the limbus of the eye. The conjunctiva is freed from the underlying fascia and insertion of the ocular muscle on the sclera, to a point well in the capsule tenons on one side, and a strabismus hook inserted under the muscle. The capsule on the other side of the muscle, where the hook presents its point, is incised and a second hook introduced from this side. Sutures may be inserted at the point chosen for division of the muscle to replace it into the new insertion.

The two hooks are separated, the muscle is divided across at a point near to its insertion in the sclera, and for recession is sutured to a new scleral insertion usually in the same meridian as the original insertion, and just behind (Fig. 22.16).

Where resection is being carried out, the amount of muscle selected for resection is removed and the shortened stump of muscle sutured to the sclera. Screw calipers are used to determine the position for the new scleral insertion (Fig. 22.17).

The conjunctiva is closed with continuous catgut, Dexon or virgin silk sutures.

Corneal transplants

DEFINITION

Transplantation of a corneal graft from an enucleated eye of another human being in the treatment of suitable corneal opacities, or irregularities such as keratoconus and keratectasis.

POSITION

Supine.

INSTRUMENTS

(These are the essential instruments required, as there are many individual instruments which may only be of use to a particular surgeon.)
Eye speculum
Lid clamps (Castroviejo)
Sponge holding forceps (Rampley), 2
Scalpel handle with No. 15 blade
Fine artery forceps, curved on flat (Mosquito), 6
Fine dissecting forceps, toothed, fixation, 2
Fine dissecting forceps, non-toothed, fixation, 2
Graft manipulators (circular spatula, iris repositor etc.)
Support for donor eye (Tudor Thomas)
Scissors, angled, sharp points
Scissors, right and left (Troutman)
Fine corneal knife (Barraquer)
Needle knife (Bowman)
Double-bladed knife or corneal trephines of various sizes
Fine needle holder (Barraquer)
Ultra fine needle holder (Troutman)
Syringe and Ryecroft cannula
Towel clips (Backhaus), 4
1 (4) White silk on small, half circle, round bodied needle for traction sutures of rectus muscles
0·7 (7/0) Silk on small curved needle with cutting edge on concavity of needle point, for cross-over suture to hold graft in place whilst final sutures are being inserted
0·2 (10/0) Purlon on small curved needle with cutting edge on convexity of needle point for sutures to secure graft in position.

OUTLINE OF PROCEDURE

There are many corneal transplant operations, but basically each consists of grafting a circular piece of healthy corneal tissue on to a prepared central area of the recipient's cornea. The operation outlined is that for a full thickness corneal graft. The donor's eye is held in a suitable stand, and a graft cut from the cornea using a trephine of appropriate size; the cornea disc remains in the trephine. The trephine is then held over the site from which the graft was taken and the central plunger screwed down to eject the graft, so that it lies with its endothelial surface bathed in the intra-occular fluid of the donor eye. The eye is covered with a piece of moistened plastic sheet, but not touching the graft.

After insertion of an eye speculum, traction sutures of white silk passed transversely through the insertions of the superior and inferior rectus muscles, are used to immobilise the eye with the centre of the cornea vertical to the ceiling.

A fine needle knife is passed into the anterior chamber at the limbus in the upper temporal quadrant, and is quickly withdrawn to avoid loss of aqueous. Sterile air is injected into the anterior chamber to reduce the risk of endothelial damage from the trephine. Transverse and vertical indirect limbal mattress sutures are inserted as Figure 22.18A to assist in the retention of the graft during its fixation by direct sutures. The epithelium of the donor cornea is normally scraped away with a scalpel blade to eliminate rejection by the recipient.

A disc of opaque cornea, corresponding with the size of the graft is cut with a trephine, gentle and even pressure being applied until the anterior chamber is entered. The trephine is gradually lifted from the circular incision, and any remaining incompletely severed tissue is cut with a fine corneal knife, or scissors. If scissors are used, these are inclined so that the posterior blade severs Descemets membrane a little wider than the circumference of the graft.

A circular spatula is manoeuvred between the cornea and the iris through the trephine hole and any remaining tags of the Descemets membrane trimmed with scissors. A peripheral iridectomy may be carried out at one or two sides of the iris.

The graft is gently manipulated into its position in the trephine opening, care being taken to avoid damage to the endothelium; the surface of the graft is flush with the surrounding cornea. The loops of the indirect limbal mattress sutures are positioned over

Fig. 22.18 Corneal graft. (A) Temporary limbal indirect graft retention sutures. (B) and (C) Application of trephine to cornea; rectus traction sutures and graft retention sutures in position. (D) and (E) Method of suturing graft. (F) Injection of sterile air into anterior chamber. (Stallard.)

the graft and drawn sufficiently taut to steady the graft. Interrupted 0·2 (10/0) Perlon sutures are inserted to unite the corneal graft to the host; these remain in position for two weeks. Sterile air is injected into the anterior chamber, and the suture line is completed with a continuous suture of Perlon, which is removed after six months.

The temporary graft retention sutures are removed and a retro-ocular injection of 1 ml of lignocaine (Xylocaine) and 15 per cent alcohol is given. The upper lid is drawn over the eye and retained in position with tullegras, an eye pad dressing and eye shield.

Iridectomy

DEFINITION

Excision of a segment of iris. This is performed for many conditions, including cysts or tumours of the iris, anti-glaucoma operations, iris prolapse, as part of cataract extraction, etc.

POSITION

Supine.

INSTRUMENTS

(Essential instruments only are listed as there are many kinds of forceps, etc., which are personal and only of interest to a particular surgeon.)
Sponge holding forceps (Rampley), 2
Eye speculuae (Clarkson-Lang and Barraquer)
Fine knife or razor fragment in holder

Fig. 22.19   Graft iris forceps.

Fig. 22.20   Morrison-Butler Lacrimal cannula.

Fig. 22.21   Arruga iris forceps.

Fig. 22.22   Bowman iris hook.

Fig. 22.23   de Wecker iris scissors.

Figs. 22.19 to 22.23   Iris instruments. (Down's Surgical Ltd.)

Keratome
Fine artery forceps, curved on flat (Mosquito), 4
Fine dissecting forceps, toothed fixation (Jayles)
Iris forceps of appropriate shape to suit a particular surgeon
Eye scissors (De Wecker)
Iris scissors, sharp points, curved and straight
Iris hook
Iris repositor (Bowman)
Fine needle holder (Barraquer)
Lacrimal cannula with 2 ml syringe for irrigation (Sodium chloride 0·9 %)
Towel clips (Backhaus), 4
1 (4) White silk on small half circle round bodied needle for traction sutures
0·5 (8/0) Virgin silk on small curved cutting needle for conjunctival sutures.

OUTLINE OF PROCEDURE

After insertion of an eye speculum, traction sutures of white silk passed transversely through the insertions of the superior and interior rectus muscles are used to immobilise the eye in the desired position. A conjunctival flap is made to protect the incision afterwards.

Fig. 22.24 Iridectomy. (A) Insertion of keratome. (B) Limbal incision. (C) Iris forceps inserted into anterior chamber in closed position. (D) Narrow iridectomy using de Wecker scissors. (E) Broad iridectomy. (F) Deposition of iris pillars. (Stallard.)

Fixation forceps are placed at a point close to the limbus and opposite the site for the limbal incision. A Keratome is inserted about 0·5 mm behind the limbus and passed slightly obliquely through the cornea. The knife is then withdrawn quickly to avoid loss of aqueous, and a conjunctival flap cut of a size to give adequate cover to the incision. An incision is made in the limbus and the anterior chamber entered. The closed tip of an iris forceps is introduced into the anterior chamber just beneath the cornea. When the iris sphincter is reached, the forceps are opened and a tiny fold of iris grasped as close to the sphincter as possible. This fold of iris is withdrawn and cut off with de Wecker's scissors held at the lips of the wound. The iridectomy may be narrow or broad (Figs. 22.24F to 22.25A); any blood from the cut iris is soaked up with a small cellulose sponge held over the incision Reposition of the iris pillars are accomplished with a repositor (Fig. 22.24F).

Any blood remaining in the anterior chamber is washed out with warm saline and the incisions are closed with virgin silk. Saline is injected into the anterior chamber, the eyelids closed and normal dressing applied.

Trabeculectomy

DEFINITION

Excision of a short length of the canal of Schlemm leaving the two cut ends of the canal open directly into aqueous humour, with no trabecular tissue intervening. Carried out for glaucoma to relieve the outflow obstruction of aqueous humour.

POSITION

Supine.

INSTRUMENTS

As for iridectomy plus
Scalpel handle No. 3, with No. 15 blade (Bard Parker)
Scleral hook (Cruise)
Anterior chamber paracentesis needle
Angled corneal splitter (Tooke)
Syringe 2 ml, and fine hypodermic needle
Hand cautery and points
0·7 (7/0) Dexon on small curved cutting needle.

OUTLINE OF PROCEDURE

After insertion of an eye speculum, a traction suture is inserted through the belly of the superior rectus muscle. A subconjunctival injection of saline, 0·2 ml, is made between the 10 and 2 o'clock meridians.

A concentric conjuctival incision is made and a flap reflected over the cornea, to expose the limbus. Episcleral tissue is scraped forwards with an angled cornea splitter. A 5 mm incision is made in the limbus and further radial incisions are made from the ends of this, posteriorly through half of the sclera.

An anterior chamber paracantesis needle may be inserted into the anterior chamber, through the limbus, and withdrawn quickly to avoid loss of aqueous.

A scleral hook is used to lift the edge of the limbus incision which is undermined posteriorly with a No. 15 scalpel blade. Sutures of Dexon are inserted and left as loops on the sclera.

Some aqueous is evacuated (to lower the intra-occular pressure) by pressing the edge of the paracentesis puncture hole. Under the highest power of the operating microscope, a 4 mm incision is made over the scleral spur to enter the anterior chamber. Using fine forceps to hold the deep corneo-scleral flap, 4 mm are excised with fine scissors.

A peripheral iridectomy is carried out. The scleral flap is replaced and secured by tightening the Dexon loops before tying. The conjunctival flap is closed with virgin silk and saline injected into the anterior chamber before applying dressings for iridectomy.

Fig. 22.25 Peripheral iridectomy. (A) The iris root is grasped with von Graefe's straight iris forceps. (B) The iris is withdrawn into the incision and peripheral iridectomy is performed with de Wecker's scissors. (C) Peripheral coloboma after replacement of the iris. (Stallard.)

Cataract extraction

DEFINITION

The removal of an 'opaque' crystalline lens.

POSITION

Supine.

INSTRUMENTS

Sponge holders (Rampley), 4
Eye speculum (Clark or Lang)
Scalpel handle No. 3, with No. 15 blade (Bard Parker)
Eyelid retractors (Desmarre), 2
Fine dissecting forceps, toothed and non-toothed, fixation
Iris scissors, curved on flat, sharp points
Iris scissors, straight, sharp points
Capsule forceps (Arruga)
Iris forceps (Barraquer)
Eye scissors (de Wecker)
Iris repositor (Bowman)

Fig. 22.26 Intra capsular cataract extraction. (A) Cutting conjunctival flap. (B and C) Snip incision in conjunctiva at 12 o'clock. Scissors spread beneath conjunctiva to limbus. Lateral and medial incisions to complete conjunctival flap. (D) Episcleral tissue stripped from limbus. (E) Half-thickness limbal incisions at 11 and 1 o'clock for pre-section corneal-scleral sutures. (F) Insertion of corneo-scleral sutures with stay-knots at 11 and 1 o'clock meridians. (Seen from above.) (G) Cryo-extraction. Corneal flap lifted. Iris retractor and guard applied. Cryo-probe indents anterior capsule. (H) Injection of sterile saline into anterior chamber. (Stallard.)

Razor fragment in holder
Angled corneal splitter (Tooke)
Corneal scissors (Castroviejo)
Vectis (Snellen)
Fine needle holder (Barraquer)
Fine needle holder (Castroviejo)
Lacrimal cannula with 2 ml syringe
Anterior chamber cannula (Ryecroft) with irrigator (Southampton) for irrigation (Sodium chloride 0·9%)
Chymar, Trypsin, Zonulysin (to digest suspensory ligaments)
Cryo-probe and cryo machine
1 (4) White silk on small half-circle round bodied needle for traction sutures.
0·7 (7/0) Dexon on small curved cutting needle for corneo-scleral sutures
0·5 (8/0) Virgin silk on small curved cutting needle for conjunctival sutures.

OUTLINE OF PROCEDURE (Intra capsular)

This operation is generally performed under local anaesthesia, consisting of 4 per cent cocaine conjunctival instillation, retrobulbar injection of 2 per cent lignocaine (Xylocaine) and facial nerve injection of 2 per cent lignocaine (Xylocaine) to prevent the patient from closing his eyelids.

After insertion of an eye speculum, a traction suture is inserted through the belly of the superior rectus muscle. The conjunctiva is incised above the limbus, undermined, and curved incisions are made on each side (Figs. 22.26A to C). A flap of conjunctiva is reflected over the limbus with a corneal splitter (Fig. 22.26D). Half thickness incisions are made in the limbus and pre-section corneo-secral sutures inserted (Figs. 22.26E and F).

The episcleral tissue just posterior to the limbus is held with forceps and an incision made with the razor fragment 2 mm posterior to the corneo-scleral junction. Three Dexon stay-sutures are inserted to facilitate closure of the corneal flap after the lens has been removed. The corneo-scleral incision is completed either with a corneal splitter or No. 15 scalpel; alternatively corneal scissors are used. A peripheral iridectomy may be performed.

A fine anterior chamber cannula is used to inject a drop of Chymar, Trypsin and Zonulysin in the vicinity of the nasal and temporal suspensory ligaments; this is left to digest the ligaments for a period between 1 minute to $3\frac{1}{2}$ minutes. The anterior chamber is then irrigated with saline to remove traces of enzymes.

Because of the greater tensile strength which can be applied, cryo-extraction of the lens, is the method of choice in preference to capsule forceps. Basically the instrument consists of a probe or stilette which can be cooled rapidly to $-35°C$ and then heated to $150°C$. Bringing this fine pointed instrument in contact with the lens causes it to adhere to the tip. The lens can then be extracted without the use of forceps. An instrument such as the Spembley Amoils cryo surgical system uses carbon dioxide or nitrous oxide gas as the refrigerant and incorporates a high-speed defrost mechanism which allows rapid detachment of the lens from the probe after it has been extracted (Figs. 22.26G and 22.30).

After the lens has been extracted the iris usually falls into position. The stay sutures are drawn together, and 0·5 per cent isotonic pilocarpine injected into the anterior chamber through a lacrimal cannula to constrict the pupil and prevent forward movement at the vitreous. The corneo-scleral incision is closed with Dexon and saline is injected into the anterior chamber (Fig. 22.26H).

The conjunctival incision is closed with virgin silk and the normal dressing applied.

Although intra capsule extraction has been described the procedure can be undertaken by extra capsular extraction or operation. Extra capsular extraction is usually indicated when the lens capsule is fragile as in elderly patients. The initial operative procedure is similar to that for intra capsular extraction. The surgeon introduces a closed pair of toothed capsule forceps into the anterior chamber, the forceps are opened slightly and the centre of the anterior lens capsule is grasped firmly; a large piece of anterior capsule is removed. Alternatively the piece of capsule to be removed is sectioned with a cystotome and then removed with forceps (Figs. 22.27A and 22.27C). The lens is delivered with a lens expressor and, the corneo-scleral stay sutures drawn tight. The anterior chamber may be irrigated with saline if any lens tissue or flecks of blood remain.

Aspiration of the lens is accomplished, first by carrying out a capsulotomy through the anterior capsule followed by aspiration with a size 17 hypodermic needle and 2 ml syringe. Alternate aspiration and injection of Ringers solution may be required to complete removal of all tissue.

Sometimes, after cataract operations the surgeon may insert a plastic lens implant into the anterior chamber. This is usually carried for patients who are unable to tolerate a contact lens and are troubled by anisometropia and diplopia. Two such operations are illustrated in Figures 22.28 to 22.30.

Fig. 22.27 Extra capsular extraction. (A) Cataract extraction. Anterior capsulectomy with toothed forceps. (B) Anterior capsulectomy with cystotome. Preliminary to extracapsular cataract extraction. (C) Right cataract extraction. Delivery of the lens by expressor and a cystotome, after which the corneo-scleral sutures are drawn tight. (Stallard.)

Fig. 22.28 Insertion of anterior chamber plastic lens. (A) Corneal flap lifted by a hook. Tip of lens directed up and to nasal side. (B) Flanges of plastic lens depressed into filtration angle by iris repositor. (C) Suture of corneal incision. (Stallard.)

Fig. 22.29 Insertion of Dannheim's lens. (A) Corneal flap held forwards with a hook. Upper Supramid loop held in two forceps. (B) Upper Supramid loop secured in corneo-scleral suture. Narrow limbal section at 6 o'clock. (C) Lower Supramid loop grasped in a blunt hook. (D) Lower Supramid loop included in corneo-scleral suture. (Stallard.)

Fig. 22.30 Cryotherapy apparatus – Amoils TCC-42. (Spembley Ltd.)

Retinal detachment

DEFINITION

Loss of continuity between the internal and external limiting membranes i.e., detachment of the retina from the choroid.

POSITION

Supine.

INSTRUMENTS

Eye speculae (Clark and Lang), 2
Fine artery forceps, curved on flat, mosquito, 10
Scalpel handle No. 3 with No. 15 blade (Bard Parker)

Fine dissecting forceps, 2/3 teeth, fixation (Lester)
Fine dissecting forceps, 1/2 teeth, fixation (Jayles), 2
Fine dissecting forceps, non-toothed, fixation (Moorfields), 2
Fine scissors, curved on flat, blunt points (Strabismus)
Iris scissors, curved on flat, sharp points
Spring scissors (Wescott)
Strabismus hooks (Grafe or Chevasse), 2
Eyelid retractors (Desmarre), 2
Eyelid retractor (Fergusson)
Dilator canaliculus (Nettleship)
Iris repositor (Bowman)
Corneal forceps (Dixey Colibri)
Caliper
Fine needle holder (Castroviejo)
Bulldog clips, 4
Hand cautery and points
Towel clips (Backhaus), 4
Cryotherapy, diathermy and catholysis apparatus
Fine pen and methylene blue (Optional)
4 (1) and 1·5 (5/0) White silk on small half-circle round bodied needle for traction sutures
1·5 (5/0) Dacron on small curved cutting needle (where silicone rod or strap prosthesis is inserted)
1 (6/0) Chromic catgut
or
0·5 (8/0) Silk on small cutting needle for conjunctiva
0·7 (6/0) Silk on small curved cutting needle for marker suture.

OUTLINE OF PROCEDURE

There are many operations for retinal detachment but the principle is to seal the retinal break or breaks. This may be accomplished by cryotherapy, or less often now by diathermy; scleral indentation; scleral encircling; or photocogulation.

Cryotherapy or diathermy: After insertion of a speculum, a marker suture of silk is inserted to identify the horizontal meridian. The conjunctiva episcleral tissues and tenons capsule are incised to expose the sclera (Fig. 22.31A) and the meridian of the retinal break is marked with a traction suture of silk inserted through the conjunctiva and episcleral tissue. Two silk sutures are inserted through the posterior edge of the conjunctival incision and are clamped with bulldog clips to hold them in position over the head towel.

Stabismus hooks are passed under adjacent rectus muscles to facilitate control of the eye rotation; alternatively, traction sutures of white silk may be utilised (Fig. 22.31B). It may be necessary to divide a rectus muscle to gain access to a retinal break in the macular region or behind the equator of the globe, especially the upper quadrant.

The two arms of the limbal suture are separated and utilising an indirect ophthalmoscope the operator visualises the site of the retinal break. A cryoprobe is applied until the tissues around the retinal break are co-agulated satisfactorily (Fig. 22.31C). If diathermy is used it is usual to raise a lamellar scleral flap to allow direct application of the electrode rather than the unpleasant effect of the current passing through the whole thickness of the sclera.

After satisfactory coagulation it is usual to drain away inter-retinal fluid, either by penetrating diathermy or scleral incision. This is a very delicate procedure. The scleral incision is closed with Dacron and silk sutures are used for the conjunctiva.

Scleral indentation. This consists of a silicone rod which is fixed to the sclera over the site of the retinal break (Fig. 22.33). The principle behind this is the fact that when the sclera is buckled and the retinal break lies against the choroid at the hump of the indentation, traffic of fluid from the vitreous is stopped and any inter-retinal fluid is absorbed through the choroid without the need for a drainage operation.

Scleral encircling. Usually undertaken in conjunction with cryotherapy the purpose is to reduce the volume of the eye, achieve mechanical block of retinal breaks, eliminate or lessen vitreous reactions, and to maintain adequate intra-ocular pressure without risk of hypotony.

A silicone strap is threaded through a lamellar tunnel cut in the sclera in four quadrants of the eye. Alternatively, it is passed under the four recti muscles. The strap is overlapped and secured with Dacron sutures as illustrated in Figure 22.34.

Fig. 22.31 Cryotherapy for retinal detachment. (A) Conjunctival incision. (B) Traction sutures passed through superior and lateral rectus muscles; arms of limbal suture separated position of retinal break and lamellar scleral flap marked with methylene blue. (C) Application of cryoprobe to sclera. (Stallard.)

Fig. 22.32 Diathermy for retinal detachment. (A) Dissection of lamellar scleral flap. (B) Diathermy applied to deepest layers of sclera. (Stallard.)

Fig. 22.33 (*Left*) Scleral indentation. Silicone rod is fixed to sclera by two Dacron mattress sutures over site of retinal break. (Stallard.)

Fig. 22.34 (*Right*) Scleral encircling. Encircling silicone band passed through lamellar scleral tunnels in the four quadrants and secured by overlapping and two Dacron mattress sutures in the lower temporal quadrant. (Stallard.)

Simple enucleation

DEFINITION

Removal of the entire eyeball for disease or injury.

POSITION

Supine.

INSTRUMENTS

Eye speculum
Fine dissecting forceps, toothed, fixation
Fine dissecting forceps, non-toothed, fixation
Scleral fixation clamps, toothed
Iris scissors, sharp points, curved and straight, 2
Scissors, curved on flat, 13 cm (5 in) (Mayo)
Muscle hook
Tonsil snare (optional)
Fine artery forceps, curved on flat mosquito, 5
Fine artery forceps, straight mosquito, 5
Fine artery forceps, straight mosquito, 5
Fine needle holder (Silcock, Kilner multiple joint)
2 (4/0) Chromic catgut or Dexon may be required for ligatures
1·5 (5/0) Dexon on a small curved cutting needle for conjunctival suture.

OUTLINE OF PROCEDURE

General anaesthesia usually administered for this operation.

The conjunctiva is incised close to the limbus and into the internal and external commissures and into the superior and interior fornices. The internal rectus, superior rectus, inferior rectus and external rectus muscles are divided in that order, utilising a muscle hook and sharp-pointed scissors. The external rectus is usually cut, leaving a small tab of muscle adherent to the sclera so that a scleral clamp or mosquito artery forceps can be applied to control the eyeball for subsequent enucleation.

The eyeball is prolapsed from the orbit utilising this clamp, and the enucleation completed either by threading a tonsil snare over the eyeball and optic nerve, or dividing the nerve with Mayo's scissors. A snare is never used if the eyeball is perforated.

The superior, inferior, medial and lateral recti are sutured together in a cross. Haemorrhage is controlled by pressure or catgut or Dexon ligatures and the conjunctiva is closed with a running suture of silk, which is not tied.

Orbital implants are now widely used following enucleation. These include Roper Hall magnetic implant and Castro Viego plastic implant.

FURTHER READING

STALLARD, H. B. (1973) *Eye Surgery*. Bristol: Wright.

23
ORTHOPAEDIC OPERATIONS

Tourniquets

Many orthopaedic operations are performed under tourniquet in a bloodless field. A correctly applied tourniquet will compress the vessels just sufficiently to stop blood flow, and no more. Excessive pressure is not only unnecessary but carries with it the danger of irreversible ischaemia in the muscles and damage to nerve fibres.

A tourniquet on the lower limb should be applied to mid-thigh, well clear of the knee joint; and for the upper limb, it should be placed at mid-biceps level well above the elbow joint. If a tourniquet is applied near a joint or over a bony prominence, there is little padding effect of muscle and fat, therefore the pressure exerted may damage vessels or nerves by compressing them directly against the bone.

Although Esmarch's rubber bandages may be used, there should be some means of measuring the pressure exerted by a tourniquet and for this reason the pneumatic type is regarded as the most satisfactory. As this pressure is applied evenly around the limb, and the chance of 'pinching' the skin or causing areas of irregular pressure is almost eliminated.

The Conn pneumatic tourniquet (Fig. 23.2) is one type which allows the pressure to be measured with an aneroid gauge.

The limb is exsanguinated with a rubber bandage applied over a towel, from extremity to the level of the tourniquet. The Conn tourniquet, which should be in direct contact with the skin and **not** applied over a towel, should then be inflated with a hand pump, and the Esmarch's bandage removed. With the Conn tourniquet the pressure applied to an arm should not exceed 275 mmHg (5 lb p.s.i.); and to a leg, 550 mmHg (10 lb p.s.i.). Although this is in excess of the usual systolic blood-pressure, it is still within safe limits and is necessary to compensate for the padding effect of muscle and fat overlying the vessel wall, when using this type of cuff.

After inflating the cuff with a hand pump, the non-return valve remains closed until release of the tourniquet is required. If the pressure should drop, e.g., due to leaks, it must be raised again with the pump which remains connected to the apparatus. In order to do this the non-return valve is opened slightly, and closed again after the correct pressure has been reached.

The Northwick Park exsanguinator and tourniquet is an apparatus which has been developed to improve the control of tourniquet pressure. This consists of a separate pneumatic sleeve and pneumatic cuff.

To exsanguinate the limb the pneumatic sleeve is drawn over the limb and covers it up to the level of the tourniquet. It is then inflated to a pressure 50 mmHg above systolic pressure and held at that pressure for one minute. The tourniquet is then inflated to a pressure of 50 mmHg above systolic pressure in the upper limb and 100 mmHg above systolic in the lower limb.

There is a double reciprocating pump attached to the tourniquet which allows rapid re-inflation should any drop in pressure occur. This is a safety device which will prevent any danger of the tourniquet going down during an operation. The cuff is deflated simply by turning the tourniquet switch to deflate.

512   Operating Theatre Technique

Fig. 23.1A The Northwick Park exsanguinator and tourniquet showing inflation of exsanguinator. (Zimmer Orthopaedic Ltd.)

Fig. 23.1B (left) The Northwick Park exsanguinator and tourniquet showing tourniquet cuff inflated. *Inset :* control apparatus.

Fig. 23.2 (right) The Conn tourniquet. (Zimmer Orthopaedic Ltd.)

The Kidde tourniquet is an apparatus which permits the rapid inflation of a tourniquet cuff to a pre-set pressure which is automatically maintained until change is desired. Variation in pressure (between a range of 0–1000 mmHg) can be achieved easily during lengthy operative procedures.

The apparatus utilises a non-toxic gas in liquid form, which is delivered from a replaceable pressurised can. The level of gas is indicated in a visible gas reservoir.

The Kidde tourniquet may be used with any pneumatic cuff although a special neoprene tourniquet secured with velcro tape is available.

Fig. 23.3 The Kidde automatically compensated tourniquet. (Howmedica U.K. Ltd.)

Generally, surgeons do not leave a tourniquet in position for too long a time. If the limb has been exsanguinated, 1 hour is within safe limits, but for operations lasting much longer than this, the surgeon may release and re-inflate the tourniquet at hourly intervals.

An efficient system of recording the application and removal of tourniquets must be in operation. A tourniquet forgotten and left in position when the patient returns to the ward can be disastrous and result in the loss of a limb.

Skeletal traction (long bones)

DEFINITION

The insertion of pins or wires through a bone in order to apply traction as an alternative to skin traction.

POSITION

Usually supine, but varies with the site for insertion.

INSTRUMENTS

As Figure 23.4
Splints, weights, pulleys, traction frame, etc.

OUTLINE OF PROCEDURE

Skeletal traction may be used as a temporary procedure for the manipulation of a fracture during operation, or as a permanent means of maintaining this reduction after operation until the fracture heals. It is used either as fixed traction, or as sliding traction with weights and pulleys, etc., in combination with a splint.

Fig. 23.4 Skeletal traction, Steinmann pin and Kirschner wire

1. Sponge-holding forceps (Rampley), 2.
2. Scalpel handle No. 9 with No. 15 blade (Bard Parker).
3. Traction pins (Steinmann) of appropriate diameter; diamond and trocar points illustrated.
4. Hand chuck for Steinmann pins.
5. Traction pin stirrups (Bohler), and corks for points of pins.
6. Traction wires (Kirschner), 3 sizes.
7. Drill with telescopic guide for insertion of Kirschner wires. (Chuck keys may be required.)
8. Swabs.
9. Towel clips, 2.
10. Gallipot containing skin antiseptic.
11. Cotton-wool for sealing around the protruding pins.
12. Mallet (Heath).
13. Nobecutane for sealing puncture wounds.
14. Traction wire stirrup (Kirschner) and key.

For average adults with a traction of up to 9 kg (20 lb) a Steinmann pin size 4 mm ($\frac{5}{32}$ in) diameter is usually adequate, although for larger patients and a greater degree of traction it may be necessary to increase this diameter to 4·8 mm ($\frac{3}{16}$ in). If the pin is to be inserted with a hand or power drill, it should have a diamond-shaped point; but if a hand chuck and mallet are used, the point needs to be of a trocar shape.

When inserting a Steinmann pin, a small skin incision is first made at the entrance and then the exit of the pin. Each end is then attached to a Bohler's stirrup and the limb is immobilised on a splint in the usual manner.

Kirschner wires are very thin in comparison with Steinmann pins. However, when these wires are maintained under tension in a special stirrup (in a manner similar to a piano wire) the degree of traction obtainable is quite considerable and as a very small hole is made, bone damage is minimal. There are three sizes of wires, 0·9 mm (0·035 in), 1·15 mm (0·045 in), 1·6 mm (0·062 in) in diameter, the middle size being the most popular. Kirschner wires are inserted with a special hand or power drill, having a telescopic attachment which is extended to support the wire. This attachment collapses as the wire is inserted, the wire is stretched taut in the special Kirschner stirrup and splints applied as before. In both cases the point at which the pin or wire enters and leaves the skin is sealed with a piece of cotton-wool and plastic skin or collodion.

For fractures of the femoral shaft, a pin or wire is passed through the upper part of the tibia; and for fractures of the tibial shaft, the pin or wire is passed through the lower end of the tibia or os calcis.

Skeletal traction (skull)

DEFINITION

Traction applied to the skull in the treatment of cervical lesions, e.g., cervical dislocations, by means of a caliper.

POSITION

Supine, with no pillow.

INSTRUMENTS

Batchelor's Zygoma Hooks
   Sponge-holding forceps (Rampley), 2
   Scalpel handle No. 3 with No. 15 blade (Bard Parker)
   Zygoma hooks (2) and frame (Fig. 23.5)
   Local anaesthetic requisites (Fig. 10.35)
   Traction cord, weights and pulleys, etc.

Fig. 23.5 Zygona hooks and traction bar. (Batchelor.)

OUTLINE OF PROCEDURE

The Batchelor's zygoma hooks are the simplest to insert and many surgeons regard them as more satisfactory, for they have little tendency to slip out after insertion.

The zygoma area is infiltrated with local anaesthetic, and a small stab incision is made sufficient for insertion of the hook. A hook is inserted under the zygoma on each side and connected to the frame to which traction is applied by weights and pulleys attached to the patient's bed.

The bone and fracture set of instruments

The basic set consists of suitable instruments for the average bone operation. The very small or large bone instruments are added as required, and do not form part of the basic set unless they are in constant use.

Bone levers, hooks and holding forceps are generally used in pairs, especially for the manipulation of fractures. Bone-cutting and nibbling or gouge forceps may have single joints; or multiple joints (compound action), which allows considerable force to be applied with the minimum of effort, and are of great value when the bone is very hard.

Open reduction of a fracture

DEFINITION

Reduction of a fracture by open operation.

POSITION

Dependent upon the location of the fracture.

INSTRUMENTS

    General set (Figs. 14.1 to 14.28)
    Cutting forceps, compound action (Horsley)
    Cutting forceps, straight (Liston)
    Cutting forceps, angled on flat (Liston)
    Elevators or levers (Bristow)
    Elevators or levers, medium size (Lane), minimum of 2
    Gouge or nibbling forceps, angled on side
    Gouge or nibbling forceps, angled on flat
    Gouge or nibbling forceps, compound action
    Holding forceps (St Thomas' Hospital)
    Holding forceps (Fergusson lion), 2
    Hooks (Lane)
    Mallet (Heath)
    Mallet (Rowland)
    Necrosis or sequestrum forceps, straight
    Necrosis or sequestrum forceps, angled on flat
    Periosteal elevators or rugines (large), (Mitchell), straight and round end
    Periosteal elevator or rugine (small), (Faraboeuf).
    (If internal fixation is contemplated, instruments for this are added. See appropriate section, e.g., plating and screwing.)
    2·5 or 3 (2/0 or 0) Plain catgut or Dexon for ligatures

Orthopaedic Operations 517

Fig. 23.6   Horsley Bone Cutting Forceps (Compound Action).

Fig. 23.7   Stamms Bone Cutting Forceps.

Fig. 23.8   Jansen-Zaufel Bone Rongeur (Compound Action).

Fig. 23.9   Wilms Gouge Forceps.

Figs. 23.6 to 23.9   Bone cutting/gouge forceps. (Zimmer Orthopaedic Ltd.)

Fig. 23.10   Liston Bone Cutting Forceps. (Chas. F. Thackray.)

518   Operating Theatre Technique

Fig. 23.11   Volkmann Curetting Spoon. (Double end. Four sizes A, B, C and D.)

Fig. 23.12   Trethowan (Ring) Bone Lever.

Fig. 23.13   Lane Bone Lever.

Fig. 23.14   Bristow Bone Lever.

Fig. 23.15   St Thomas' Bone Levers.

Fig. 23.16   Bone Hook. (Chas. F. Thackray Ltd.)

Fig. 23.17   Faraboeuf Rugine.

Figs. 23.11 to 23.17   Bone levers, rugines, hook, and curetting spoon.

Orthopaedic Operations

Fig. 23.18 Lane Bone Holding Forceps.

Fig. 23.19 Necrosis Forceps (Straight).

Fig. 23.20 Fergusson Lion Bone Holding Forceps.

Fig. 23.21 Hey Groves Bone Holding Forceps with Self-Retaining Screw.

Fig. 23.22 Burns Bone Holding Forceps.

Fig. 23.23 Lowman Self-Retaining Bone Holding Clamps.

Figs. 23.18 to 23.23 Bone holding forceps. (Zimmer Orthopaedic Ltd.)

3, 4 or 5 (0, 1 or 2) Plain or chromic catgut or Dexon sutures on appropriate needle for that area of the body

2·5 or 3 (2/0 or 0) Silk or nylon on a curved or straight cutting needle for skin sutures.

OUTLINE OF PROCEDURE

The open reduction of a fracture is performed when adequate reduction by closed methods has been unsuccessful or is impossible; when displacement, angulation or deformity are likely following closed reduction, e.g., fractures of the patella; to promote union and reduce stay in hospital, e.g., internal fixation of fractures of the middle and upper femoral shaft; to reduce mortality, e.g., internal fixation of femoral neck fractures and intertrochanteric fractures.

Fig. 23.24   Nylon Faced Mallet.   Fig. 23.25   Heath Mallet.

Figs. 23.24 and 23.25   Orthopaedic mallets. (Zimmer Orthopaedic Ltd.)

The fracture is exposed through a skin incision which is sufficiently long to provide adequate exposure with minimal retraction of soft tissues. This incision is generally not placed directly over bony prominences, and the fracture is approached through intermuscular planes rather than through muscle bellies.

The bone is exposed by minimal periosteal stripping and reduction is accomplished with bone levers, hooks or bone-holding forceps. If internal fixation is contemplated, the reduction may be maintained with ordinary bone-holding forceps or the self-retaining kind.

If the fracture has not been fixed internally some type of external splintage will be needed (Chapter 29). Occasionally internal fixation may be combined with external splintage as a temporary measure.

Drills, plates and screws

Internal fixation for bone surgery can take the form of a plate screwed into position on the surface of a bone; a screw passing through the bone to transfix the fracture; or an intramedullary nail or pin inside the bone.

There are very few metals which can be left inside the body without causing at least a severe reaction, if not complete corrosion. The 'noble' metals including gold and silver may be used, but are very expensive and often mechanically weak. It must be mentioned that tantalum is another metal which has been used for implants, but it has been shown that this metal can cause severe tissue reaction (not corrosion) and its use is now rather limited.

There are three metals which have been found suitable for surgical implants, although none of these is regarded as perfect. The three implant metals are: special stainless-steel of the SMo or EN58J type; Vitallium or Vinertia; and Titanium.

The SMo or EN58J is called an austenitic stainless-steel containing about 18 per cent of chromium, 10 to 13 per cent nickel and 2 to 3 per cent molybdenum, in addition to iron residue and traces of other elements. It has excellent corrosion resistant properties, great toughness and can be worked by machine.

Austenitic stainless-steel is non-magnetic, but may become slightly magnetic as a result of cold working such as the drawing process used to manufacture Kirschner wires, Kuntscher nails and Steinmann pins. It cannot be hardened much more than a Rockwell C35 (a degree of hardness determined with a special testing machine) and is therefore not suitable for osteotomes which require a lasting sharp edge.

The resistance of austenitic stainless-steel to corrosion lies in its 2 to 4 per cent addition of molybdenum, but equally important are the highly polished surface finish, careful cleansing process, the creation of an oxide surface layer and removal of debris left in the implant during the polishing operations by 'passivating' the implant in a chemical bath, and adequate inspection after manufacture of detect flaws. It is interesting to note that the most satisfactory method of polishing implants is by reverse plating. In this method, which is the exact opposite of electrolytic plating (e.g., chromium plating), debris is 'thrown' off the implant even from the most inaccessible areas such as the threads of screws and cannulations of pins.

Under normal circumstances the protective oxide layer is self-sealing if the surface of an implant becomes slightly scratched. In spite of this, care must be taken to avoid scratching any implant during handling, as a point of corrosion may be set up which could cause severe reaction in the tissues.

It is appropriate here to mention the martensitic stainless-steels which are used in the manufacture of most surgical instruments. These stainless-steels are magnetic and can be hardened to a Rockwell C56 to C60 which is adequate for osteotomes and chisels, etc. Ordinary plated carbon steel can be hardened to a Rockwell C55 to C65 and for this reason some surgeons contend that carbon steel osteotomes retain a better edge than stainless-steel osteotomes. However, with improved manufacturing techniques, stainless-steel is fast approaching carbon steel in quality from this point of view.

Martensitic stainless-steel is rust resistant but it corrodes if left in the tissues and is therefore entirely unsuitable for internal use. A surgeon will take steps to remove a fragment of martensitic stainless-steel which has 'flaked off' from a surgical instrument and become embedded in the tissues.

Vitallium (American), Alivium, Coballoy (British) are non-ferrous alloys (they do not rust) containing 57 to 63 per cent cobalt, 27 to 30 per cent chromium and 5 to 7 per cent molybdenum, with traces of other elements. The metal is virtually inert in the body tissues and is very strong but very difficult to work by machine. Most implants, even screws, are cast from molten metal because of this difficulty. The tensile strength is in the order of 63 to 66 kgf per mm^2 (40 to 42 tons per in^2).

Non-ferrous alloys do not rely upon a high surface polish for part of their corrosion resistance, and slight damage to the surface is not quite so important as with the stainless-steels. But this does not mean that any less care should be taken during handling, for a highly polished smooth surface of an implant may be essential, e.g., for arthroplasty of joints.

Titanium alloy used for surgical implants contains about 90 per cent pure Titanium, the remaining elements varying in proportion according to the type of implant. Where high loadings and wear may be expected the alloy contains tin 2 per cent, Molybdenum 4 per cent, aluminium 4 per cent and silicon 0·5 per cent. For bone screws the trace elements are aluminium 6 per cent, Vanadium 4 per cent, iron 0·3 per cent and hydrogen 0·01 per cent.

Unlike austenitic stainless-steels such as SMo, Titanium cannot be 'work hardened' by machining or cold drawing, so that the high tensile strength achieved in cold drawn stainless-steel wire as used for staples, Kirschner wires, Steinmann pins, Rush type pins cannot be reproduced in Titanium. However those implants usually made from the annealed material of stainless-steel, have less tensile strength and yield point (or ductility) as compared with Titanium before permanent deformation of the implant occurs under stress.

Implants suitable for manufacture in Titanium include, hip prostheses, hip nails, bone plates and screws. For its strength the metal is exceptionally light being about half the weight of the equivalent size in stainless-steel. It is extremely inert and resistant to corrosion by body tissue and fluids. Its ultimate tensile strength can be as high as 95 kgf per mm^2 (60 tons per in^2) but on average is in the region of 70 kgf to 79 kgf per mm^2 (44 to 50 tons per in^2). Titanium has been used clinically since 1957 and as a result of many papers on its successful use it is for some purposes replacing the other metallic implant materials.

To use different metals in contact with one another in the body is very undesirable. Although all three metals described are relatively inert when used alone, severe reactions can occur if, for instance, a stainless-steel screw is used in contact with a Vitallium plate. This reaction is said to be partially an electrolytic and partially a chemical process. Whatever the cause, the end result is corrosion of the implant, and often non-union of the fracture or a discharging wound. *The scrub nurse must ensure that she does not give the surgeon implants made from different metals and which are to be used in contact with one another in the tissues.*

It is possible for small fragments of metal to 'flake off' from instruments used for the insertion of implants. For this reason, it is desirable that all instruments used for handling implants are made from or tipped with the same metal as the implant; otherwise small fragments of metal may be transferred from the insertion instruments and set up local points of corrosion in the tissues. This is especially so with screwdrivers, which may slip off the screw during insertion.

Drills

Bone drills are made from three materials, martensitic stainless-steel, Vitallium and plated carbon steel. The first two types of drills are sterilised by steam, but the carbon steel drills must be dry-heat sterilised.

Drill points must be kept sharp and at slightly less than the 45 degrees angle point of the conventional industrial drills. If the drill shaft is not straight, or has been incorrectly aligned in the drill chuck, the result will be an oval hole in the bone. Correct alignment is checked by looking along the drill shaft as the chuck is rotated. A drill end (up to 6·4 mm ($\frac{1}{4}$ in) in diameter) should appear as a point about the size of a full stop on this page. A blunt drill appears as a larger point, and a wobbling drill as an oval-shaped point. In this case the drill must be re-aligned in the chuck, or discarded for straightening and re-sharpening before further use.

Vitallium drills appear to have several advantages over the other two types. They are rustless, have lasting sharpness and the ability to bend 90 degrees without breaking.

Screws

Bone screws have fine or coarse threads which either extend for the full length of the screw or for only three-quarters of the length.

The screw slot varies in shape within three varieties: the plain slot, the Phillip's recessed head/Duodrive and the cruciform or cross slot. A standard shape of screwdriver is used for the first variety but a special 'cross point' screwdriver must be used for the other two.

Fig. 23.26 Sherman Bone Screws. (Full size approx.)

S.Mo. (EN 58J). Stainless steel, Titanium or Vitallium.

Fine and coarse thread, with self-tapping point and single or cross slotted head.

Supplied in two diameters: 3·6 mm($\frac{9}{64}$ in) and 4 mm ($\frac{5}{32}$ in).
Lengths available in 10 mm to 51 mm in approx. 3 mm steps, 57 mm, 64 mm, 70 mm, 76 mm, 83 mm, 89 mm, 95 mm and 102 mm
$\frac{3}{8}$ to 2 in, in $\frac{1}{8}$ in steps, $2\frac{1}{4}$, $2\frac{1}{2}$, $2\frac{3}{4}$, 3, $3\frac{1}{4}$, $3\frac{1}{2}$, $3\frac{3}{4}$ and 4 in.

Technical Data—

$\frac{9}{64}$ in (3·6 mm) diameter screws:

   Head diameter: $\frac{15}{64}$ in (·234 in or 5·9 mm).
   Outside thread diameter: $\frac{9}{64}$ in (·140 in or 3·6 mm).
   Root thread diameter: $\frac{7}{64}$ in (·109 in or 2·8 mm).
   Threads per inch (fine thread): 32
   Threads per inch (coarse thread): 20
   Recommended drill size: No. 31 (·120 in or 3 mm).

$\frac{5}{32}$ in (4 mm) diameter screws:

   Head diameter: $\frac{9}{32}$ in (·281 in or 7·1 mm).
   Outside thread diameter: $\frac{5}{32}$ in (·156 in or 4 mm).
   Root thread diameter: just under $\frac{1}{8}$ in (·116 in or 2·9 mm).
   Threads per inch (fine thread): 32.
   Threads per inch (coarse thread): 20.
   Recommended drill size: $\frac{9}{64}$ in (·140 in or 3·6 mm).

Fig. 23.27 Varieties of Screw Heads (Enlarged Views).

A. Single slot, available in all varieties of screws both S.Mo. (EN 58J). Stainless steel, Titanium and Vitallium.
B. Cross slot, available in Sherman screws S.Mo. (EN 58J). Stainless steel and Titanium.
C. Hexagonal recessed slot.
D. Phillips recessed head, available in Phillips screws Vitallium, which have an identical shaft to $\frac{9}{64}$ in diameter Sherman screws. (These are now available as Duo Drive screws on which a single slot, suitable for an ordinary screwdriver, is superimposed over the cross recess.

Fig. 23.28 Transfixion Screw.

S.Mo. (EN 58J). Stainless steel, Titanium or Vitallium.

Partially coarse thread with self-tapping point and single slotted head.

Supplied in one diameter: 4·4 mm ($\frac{11}{64}$ in).
Lengths available: 45 mm ($1\frac{3}{4}$ in), 51 mm (2 in), 57 mm ($2\frac{1}{4}$ in), and 64 mm ($2\frac{1}{2}$ in), (Vitallium); 45 mm ($1\frac{3}{4}$ in), 51 mm (2 in), 57 mm ($2\frac{1}{4}$ in), 64 mm ($2\frac{1}{2}$ in), 70 mm ($2\frac{3}{4}$ in), and 76 mm (3 in), S.Mo. (EN 58J).

Technical data—

   Head diameter: $\frac{9}{32}$ in (·116 in or 2·9 mm).
   Outside thread diameter: just over $\frac{11}{64}$ in (·177 in or 4·5 mm).
   Root thread diameter: just under $\frac{9}{64}$ in (·135 in or 3·4 mm).
   Threads per inch: 20 (S.Mo.); 18 (Vitallium).
   Recommended drill size: $\frac{9}{64}$ in (·140 in or 3·6 mm).

Figs. 23.26 to 23.28 Bone screws. (Zimmer Orthopaedic Ltd.)

Fig. 23.29   Wood Type Thread Bone Screws

S.Mo. (EN 58J). Stainless steel, Titanium or Vitallium.

Fully and partially coarse threaded with tapered point, single slotted head.

Supplied in two diameters: 2·8 mm ($\frac{7}{64}$ in) Vitallium, and 3·6 mm ($\frac{9}{64}$ in) S.Mo. (EN 58J), stainless steel Titanium or Vitallium.

Lengths available: 2·8 mm ($\frac{7}{64}$ in) diameter, 10 mm ($\frac{3}{8}$ in), 13 mm ($\frac{1}{2}$ in), 16 mm ($\frac{5}{8}$ in) and 19 mm ($\frac{3}{4}$ in); 3·6 mm ($\frac{9}{64}$ in) diameter, 19 mm ($\frac{3}{4}$ in), 22 mm ($\frac{7}{8}$ in), 25 mm (1 in), 29 mm ($1\frac{1}{8}$ in), 32 mm ($1\frac{1}{4}$ in), 38 mm ($1\frac{1}{2}$ in) and 38 mm ($1\frac{1}{2}$ in) and 45 mm ($1\frac{3}{4}$ in).

Technical Data—

2·8 mm ($\frac{7}{64}$ in) diameter screws:
Head diameter: $\frac{1}{4}$ in (·25 in or 6·4 mm).
Outside thread diameter: $\frac{7}{64}$ in (·109 in or 2·8 mm).
Root thread diameter: $\frac{5}{64}$ in approx. (·078 in or 2 mm).
Threads per inch: 22.
Recommended drill size: $\frac{3}{32}$ in (·093 in or 2·4 mm).

3·6 mm ($\frac{9}{64}$ in) diameter screws:
Head diameter: $\frac{15}{64}$ in (·234 in or 5·9 mm).
Outside diameter:– in (·140 in or 3·6 mm).
Root thread diameter: just under $\frac{7}{64}$ in (·100 in or 2·5 m).
Threads per inch: 20.
Recommended drill size: $\frac{7}{64}$ in (·109 in or 2·8 mm).

Fig. 23.30   Johannson Lag Screw

S.Mo. (EN 58J). Stainless steel or Vitallium.

Very coarse thread for one-third of shaft approximately tapered point, single slotted hexagon head.

Supplied in one shaft diameter: 4 mm ($\frac{5}{32}$ in).
Lengths available: 41 mm ($1\frac{5}{8}$ in), 57 mm ($2\frac{1}{4}$ in) and 76 mm (3 in).

Technical Data—

Head diameter: $\frac{5}{16}$ in A/f hexagon (·312 in or 8 mm).
Outside thread diameter: $\frac{11}{32}$ in (·343 in or 8·7 mm) tapering to about $\frac{3}{16}$ in (·187 in or 4·8 mm).
Root thread diameter (shaft): $\frac{5}{32}$ in (·156 in or 3·9 mm).
Threads per inch: 10.
Recommended drill size: $\frac{3}{16}$ in (·187 in or 4·8 mm) for about $\frac{1}{8}$ in through the bone cortex followed by $\frac{5}{32}$ in (·156 in or 4 mm) for total depth of screw being inserted.

Figs. 23.29 and 23.30   Bone screws (*cont'd.*)

Screws used for holding bone plates in position are of two main diameters, 3·6 mm ($\frac{9}{64}$ in) and 4 mm ($\frac{5}{32}$ in). Sherman, Phillips and cruciform are 3·6 mm ($\frac{9}{64}$ in) and 4 mm ($\frac{5}{32}$ in) diameter.

As the screw always passes through both cortices in the fixation of bone plates, this type of screw is fully threaded in order that the threads may gain the greatest purchase in both sides of the bone.

Screws used alone for the fixation of bone fragments are partially threaded and termed 'wood or transfixion' screws. In this case the screw is usually inserted through the fragment and into the area of cancellous bone adjacent, e.g., fracture of the medial malleolus. The partially threaded portion of the screw near the head allows the surgeon to 'draw up' the loose fragment against the larger one without causing the bone to split.

Fig. 23.31 Fracture of the olecranon. (Robinson.)

(A) The displacement due to the pull of the triceps.
(B) Internal fixation by a screw.

Fig. 23.32 Direction of cortex screws in spiral or long oblique fractures.

At least one screw should be inserted perpendicular to the shaft of the bone. The other screws should be inserted in such a way that some will come to lie anteriorly and others posteriorly to the middle screw in order to exert interfragmental compression at right angles to the fracture plane and overcome all shearing or torsional stresses.

Cross-section demonstrates why screws placed in different directions effect the best compression between fragments. (Hall.)

The holding power of a screw is almost at its maximum in bone when the size of the hole drilled is approximately equivalent to half the distance between the outside diameter and root diameter of the screw threads. Therefore, the hole drilled in cortical bone should approximate 85 per cent of the outside diameter of the screw. This obviates both the weak holding power of larger holes and the tendency of the screws to split the bone with smaller holes. However, when the bone is of a soft composition, i.e., cancellous bone, the hole drilled should be only slightly larger than the root diameter of the threads.

For a 2·8 mm ($\frac{7}{64}$ in) diameter screw, size No. 9, 2·4 mm ($\frac{3}{32}$ in) diameter drill is used; 3·6 mm ($\frac{9}{64}$ in) diameter screws require a size No. 31 approx. 2·8 mm ($\frac{7}{64}$ in) diameter drill; 4 mm ($\frac{5}{32}$ in) diameter screws require a 3·6 mm ($\frac{9}{64}$ in) or 3·2 mm ($\frac{1}{8}$ in) diameter drill; and 4·5 mm approx. ($\frac{11}{64}$ in) diameter screws require a 4 mm ($\frac{5}{32}$ in) or 3·6 mm ($\frac{9}{64}$ in) diameter drill.

Fig. 23.33 Williams improved automatic screwdriver. (Chas F. Thackray Ltd.)

The upper illustration shows the screwdriver ready for use; the spring-loaded driving shaft has been pushed forward to engage the slot of the screw head; the lower illustration shows the lever (A) open and the screw head disengaged. The lever (A) is closed or opened to fix or release a screw from the shaped sleeve (B) in the end of the tubular shaft.

Standard screws such as Sherman's or Lane's patterns can be used with this instrument, up to 4 mm ($\frac{5}{32}$ in) external diameter of thread with a head diameter of 7·1 mm ($\frac{5}{32}$ in). The shaped sleeve at the distal end accommodates a wide variation in shapes of screw heads.

It is possible to use the instrument to drive a screw fully home after it has been released, and in this case the lever (A) is closed so that the screwdriver protrudes from the sleeve. However, some surgeons use an ordinary Lane's screwdriver to complete this manoeuvre.

A special feature of the instrument is the adjusting screw (C) in the base of the handle. This screw is adjusted to give the lever (A) a firm fixation on the screw head. Once this screw is set correctly it need not be altered unless a screw with a larger or smaller head is required.

The use of this instrument was described in the *Lancet*, June 15, 1957, p. 1225.

After drilling a hole the surgeon measures its depth with a screw measure. This measure has a hooked end with which he feels the outer edge of the hole in the opposite cortex. The handle of the instrument is then slid down to touch the proximal cortex and the depth read off against a scale engraved on the handle.

If the surgeon does not wish to drill right through the bone, the depth of the hole is determined by probing the bottom with his measure and reading off the scale as before.

A self-retaining or automatic screwdriver is used to insert the screw up to 6·4 mm ($\frac{1}{4}$ in) from the head. The Williams or Burns are probably the ones most popular for standard single-slot screws. Alternatively there are a number of power operated screwdrivers including the Stryker bit which fits into the Stryker power tool and the 3M Air Driver.

The Williams screwdriver is adjustable for various sizes of screw heads by means of the large screw connected to the retaining lever on the handle (illustrated in Figs. 23.33 and

Sizes available (holes are same specification as venable plates)

Number	Length, S.Mo.	Length, Vitallium	No. of holes
00	140 mm (5½ in)	135 mm (5 5/16 in)	8 (Not ill.)
0	140 mm (5½ in)	135 mm (5 5/16 in)	6
1	117 mm (4 5/8 in)	114 mm (4½ in)	6
2	117 mm (4 5/8 in)	114 mm (4½ in)	6
3	117 mm (4 5/8 in)	114 mm (4½ in)	6
4	92 mm (3 5/8 in)	89 mm (3½ in)	6
5	79 mm (3⅛ in)	76 mm (3 in)	4
6	79 mm (3⅛ in)	76 mm (3 in)	4
6½	76 mm (3 in)	76 mm (3 in)	4
7	57 mm (2¼ in)	60 mm (2 3/8 in)	4
8	51 mm (2 in)	48 mm (1 7/8 in)	4
10	45 mm (1¾ in)	41 mm (1 5/8 in)	3
11	35 mm (1 3/8 in)	35 mm (1 3/8 in)	3
12	32 mm (1¼ in)	29 mm (1⅛ in)	2

Fig. 23.34 Sherman Bone Plates. S.Mo. (EN 58J). Stainless Steel or Vitallium.

23.49). When loading screws, care must be taken to avoid force as the lever is closed. The adjusting screw must be altered until the lever closes easily with the screw in position. Failure to do this will result in breakage of the sleeve which supports the screw head. Both the Williams and the Burns screwdrivers must be dismantled, cleaned, lubricated regularly and sent for repair when the tip becomes worn and does not fit snugly into the screw head.

The screw is finally tightened home with a plain-end screwdriver, such as Lane's which must fit tightly into the screw slot. Nothing is more irritating than a screwdriver

528   Operating Theatre Technique

Fig. 23.35 Egger Bone Plates. S.Mo. (EN 58J). Stainless steel, Titanium or Vitallium.

Technical Data—

Sizes available:

Plates (with slots to accommodate $\frac{9}{64}$ in (3·6 mm) diameter screws):

S.Mo. (EN 58J). Stainless steel, Titanium or Vitallium: Width, $\frac{1}{2}$ in (0·5 in or 12·8 mm); thickness, $\frac{1}{8}$ in (·125 in or 3·2 mm); lengths of 4, 5 and 6 in (wide).

S.Mo. (EN 58J). Stainless steel and Titanium: Width, $\frac{3}{8}$ in (·375 in or 9·5 mm); thickness, $\frac{1}{8}$ in (·125 in or 3·2 mm); lengths of 3 or 4 in (narrow).

Vitallium: Width, $\frac{13}{32}$ in (·406 in or 10·3 mm); thickness, $\frac{1}{8}$ in (·125 in or 3·2 mm); lengths of 3 or 4 in (narrow).

Fig. 23.36 Hicks Lugged Antirotation Bone Plates.

S.Mo. (EN 58J). Stainless Steel or Vitallium. For fractured shaft of ulna or radius.

Technical data—

Length: 76 mm (3 in). Left and right hand.

Figs. 23.35 to 23.36 Egger and Hicks bone plates. (Zimmer Orthopaedic Ltd.)

Fig. 23.37 Muller-type compression bone plating set (reduced size) Titanium. (Down Bros.)

Heavy Duty Femur Plates:

A size 8 in × 12 hole × 6 s.w.g. (1 only).
 size 7 in × 10 hole × 6 s.w.g. (1 only).
 size 6 in × 8 hole × 6 s.w.g. (1 only).

Normal Duty Femur Plates:

B size 6 in × 8 hole × 9 s.w.g. (2 only).
C size 5 in × 7 hole × 9 s.w.g. (2 only).
D size 4½ in × 6 hole × 9 s.w.g. (2 only).

Tibial Plate:

E size 4$\frac{5}{8}$ in × 7 hole × 10 s.w.g. (2 only).
F size 4 in × 6 hole × 10 s.w.g. (2 only).
G size 3$\frac{3}{8}$ in × 5 hole × 10 s.w.g. (2 only).
H size 2$\frac{3}{4}$ in × 4 hole × 10 s.w.g. (1 only).

I Fitzgerald Screws, thread 4·5 mm diam. (outside): sizes 25 mm (1 in) to 50 mm (2 in).

Instruments:

J Co-aptation Device.
K Fitzgerald Screwdriver with hexagonal end.
L Drill guide for use with $\frac{5}{32}$ in drill.
M Tap for bone screws 4·5 mm diam. 20 tpi.
N Wire tightener.
O Box spanner with universal joint for use with co-aptation device.
P Six only 11 in lengths Titanium wire 20 gauge.
Q Twist Drills $\frac{5}{32}$ in diam. 3 in and 5 in long.

Fig. 23.38 Illustration of compression plating. (A) The compression device hooked into the lowest hole of plate but fracture not yet compressed. (B) Compression applied while lower half of the plate is screwed to the lower fragment.

which keeps slipping out of the slot as the screw is driven home, and in addition, there is a grave danger of scratching the screw, with risk of corrosion.

Plates

Bone plates are designed to provide maximum strength with minimal dimensions, although no plate will take full weight bearing until the fracture has almost healed. Plates may be contoured slightly to accommodate the curvature of a bone, but if great angles are needed, the manufacturer will incorporate these when the implant is cast or machined. Once a plate has been contoured, it must not be re-bent in the reverse direction, otherwise metal fatigue may occur.

Plates such as Sherman's, Venable's and Lane's have holes for screw fixation, but there are other types including the Egger's contact plates which have slots instead. Slotted bone plates are designed to permit the fractured ends of the bone to move together slightly under the plates after they have been inserted. This allows constant contact of the bone ends (due to muscular pressure) while slight necrosis, absorption, and osteogenesis at the traumatised ends occurs. The other advantage is that the surgeon is able to insert his screws at any selected position along the slot.

The Hicks plates have lateral lugs in which the screw holes are positioned and which prevent rotation of the fragments after insertion of the plate (Fig. 23.36).

In order to minimise bacterial contamination of implants such as screws and plates, etc., these should always be handled with sterile forceps and not the gloved hands.

Fig. 23.39

(A) Forceps.
(B) Clamping device.
(C, D and E) Three pairs of jaws.
(F) Pair of hooked jaws.
(G) One 'peg'.

Fig. 23.40 Grooved Jaws Pivoted at their Attachment

Used for gripping long bones in bone grafting or plating.

Fig. 23.41 Hooked Jaws.
Used to grip a fractured patella.

Fig. 23.42 Hooked Jaw and 'Peg'.
Used to grip a fractured olecranon.

Figs. 23.39 to 23.42 Charnley adjustable bone holding forceps with range of detachable jaws.
(Chas. F. Thackray Ltd.)

Fig. 23.43 Desoutter Air Driven Bone Saw. (Desoutter.)

Fig. 23.44 Screw-Holding Forceps.

Fig. 23.45 Lane Plate-Holding Forceps.

Fig. 23.46 Screw Depth Gauge.

This is used to determine the length of the screw needed to penetrate the bone. The end of the gauge is inserted in the drilled hole and hooked over the bone surface. By releasing the thumb screw, the sleeve may be advanced snugly against the bone or bone plate. When the screw is tightened, the sleeve will remain in position as the gauge is withdrawn. Calibrations on the stem barrel indicate the length of screw required.

Fig. 23.47 Pistol-Grip Hand Drill with Jacobs Chuck.

This drill has a 2-to-1 gear ratio and is cannulated for the entire length to accommodate Steinmann pins, Kirschner wires, long-shank drills and screwdriver bits. Release of the thumb-operated lever at the top of the drill instantly stops the turning of the gears and locks the chuck.

Figs. 23.43 to 23.47 Screwing and plating instruments. (Zimmer Orthopaedic Ltd.)

Plating and screwing

DEFINITION

Internal fixation of a fracture by means of plates and screws.

POSITION

Generally supine, but dependent upon the location of the fracture.

INSTRUMENTS

General set (Figs. 14.1 to 14.28)
Bone and fracture instruments (p. 516)
2·5 or 3 (2/0 or 0) Plain catgut or Dexon for ligatures
3, 4 or 5 (0, 1 or 2) Plain or chromic catgut or Dexon sutures, on appropriate needle for that area of the body
2·5 or 3 (2/0 or 0) Silk or nylon on a small, medium or large cutting needle for skin sutures
Plaster of Paris or splints may be required
Bone clamp, self-retaining (Hey Grove), 2
Bone clamp, adjustable and self-retaining (Charnley) (Fig. 23.39)
Bone clamp, self-retaining (Lowman)
Bone clamps, self-retaining (Sinclair), large and small
Bone plates, appropriate size
Ordinary screwdriver (Lane)
Automatic screwdriver (Williams)
Plate benders, 2
Plate-holding forceps
Screw-holding forceps
Screw measuring device (Crawford Adams)
Set of screws and drills
Power drill and chuck key
Rubber air hose or drive-cable for power drill.

OUTLINE OF PROCEDURE

The fracture is exposed and reduced. If plating is to be performed, the plate is adjusted to the correct contour and applied to the bone subperiosteally, and screwed in position. If screw fixation only is required, one or more screws are introduced obliquely across the fracture line.

The wound is closed in the usual manner and temporary splints applied if required.

Wiring

DEFINITION

Internal fixation of a fracture by means of cerclage wire loops.

POSITION

Generally supine, but dependent upon the location of the fracture.

INSTRUMENTS

General set (Figs. 14.1 to 14.28)
Bone and fracture instruments (p. 516)
Wiring set (Fig. 23.48)
Bone clamps illustrated on pages 519 and 531 may be required
Bone awl or drill

Fig. 23.48   Instruments for wiring.

1. Wire knot-tying forceps (Harris).
2. Wire-cutting forceps, compound action.
3. Pliers and wire-cutting forceps combined.
4. Wire-twisting apparatus (Hey Grove).

2·5 or 3 (2/0 or 0) Plain catgut or Dexon for ligatures
3, 4 or 5 (0, 1 or 2) Plain or chromic catgut or Dexon sutures on appropriate needles for that area of the body
2·5 or 3 (2/0 or 0) Silk or nylon on a small, medium or large cutting needle for skin sutures
Plaster of Paris or splints may be required.

OUTLINE OF PROCEDURE

The fracture is exposed and reduced. Austenitic stainless-steel wire within the range of 29 SWG and 18 SWG (Chapter 7) is generally used, although sizes 20, 24 and 28 SWG are the most useful.

The fracture may be immobilised by a circumferential wire loop, e.g. a butterfly fracture of a bone shaft; or a loop is passed through holes drilled in each fragment, e.g., fracture of the patella.

The surgeon will require a bone awl or drill if holes are needed in the bone fragment. If the wire is sufficiently stiff it is passed directly round the bone or through the holes made. If a smaller gauge of wire is used, it is first threaded on to a large suture needle and is twisted back upon itself for about one inch. Alternatively, an aneurysm needle or wire passer (e.g., Sharps) may be used and the wire is threaded through the eye but not twisted back upon itself. Sometimes the surgeon may find it easier to pass the aneurysm needle round the bone first and then thread the wire through the terminal hole.

When the wire is in position, a final check is made on correct alignment of the fragments and the wire is twisted or tied in a knot. If the wire is to be twisted, this is accomplished either with special twisting forceps or two pairs of pliers. If a knot is being tied and unless the wire is very fine, a special forceps for tying wire knots is needed. Fine wire is then cut with heavy scissors reserved for the purpose and heavy wire with wire-cutting forceps.

It is essential the scrub nurse ensures that wire is free from kinks before she hands it to the surgeon. A kink is a weak point and is very liable to break, either during insertion or after operation.

The wound is closed in the usual manner and splints or plaster of Paris may be applied.

Internal fixation by nail or pin. Femoral neck fractures, Smith Petersen nail

DEFINITION

The internal fixation of a subcapital or transcervical fracture of the femoral neck with a trifin pin. This procedure may be used also to immobilise a slipped upper femoral epiphysis in adolescents.

POSITION

Immobilised on a fracture table (Fig. 4.19).

INSTRUMENTS

General set (Figs. 14.1 to 14.28)
Bone and fracture instruments (p. 516)
Set of trifin nails (Smith Petersen) (Fig. 23.49), or four flange nails
Steel rule, 15 cm (6 in)
Plate blenders, 2
3 (0) Plain catgut or Dexon for ligatures
3 or 4 (0 or 1) Plain catgut or Dexon on a medium half-circle cutting or Mayo needle with a trocar point for muscle sutures
2·5 or 3 (2/0 or 0) Silk or nylon on a medium curved cutting needle for skin sutures.

OUTLINE OF PROCEDURE

The patient is immobilised on a fracture table and if necessary the fracture is manipulated and reduced. This fracture table may be similar to that illustrated in Fig. 4.19, Bell, Albee or Hawley table, Shropshire horse, or a special attachment on a general operation table. The position of the patient's legs is adjusted to maintain reduction of the fracture during operation, and this usually means in abduction and extension with some degree of internal rotation of the affected limb.

X-ray apparatus is positioned to give anterior and lateral position films during the course of operation.

An incision is made about 25 mm (1 in) below the tip of the trochanter, and is carried 5 cm to 8 cm (2 to 3 in) down the lateral aspect of the thigh parallel with the femoral shaft. Dissection is made down to the fascia lata which is incised and split with scissors

Fig. 23.49 Femoral neck fracture, Smith Petersen nail

1. Three guide wires of exactly the same diameter and length 2·3 cm × 25 cm ($\frac{3}{32}$ in × 10 in).
2. Guide wire hand chuck (Watson-Jones).
3. Fracture impactor (Smith Petersen).
4. Box spanner for bolt (Smith Petersen).
5. Driver/extractor for trifin nail (Smith Petersen).
   A. Tommy bar for additional leverage on capstan during extraction of nail.
   B. Extractor barrel.
   C. Driver/extractor, threaded bar.
   D. Extraction capstan.
6. A. Trifin nail of appropriate size (Smith Petersen), sterile in packet.
   B. Showing Smith Petersen trifin nail.
   C. Small retaining plate (Coventry).
   D. Bolt and spring washer for attaching plate to nail (Coventry).
7. Set of screws and drills in fabric wallet.
8. Trifin nail starter (Smith Petersen).
9. Automatic screwdriver (Williams).
10. Ordinary screwdriver (Lane).
11. Screw measuring device (Crawford Adams).
12. Plate-holding forceps.
13. Screw-holding forceps.
14. Power drill (Desoutter compressed air drill).
15. Rubber air hose for power drill, and chuck key.

Fig. 23.50 The 3M Air Driver II with attachments. (Surgical Products 3M United Kingdom Ltd.)

A The handpiece is an air vane motor with a maximum speed of 20,000 r.p.m. There is a speed selector ring which can be used to vary the speed and also to select forward or reverse drive. The speed can be further controlled by the throttle lever, which incorporates a safety catch. The Air Driver II, which runs on compressed air at 90–110 p.s.i., has a bayonet connection for the hose with a swivel to prevent the hose from twisting.
B Return air hose with exhaust diffuser at the end connecting with the air cylinder.
C Osteotomy saw attachment (oscillating), with blades which can be set at five different angles. This saw is particularly useful for difficult osteotomies where the bone is deep in the tissues.
D Reciprocating saw attachment, with blades.
E Oscillating saw attachment, with blades.
F 1,000 r.p.m. drive attachment (geared), with Jacobs chuck, self-retaining screwdrivers and twist drills.
G 300 r.p.m. drive attachment (geared), with acetabulum reamer. This attachment provides the high torque necessary for heavy duty work.
H 500 r.p.m. 90° drive 90° drive attachment (geared), with flexible intramedullary reamer. It is fully cannulated for reaming, driving Steinmann pins etc.
I Stainless steel autoclave case.

in line with the skin incision. The fascia lata is retracted to expose the vastus lateralis which is incised and retracted away from the femur with bone levers. Further blunt dissection with a periosteal elevator exposes the region of the trochanter.

A Smith Petersen nail, like many implants used for the fixation of fractures in the femoral neck region, has a central cannulation to accommodate a guide wire. It is important that a guide wire is checked for correct size by passing it through the cannulation of the nail. If the wire is too tight, or does not run smoothly through it (perhaps due to a bent wire or some manufacturing error), either the wire or the nail must be replaced.

Fig. 23.51 Types of fractures of the upper end of the femur.

Fig. 23.52 Fixation of the fracture with a nail plate.

There is grave danger of a tight wire being carried through into the pelvis as the nail is driven home.

After drilling a 4·8 mm ($\frac{3}{16}$ in) to 6·4 mm ($\frac{1}{4}$ in) hole in the bone about 25 mm (1 in) below the trochanter along the shaft, the guide wire is inserted into the femoral neck and an X-ray taken to confirm its position. The guide wire may require several adjustments before the correct position is achieved.

The length of the nail required is determined by placing another identical guide wire alongside the portion of the wire which projects from the bone, and the amount projecting is deducted by measurement from the total length of the guide wire. This measurement is the same as that in the femoral neck.

If a small plate is to be used to retain the nail in position, it is usual to add a 6·4 mm ($\frac{1}{4}$ in) to the required measurement of nail.

A three or four flange nail of appropriate length is hammered home over the guide wire within 13 mm ($\frac{1}{2}$ in) of the cortex. The guide wire is then removed, and the fracture impacted with a blow on a Smith Peterson impactor positioned over the head of the

Orthopaedic Operations

A. McLaughlin Plate

B. Locking Collar – Self Locking Nut

C. McLaughlin Nail

Fig. 23.53   McLaughlin Plate Assembly (for nails with external thread).

Includes:
Plate Lengths: 38 mm (1½ in), 57 mm (2¼ in), 82·5 mm (3¼ in), 95 mm (3¾ in), 114 mm (4½ in), 133 mm (5¼ in), 203 mm (8 in).
Holes: 2, 3, 4, 5, 6, 7, 12.

Nail Lengths: 76 mm (3 in), 82·5 mm (3¼ in), 89 mm (3½ in), 95 mm (3¾ in), 102 mm (4 in), 108 mm (4¼ in), 114 mm (4½ in), 121 mm (4¾ in), 127 mm (5 in), 133 mm (5¼ in), 140 mm (5½ in), 146 mm (5¾ in), 152 mm (6 in).
The Vitallium McLaughlin nail is four-flanged and cannulated to accept a 2·4 mm ($\frac{3}{32}$ in) guide wire.

Enlarged

Fig. 23.55   McLaughlin Plate Assembly (for nails with internal thread).

Fig. 23.54   Thornton Nail, Smith-Petersen type.

Plate Lengths: 38 mm (1½ in), 57 mm (2¼ in), 82·5 mm (3¼ in), 95 mm (3¾ in), 114 mm (4½ in), 133 mm (5¼ in), 203 mm (8 in).
Holes: 2, 3, 4, 5, 6, 7, 12.

Nail Lengths: 76 mm (3 in), 82·5 mm (3¼ in), 89 mm (3½ in), 95 mm (3¾ in), 102 mm (4 in), 108 mm (4¼ in), 114 mm (4½ in), 121 mm (4¾ in), 127 mm (5 in), 133 mm (5¼ in), 140 mm (5½ in), 146 mm (5¾ in), 152 mm (6 in).
The Vitallium Thornton nail is designed with a serrated head and is cannulated to accept a 2·4 mm ($\frac{3}{32}$ in) guide wire.

Figs. 23.53 to 23.55   Femoral neck nails and plates. (Howmedica, U.K., Ltd.)

Fig. 23.56 Pugh Hip Nail (Self-Adjusting). (Zimmer Orthopaedics Ltd.)
S.Mo. (EN 58J). Stainless Steel.

Plate Lengths: 25 mm (1 in), 51 mm (2 in), 76 mm (3 in), 102 mm (4 in), 127 mm (5 in) and 152 mm (6 in).
Angle 135°
Machined from 13 mm (·5 in) diameter material, cannulated for 2·4 mm ($\frac{3}{32}$ in) guide wire.

This technique has been devised to give a more desirable and adequate fixation of the nail and plate combination for fractures of the neck of the femur, inter and subtrochanteric fractures, with additional advantages over the commonly used nails or nail and plate combinations. The nail is designed to telescope within the tube, thereby keeping the fracture constantly impacted. To accomplish this, the nail must have sufficient clearance to slide readily, but at the same time, must have enough resistance to prevent the nail from falling out of the head should a little absorption occur at the trifin portion at the end of the nail. The resistance is furnished by means of a friction ring so constructed that the nail will not slide unless a few pounds of pressure is exerted on the end of the nail. This ensures sliding action without binding.

Fig. 23.57 Modified Jewett Nail Plate. (Howmedica, U.K., Ltd.)
Vitallium. S.Mo. (EN 58J). Stainless steel, Titanium.

Sizes available:

Plate Length: 102 mm (4 in). 4 Holes.
Angles: 120°, 125°, 130°, 135°, 140°, 150°, 160°.
Nail Length: 76 mm (3 in), 82·5 mm (3¼ in), 89 mm (3½ in), 95 mm (3¾ in), 102 mm (4 in), 108 mm (4¼ in), 114 mm (4½ in), 121 mm (4¾ in), 127 mm (5 in).

Plate Length: 127 mm (5 in). 5 Holes.
Angles: 130°, 135°, 140°, 150°.
Nail Length: 76 mm (3 in), 82·5 mm (3¼ in), 89 mm (3½ in), 95 mm (3¾ in), 102 mm (4 in), 108 mm (4¼ in), 114 mm (4½ in), 121 mm (4¾ in), 127 mm (5 in).

Plate Length: 152 mm (6 in). 6 Holes.
Angles: 130°, 135°, 140°, 150°.
Nail Length: 76 mm (3 in), 82·5 mm (3¼ in), 89 mm (3½ in), 95 mm (3¾ in), 102 mm (4 in), 108 mm (4¼ in), 114 mm (4½ in), 121 mm (4¾ in), 127 mm (5 in).

Plate Length: 203 mm (8 in). 7 Holes.
Angle: 130°.
Nail Length: 76 mm (3 in), 82·5 (3¼ in), 89 mm (3½ in), 95 mm (3¾ in), 102 mm (4 in).

Plate Length: 254 mm (10 in). 9 Holes.
Angle 130°.
Nail Length: 76 mm (3 in), 82·5 mm (3¼ in), 89 mm (3½ in), 95 mm (3¾ in), 102 mm (4 in).

Diameter of Nail 12·7 mm (½ in). Thread ¼ in-20.
The Jewett nail-plate has a three-flanged nail. It is cannulated to accept a 2·4 mm ($\frac{3}{32}$ in) guide wire.

Figs. 23.56 and 23.57 Femoral neck nails (*cont'd.*).

Orthopaedic Operations 541

Fig. 23.58 McKee Trifin Nail and Interochanteric Plate. (Zimmer Orthopaedic Ltd.)
S.Mo. (EN 58J). Stainless steel, Titanium or Vitallium.

Sizes of nail available:
75 mm to 150 mm lengths in 5 mm steps. Nail: 3 to 6 in lengths in $\frac{1}{4}$ in steps; diameter, 13 mm (·5 in).
Plates: Available with a single slot, four slots, four holes or six holes. The nail is cannulated to receive a 2·4 mm ($\frac{3}{32}$ in) guide pin and the male screw thread is 7 mm diameter, 1 mm pitch to take a locking nut.

protruding nail. The nail is then driven home either flush with the femoral cortex (no retaining plate) or with approx 6 mm ($\frac{1}{4}$ in) left projecting (small, one hole retaining plate).

If required, the small retaining plate may then be secured to the nail with a threaded bolt and screwed to the femoral shaft.

The wound is closed in layers and the patient may require a plaster boot which incorporates a short splint across the heel and at right angles to the leg to prevent rotation of the foot after operation.

There are many other types of appliances for immobilising femoral neck fractures, these include sliding nails (Pugh) and compression screws (Charnley, Garden).

Internal fixation by nail or pin. Femoral trochanteric fractures, McLaughlin and McKee

DEFINITION

The internal fixation of a basal, petrochanteric or subtrochanteric fracture of the upper femur.

POSITION

As for Smith Petersen nail (Fig. 4.19).

INSTRUMENTS

McLaughlin Appliance
   General set (Figs. 14.1 to 14.28)
   Bone and fracture set (p. 516)
   Femoral neck fracture set (Fig. 23.49)
   Set of trifin nails (Smith Petersen) (p. 539)
   Intertrochanteric plate, five or seven hole, with bolt and locking washer (McLaughlin)
   Ligatures and sutures as for Smith Petersen nail

McKee Nail and Plate
   General set (Figs. 14.1 to 14.28)
   Bone and fracture set (p. 516)
   Femoral neck fracture set (Fig. 23.49 minus items 4, 5 and 6)

Fig. 23.59 Insertion of Jewett nail plate. Drilling femoral cortex, insertion of guide wire, insertion of nail plate, securing plate to femoral shaft with screws. (Hall.)

Driver/extractor (McKee)
Box spanner (McKee)
Trifin nail of appropriate size (McKee), (Fig. 23.58)
Intertrochanteric plate (McKee), (Fig. 23.58)
Plate benders, 2
Ligatures and sutures as for Smith Petersen nail

Jewett Nail-Plate
General set (Figs. 14.1 to 14.28)
Bone and fracture set (p. 516)
Femoral neck fracture set (Fig. 23.49, minus items 4, 5 and 6)
Driver/extractor (Jewett)
Nail-plate of appropriate size (Jewett)
Ligatures and sutures as for Smith Petersen nail.

OUTLINE OF PROCEDURE

The initial stages of the immobilisation of the patient, fracture reduction and incision are similar to that for Smith Petersen nail. In the case of the McLaughlin appliance and McKee plate, however, the incision extends several centimetres further down the femoral shaft in order to provide adequate exposure to insert the longer plate.

A McLaughlin Plate is bolted to a Smith Petersen nail which is inserted as described previously, with 6 mm ($\frac{1}{4}$ in) of the nail head left protruding from the bone. The plate is secured to the femoral shaft with five or seven screws, depending upon the length of the plate. The design of this plate, which has a curved shoulder, allows adjustment of the angle between the nail and plate without having to actually bend the plate itself.

A McKee Plate is bolted to a McKee nail which is inserted in a manner similar to a Smith Petersen nail. The difference between the two nails is, that whereas the Smith Petersen nail has a threaded hole in the head portion, the McKee nail has a threaded projection. The plate is fitted over this threaded projection and secured with a hexagonal nut. However, this type of plate may first require adjustment of its angle with the plate benders, in order that the plate lies flush along the shaft when bolted to the nail. The plate is then secured to the shaft by four or six screws, depending upon the length of plate selected.

A Jewett nail plate is a one-piece appliance used as an alternative to separate nails and plates. The initial stages follow those described previously. The nail plate is driven home over the guide wire and the plate screwed to the femoral shaft. The wound is closed in layers in the usual manner.

Slipped upper femoral epiphysis

It has been mentioned that the Smith Petersen trifin nail can be used to immobilise a slipped upper femoral epiphysis. Alternatively, Austin Moore pins, Knowle's pins or fine Steinmann pins may be used for this procedure.

These pins resemble guide wires but are made from austenitic stainless steel or Vitallium. The procedure is similar to Smith Petersen nail up to the insertion of the guide wire, but in this case an Austin Moore pin, Knowle pin or Steinmann pin is drilled into the femoral neck and across the epiphyseal line.

The position and length of the pin are checked radiologically and when satisfactory, several other pins, up to four, may be inserted alongside the first pin within the neck but generally at slightly different angles. Any excess pin projecting from the bone is cut off and the wound is closed in the usual manner.

One of the advantages of this technique is said to be that these pins occupy less space within the femoral neck than the conventional trifin nail, and there is consequently less interference with bone formation (it is also less traumatic).

Intramedullary fixation of the femoral shaft fracture, Kuntscher nail

DEFINITION

Intramedullary fixation of fractures of the middle and upper shaft of the femur.

POSITION

Either supine, with a sandbag under the affected buttock, or full lateral.

Fig. 23.60 Femoral shaft fracture, Kuntscher nail

1. Extractor for Kuntscher nails (Brigden).
   A. Extractor barrel.
   B. Extension tube for extractor barrel (long nails).
   C. Threaded extractor bar.
   D. Extractor hook.
   E. Sleeve designed for contact with trochanter or end of fractured bone.
   F. Extractor capstan.
2. Drivers and set for Kuntscher nails, one driver for each diameter of nail in use.
3. Retractor, self-retaining (Adson).
4. Large bone-levers (Lane), 2.
5. Bone clamp, self-retaining (Hey Grove), 2.
6. Large bone-holding forceps (Lane), 2.
7. Guide for Kuntscher nails.
8. Reamer for Kuntscher nails.
9. Nail bender.
10. Femoral shaft nail (Kuntscher). Those illustrated show 8·5 mm, 9 mm and 9·5 mm diameter.

Orthopaedic Operations

CLOVERLEAF SECTION
Kuntscher Medullary Nails are produced with a cloverleaf profile to achieve axial and longitudinal elasticity.

TAPERED ENDS
Specially tapered conical points encourage a free passage through the medullary canal and reduce the possibility of impacting.

SLOT IN THE ENDS
To provide an adequate slot, for extraction, with minimum weakening of the section, Zimmer Kuntscher Nails are *punched* and not milled.

ELECTRIC ETCHING
Diameter and length are marked by an electric etching process, which is chemically clean.

Cross section.   Characteristics.

Fig. 23.61   Kuntscher Intramedullary Femoral Nails. (Zimmer Orthopaedic Ltd.)

S.Mo. (EN 58J). Stainless steel

A. Single slot
B. Slotted and pointed each end.

These are clover-leaf in section and are supplied either slotted and pointed at one or both ends, the latter being essential if the nails are to be inserted by the retrograde method.

Standard sizes available:
    12 mm width; lengths of 36 to 52 cm in 2 cm steps.
    9, 10 and 11 mm width; lengths of 32 to 52 cm in 2 cm steps.
    8 mm width; lengths of 14 to 42 cm in 2 cm steps.
    6 mm width; lengths of 14 to 34 cm in 2 cm steps.

INSTRUMENTS

General set (Figs. 14.1 to 14.28)
Bone and fracture set (p. 516)
Kuntscher nail set (Fig. 23.60)
Diathermy leads, electrodes and lead anchoring forceps
Power drill
Intramedullary reamers, appropriate size
3 and 4 (0 and 1) plain catgut or Dexon for ligatures
4 or 5 (1 or 2) Chromic catgut, Dexon or silk, etc., on a large half-circle cutting or Mayo's needle with a trocar point for muscle sutures
3 (0) Silk or nylon on a large curved or straight cutting needle for skin sutures.

Fig. 23.62 Reaming of the upper femoral fragment before inserting Kuntscher nail. (Hall.)

Fig. 23.63 Nail being driven from upper end of femur into lower fragment. (Hall.)

OUTLINE OF PROCEDURE

There are several surgical approaches to the femur but the one most used for Kuntscher nailing is the lateral approach.

The leg is angulated at the fracture site, and a short incision made over the fracture on a line which extends between the greater trochanter and the external condyle of the femur. The superficial and deep fascia are incised and the vastus lateralis and vastus intermedius are divided in the direction of their fibres.

The upper and lower fragments of the fracture are exposed by retraction with bone levers, and the fracture is reduced. The fracture is then disimpacted and the upper fragment elevated out of the wound. Some surgeons ream out the medullary canal with a hand or power-reamer before inserting the nail to obviate a tendency for the nail to jam (Fig. 23.62). A clover leaf nail, slotted and pointed at both ends and of appropriate length, is inserted into the upper fragment. This nail is driven through the trochanter into the buttock and through a small skin incision made overlying, until the distal end is flush with the fracture surface. The fracture is then reduced and the nail driven from the upper end into the lower fragment (Fig. 23.63). The nail is inserted so that the slot at the upper end just projects above the trochanter for removal of the nail at a later date.

The wound is closed in layers and the patient may be immobilised temporarily on a Thomas splint.

Intramedullary fixation of tibial shaft fractures, Kuntscher nail

DEFINITION

Intramedullary fixation of tibial shaft fractures with a nail.

POSITION

Supine, with leg flexed over a triangular support (optional).

INSTRUMENTS

General set (Figs. 14.1 to 14.28)
Bone and fracture set (p. 516)
Kuntscher nail set (Fig. 23.60)
Power drill
9·6 mm ($\frac{3}{8}$ in) diameter twist drill
Intramedullary reamers, appropriate size
3 (0) Plain catgut or Dexon for ligatures
4 (1) Plain catgut or Dexon on a medium half-circle cutting or Mayo needle with a trocar point for muscle and fat sutures
2·5 (2/0) Silk or nylon on a medium curved or straight cutting needle for skin sutures.

OUTLINE OF PROCEDURE

Some surgeons perform this operation as a 'blind' procedure by inserting the nail into the upper end of the tibia and controlling the position of the fracture and insertion of the nail radiologically. However, the method generally used is to expose and reduce the fracture before 'nailing'.

A curved incision is made over the fracture site on either side of the anterior border of the tibia. The skin is reflected and the periosteum incised and retracted with bone levers. The fracture is reduced under direct vision and the reduction maintained with bone clamps.

A small incision is made medially at the upper part of the tibia and a 10 mm ($\frac{3}{8}$ in) hole is drilled with the drill pointing in the direction of the tibial tubercle. The nail is inserted and driven along the inside of the tibial shaft past the fracture and into the lower fragment. The nail may be bent slightly before insertion. The wounds are closed in the usual manner.

A useful bending tool can be fabricated from two lengths of tubular stainless-steel.

A splint is generally unnecessary until the patient commences weight bearing, and then a light plaster cast may be applied.

Osteotomy – McMurray's osteotomy of the femur

DEFINITION

Division of the upper shaft of the femur and displacement in order to alter the line of weight bearing of the extremity, e.g., in cases of osteoarthritis and certain femoral neck fractures.

POSITION

Supine, with leg abducted and supported by an assistant, or as Figure 4.19, Smith Petersen nail.

INSTRUMENTS

General set (Figs. 14.1 to 14.28)
Bone and fracture set (p. 516)
Power drill or hand drill
Twist drills, 3·2 mm ($\frac{1}{8}$ in) to 4·8 mm ($\frac{3}{16}$ in) diameter
Osteotomes 16 mm ($\frac{5}{8}$ in), 19 mm ($\frac{3}{4}$ in) and 38 mm ($1\frac{1}{2}$ in)
Bone punches (Smillie straight and angled), 2
(A high-speed airturbine and burr may be used for performing the osteotomy (similar to Fig. 23.64))
3 (0) Plain catgut or Dexon for ligatures
4 or 5 (1 or 2) Plain or chromic catgut or Dexon on a medium half-circle cutting or Mayo needle with trocar point for muscle sutures
2·5 or 3 (2/0 or 0) Silk or nylon on a large curved or straight cutting needle for skin sutures.

Osteotomes, chisels and gouges generally are made from carbon or martensitic stainless-steel. Although carbon steel is the better material for a sharp edge, stainless-steel is less brittle, and there is less risk of a fragment breaking off during use (p. 521).

These cutting instruments are made in a variety of shapes and sizes as can be seen from Figure 23.65, but are classed according to the basic shape of the blade. An ostetome has two bevelled sides curving towards the cutting edge; a chisel has one flat side and one bevelled side; and a gouge has a curved cutting edge and is hollowed or grooved in section, being concave on one side and convex on the other.

Theoretically an osteotome is used for splitting as in the procedure of osteotomy, and a chisel for slicing; but many surgeons use a thick blade osteotome for splitting and a thin blade type for slicing. A gouge is used for grooving or hollowing and is of special use when saucering an osteomyelitis cavity or cyst.

If Plate Fixation is Contemplated
Twist drill, No. 31 for 3·6 mm ($\frac{9}{64}$ in) screws, or 3·6 mm ($\frac{9}{64}$ in) for 4 mm ($\frac{5}{32}$ in) screws
Set of bone screws
Screw measure
Plate and screw-holding forceps, 2
Various bone clamps (Figs. 23.39 to 23.42 and 23.60)
Automatic screwdriver (Williams or Burns)
Plain screwdriver (Lane)
Osteotomy plates (Wainwright, Wainwright-Hammond, Moore/Blount, etc., Figs. 23.70 to 23.74)
Appropriate osteotomy driver/extractor.

Orthopaedic Operations 549

Fig. 23.64 A high-speed airturbine and burr being used for osteotomy of metatarsal.

Fig. 23.65 Gouges, chisels and osteotomes

1a. Hahn gouge.
1b. Jones gouges, medium and large.
1c. Smith Petersen hip gouge.
2a. MacEwan chisel, side view.
2b. Hahn chisel.
3a. Whitchurch Howell osteotome, large.
3b. Bristow osteotome, medium.
3c. Whitchurch Howell osteotome, small.
3d. MacEwan osteotome, medium.
3e. MacEwan osteotome, small.
3f. MacEwan osteotome, side view.
3g. Platt osteotome, curved on flat.

OUTLINE OF PROCEDURE

The trochanteric region of the femur is exposed as previously described for Smith Petersen nail.

A hole is drilled across the shaft below the level of the trochanter but just above the level of the lesser trochanter. Sometimes this drill is left in position whilst a radiographic check is made. Several holes are then drilled in the line of the osteotomy and the femur is cleanly divided with an osteotome. Alternatively, the femoral shaft is divided with a high-speed turbine and burr.

The leg is abducted and pressure applied to the proximal portion of the lower fragment until the shaft is displaced inwards. If no plate is being inserted, the wound is closed and the patient immobilised in a double plaster of Paris spica.

Some surgeons utilise metallic blade plates to fix the osteotomy, and these are driven into the upper fragment and screwed to the femoral shaft. The plate may incorporate a compression device to draw together the fragments on either side of the osteotomy, e.g., Wainwright-Hammond osteotomy plate Figures 23.75 to 23.86, Coventry Infant lag screw and plate for varus osteotomy in children. If this fixation is secure, the plaster spica is omitted.

Osteotomy of the tibia, with metallic fixation

DEFINITION

Division of the shaft of tibia and excision of a wedge in order to alter the line of the shaft (especially performed for tibial deformities) and fixation with a plate or screws.

POSITION

Supine.

INSTRUMENTS

General set (Figs. 14.1 to 14.28)
Bone and fracture set (p. 516)
Plating and screwing set (p. 523)
Circular saws
Osteotomes 16 mm ($\frac{5}{8}$ in), 19 mm ($\frac{3}{4}$ in) and 38 mm ($1\frac{1}{2}$ in)
3 (0) Plain catgut for ligatures
4 (1) Plain catgut or Dexon on a medium half-circle cutting or Mayo needle with a trocar point for muscle sutures
2·5 (2/0) Silk or nylon or a medium curved or straight cutting needle for skin sutures.

OUTLINE OF PROCEDURE

The area for osteotomy is exposed with minimal periosteal stripping. A wedge of bone is excised, either with a circular saw or an osteotome, and the tibial shaft is re-aligned. The osteotomy is fixed by screws alone, or a plate contoured to the shape of the tibial shaft and secured with several screws.

The wound is closed in the usual manner; plaster of Paris may or may not be applied. This technique can be used for almost any bone shaft where it is necessary to excise a wedge of bone in order to alter the contour of the shaft.

Femoral and tibial epiphyseal arrest

DEFINITION

Arrest of epiphyseal growth by inserting staples across the epiphyseal line of the lower femur and upper tibia. This retards growth of a normal leg in a child so that the short leg is allowed to grow and the two are equal in length when maturity is reached.

POSITION

Supine.

Fig. 23.66   Staple Driver/Inserter.

Fig. 23.67   Staple Punch or Set.

Fig. 23.68   Müller Staple Driver Inserter. (Staple fitted in position for insertion.)

Fig. 23.69   Staple Extractor.

S.Mo. (EN 58J) Stainless steel

2·4 mm ($\frac{3}{32}$ in) diameter
16 mm ($\frac{5}{8}$ in) width × 19 mm ($\frac{3}{4}$ in) length
22 mm ($\frac{7}{8}$ in) width × 19 mm ($\frac{3}{4}$ in) length

1·2 mm ($\frac{1}{16}$ in) diameter
16 mm ($\frac{5}{8}$ in) width × 19 mm ($\frac{3}{4}$ in) length
22 mm ($\frac{7}{8}$ in) width × 19 mm ($\frac{3}{4}$ in) length

Vitallium

16 mm ($\frac{5}{8}$ in) width × 16 mm ($\frac{5}{8}$ in) or 22 mm ($\frac{7}{8}$ in) length
22 mm ($\frac{7}{8}$ in) width × 16 mm ($\frac{5}{8}$ in) or 22 mm ($\frac{7}{8}$ in) length
10 mm ($\frac{3}{8}$ in) width × 16 mm ($\frac{5}{8}$ in), 22 mm ($\frac{7}{8}$ in) or 29 mm ($1\frac{1}{8}$ in) length

Figs. 23.66 to 23.69   Epiphyseal staple sizes and insertion instruments.

INSTRUMENTS

General set (Figs. 14.1 to 14.28)
Bone and fracture set (p. 516)
Staples, stainless-steel or Vitallium (Müller)
Staples driver/inserter
2·5 mm (2/0) Plain catgut or Dexon, for ligatures
3 (0) Plain catgut or Dexon on a medium half-circle cutting needle for deep sutures
2·5 (2/0) Silk or nylon on a medium curved cutting needle for skin sutures.

Fig. 23.70 Wainwright-Hammond osteotomy blade plates.

By means of minor modifications and the addition of a transfixing transverse screw, a well tried and highly successful blade plate for high femoral osteotomy can provide complete rigidity of fixation in compression which is ideal for rapid union. The advantages of the Wainwright-Hammond Osteotomy Blade Plate include maximum stability, the possibility of early postoperative mobilisation and minimal pain combined with absolute safety and the reduction of blood loss from divided bone surfaces.

Long – Blade length 57 mm (2¼ in). Plate length 76 mm (3 in).
Standard – Blade length 51 mm (2 in). Plate length 76 mm (3 in).
Small – Blade length 45 mm (1¾ in). Plate length 76 mm (3 in).
Transverse Screws – Lengths 51 mm (2 in), 57 mm (2¼ in), 64 mm (2½ in), 70 mm (2¾ in).

Screw head – Phillips recessed.

Fig. 23.71 Drilling with Phoenix jig attached to Wainwright-Hammond osteotomy plate.

Orthopaedic Operations

Fig. 23.72
Harris Modified Müller osteotomy plate.
S.Mo. (EN 58J). Stainless Steel.

Sizes available:
41 mm (1⅝ in), 45 mm (1¾ in), 48 mm (1⅞ in), 51 mm (2 in), 54 mm (2⅛ in).

Fig. 23.74 Post-operative radiograph.

Fig. 23.73

1 Insertion of Guide Wire. Note wedge to be removed for varus osteotomy.

2 Appliance inserted parallel to proximal cut surface of the osteotomy and at least 2·5 cm (1 in) above it.

3 Müller clamp in position. Note the gap at the osteotomy.

4 Osteotomy compressed.

Figs. 23.72 to 23.73 Harris modified Müller osteotomy plate and insertion of plate. (Zimmer Orthopaedic Ltd.)

D. HOWSE & CO.

Fig. 23.75 Cannulated Cortex Reamer.
Overall Length 102 mm (4 in).

Fig. 23.77 Cannulated T-wrench.
Overall Length 254 mm (10 in).

Fig. 23.79 C-Spanner.
Overall Length 102 mm (4 in). *For holding Lag Screw whilst tightening Nut*

Fig. 23.80 Cannulated Threaded Handle.
Overall Length 152 mm (6 in).

Fig. 23.82 Guide Wire. Diameter ·062 in. Length 102 mm (4 in).

Fig. 23.84 Plate Benders.
TUFNOL handle. Overall Length 216 mm ($8\frac{1}{2}$ in) (2 parts).

Fig. 23.85 Cannulated Lag Screw with Nut.
Thread Diameter 6·3 mm (·250 in). Core diameter 4 mm (·160 in).
Lengths: 19 mm ($\frac{3}{4}$ in), 22 mm ($\frac{7}{8}$ in), 25 mm (1 in).

Fig. 23.76 Cannulated Lag Screw with Nut.
Thread Diameter: 6·3 mm (·250 in). Core Diameter 6·3 mm (·16 in).
Shank Diameter: 5·1 mm (·21 in).
Lengths: 29 mm ($1\frac{1}{8}$ in), 32 mm ($1\frac{1}{4}$ in), 35 mm ($1\frac{3}{8}$ in), 38 mm ($1\frac{1}{2}$ in), 41 mm ($1\frac{5}{8}$ in), 45 mm ($1\frac{3}{4}$ in), 48 mm ($1\frac{7}{8}$ in), 51 mm (2 in), 57 mm ($2\frac{1}{4}$ in), 64 mm ($2\frac{1}{2}$ in).

Fig. 23.78 Standard Plate.
used with 2·8 mm ($\frac{7}{64}$ in) screws.
Sizes:
2 hole × 51 mm (2 in) overall;
3 hole × 60 mm ($2\frac{3}{8}$ in) overall;
4 hole × 76 mm (3 in) overall.

Fig. 23.81 Standard Plate – Straight.
used with 2·8 mm ($\frac{7}{64}$ in) screws.
Sizes:
2 hole × 51 mm (2 in) overall;
3 hole × 60 mm ($2\frac{3}{8}$ in) overall;
4 hole × 76 mm (3 in) overall.

Fig. 23.83 Heavy Duty Plate
used with 3·6 mm ($\frac{9}{64}$ in) or 4 mm ($\frac{5}{32}$ in) screws.
Sizes:
2 hole × 51 mm (2 in) overall;
3 hole × 60 mm ($2\frac{1}{2}$ in) overall;
4 hole × 76 mm ($3\frac{3}{8}$ in) overall.

Fig. 23.86 Heavy Duty Plate – Straight.
used with 3·6 mm ($\frac{9}{64}$ in) or 4 mm ($\frac{5}{32}$ in) screws.
Sizes:
2 hole × 51 mm (2 in) overall;
3 hole × 60 mm ($2\frac{1}{2}$ in) overall;
4 hole × 76 mm ($3\frac{1}{8}$ in) overall.

Figs. 23.75 to 23.86 Coventry Infant Lag Screw S.Mo. (EN 58J) Stainless steel (Reduced size)
Developed by R. J. Brigden for Mr J. H. Penrose, FRCS, consultant orthopaedic surgeon at Coventry and Warwickshire Hospital, England.

The use of a rigid blade plate for varus and valgus osteotomies in children has two disadvantages. Firstly the blade component has to be hammered home into the neck which is unnecessarily traumatic in a child, and secondly when performing a varus osteotomy the osteotomy has to be completed first. This subsequently involves driving the blade into the now mobile upper fragment which can prove difficult. Both these difficulties can be overcome by the use of a coarse threaded screw and plate as illustrated. The screw is cannulated and can be introduced over a guide wire if desired. When the screw has been satisfactorily placed in the neck the osteotomy is performed.

During the application of the plate complete control of the angle of the upper fragment can be maintained by temporarily screwing a threaded handle on to the screw in place of the nut. When the plate has been screwed onto the shaft of the femur the handle is removed and the nut applied, giving rigid fixation. No hammering is necessary and the ease of application and subsequent removal is striking.

The guide wire is inserted in the desired position

The hole in the cortex is cut with the cannulated cortex reamer over the guide wire

The lag screw is inserted over the guide wire with the cannulated T-wrench

The angle of the upper fragment is controlled by temporarily screwing the threaded handle on to the lag screw in place of the nut

Holding the lag screw with the C-spanner the nut is tightened with the T-wrench

Fig. 23.87 Insertion technique for Coventry infant lag screw and plate. (D. Howse & Co.)

Fig. 23.88 Radiograph taken after insertion of Coventry infant lag screw and plate.

OUTLINE OF PROCEDURE

The epiphyseal lines of the lower end of the femur, upper end of the tibia and fibula are exposed through medial and lateral incisions which extend above and below the joint line on each side.

A 4 to 5 cm (1½ to 2 in) longitudinal incision is made along the central axis of the bone over the epiphyseal line, and the periosteum is reflected slightly. Two or more staples are inserted so that they bridge the epiphyses. This procedure is repeated on the other side of the femur and at both sides of the upper tibial epiphyses. The number of staples inserted, and whether femoral and tibial epiphyses are dealt with at the same operation, depends upon the degree of shortening required. The epiphyseal line of the proximal fibula may be curetted to obliterate the growth centre. This operation is generally performed under X-ray control.

The wound is closed in the usual manner. Growth of the bone continues after the staples are removed at a later date.

Bone grafts

Autogenous Bone Grafts (from the patient himself) are usually removed from either the tibia, fibular or ilium. These three provide cortical grafts, whole bone transplants or cancellous chips and strips respectively, although, of course, there is some of each type of bone in all.

Homogenous Bone Grafts (from another human donor) are obtained usually from non-infected amputated limbs and are stored in deep freeze, or are freeze dried in pieces of a size suitable for grafting.

In deep freeze, grafts are stored at $-15°C$ and then thawed in warm saline just before use. A small fragment of bone must be cultured a few days before use to confirm sterility of the specimen.

In the case of freeze dried specimens these are reconstituted by submerging in sterile saline before use.

In all cases, before the bone is stored, all soft tissue and cartilage is removed from the specimen and a Wassermann reaction performed on the donor, together with a check on the medical history.

Autogenous onlay graft, tibia to other long bone

DEFINITION

The removal of a cortical bone graft from the anterior surface of the tibia for transplantation as an only graft, which is screwed into position to bridge a non-united fracture of another long bone. This type of graft may be used also for other procedures such as spinal fusion.

POSITION

Generally supine.

INSTRUMENTS

General set (Figs. 14.1 to 14.28)
Bone and fracture set (p. 516)
Bone grafting set (Fig. 23.91)

Fig. 23.89 Classical methods of cortical bone grafting. Inlay, diamond inlay, intramedullary peg, onlay sliding onlay, and double onlay grafts. A, B – inlay grafting by the Albee technique; C – diamond inlay grafting; D – sliding inlay grafting; E – intramedullary peg grafting; F – sliding intramedullary peg grafting; G – onlay grafting; H, J – sliding onlay grafting; K – double onlay grafting. (Wilson – *Watson – Jones*.)

Fig. 23.90 Technique of massive onlay grafting of bone. The ends of the fractured bone are freshened and a bed is prepared on the surface of each fragment with a chisel (A). The graft cut from the tibia may include one or both cortical margins (B, C). The graft is fixed to the host bone by screws inserted after a track has been drilled (D). The screws must engage the opposite cortex (F) and the length should be measured accurately. Incorrect fixation with screws only engaging one cortex is also shown (E). (Wilson – *Watson – Jones*.)

Bone clamps shown in Figure 23.39a
Twist drill of appropriate size
Set of bone screws
Screw measure
Screw-holding forceps
Automatic screwdriver (Williams or Burns)
Plain screwdriver (Lane)
2·5 or 3 (2/0 or 0) Plain catgut or Dexon for ligatures
Appropriate size of catgut or Dexon and needles for muscle sutures in that area of the body
2·5 or 3 (2/0 or 0) Silk or nylon on a medium curved or straight cutting needle for skin sutures
Plaster of Paris.

OUTLINE OF PROCEDURE

The tibia is exposed through a curved incision and the periosteum is stripped off carefully from the graft area.

Fig. 23.91 Bone-grafting instruments

1. Irrigation syringe.
2. Bone punch, angled (Smillie).
3. Bone punch, straight (Smillie).
4. Bone rasp (Tubby).
5. Bone file (Tubby).
6. Circular saws, twin and single.
7. Power drill (Desoutter compressed air).
8. Rubber air hose for power drill and chuck key.

An oblong graft is removed from the anterior surface of the tibia with a circular or oscillatory bone saw. Ordinarily the borders are not violated as this would considerably weaken the tibia. The circular saw is driven by a power drill, and may be a medium 38 mm ($1\frac{1}{2}$ in) to 40 mm ($1\frac{5}{8}$ in) single or twin blade for the sides, and a small 19 mm ($\frac{3}{4}$ in) to 20 mm ($\frac{3}{4}$ in+) single blade for the ends. Saline irrigation provides lubrication for the saw, and the assistants must ensure that swabs and their hands are kept as far away from the blade as possible. In the first case, the gauze may foul the saw and become entwined with it; and in the second case, the saw may jerk during use with risk of injury to the assistant's hand. The use of an oscillatory bone saw reduces the danger of the blade 'jumping'. The oscillating movement of the blade from side to side permits cuts in either direction in bone but does not tear soft tissue, which if touched moves with the blade. Furthermore, it is considered that the amount of burning of the bone due to friction is reduced considerably.

The wound is closed in layers and the limb may be placed in a plaster cast. Sometimes if two teams are operating, one may cut the graft and the other insert it to reduce the operating time. In this case the instruments are split into two sets.

The non-united fracture area is exposed and the periosteum stripped off for the extent of the graft. The fracture ends are freshened, the bone re-aligned, and the cortical graft screwed in position on either side with two or more screws. The wound is closed in layers and a plaster cast applied.

Autogenous inlay or sliding graft

DEFINITION

Sliding an oblong-shaped graft cut from the affected bone itself across a non-united fracture.

POSITION

Generally supine.

INSTRUMENTS

As for onlay graft.

OUTLINE AND PROCEDURE

The fracture area is exposed and the periosteum stripped off for the extent of the graft. The fractured ends are freshened and fibrous tissue excised.

Using a twin saw, the surgeon cuts an oblong slot about 13 mm ($\frac{1}{2}$ in) wide, with one-third of its length at one side of the fracture line and two-thirds at the other. The grafts are levered from their bed and are re-inserted into the slot, but reversed so that the longer of the two bridges the fracture line. The two grafts are secured with screws and the wound is closed in the usual manner.

Either a plaster of Paris cast or a splint is applied.

Autogenous cancellous iliac grafts

DEFINITION

The removal of cancellous strips or wedges from the ilium as a bone graft for non-united fractures or in fusion procedures, e.g., spine.

Orthopaedic Operations

Fig. 23.92 Cancellous chip grafting of bone. Cancellous chip grafts should usually be cut from the ilium in the region of the posterior superior spine and the crest (A) or from near the anterior superior spine (B). The crest is reflected with its attached muscles and the grafts are then cut with a gouge (C). (Wilson – *Watson – Jones*.)

POSITION

Supine.

INSTRUMENTS

General set (Figs. 14.1 to 14.28)
Bone and fracture set (p. 516)
Osteotomes, 16 mm ($\frac{5}{8}$ in), 19 mm ($\frac{3}{4}$ in) and 25 mm (1 in)

Fig. 23.93 Bone for Phemister grafting should be cut as cancellous strips from the anterior part of the iliac crest (A), the cortical top of the crest being discarded. Both sides of the crest must be displayed (B). To close the donor site the gluteal muscles are sutured to the abdominal muscles. Suction drainage should be used for 24 to 48 hours after taking the graft. (Wilson – Watson – Jones.)

Diathermy leads, electrodes and lead anchoring forceps
Suction tubing, nozzles and tube anchoring forceps
Power saw may be required
Corrugated drainage tubing
4 (1) Plain catgut or Dexon for ligatures
4 or 5 (1 or 2) Plain or chromic catgut or Dexon on a large half-circle cutting or Mayo needle with a trocar point for muscle sutures
2·5 or 3 (2/0 or 0) Silk or nylon on a large curved cutting needle for skin sutures.

OUTLINE OF PROCEDURE

An incision is made along the subcutaneous border of the iliac crest and carried down to bone. The muscles are reflected off the bone subperiosteally to expose the graft area.

For sliver or chip grafts, these are removed with an osteotome parallel to the iliac crest. For wedge grafts, the graft is outlined with an osteotome and then peeled up with slight prying movements of a broad osteotome.

The wound is closed in the usual manner, occasionally with drainage. The graft is then transferred to the host area either as strips, chips, or a wedge which may be screwed into position.

Aspiration of a joint

DEFINITION

The removal of fluid from a joint by suction, using a syringe and hollow needle.

Fig. 23.94 Aspiration of a joint

1. Sponge-holding forceps (Rampley), 2.
2. Scalpel handle No. 9 with No. 15 blade (Bard Parker).
3. Towel clips, 2.
4. Aspiration syringe (Martin).
5. Wide-bore needles for Martin aspiration syringe, 3 assembled needles and 1 dismantled to show needle and obturator.
6. Nobecutane for sealing puncture wound.
7. Specimen bottle.
8. Swabs.
9. Gallipot containing skin antiseptic.
10. Cotton-wool for sealing over puncture wound.
11. 20 ml syringe and aspiration needles.

POSITION

Depends upon the joint being aspirated.

INSTRUMENTS

As Figure 23.94.

OUTLINE OF PROCEDURE

Basically the same set of instruments is required for the aspiration of any joint. Wide-bore aspirating needles are used with a syringe of at least 20 ml capacity.

The area is prepared and draped, and the needle attached to the syringe is inserted into the cavity. If the needle is large, a scalpel will be used to make a stab incision. The fluid is aspirated and a specimen sent to the laboratory for microbiological examination. The puncture wound is sealed with cotton-wool and Nobecutane, and a pressure dressing may be applied in conjunction with a splint or guarding plaster.

Arthroscopy

DEFINITION

Endoscopic examination of a joint; generally the knee joint.

POSITION

Supine with leg straight or flexed over the bottom section of the operation table, which is lowered or removed.

Fig. 23.95 Arthroscope in knee joint with filling tube plus drainage tube.

Fig. 23.96 Viewing medial meniscus. (Down's Surgical Ltd.)

Fig. 23.97 Arthroscope, sleeve with telescope. (Down's Surgical Ltd.)

INSTRUMENTS

Sponge-holding forceps (Rampley), 3
Scalpel handle No. 3 with No. 10 blade (Bard Parker)
Artery forceps, curved on flat (Dunhill), 2
Dissecting forceps, toothed fine (Gillies)
Scissors, straight, 15 cm (6 in) (Mayo)
Needle holder (Kilner)
Arthroscope, fibre light cable, irrigation tube, trocar and cannulae for arthroscope, and biopsy forceps
Biopsy forceps

Irrigation fluid in plastic bag (sodium chloride, 0·9 per cent) and irrigation set
Aspiration needles, 14 g, 7·5 cm (3 in)
Plastic or rubber tubing, 60 cm (24 in), 2
Towel clips (Backhaus), 6
Syringes, 250 ml, 2
2·5 (2/0) Silk or nylon on a small curved cutting needle for skin sutures.

OUTLINE OF PROCEDURE

The operation is performed under tourniquet; the area is prepared and the lateral aspect of the knee covered with a plastic skin drape (Steridrape, Vi drape or Opsite). The tubing is connected to the irrigation set and occluded with clamps; the other tubing is occluded at one end and secured near the operation site; the arthroscope is connected to the light source and checked.

Sodium chloride, 0·9 per cent (80 ml), is injected to distend the knee joint, the syringe removed, and the occluded drainage tubing attached to the needle remaining in the knee joint. A small incision is made in the intra-patella region, and the trocar and cannula inserted into the joint-space through this incision. The trocar is removed, clip taken off the drainage tubing and the arthroscope inserted through the cannula, followed by commencement of the drip irrigation.

The patella-femoral articulation and the supra condylar pouch are examined. The medial compartment, lateral femoral tibial articulation and medial meniscus are readily visualised by flexing the knee with a valgus strain. If a biopsy is required, it is usual to insert a second trocar and cannula through which a pair of biopsy forceps can be introduced, so that a biopsy can be undertaken under direct vision. Alternatively, the arthroscope can be removed, and a blind biopsy undertaken through the arthroscopic cannula. A camera can be attached to the eyepiece to take photographs at any stage of the procedure.

At the end of the procedure the knee joint is drained of fluid, the drainage needle removed and the small incision(s) closed with a suture, if not proceeding to an arthrotomy. A plaster wool and crêpe bandage is applied.

Arthrotomy, meniscectomy or removal of loose bodies (knee)

DEFINITION

Removal of a torn semilunar cartilage, or removal of loose bodies which are usually osteocartilaginous in nature.

POSITION

Supine, with leg straight or flexed over the bottom section of the table, which is lowered or removed.

INSTRUMENTS

Sponge holding forceps (Rampley), 5
Scalpel handles No. 4 with No. 20 blades (Bard Parker), 2
Dissecting forceps, toothed (Lane), 2
Dissecting forceps, non-toothed, 15 cm (6 in), 2
Scissors, straight, 15 cm (6 in) (Mayo)
Scissors, curved on flat, 15 cm (6 in) (Mayo)
Retractors, double hook, 2

Fig. 23.98 Meniscectomy

1. Cartilage knives (Smillie).
   A. Chisel-shaped blade.
   B. and C. With probe-shaped lateral projections.
2. Meniscectomy knives (Fairbank).
   A. Blade for cutting to the left.
   B. Blade for cutting to the right.
3. Cartilage knife (Munro).
4. Cartilage-holding forceps.
5. Cartilage-holding forceps (Martin).
6. A. Cartilage-holding forceps, curved on flat (Mayo-Oschner), 3.
   B. Cartilage-holding forceps, straight (Kocher), 2.
7. Cartilage retractors (Smillie), set of 3.
8. Cartilage retractors (Jackson Burrow).

Small retractors, single hook, 2
Artery forceps, curved on flat (Kilner), 5
Tissue forceps (Allis), 5
Needle holder (Kilner)
Meniscectomy set (Fig. 23.98)
2·5 (2/0) Plain catgut or Dexon for ligatures
3 or 4 (0 or 1) Plain catgut or Dexon on a medium half-circle cutting needle for deep sutures
2·5 (2/0) Silk or nylon on a medium curved cutting needle for skin sutures.

OUTLINE OF PROCEDURE

The long slender knives used for removing a torn cartilage need to be resharpened frequently. However, care must be taken to ensure that the knife is discarded when its dimensions and strength have been reduced considerably by grinding. A very thin, weak knife is dangerous in the knee joint, for if it breaks in the back of the knee, the

Fig. 23.99 The upper end of tibia and menisci. (A) The medial meniscus is attached to the medial ligament. (B) Anterior horn tear. (C) Posterior horn tear. (D) Bucket-handle tear. (Macfarlane.)

Fig. 23.100 Removal of semilunar cartilage of the knee. The cartilage is first freed from its peripheral attachment (A), and at its anterior end. It is then dislocated, if possible, into the intercondyloid space (B), before being detached posteriorly. (Top inset) Incision. (Farquharson and Rintoul.)

surgeon may have to make an additional incision in order to remove the broken piece.

A curved or straight incision is made just medial or lateral to the patella, depending upon the location of the torn meniscus or loose bodies. Occasionally it may be necessary to make a posterior approach from the back of the knee. The incision is deepened through the fascia and the capsule and synovium is incised.

In the case of meniscectomy, the semilunar cartilage is detached from the tibial plateau, utilising the special clamps and cartilage knives. In the case of loose bodies, these are removed with forceps or a curetting spoon.

The wound is closed in layers and the knee is immobilised with a padded metal back splint, wool and bandages.

Synovectomy (knee joint)

DEFINITION

Excision of a diseased synovial membrane.

POSITION

Supine.

INSTRUMENTS

General set (Figs. 14.1 to 14.28)
Tissue forceps, curved (Fagge), 5
Long scalpel, solid variety
Scissors, curved on flat 15 cm (6 in) (Mayo)
3 (0) Plain catgut or Dexon for ligatures
4 (1) Plain catgut or Dexon on a large half-circle cutting or Mayo needle with trocar point for capsule sutures
4 or 5 (1 or 2) Chromic catgut, Dexon or silk on a large half-circle cutting or Mayo needle with trocar point for muscle sutures
3 (0) Silk or nylon on a large curved cutting needle for skin sutures.

OUTLINE OF PROCEDURE

The joint is exposed through an anteromedial incision, which generally commences about 10 cm (4 in) above the knee joint on the medial border of the quadriceps tendon, curves round the inner border of the patella, and continues in the midline down to or below the tibial tubercle. The fascia is incised and retracted and the capsule exposed by dissection between the medial border of the quadriceps tendon and the vastus medialis muscle. The capsule and synovial membrane are incised and the patella retracted laterally.

The entire synovial membrane is excised by block dissection from the inner, outer and anterior aspects of the joint. The prepatellar pad of fat is excised and any other pathological tissue on the femoral condyles is removed with a scalpel or gauze swab. Care is taken to avoid damage to the posterior capsule of the knee and the popliteal vessels in the midline.

After all the pathological tissue has been excised the wound is closed. If the ligaments have been divided they are apposed and sutured. The capsule is sutured, followed by the fascia and skin. The leg is immobilised either with a padded metal back splint, wool and bandages, or a plaster of Paris cast.

Patellectomy

DEFINITION

Excision of the patella for hypertrophic arthritis and fractures.

POSITION

Supine.

INSTRUMENTS

As for synovectomy
Bone-holding forceps (St Thomas')

Bone awl
Ligatures and sutures as for synovectomy.

OUTLINE OF PROCEDURE

A longitudinal or transverse incision is made over the patella and deepened down to the bone. The whole patella (or fragments in the case of a fracture) is dissected free from the tendon.

The knee is closed in the usual manner, repairing the defect in the quadriceps mechanism by overlapping the tendon with chromic catgut, Dexon or silk sutures. The leg is immobilised in a plaster of Paris cast.

Arthrodesis of toes

DEFINITION

Fusion of the proximal phalangeal joints of the toes.

POSITION

Supine.

INSTRUMENTS

Sponge-holding forceps (Rampley), 5
Towel clips, 5
Scalpel handles No. 3 with Nos 10 and 15 blades (Bard Parker), 2
Scalpel, solid variety
Fine dissecting forceps, toothed (Gillies), 2
Fine dissecting forceps, non-toothed (McIndoe)
Fine retractors, double hook, 2
Scissors, curved on flat, 13 cm (5 in) (Mayo)
Small bone cutting forceps (Liston)
Small bone nibbling forceps, curved
Bone levers (Trethowan ring spikes), 2
Small rugine (Faraboeuf)
Small gouges, 6 mm, 10 mm and 12 mm (Jenkins or Hahn), 3
Small mallet (Rowland)
Bone awl (optional)
Austenitic traction wires (Kirschner), 1·6 mm (0·062 in) diameter, 9 cm ($3\frac{1}{2}$ in) long, and sterile corks
Hand chuck or Kirschner wire drill, if wires are to be used
Wire-cutting forceps
Small needle holder
2 (3/0) Silk or nylon on a small curved cutting needle for skin sutures
Ribbon gauze and plastic dressing (Nobecutane) to form individual toe splints.

OUTLINE OF PROCEDURE

A transverse or longitudinal incision is made over the joint to be fused. The joint is exposed and the cartilage removed from the bone surfaces with bone cutters, gouges or the solid scalpel. Fusion is achieved either with a 'spike' arthrodesis or intramedullary wires.

With a 'spike' arthrodesis, the distal end of the proximal or middle phalanx is fashioned into the shape of a spike and a hole made with an awl in the proximal end of the middle or distal phalanx. This spike is wedged into the hole and the skin incision sutured before immobilising the toe with a Nobecutane splint.

For Kirschner wire fixation, the wire is drilled retrograde fashion from the joint through the distal phalanx and out through the toe pulp just below the nail, so that one end is flush with the joint surface being fused. The two bone ends are brought into apposition and the wire is drilled back across the joint surface and into the proximal phalanx. If an excess amount of wire is left protruding from the toe, this is cut short or turned over before attaching a cork to cover the point. The skin incision is sutured and the toe immobilised further with a Nobecutane splint.

Arthrodesis of ankle (sliding fibula graft)

DEFINITION

Fusion of the ankle utilising fibula graft.

POSITION

Supine, with a sandbag placed under the buttock on the affected side.

INSTRUMENTS

General set (Figs. 14.1 to 14.28)
Bone and fracture set (p. 516)

Fig. 23.101 Arthrodesis of ankle. (A) White area outlines the bone to be removed. The part of the fibula depicted by the broken line is preserved for use as an onlay graft. (B) The operation completed. The lower part of the tibia and the talus are sandwiched between the two bone grafts. (Crawford Adams.)

Fig. 23.102 Triple arthrodesis of the ankle carried out with air tool and burr. (A) Excision of head of talus. (B) Removing navicular cartilage. (C) Excision of bone from both surfaces of calcaneo cuboid joint. (D) Removal of both surfaces of subtalar joint. (E) Osteotomy of calcaneus. (F) Completed operation. (Hall.)

Plating and screwing set (p. 533)
Osteotomes, 13 mm ($\frac{1}{2}$ in), 16 mm ($\frac{5}{8}$ in) and 19 mm ($\frac{3}{4}$ in)
Gouges, 13 mm ($\frac{1}{2}$ in), 16 mm ($\frac{5}{8}$ in) and 19 mm ($\frac{3}{4}$ in)
Circular saws, medium and small, single blades
Wire saw and handles (Gigli or Olivecrona), optional
2·5 (2/0) Plain catgut or Dexon for ligatures
3 or 4 (0 or 1) Plain catgut or Dexon on a medium half-circle cutting or Mayo needle with a trocar point for muscle sutures
2·5 (2/0) Silk or nylon on a medium curved cutting needle for skin sutures
Plaster of Paris.

OUTLINE OF PROCEDURE

An incision is made along the line of the fibula starting about 15 cm (6 in) above the ankle joint, curving slightly as it reaches the heel.

The superficial and deep tissues are incised to expose the fibula and ankle joint. The fibula is divided across about 13 cm (5 in) above the external malleolus and excised, and is placed in a sterile saline. The cartilage is excised from the joint surfaces of the tibia and talus. The lateral surface of the tibia adjoining the excised portion of the fibula is roughened and a groove cut in the lateral surface of the talus bone.

All periosteum and cartilage is removed from the fibula graft and the medial aspect is smoothed to ensure a close fit when the fibula is re-inserted below its original position. This graft is then screwed to the tibia and talus and any gaps which may be left are packed with cancellous bone chips which can be obtained either from the bone bank or the patient's iliac crest.

The wound is closed in the usual manner and the leg is immobilised in a plaster of Paris cast.

Triple Arthrodesis. Stabilisation of the foot

DEFINITION

Stabilisation of the foot by removing the cartilaginous surfaces of the subtaloid, calcaneocuboid and talonavicular joints.

POSITION

Supine, with a sandbag under the buttock on the affected side.

INSTRUMENTS

General set (Fig. 14.1 to 14.28)
Bone and fracture set (p. 516)
Osteotomes, 16 mm ($\frac{5}{8}$ in), 19 mm ($\frac{3}{4}$ in) and 25 mm (1 in)
Gouges, 16 mm ($\frac{5}{8}$ in), 19 mm ($\frac{3}{4}$ in) and 25 mm (1 in)
2·5 (2/0) Plain catgut or Dexon for ligatures
3 or 4 (0 or 1) Plain catgut or Dexon on a medium half-circle cutting or Mayo needle for deep sutures
2·5 (2/0) Silk or nylon on a medium curved cutting needle for skin sutures.

OUTLINE OF PROCEDURE

The subtaloid, talo-navicular and calcaneo-cuboid joints are generally exposed through a curved dorsolateral incision which is deepened through the fascia and ligaments. The foot is dislocated medially at mid-tarsal level.

The cartilage is removed from the joint surfaces in such a manner that the three bones can be brought in good contact with each other in the position chosen for fusion. The wound is closed and a plaster of Paris cast applied to the leg.

Some surgeons utilise metallic staples across the calcaneocuboid joint.

Arthrodesis of knee (Charnley's operation)

DEFINITION

Fusion of the knee joint by compression arthrodesis.

POSITION

Supine.

INSTRUMENTS

General set (Figs. 14.1 to 14.28)
Bone and fracture set (p. 516)
Amputation saw with detachable guard (Sergeant) or power driven saw
Large tissue forceps (Fagge or Lane), 4
Traction pins (Steinmann), 2 of size 4·8 mm ($\frac{3}{16}$ in) diameter by 20 cm to 25 cm (8 to 10 in) long, with diamond points and square or triangular chuck ends
Hand or power drill
Compression clamps (Charnley), 2
Pin caps or small corks, 2
3 (0) Plain catgut or Dexon for ligatures
4 and 5 (1 and 2) Plain catgut or Dexon on a medium half-circle cutting or Mayo needle with a trocar point for capsule, etc.
2·5 or 3 (2/0 or 0) Silk or nylon on a medium curved or straight cutting needle for skin sutures.

OUTLINE OF PROCEDURE

The joint is exposed through a longitudinal anterolateral incision or a transverse incision similar to patellectomy but with wider exposure.

The patella is either excised or the cartilage from the undersurface is removed with the amputation saw. The joint is flexed and a small amount of the upper end of the tibia and condyles at the lower end of the femur, together with the joint cartilage, are removed with the saw. The saw cuts are placed almost parallel to each other so that when the raw surfaces of the two bones are brought together, the knee is in the correct position for fusion (that is usually with about 10 degrees of flexion).

Two stout Steinmann's pins are inserted parallel to each other through the lower end of the femur and the upper end of the tibia. These are clamped together with Charnley's compression clamps on the medial and lateral aspect of the leg, with sufficient compression to maintain good contact between the two surfaces of raw bone.

The wound is closed and the leg is immobilised on a Thomas splint or in a plaster of Paris cast.

574   Operating Theatre Technique

Fig. 23.103 Arthrodesis of knee (Charnleys operation). (A) Incision over joint. (B) Excision of bone wedge from superior aspect of upper tibia. (C) Similar amount of bone excised from lower end of femur so that both surfaces fit together with the knee in 10 degrees of flexion to full extension. (D) Steinmans pins inserted and compression clamps applied. (Hall.)

INSTRUMENTS

General set (Figs. 14.1 to 14.28)
Bone and fracture set (p. 516)
Artery forceps, curved on flat (Kelly Fraser), 20
Large tissue forceps (Fagge or Lane), 5
Large retractors (Hibb), 2
Scissors, heavy, curved on flat, 20 cm (8 in) (Mayo)
Long scalpel, solid variety
Osteotomes, 16 mm ($\frac{5}{8}$ in), 22 mm ($\frac{7}{8}$ in) and 38 mm ($1\frac{1}{2}$ in)
Osteotomes, 13 mm ($\frac{1}{2}$ in) and 16 mm ($\frac{5}{8}$ in) (curved)
Gouges, 13 mm ($\frac{5}{8}$ in), 22 mm ($\frac{7}{8}$ in) and 38 mm ($1\frac{1}{2}$ in)
Hip levers (Judet), 2
Reamers for shaping the femoral head (32 mm [$1\frac{1}{4}$ in] and 38 mm [$1\frac{1}{2}$ in]. Crawford Adam head shapers are suitable)
Perforator drills for acetabular hole (32 mm [$1\frac{1}{4}$ in] and 38 mm [$1\frac{1}{2}$ in])
Hip brace
Irrigation syringe and warm sterile saline
Suction tubing, wide nozzles and tube anchoring forceps
Diathermy leads, electrodes and lead anchoring forceps
3 and 4 (0 and 1) Plain catgut or Dexon for ligatures
4 or 5 (1 or 2) Chromic catgut or Dexon or silk on a large half-circle cutting needle for muscle sutures
3 (0) Silk or nylon on a large curved cutting needle for skin sutures.

OUTLINE OF PROCEDURE

There are several approaches to the hip joint, including anterior, lateral or posterior. Only one approach will be described to avoid confusion, and that is the anterolateral approach.

An incision is made commencing about 8 cm (3 in) below the trochanter, continuing to a point over the trochanter where it curves anteriorly to complete the flap. The fascia lata is incised in line with the longitudinal portion of the wound and the gluteus medius and minimus are divided transversely. The capsule of the hip joint is incised and the hip dislocated forwards.

The size of the femoral head is reduced to that of the femoral neck by gouging and planing away the cartilage and cortex of the bone. A hole of corresponding size is drilled in the acetabulum and all joint cartilage is removed. The cavity is irrigated to remove debris and the hip is returned to its normal position, but with the reconstructed head and neck jammed in the hole made in the acetabulum. Any gaps remaining in the joint cavity are filled with bone shavings obtained when drilling the acetabular hole.

The wound is closed with the leg supported in the optimum position for fusion, and a double hip plaster spica is applied for immobilisation.

Arthrodesis of shoulder (Smith Petersen trifin nail)

DEFINITION

Fusion of the shoulder joint with fixation obtained by the insertion of a Smith Petersen trifin nail across the joint.

POSITION

Supine, with a sandbag placed under the scapula on the affected side.

Arthrodesis of hip (Brittain extra-articular fusion)

DEFINITION

Extra-articular fusion of the hip by means of cortical bone graft which is driven through an osteotomy of the upper femur and into the ischium.

POSITION

As for Smith Petersen nail (Fig. 4.19).

INSTRUMENTS

General set (Figs. 14.1 to 14.28)
Bone and fracture set (p. 516)
Bone grafting set (Fig. 23.91)
Osteotomes, 13 mm ($\frac{1}{2}$ in), 25 mm (1 in) and 38 mm ($1\frac{1}{2}$ in)
Twin chisels (Brittain) for positioning of graft (optional)
Twist drills, 4·8 mm ($\frac{3}{16}$ in) and 6·4 mm ($\frac{1}{4}$ in) diameter, 13 cm (5 in) long
Bone punches (Smillie), angled and straight, 2
3 (0) Plain catgut or Dexon for ligatures
4 (1) Plain or chromic catgut or Dexon on a large half-circle cutting or Mayo needle with trocar point for muscle sutures
3 (0) Silk or nylon on a large curved or straight cutting needle for skin sutures.

OUTLINE OF PROCEDURE

The upper third of the femur is exposed through a lateral longitudinal incision as for Smith Petersen nail. A drill is introduced at a predetermined point through the femur and into the ischium. Its position is verified radiologically and, if correct, a number of holes are drilled along a transverse line each side of it.

Either a suitable piece of cortical bone about 13 mm ($\frac{1}{2}$ in) wide by 15 cm (6 in) long is cut from the tibia (see bone grafting) or removed from the bone bank. The graft is bevelled to a point at one end and denuded of any adherent soft tissue. An osteotomy of the femur is made in line with the drill holes and the osteotome is driven on until it has penetrated the ischium. A slot is created in the ischium by levering the osteotome backwards and forwards and the graft is inserted along the blade until it enters this slot. The osteotome is then removed and the graft is driven home. Some surgeons use the Brittain twin chisel to assist this manoeuvre but in either case the graft is inserted so that its endosteal portion lies distally.

The distal portion of the femur just below the osteotomy is then displaced inwards with the bone punch and the wound is closed in layers. The patient is immobilised in a double hip spica.

Arthrodesis of the hip (Charnley's central dislocation fusion)

DEFINITION

Intra-articular fusion of the hip by planing the head and neck of the femur into a tubular shape which fits into a corresponding size of hole in the acetabulum.

POSITION

Supine.

INSTRUMENTS

> General set (Figs. 14.1 to 14.28)
> Bone and fracture set (p. 516)
> Artery forceps, curved on flat (Kelly Fraser), 20
> Large tissue forceps, curved (Fagge), 5
> Osteotomes, 13 mm ($\frac{1}{2}$ in), 16 mm ($\frac{5}{8}$ in) and 19 mm ($\frac{3}{4}$ in) (straight)
> Osteotomes, 13 mm ($\frac{1}{2}$ in) and 16 mm ($\frac{5}{8}$ in) (curved)
> Gouges, 13 mm ($\frac{1}{2}$ in), 16 mm ($\frac{5}{8}$ in) and 19 mm ($\frac{3}{4}$ in)
> Scalpel, solid variety
> Set of trifin nails (Smith Petersen)
> Driver/extractor (Smith Petersen)
> Guide wires, 20 cm (8 in), 2
> Guide wire hand chuck (Watson-Jones)
> Steel rule, 15 cm (6 in)
> Twist drill 4·8 mm ($\frac{3}{16}$ in)
> Hand drill
> Diathermy leads, electrodes and lead anchoring forceps
> Suction tubing, nozzles and tube anchoring forceps
> 2·5 and 3 (2/0 and 0) Plain catgut or Dexon for ligatures
> 3 or 4 (0 or 1) Chromic catgut, Dexon or silk on a small half-circle cutting or Mayo needle with trocar point for muscle sutures, etc.
> 2·5 (2/0) Silk or nylon on a medium curved cutting needle for skin sutures.

OUTLINE OF PROCEDURE

The chest portion of a shoulder spica is applied before operation. The shoulder joint is generally approached through an anterior incision which may curve laterally over the point of the shoulder.

The deltoid muscle is divided and the capsule exposed either by retraction or division of the muscle overlying the joint. The capsule is opened and the head of the humerus visualised by external rotation of the arm. Cartilage is excised from the head of humerus and glenoid cavity, and the arm is placed in the optimum position for fusion.

A hole is drilled just below the humeral neck and a guide wire is inserted into the glenoid and neck of the scapula. The position of this guide wire may be checked radiologically, and when correct, a Smith Petersen nail of appropriate length is driven across the joint and into the scapula. The guide wire is removed and the wound closed in layers. The acromium may be used to reinforce the fusion by being attached to the tubercle.

The plaster of Paris spica is completed to immobilise the arm until fusion takes place.

Arthrodesis of the wrist (Brittain fusion)

DEFINITION

Fusion of the wrist by inserting a bone graft between the lower end of the radius and the base of the third metacarpal bone.

POSITION

Supine, with affected arm extended on an arm table.

INSTRUMENTS

> General set (Figs. 14.1 to 14.28)
> Bone and fracture set (p. 516)

Bone grafting set (p. 516)
Power driven burr may be used
2·5 (2/0) Plain catgut or Dexon for ligatures
3 (0) Plain catgut or Dexon on a small half-circle cutting needle for deep sutures
2·5 (2/0) Silk or nylon on a medium curved cutting needle for skin sutures.

Fig. 23.104 (A) Arthrodesis of wrist. Preparation of graft bed in distal radius and carpals. (B) Removal of graft from ilium and insertion of graft in wrist to maintain arthrodesis. (Hall.)

OUTLINE OF PROCEDURE

A longitudinal incision is made on the dorsal aspect of the wrist extending just distal to the base of the third metacarpal to about 8 cm (3 in) above the lower end of the radius. This incision is deepened and the tendons retracted to each side.

A circular saw or burr is used to cut a longitudinal slot for the graft, extending from a point 5 cm (2 in) above the end of the radius to the proximal third of the third metacarpal bone. This graft bed, which is prepared about 13 mm ($\frac{1}{2}$ in) in width, includes the carpal bones between the radius and third metacarpal without respect to their identity. A small osteotome is introduced into each end of the bed of the graft to open the medullary cavity for about 10 mm ($\frac{3}{8}$ in).

A graft is taken from the bone bank or cut from the tibia and is the same width as the graft bed, but 13 mm ($\frac{1}{2}$ in) longer. This graft is pointed at both ends before introducing it into the radius for about 6 mm ($\frac{1}{4}$ in). Traction is exerted on the fingers and the other end of the graft is levered into the prepared hole in the third metacarpal bone. Release of traction will ensure a snug fit and good immobilisation of the graft.

The wound is closed in layers and a plaster of Paris cast is applied.

Arthroplasty of the hip (Austin Moore, Thompson, McKee Farrar, Howse and Charnley operations)

DEFINITION

The reconstruction of new joint surfaces in the hip by replacing the femoral head with a plastic or metallic prosthesis.

POSITION

Lateral or supine, with a sandbag under the buttock on the affected side.

Fig. 23.105 Basic arthroplasty instruments

1. Measuring calipers.
2. Steel rule 15 cm (6 in).
3. Large gouge or skid (for reduction of hip).
4. Straight osteotomes 16 mm ($\frac{5}{8}$ in), 19 mm ($\frac{3}{4}$ in), 25 cm (1 in).
5. Impactor (with nylon insert) for prosthesis.
6. Box chisel.
7. Template guide.
8. Tommy-bar for shaft of rasps.
9. Thompson rasp for femoral shaft.
10. Thompson prosthesis.
11. Austin Moore prosthesis, standard stem.
12. Austin Moore prosthesis modified, narrow stem.
13. Austin Moore rasp.
14. Hacksaw.
15. Hip Levers (Judet).
16. Femoral head skid (Smith Petersen).
17. Wire saw (Gigli) with handles.
18. Auger for extracting femoral head (Judet).
19. Acetabular reamer (Duthie).
20. Brace for acetabular reamer.
21. Extractor for Austin Moore heads.

Fig. 23.106 Additional instruments for McKee Farrar prosthesis.

1. Automatic screwdriver (Williams).
2. Pistol grip hand drill.
3. Key for Jacobs' chuck.
4. Sherman screws, Vitallium 32 mm (1¼ in).
5. Ordinary screwdriver (Lanes).
6. Bone cement powder.
7. Bone cement liquid.
8. McKee Farrar prosthesis.
9. Mixing bowl and spoon for bone cement.
10. Instrument for holding acetabular cup in position during setting of bone cement.
11. Twist drills, No. 32 (for screws) 6·4 mm (⅜ in), 9 mm (5/16 in), 10 mm (⅜ in).

INSTRUMENTS

General set (Figs. 14.1 to 14.28)
Bone and fracture set (p. 516)
Arthroplasty set (Fig. 23.105)
Additional instruments for McKee Farrar operation if required (Fig. 23.106). Howse operation (Fig. 23.108) or Charnley operation (Fig. 23.107D)
Artery forceps, curved on flat (Kelly Fraser), 20
Large tissue forceps, curved (Fagge), 5
Deep retractors (Hibb), 2
Osteotomes, 16 mm (⅝ in), 19 mm (¾ in) and 38 mm (1½ in) (straight)
Osteotomes, 16 mm (⅝ in) and 19 mm (¾ in) (curved)
Gouges, 16 mm (⅝ in), 19 mm (¾ in) and 38 mm (1½ in)
Wire saw and handles (Gigli or Olivecrona), optional

A McKee-Farrar Total Hip Prosthesis (Micro-fitting) (Howmedica U.K. Ltd.)

Thompson Type Stem

	Femoral Portion				**Acetabular Portion**			
Size		Head Size		Inside dia.		Outside dia.		Style
mm	in	mm	in	mm	in	mm	in	
$1\frac{3}{8}$		35	$1\frac{3}{8}$	35	$1\frac{3}{8}$	44·5	$1\frac{3}{4}$	4
$1\frac{3}{8}$H*		35	$1\frac{3}{8}$	35	$1\frac{3}{8}$	47·5	$1\frac{7}{8}$	2
$1\frac{9}{16}$ H*		39·5	$1\frac{9}{16}$	39·5	$1\frac{9}{16}$	51	2	1

Long neck. The neck of this unit has been elongated by 6·4 mm ($\frac{1}{4}$ in).

| $1\frac{3}{8}$ | | 35 | $1\frac{3}{8}$ | 35 | $1\frac{3}{8}$ | 44·5 | $1\frac{3}{4}$ | 5 |
| $1\frac{3}{8}$ H* | | 35 | $1\frac{3}{8}$ | 35 | $1\frac{3}{8}$ | 47·5 | $1\frac{7}{8}$ | 3 |

*The 'H' designation indicates a thicker cup

The McKee-Farrar Total Hip Prosthesis provides the surgeon with a technologically sophisticated appliance designed to replace both sides of the hip joint. It consists of a Vitallium femoral prosthesis and a Vitallium acetabular cup. The cup and stem are designed for fixation by means of quick-acting Surgical Simplex P cement.

Micro-fit interchangeable components

The articulating surfaces of the McKee-Farrar components are manufactured by proprietary techniques to close tolerances and an extremely fine surface finish. These new techniques permit interchangeability of components of identical cup and head size . . . thus providing to the surgeon the convenience of selecting the proper femoral stem and neck length *after* the acetabular component is firmly fixed.

B McKee-Farrar Total Hip Prosthesis (Minneapolis stem) (Howmedica U.K. Ltd.)

Sizes available:

	Femoral Portion				**Acetabular Portion**		
Size		Head Size		Inside dia.		Outside dia.	
		mm	in	mm	in	mm	in
$1\frac{5}{8}$		41·5	$1\frac{5}{8}$	41·5	$1\frac{5}{8}$	51	2

The femoral component consists of a Minneapolis hip prosthesis. It is normally restricted to cases where an osteotomy has been performed and pain has not been relieved. It can also be used where the upper part of the femoral shaft is damaged.

C Austin Moore Self Locking Hip Prosthesis (Howmedica U.K. Ltd.)

Vitallium. S.Mo. (EN 58J)
Stainless steel. Titanium.

Head Diameter		Stem Length Vitallium		Stem Length S.Mo. (EN 58J)	
mm	in	mm	in	mm	in
38	$1\frac{1}{2}$	127	5		
41	$1\frac{5}{8}$	127	5	127	5
43	$1\frac{11}{16}$	127	5		
45	$1\frac{3}{4}$	127	5	127	5
46	$1\frac{13}{16}$	140	$5\frac{1}{2}$		
48	$1\frac{7}{8}$	140	$5\frac{1}{2}$		
49	$1\frac{15}{16}$	140	$5\frac{1}{2}$	140	$5\frac{1}{2}$
51	2	152	6		
52	$2\frac{1}{16}$	152	6	140	6
54	$2\frac{1}{8}$	152	6		
57	$2\frac{1}{4}$	152	6	140	6
60	$2\frac{3}{8}$	152	6		
64	$2\frac{1}{2}$	152	6		

Seat width 25 mm (1 in). Stem thickness 10 mm ($\frac{1}{8}$ in).

D Charnley Total Hip Prosthesis (Chas. F. Thackray)

	Head Diameter		Stem Length		Cup O.D.	
	mm	in	mm	in	mm	in
	22	$\frac{7}{8}$	117	$4\frac{5}{8}$	43	$1\frac{11}{16}$
w/small Cup	22	$\frac{7}{8}$	117	$4\frac{5}{8}$	40	$1\frac{9}{16}$
straight narrow stem	22	$\frac{7}{8}$	121	$4\frac{3}{4}$	43	$1\frac{11}{16}$
straight narrow stem small cup	22	$\frac{7}{8}$	121	$4\frac{3}{4}$	40	$1\frac{9}{16}$

The Charnley Type Total Hip Prosthesis is a low friction replacement prosthesis for arthroplasty of the hip joint. A two-piece appliance, it combines the tissue compatibility of a Vitallium femoral prosthesis with the low friction characteristics of an ultra-high molecular weight polyethylene cup. The femoral head portion is ground to a virtually perfect spherical shape and polished to an optical mirror finish. The cup is double wrapped and sterilized by gamma radiation. A radiopaque Vitallium wire over the cup permits determination of the position of the cup post-operatively.

Fig. 23.107   Hip prosthesis for arthroplasty operations.

Sizes available

No. 607S small   No. 607E small, extended neck   No. 607L large

S.Mo. (EN 58J). Stainless Steel.

The Howse Prosthesis is a metal-to-plastic bearing prosthesis. The femoral part is made of stainless steel EN 58J, the acetabular cup of high density polyethene (RCH 1000). The combination of these two materials has proved the best for bearing surfaces. The femoral head is subjected to a special optical lapping and polishing process and is truly spherical with a superfinish in terms of micro-inches.

The cup is larger than half a sphere. The depth of its internal surface, spherically shaped, is greater than the radius of the sphere of the femoral head. A slight decrease in the thickness of the external wall of the collar allows the introduction of the head, which is held firmly by the cup after reduction. This characteristic of the prosthesis avoids post-operative dislocation and allows immediate mobilisation of the hip.

The Howse sockets are fitted with a radio-opaque marker.

The size of the internal surface of the cup has been calculated to meet exactly the size of the head at 37°, that is why at room temperature there seems to be too tight a fit between the two parts.

The prosthesis, received assembled and sterilised by gamma radiation, is ready for immediate use, thus avoiding possible damage during sterilisation. However, should the prosthesis be exposed to infection, the cup can be re-sterilised by formaldehyde solution or ethylene oxide gas (it should not be autoclaved) it is inadvisable to re-sterilise by a second exposure to gamma radiation.

Fig. 23.108   The Howse total hip prosthesis. (D. Howse & Co.)

Orthopaedic Operations 583

(A) Cup holder. Stainless steel. *TUFNOL* handle. Overall length 35 cm.

(B) Adaptors. To screw on holder. Nylon (may be sterilised by autoclaving). The cup clips onto the adaptor and can be held firmly without fear of dropping off.

(C) Socket size gauges. *TUFNOL*. With detachable heads for screwing onto cup holder if desired.

(D) Test femoral stem. Stainless steel.

(E) Left and right broaches with Tommy bar. Stainless steel. Overall length 25 cm.

(F) H. Harris Bone curette. Stainless steel. *TUFNOL* handle. Overall length 29 cm.

(G) Femoral pusher. *TUFNOL*. Overall length 15 cm.

(H) Twist drills. Stainless steel. 6·6 mm × 250 mm long. 11 mm × 250 mm long.

(I) Braddock retractor. Stainless steel handle. Overall length 28 cm. This retractor has a serrated claw edge that grips the back of the acetabulum.

Fig. 23.109 Additional instruments for insertion of Howse Total Hip Prosthesis.

Fig. 23.110 Additional instruments for Charnley low friction arthroplasty of the hip. (Chas. F. Thackray Ltd.)

1. Brace, wide throw.
2. Starting drill, 12·5 mm (½ in) diameter with centering ring.
3. Deepening reamer, spigot is 12·5 mm (½ in) diameter and engages with the pilot hole made by the starting drill in the floor of the acetabulum. The reamer produces a concave surface of 25 mm (1 in) radius.
4. Expanding reamer, this completes the cutting of a 5 cm (2 in) hemisphere after the deepening reamer has thinned the floor of the acetabulum. The profile of the hemisphere is a circle of 2·5 cm (1 in) radius with a 6·25 mm (¼ in) parallel section near the mouth.
5. Socket size gauge, small and large size gauges are used. 6. Cement restrictor.
7. Socket holder and guide, the plastic socket both small and large is held in position by an interference fit with three pins on the holder. The holder permits an orientation of 45° of the face of the socket to be made with precision. The plastic socket is clipped to the holder with the plane of the radiological marker in the same plane as the introducer handle. This enables the orientation of the radiological marker to be correct is an anteroposterior radiograph.

Arthroplasty of hip, instruments cont'd.

Femoral neck saw
Scissors, curved on flat 20 cm (8 in) (Mayo)
Long scalpel, solid variety
Syringe 20 ml, and 18 gauge filling needle
Simplex bone cement
Diathermy leads, electrodes and lead anchoring forceps
3 and 4 (0 and 1) Plain catgut or Dexon for ligatures

OUTLINE OF PROCEDURE

There are a number of alternative approaches to the hip joint. The approach may be postero-lateral for a McKee Farrar procedure (Figs. 23.111 to 23.112b), antero-lateral for a Howse prosthesis or lateral for a Charnley prosthesis. The surgeon may dislocate the hip and remove the femoral head with a saw or large osteotome, or may prefer to divide the femoral neck before dislocation, and extract the head with a large corkscrew instrument. This latter method is applicable when a prosthesis is being inserted for the treatment of a subcapital fracture of the femoral neck which is not suitable for nailing, and when the head is separated and loose in the acetabulum.

The extent to which the acetabulum is prepared depends on whether a 'total hip replacement' is to be carried out; if not an Austin Moore or Thompson prosthesis is generally inserted. With this type of prosthesis, which is made from stainless steel or Vitallium, the stem projects along the femoral neck and curves into the femoral shaft. The femoral channel is made with a long curved rasp and small gouges.

The McKee Farrar total hip prosthesis. This consists of a two-part ball and socket appliance; the femoral part being basically similar to a Thompson prosthesis, and the acetabular part a hemispherical cup, lapped to fit the head of the Thompson prosthesis, thus forming a pair which should only be used as such. The outer surface of the cup is covered with small studs and the edge of the cup fashioned with a lip. The purpose of these studs is to provide a positive hold when the cup is embedded in acrylic cement in the acetabulum. Both parts of the prosthesis are manufactured from Vitallium.

Fig. 23.110   *Continued.*

8. Socket pusher, is used to exert pressure in the centre of the socket holder where it engages in a depression. It enables the acrylic cement to be impacted in the cancellous bone by two blows of a mallet delivered through the socket pusher. This is done when the cement is nearly hard, and coins the cement to the cancellous bone and gets rid of any blood clot which may be interposed.
9. Pin retractor, used in the superior lip of the acetabulum to 'stake' back the abductor muscles improving the exposure of the acetabulum. Instruments used for reattachment of the trochanter (Nos. 10–14).
10. Wire holding forceps. 11. Wire passer.
12. Drill and wire guide forceps for trochanter.
13. Lightweight brace with female trochanter reamer.
14. Male trochanter reamer, used on the inner surface of the detached trochanter in preparation for reattachment in the correct position. Instruments required in the preparation of the acetabulum site and cementing of the plastic socket (Nos. 15–20).
15. Femoral prosthesis punch, designed to avoid damage to surface of head.
16. Femoral prosthesis pusher. 17. Femoral prosthesis with standard prosthesis mounted.
18. Tommy bar for broach. 19. Femoral broach.
20. Taper reamer for medullary canal.

Fig. 23.111 Postero-lateral approach to the hip.

(A) The gluteus maximus is split in the direction of its fibres. The dotted outline shows the underlying bony landmarks.
(B) The short transverse lateral rotator muscles deep to the gluteus maximus. Note that the sciatic nerve lies upon the superficial aspect of the obturator internus, gemelli and quadratus femoris, but deep to the piriformis.
(C) The piriformis, obturator internus and gemelli have been divided close to the greater trochanter and reflected backwards, thus protecting the sciatic nerve. (In most cases sufficient access can be gained without reflecting the piriformis.) (Crawford Adams.)

Fig. 23.112 Insertion of Austin Moore prosthesis. (A) Femoral head dislocated, division of femoral neck. (B) Reaming femoral shaft. (C) Insertion of prosthesis. (D) Hip reduced. (Hall.)

The acrylic cement mix consists of two parts, a powder (the polymer) and a liquid (the monomer). These are available as a sterile pack containing the correct amount of each. They are mixed together in a metal bowl with a spoon until within 2 or 3 minutes the plastic assumes a soft, workable consistency and no longer sticks to the gloves. The dough mix is pushed into the prepared acetabulum and the cup inserted in the correct position. The cup is held firmly by a special dome-shaped instrument until the cement has set, usually about 5 minutes. Care must be taken to clean the mixing bowl with a small quantity of acetone immediately before the remnants of cement have set. Alternatively an injection gun is available to facilitate introduction of cement into bone cavities.

Fig. 23.113   McKee-Farrar total hip prosthesis. (Hall.)

(A) Exposure of acetabulum and femoral neck.
(B) Excision of femoral head with osteotomy saw.
(C) Preparation of acetabulum, soft tissue excised, 9·3 mm ($\frac{3}{8}$ in) holes drilled in acetabulum.
(D) Cement applied to acetabulum, insertion of cup.
(E) Cement inserted in femoral medullary cavity, prosthesis being driven home so that shaft of prosthesis sits firmly upon the femoral neck.
(F) When cement is firmly set artificial joint is reduced.

Fig. 23.114 Preparation of Simplex acrylic cement. (Howmedica U.K. Ltd.)

(A) The outer plastic pouch has been peeled open, the inner plastic bag is removed and cut open with scissors, the powder is then gently poured and tapped into the bowl.
(B) A 20 ml syringe and 18 gauge needle is used to draw up the liquid monomer.
(C) Powder and liquid are stirred, either with a tongue blade or sterile spoon until the entire mass can be lifted from the bowl in one lump.
(D) The ball of cement is kneaded in the hands until it is doughy. (Alternatively, cement can be mixed within the barrel of a cement syringe and then injected into bone cavities – Exeter system.)

The Howse total hip prosthesis. This is a ball and socket, metal to plastic-bearing prosthesis. The femoral part of the appliance is made from stainless steel and resembles a Thompson prosthesis; the acetabular cup is made from high density polyethylene (RCH 1000) incorporating a radio-opaque marker.

During manufacture, the components are subjected to special optical lapping and polishing processes to ensure accuracy of fit. The acetabular cup is larger than a hemisphere and the depth of its internal surface, spherically-shaped, is greater than the radius of the sphere of the femoral head. This creates a vacuum effect which holds the prosthesis, and reduces the risk of subsequent dislocation. The prosthesis has the characteristics of low friction and low wear.

With the exception of detachment of the great trochanter, the operative procedure is similar to that for the Charnley prosthesis described on the following page. After preparation of the acetabulum, it is thickly lined with acrylic cement, care being taken to push the cement into the anchoring holes. The cup is inserted with the cup inserting instrument (Fig. 23.113d); the cup and its collar need to be entirely covered with cement.

The femoral neck is prepared as for insertion of a Thompson prosthesis. The femoral shaft is prepared with a rasp, the medullary cavity filled with cement and the femoral prosthesis pushed in, utilising the metal flat provided below and behind the actual head of the prosthesis.

Fig. 23.115 Separation of the two components of a Howse total hip prosthesis before insertion. This is done by fully flexing the femoral component within the cup, until the neck of the component touches the rim of the cup, and then levering the head out of the cup. (D. Howse & Co.)

The Charnley total hip prosthesis. This also is a metal to plastic bearing prosthesis which was the original design of this type. It is manufactured from the same materials and to the same exacting standards as the Howse prosthesis.

The essential difference between this and the Howse is that the Charnley femoral head component is smaller and does not have the Thompson type extended seating area at the base of the neck.

During preparative stages the Charnley technique consists of detaching the great trochanter which subsequently is reattached after the prosthesis has been inserted. This together with the lateral approach to the hip is said to prevent dislocation after operation.

The acetabulum is prepared by removing all remnants of articular cartilage and roughening the walls with a gouge. Three or four 6 mm ($\frac{1}{4}$ in) to 10 mm ($\frac{3}{8}$ in) wide holes are made with a drill. These holes provide anchoring points for the acrylic cement. The outer cortex of the ilium immediately above the acetabulum is cleaned of soft-tissue attachments and in the case of the McKee Farrar procedure, two screws are inserted parallel to the roof of the acetabulum. These are left projecting 6 mm ($\frac{1}{4}$ in) and provide further anchoring points for the acrylic cement.

The femoral neck is prepared in the usual way with gouges and a rasp, although care is taken that the stem of the prosthesis lies accurately within the femoral shaft with adequate room for introduction of the acrylic cement.

The femoral stem of the prosthesis is inserted and a trial reduction of the hip performed. After removing the prosthesis, a second mix of acrylic cement is made and inserted into the femoral shaft. The prosthesis is re-inserted and the cement allowed to set. The hip is then finally reduced.

Following insertion of the prosthesis the wound is closed in layers. Some surgeons may tie the legs together until the patient recovers consciousness. Russell traction of 3·2 to 4·5 kg (7 to 10 lb) may then be applied to the affected limb.

There are many types of arthroplasty of hip but the reader will find that these are probably the ones used by most surgeons at present. It must be understood that only an outline of the procedures has been described. Each of the operations requires a special technique and the reader is recommended to consult the appropriate literature for further information.

Arthroplasty of the knee

DEFINITION

The reconstruction of the new joint surfaces in the knee by replacing the femoral condyles and tibial plateau with a metallic/plastic prosthesis.

POSITION

Supine.

INSTRUMENTS

General set (Figs. 14.1 to 14.28)
Bone and fracture set (p. 516)
Osteotomes, 39 mm (1½ in) and 26 mm (1 in)
Power driven saw (optional)
Large tissue forceps (Fagge or Lane), 4
Irrigation syringe and saline
Suction tubing, nozzles and tube anchoring forceps
Venting tubes
Mixing bowl and spoon for cement
Simplex bone cement
Syringe 20 ml, and 18 gauge filling needle
3 (0) Plain catgut or Dexon for ligatures
4 and 5 (1 and 2) Plain catgut or Dexon on a medium half-circle cutting or Mayo needle with a trocar point for capsule etc.
2·5 or 3 (2/0 or 0) Silk or nylon on a medium curved or straight cutting needle for skin sutures.

OUTLINE OF PROCEDURE

Although arthroplasty of the knee can be accomplished by simply using a tibial plateau replacement prosthesis, such as Mackintosh, most operations consist of either a hinged or a gliding prosthesis.

The hinged prosthesis consists of two components which can be disassembled for insertion into the femoral and tibial shafts and then reconnected to form a hinged joint. The gliding prosthesis also consists of two components, one of which is either inserted into the femoral shaft or fitted over the femoral condyles, and the other fitted in place of the tibial plateau.

It would not be practicable to describe the multitude of operations available, the description of the procedure will therefore be confined to the Stanmore total knee replacement. The operation is performed under tourniquet.

The knee joint is exposed through a lateral para-patella skin incision and a medial para-patella incision in the joint capsule. The stem of the femoral component is aligned with the femoral shaft and the femoral condyles resected (Fig. 23.117a).

The articular surface of the tibia is resected immediately above the tibial tubercle (Fig. 23.117b) and a gauge block is used to check that the correct amount of bone has been resected. Sufficient cancellous bone is curetted from both bone surfaces to take the stems of the prosthesis and the cement. A trial reduction is made, after inserting the femoral and tibial components and connecting them with a temporary axle. A check is made that the joint will flex through its full range of flexion/extension movements; if necessary additional bone is trimmed from the tibia (Fig. 23.117c).

592 Operating Theatre Technique

Debris is washed away from the medullary and joint cavities. Both medullary cavities are then packed with cement (see page 587 for preparation) using venting tubes connected to suction. The tibial and femoral components are inserted whilst the cement is still soft, and the temporary axle used to check articulation. The trial axle is replaced with the permanent axle, which is secured with a special circlip (Fig. 23.116d).

Fig. 23.116 Stanmore Titanium total knee prosthesis.

(A) Left and right prosthesis.
(B) Components joined with axle, circlip fixing device ready for insertion.
(C) Circlip being positioned.
(D) Circlip in position and instrument removed. (Zimmer Orthopaedic Ltd.)

Fig. 23.117 Insertion of Stanmore Total knee prosthesis.
(A) and (B) Resection of femoral condyles.
(C) Resection of tibial plateau.
(D) Application of gauge block to check extent of resection.
(E) Trial reduction.
(F) Prosthesis inserted, locking axle (see also Fig. 23.116A to D). (Zimmer Orthopaedic Ltd.)

The incision is closed in the normal way and a Redivac suction drain inserted. Before the tourniquet is removed, a pressure bandage is applied over cotton wool and a plaster of Paris or polyethylene back splint applied.

Congenital dislocation of hip (shelf operation)

DEFINITION

To deepen the acetabulum by constructing a shelf of bone over the top of the femoral head.

POSITION

Lateral or supine, with a sandbag under the buttock on the affected side.

INSTRUMENTS

As for Charnley's central dislocation arthrodesis of the hip
As for skeletal traction, insertion of Steinmann pin or Kirschner wire (Fig. 23.4).

Fig. 23.118 Modified Gill operation for congenital dislocation of the hip. (A) Iliac crest exposed, reflection of the iliac apophysis. (B and C) Subtotal capsulectomy, outline of shelf made with drill holes. (D) Cutting of bone shelf from ilium. (E) A 12 mm ($\frac{1}{2}$ in) osteotome is used to turn down bone flap which is sutured to margin of capsule with catgut or Dexon. (F) Wedge graft removed from iliac crest. (G) Wedge graft in position, held with fine Steinman pin through inner table of ilium, pin cut off subcutaneously. (Hall.)

OUTLINE OF PROCEDURE

The hip joint is exposed through an anterolateral or lateral incision; the head of the femur is stripped of soft tissue structures which interfere with mobility.

(After shelf operations, it is essential that continuous traction be applied to the leg until the bone shelf has healed, as the femoral head tends to displace the grafts. This may be accomplished by skin or skeletal traction which is sometimes applied before operation.)

The shelf of bone on the acetabular rim may be constructed in several ways. The Albee technique involves the division of the acetabular rim with a thin blade osteotome in a semi-circular line following the natural curve of the acetabulum. This segment of bone is pried outward and downward and secured with triangular shaped cortical grafts from the tibia or bone bank.

The Gill operation is similar, but the shelf is made by turning down a bone flap from the outer table of the ilium, sufficiently wide to cover the portion of the femur which projects beyond the acetabulum. This flap is secured with bone wedges from the crest of the ilium or bone bank (Fig. 23.118).

The wound is closed in layers and the patient is immobilised in a double plaster of Paris hip spica with traction on the affected limb.

Recurrent dislocation of the shoulder (Bankart's and Putti-Platt capsulorraphy)

DEFINITION

A plastic procedure on the capsule and ligaments of the shoulder joint to prevent recurrent dislocation.

POSITION

Supine, with a sandbag under the scapula on the affected side.

INSTRUMENTS

General set (Figs. 14.1 to 14.28)
Bone hooks, 2
Small bone levers (Lane), 2
Small mallet (Rowland)
Small rugine, curved (Farabeouf)
Osteotome, 13 mm ($\frac{1}{2}$ in)
Bone awl
Contra-angle power drill (Bankart's operation only)
Bone graft set. (Instruments as in Fig. 23.91 may be required for graft to deficient glenoid rim.)
Staples and insertion punch, optional
Diathermy leads, electrodes and lead anchoring forceps
Suction tubing, nozzles and tube anchoring forceps
2·5 and 3 (2/0 and 0) Plain and chromic catgut or Dexon for ligatures
3 or 4 (0 or 1) Silk, etc., chromic catgut or Dexon on a small fish hook, half-circle cutting 6, or Mayo needle with trocar point for capsulorrhaphy, etc.
3 or 4 (0 or 1) Chromic catgut or Dexon on a medium half circle cutting needle for deltoid muscle sutures
2·5 (2/0) Silk or nylon on a medium curved cutting needle for skin sutures.

Fig. 23.119 Anterior exposure of shoulder. (A) The skin incision. (B) After separation of the deltoid and pectoralis major the conjoined coracobrachialis and biceps muscles are seen attached to the coracoid process. Deep to them lies the subscapularis, the fibres of which become tendinous as they approach their insertion into the humerus. The broken line shows the position of the head of the humerus. (Crawford Adams.)

OUTLINE OF PROCEDURE

Bankart Operation. An incision is made commencing at the outer border of the clavicle, curving medially to the coracoid process and continuing along the inner border of the deltoid muscle in line with the cephalic vein.

The interval between the deltoid and the pectoralis muscle is developed and the cephalic vein is retracted medially after dividing branches which may interfere with the exposure of the joint. The deltoid origin is reflected from the clavicle and the muscle retracted laterally. A hole about 3 mm ($\frac{1}{8}$ in) by 25 mm (1 in) deep may be drilled in the coracoid process with an awl or twist drill, to facilitate subsequent suture. The coracoid process is divided with an osteotome, and its tip, together with muscle attachments, is retracted medially and downwards.

The shoulder is then placed into external rotation and the subscapularis tendon is identified. A plexus of veins on the lower border of the tendon is usually ligated or diathermised and divided. Two silk sutures are placed in the medial part of the tendon and are left long for retraction. The tendon is incised, and medial portion of the tendon allowed to retract, and the capsule then opened by a vertical incision 6 mm ($\frac{1}{4}$ in) lateral to the glenoid rim.

The glenoid rim is freshened with a curette and three holes are drilled in it with an angled drill. The shoulder is placed in internal rotation and abduction, and the cartilaginous labrum which is invariably detached from the glenoid rim is sutured (or stapled) back to its original position, utilising the three holes in the bone. In order to reinforce this, the medial part of the capsule *may* be plicated over the area of repair as in the Putti-Platt procedure. The subscapularis tendon is approximated with sutures, the coracoid process is re-attached, and the rest of the wound closed in layers. The arm is immobilised to the chest with cotton-wool and crêpe bandages.

Fig. 23.120 Bankhart's operation for recurrent dislocation of the shoulder. (Wilson – *Watson – Jones.*)

(A) Division of coracoid process of deltoid with an osteotome.
(B) Division of subscapularis tendon.
(C) Incision of joint capsule.
(D) Three holes are made in glenoid rim, either using an angled drill or towel forcep.
(E) Reattachment of cartilaginous labrum with sutures which utilise holes in glenoid rim.
(F) Reattachment of coracoid process with sutures.

Fig. 23.120 (cont'd.) E F

Fig. 23.121 Putti-Platt operation for recurrent dislocation of shoulder.
(A) The coraco-brachialis has been divided by osteomising the coracoid process (as in Fig. 23.120).
(B) The medial part of scapularis and the capsule being retracted inwards, the detachment of the glenoid labrum (Bankhart's lesion) is exposed.
(C) The tissues in front of the neck of the scapula, including labrum periosteum and deep capsule, are sutured to the lateral stump of subscapularis.
(D) The four or five sutures have been tied while the limb was in internal rotation. The medial part of the capsule and subscapularis are then overlapped and sutured to the region of the tuberosity. After repair of the coraco-brachialis and the closure of the wound the limb is held in internal rotation for four weeks. (Sir Henry Osmond-Clarke.)

Putti-Platt Operation. The exposure is essentially the same as the Bankart's operation as far as the subscapularis tendon. This tendon is incised about 25 mm (1 in) medial to its insertion, and the joint is opened. The lateral portion of the subscapularis tendon is sutured either to the anterior rim of the glenoid cavity or the deep surface of the stripped capsule and subscapularis. The medial portion of the capsule is plicated over this lateral part of the subscapularis tendon, and finally the medial portion of the subscapularis tendon is plicated over all the previous suture lines, being attached to the bicipital groove or tendinous cuff over the greater tuberosity. This is in effect an overlapping of the medial and lateral parts of the capsule and subscapularis tendon so that a barrier to redislocation is formed.

The wound is closed as before, with immobilisation of the arm to the side.

Spinal fusion

DEFINITION

Fusion of the spine in the treatment of tuberculosis, spondylolisthesis, scoliosis and some fracture dislocations.

POSITION

Knee/elbow, as Figure 4.17, or prone position of extension similar to the application of a spinal jacket illustrated in Chapter 31.

INSTRUMENTS

As in laminectomy (Chapter 23, Neurosurgery, page 502)
Bone grafting set (Fig. 23.91)
Spinal rasps (Wheeler and Tubby), 2

Fig. 23.122 H-shaped graft for posterior lumbar fusion. The graft is retained in position by cross pins transfixing the spinous processes. (Crawford Adams.)

Fig. 23.123 Meurig Williams Spinal Plates.
Patent No. 780652. S.Mo. (EN 58J). Stainless steel.
(Zimmer Orthopaedic Ltd.)

(A and B) Spinal plates, straight, 5 and 6 in.
(C) Spinal plates, curved, for lumbosacral fusion, available in sizes 102 mm (4 in), 127 mm (5 in) and 152 mm (6 in).
(D) Spinal bolts with serrated nuts and washers, length, $\frac{3}{4}$ in.

Bolts:
Outside diameter of thread: $\frac{1}{8}$ in. (·125 in or 3·2 mm).
Threads per inch: 32.
Diameter of hexagon nut: $\frac{5}{16}$ in. A/f hexagon (·312 in or 8 mm).
Recommended drill size: Usually right-angled awl or contra-angle dental drill, size $\frac{1}{8}$ in (·125 in or 3·2 mm).

To hold a dislocation of the spine in the reduced position it is desirable to obtain the maximum fixation which is possible only if all the bolts are anchored through bone. It is therefore essential to select plates of sufficient length to extend along at least five vertebrae, allowing the bolts to pass through two of the spinous processes above and two below the affected vertebra for preference, which then becomes the central point of fixation.

The Meurig Williams plates are said to have a distinct advantage over conventional plates because, being slotted over almost the entire length, it is possible to introduce all the fixation bolts through bone. This is not always possible with conventional plates due to the difficulty of lining up the holes in the plates opposite the spinous processes. Very often two bolts have to be introduced through the interspinous ligaments with consequent risk of the plates cutting out.

This apparatus enables serrated washers and nuts with bolts matching the serrations in the plates to be used in order to ensure that a positive fixation is obtained, thereby overcoming the natural tendency for longitudinal movement in the slotted plates, so that the spine remains stable in the reduced position.

Fig. 23.124 Kellers operation using power saw. (A) Area of bone to be removed. (B) Excision of base of proximal phalanx. (C) Removal of exostosis. (D) Smoothing plantar surface of metatarsal. (Hall.)

Osteotomes, 13 mm ($\frac{1}{2}$ in), 16 mm ($\frac{5}{8}$ in), 19 mm ($\frac{3}{4}$ in) and 38 mm ($1\frac{1}{2}$ in) (straight)
Osteotomes, 13 mm ($\frac{1}{2}$ in), 16 mm ($\frac{5}{8}$ in) and 19 mm ($\frac{3}{4}$ in) (curved)
Gouges, 16 mm ($\frac{5}{8}$ in), 19 mm ($\frac{3}{4}$ in) and 25 mm (1 in).

For Wire Fixation
  Wiring set (Fig. 23.48)

For Plating or Screw Fixation
  Spinal plates (set of Wilson or Meurig Williams, small medium and large), 2 of each
  Spinal bolts, nuts and washers (Wilson or Meurig Williams), various lengths
  Angled awl or contra-angle drill
  Set of suitable spanners for bolts
  Plating and screwing set (p. 533), optional
  Ligatures and sutures as for laminectomy.

OUTLINE OF PROCEDURE

The initial stages of the operation follow that for laminectomy, but with a wider exposure at both sides of the vertebrae. For disease of the spine, usually two vertebrae above and two below the lesion are fused.

Fusion is accomplished by a bone graft which can be taken from the patient himself or the bone bank. Cortical grafts, i.e., from the tibia, may be screwed or bolted in position either singly or as a twin graft on each side of the spine. The spinous processes and laminae are carefully prepared before the graft is inserted by removing periosteum and generally freshening the bone surfaces. Sometimes the spinous processes are removed completely and the area bridged with an 'H' bone graft. In addition to preparing the graft bed, the surgeon may perform a laminectomy and explore the intervertebral disc spaces.

Following the insertion of a cortical graft, the area is packed with cancellous bone chips or strips. Alternatively, especially in the treatment of fractures, metallic spinal plates may be used to bridge the affected vertebrae. These plates can be used as pairs, one on each side; or in combination with a cortical graft to stimulate osteogenesis. The plates are bolted or screwed in position and cancellous strips or chips inserted as before. Wire loops may be used also, in conjunction with cortical or cancellous bone grafts.

Another method of spinal fusion consists of removing soft tissue from the lamellae surfaces, excising the tips of the spinous processes and packing a large quantity of cancellous bone chips and shavings in the graft bed.

The wound is closed in the usual manner and the patient immobilised on a plaster of Paris bed which has been prepared to measurement before operation.

Hallux valgus (Keller's operation)

DEFINITION

Removal of an exostosis of the first metatarsal head and a portion of the proximal phalanx in the treatment of hallux valgus or bunions.

POSITION

Supine.

INSTRUMENTS

Sponge-holding forceps (Rampley), 5
Towel clips, 5

Scalpel handles No. 3 with No. 10 blades (Bard Parker), 2
Scalpel, solid variety
Dissecting forceps, toothed (Lane), 2
Scissors, curved on flat, 13 cm (5 in) (Mayo)
Scissors, straight, 13 cm (5 in) (Mayo)
Small retractors, double hook, 2
Artery forceps, curved on flat (Kilner), 5
Tissue forceps (Allis), 5
Bone levers (Trethowan), 2
Small rugine (Faraboeuf)
Bone-cutting forceps, compound action (Horsley)
Small bone-cutting forceps, single action (Liston)
Bone hook (Lane)
Mallet (Heath)
Osteotomes, 13 mm ($\frac{1}{2}$ in) and 16 mm ($\frac{5}{8}$ in)
Small needle holder (Kilner)
2·5 (2/0) Plain catgut or Dexon for ligatures
3 (0) Plain catgut or Dexon on a small half-circle cutting needle for subcutaneous structures
2 (3/0) Silk or nylon on a small curved cutting needle for skin sutures.

OUTLINE OF PROCEDURE

A curved incision is made over the medial aspect of the first metatarsophalangeal joint, and the skin reflected with bone levers placed on either side of the base of the proximal phalanx.

The base of the phalanx is divided with bone-cutting forceps and removed. The bursa which usually lies over the bunion is excised and the exostosis on the medial aspect of the first metatarsal is removed with an osteotome.

The subcutaneous structures are approximated with catgut or Dexon and the skin closed in the usual manner.

Arthroplasty of the metcarpophalangeal and proximal interphalangeal joints (Nicolle operation)

DEFINITION

Excision of the metacarpophalangeal joint or interphalangeal joint and replacement with an intramedullary prosthesis having an integral hinge joint.

INSTRUMENTS

Sponge-holding forceps (Rampley), 5
Towel clips, 5
Scalpel handles No. 3 with No. 10 blades (Bard Parker), 2
Scalpel handle No. 9 with No. 15 blade (Bard Parker)
Scalpel, solid variety
Dissecting forceps, toothed 13 cm (5 in) (Lane), 2
Dissecting forceps, fine toothed (Gillies), 2
Scissors, curved on flat 13 cm (5 in) (Mayo)
Scissors, curved on flat, 14·5 cm (5$\frac{3}{4}$ in) (Lahey)
Small retractors, double hook (Lane rake), 2
Skin hooks, single hook (Gillies), 2

Artery forceps, curved on flat (Kilner), 5
Tissue forceps (Allis), 5
Bone levers (Trethowan), 2
Small rugine (Faraboeuf)
Small bone-cutting forceps (Stamms)
Nicolle reamer (Fig. 23.125A)
Nicolle prosthesis impactor/extractor, large and small (Fig. 23.125B and C)
Nicolle finger joint prosthesis (appropriate size – 7 available) (Fig. 23.125D)

Fig. 23.125 Instruments for Nicolle finger joint prosthesis. (A) Finger joint reamer. (B and C) Finger joint impactor/extractor, large and small. (D) Nicolle finger joint prosthesis. (E) Trial prosthesis stems. (Zimmer Orthopaedic Ltd.)

Fig. 23.126 Nicolle finger joint prosthesis. (A and B) X-ray appearance and hand before surgery. (C) Exposure of metacarpal phalangeal joints. (D) Prosthesis inserted. (E) Suture complete. (F) X-ray appearance of hand four months after surgery. (Zimmer Orthopaedic Ltd.)

Nicolle trial prosthesis stem (Fig. 23.125E)
Power bone saw or Hall drill
Small needle holder (Kilner)
2·5 (2/0) or 2 (3/0) plain catgut or Dexon for ligatures
2 (3/0) or 1·5 (4/0) white braided nylon, Dacron or polyester on small curved cutting needle for extensor expansion and capsular tissues
1·5 (4/0) or 1 (5/0) silk, nylon or polyester on small curved cutting needle for skin sutures
2 ml syringe and needle for antibiotic
Malleable aluminium or plaster of Paris splints.

OUTLINE OF PROCEDURE

Metacarpophalangeal joint replacement.

Metacarpophalangeal joints are exposed through a 4 cm dorsal longitudinal incision in the skin and extensor expansion. The extensor tendon is retracted medially and the metacarpal head is excised just distal to the tubercles.

The bone ends are reamed out to receive the intramedullary stems of the prosthesis. The appropriate size of joint is determined by a set of six trial prostheses. A size of joint should be selected which fits snugly within the intramedullary canal and does not rotate.

Using a joint impactor the individual halves of the prosthesis may be inserted firmly without damage to the surfaces of the prosthetic joint. To insert the prosthetic joint the appropriate size is first separated into two halves and the larger proximal end then inserted. Simultaneous distraction and flexion of the bone ends will then facilitate insertion of the distal half, care being taken not to damage the capsule while the two bearing surfaces of the joint are allowed to come together. If correctly inserted the joint will allow full passive range of extension and flexion of at least 90°. If the joints cannot be fully extended passively, release of the ulnar collateral ligaments or volar plate is indicated and if necessary additional length of the metacarpal head can be removed. When reaming out the proximal bone end it is desirable to employ a burr to hollow out the residual portion of the metacarpal head so that the prosthesis seats well into the bone, which also contributes to a fuller range of passive extension.

Extensor indicis proprius transfer and imbrication of the slack tissue in the dorsal capsule is next completed, followed by skin closure with fine mattress sutures. Rebalancing of the soft tissue mechanism is essential to the success of prosthetic joint replacement.

A padded dressing with volar plaster of Paris slab maintains the fingers in almost complete extension at the metacarpophalangeal joints. Early active finger tip movement within the dressing is encouraged.

There are several other plastic finger joint prostheses, some of which are suitable also for proximal inter phalangeal joints. The Harrison-Nicolle polypropylene intramedullary pegs are of one-piece construction with the inherent property of being able to withstand almost indefinite flexion and extension without fatigue. The technique of insertion is similar to the Nicolle prostheses.

Exostosectomy

DEFINITION

The excision of an abnormal bony prominence.

POSITION

Dependent upon the location of the exostosis.

INSTRUMENTS

> General set (Figs. 14.1 to 14.28)
> Bone and fracture set (p. 516)
> Osteotomes, 13 mm ($\frac{1}{2}$ in), 19 mm ($\frac{3}{4}$ in) and 25 mm (1 in)
> Appropriate ligatures and sutures for that area of the body.

OUTLINE OF PROCEDURE

The exostosis is exposed and the periosteum elevated. An osteotome is used to excise the bony prominence and the wound is closed in the usual manner.

Bone tumours

The technique involved depends upon the location and extent of the lesion. If amputation of a limb is contraindicated, the surgeon may excise the tumour and replace the defect with a bone graft. This graft may be purely a question of filling in a cavity with cancellous chips, or may mean transplant of a large wedge of bone.

Instruments required vary but as a guide the surgeon will probably require a general set (Figs. 14.1 to 14.28); a bone and fracture set (p. 516); with the possible addition of instruments for bone grafting (Fig. 23.91) and instruments for plating and screwing (p. 533).

Amputation, forearm

DEFINITION

Amputation through the forearm, preferably at a level which is a few centimetres above the wrist.

POSITION

Supine, with the affected arm extended on an arm table.

INSTRUMENTS

> General set (Figs. 14.1 to 14.28)
> Rugine (Mitchell)
> Bone-cutting forceps, compound action (Horsley)
> Amputation saw (Sergeant) or power driven saw/cutting burr, connecting tubing or drive cable
> Bone levers, small (Lane), 4
> Fine rubber or plastic drainage tubing
> Redivac suction drainage bottle, optional
> 2·5 and 3 (2/0 and 0) Plain and chromic catgut or Dexon for ligatures
> 3 (0) Silk, etc., for ligatures
> 2·5 (2/0) Silk or nylon on a medium curved cutting needle for skin sutures.

OUTLINE OF PROCEDURE

Equal anterior and posterior skin flaps are cut, together with the underlying fat and muscle fascia. These are reflected up and the radial and ulnar nerves are sectioned above the level for dissection of the bone.

Fig. 23.127 Amputation through the forearm using a power driven cutting burr. (Hall.)

The muscles are divided across just below the level of bone resection and are retracted proximally. The radius and ulna are divided across with a saw and the hand removed. The major vessels are identified and ligated with catgut, Dexon or silk and the two fascial flaps are approximated with catgut or Dexon sutures. If the operation is being performed without a tourniquet, the major vessels are identified and clamped before transection of the muscles and bone.

A drain may or may not be inserted and the wound is closed.

Amputation through the humerus

DEFINITION

Amputation of the arm through the humerus.

POSITION

Supine, with affected limb extended on an arm table initially.

INSTRUMENTS

As for amputation of forearm.

OUTLINE OF PROCEDURE

Equal anterior and posterior skin flaps are cut, but may be modified in order to effect a plastic closure. These flaps are reflected with the fat and muscle fascia, and the anterior muscles are divided across just below the level for bone section. The major vessels are identified and clamped, and the posterior muscles are divided. The bone is divided with a saw and the arm removed.

The nerves are divided at the level of bone section and the major vessels are ligated with double ligatures. The muscles are bevelled to form a thin myofascial flap and are approximated with catgut or Dexon sutures. A drainage tube is inserted and the skin closed in the usual manner.

Amputation below the knee

DEFINITION

Amputation of the leg through the upper or middle tibia.

POSITION

Supine.

INSTRUMENTS

General set (Figs. 14.1 to 14.28)
Large tissue forceps (Fagge or Lane), 5
Rugine (Mitchell)
Bone-cutting forceps, compound action (Horsley)
Amputation saw (Sergeant)
Bone file (optional)
Wire saw and handles (Gigli or Olivecrona), or rib shears optional
Amputation knife
Bone-holding forceps (Fergusson lion)
Medium rubber or plastic drainage tubing
Redivac suction drainage bottle, optional
2·5 and 3 (2/0 and 0) Plain catgut or Dexon for superficial ligatures
3 and 4 (0 and 1) Chronic catgut, Dexon or silk for deep ligatures
4 (1) Plain catgut on a medium half-circle cutting needle for muscle sutures
2·5 (2/0) Silk or nylon on a medium curved cutting needle for skin sutures.

OUTLINE OF PROCEDURE

Unequal skin flaps are cut, with the anterior flap slightly longer than the posterior one at the selected level for amputation.

These incisions are carried down to muscle fascia and the flaps are reflected up on each aspect. The periosteum overlying the point for division of the bone is reflected and the anterior muscles are sectioned. During this stage the anterior tibial vessels are ligated and divided and the superficial perioneal and tibial nerves are divided at the level of bone section.

The tibia and fibula are sawn across about a quarter of an inch proximal to the divided anterior muscles. The posterior muscles are divided with an amputation knife and the posterior vessels identified, clamped and divided. The leg is removed and the vessels ligated. The fibula is exposed by subperiosteal dissection and is divided with bone-cutting forceps, a Gigli saw or rib shears at a point which is about 25 mm (1 in) to 40 mm ($1\frac{1}{2}$ in) above the level of the sectional tibia. The crest of the tibia is bevelled with a saw or file to prevent a sharp edge pressing on the skin. A flap of fascia is sutured over the stump, a drain is inserted and the skin closed in the usual manner.

Amputation, mid-thigh

DEFINITION

Amputation of the leg through the middle part of the femur.

POSITION

Supine, or with the knee flexed over the lower part of the table which is lowered or removed.

INSTRUMENTS

General set (Figs. 14.1 to 14.28)
Mid-thigh amputation set (Fig. 23.128)
Rugine (Mitchell)
Bone hook (Lane)
2·5 and 3 (2/0 and 0) Plain catgut or Dexon for superficial ligatures
3 and 4 (0 and 1) Chromic catgut, Dexon or silk for deep ligatures
4 (1) Chromic catgut or Dexon on a large half-circle cutting needle for muscle sutures
3 (0) Silk or nylon on a large curved or straight cutting needle for skin sutures.

OUTLINE OF PROCEDURE

Equal skin flaps are cut at the level for amputation and are reflected up with the fascia. If a tourniquet is in position, the muscles are severed by the circular sweep of an amputation knife which commences its cut on the anteromedial aspect of the thigh, cuts posteriorly, then laterally and finally anterolaterally. The muscles are then retracted with the amputation shield to a point about 25 mm (1 in) above the level for bone section.

Fig. 23.128 Mid-thigh amputation.

1. Amputation shield.
2. Amputation knife (Liston).
3. Tissue forceps (Lane or Fagge).
4. Artery forceps, straight, 20 cm (8 in) (Spencer Wells).
5. Long drainage tube, plastic, pre-packed sterile for use with Redivac or similar suction device.
6. Amputation saw.

The femur is sawn across and the leg removed. The major vessels are picked up with forceps and ligated before release of the tourniquet. The tourniquet is released, hot packs applied and the smaller vessels picked up and ligated. The sciatic nerve is divided at the level of bone section.

Fig. 23.129 Amputation through the middle third of the thigh. (Farquharson and Rintoul.)

If a tourniquet cannot be used, perhaps due to a high level of amputation, the femoral vessels are identified, ligated and divided before the muscles are cut across. The procedure then follows that described previously.

The muscles and fascia are sutured together over the end of the femur, a drain is inserted and the skin closed in the usual manner.

(*Alternatively the limb may be amputated by disarticulation through the knee joint. In this procedure the skin flaps are fashioned at a lower level, but the basic technique is similar to that described.*)

Tendon suture (end to end anastomosis and free grafts)

DEFINITION

The repair of a divided tendon either as an end to end anastomosis with or without tendon lengthening or transplant; free tendon grafts.

POSITION

Supine, with affected hand extended on an arm table.

INSTRUMENTS

Sponge-holding forceps (Rampley), 5
Scalpel handles No. 3 with No. 10 blades (Bard Parker), 2
Scalpel handles No. 9 with No. 15 blades (Bard Parker), 2
Fine artery forceps, straight, mosquito, 5
Fine artery forceps, curved on flat, mosquito, 10
Fine dissecting forceps, toothed (Gillies), 2
Fine dissecting forceps, non-toothed (McIndoe), 2
Fine scissors, curved on flat, 10 cm (4 in) (Kilner)
Fine scissors, straight, 10 cm (4 in) (Strabismus)
Scissors, stitch, 13 cm (5 in)
Fine tissue forceps (McIndoe), 6
Fine retractors, double end, 'rake' (Lane), 2
Skin hooks (Gillies or McIndoe), 4
Probe, malleable silver
Crocodile or tendon passing forceps

Fig. 23.130 (A to D) The classical method of tendon suture. Note the manner in which the suture material, with a needle at each end, is 'spliced' into the tendon, and that the knots are buried between the cut ends. (E and F) Tendon repair by the use of withdrawable sutures of stainless steel wire (*After Bunnell*). (Farquharson and Rintoul.)

Fine bowl awl
Fine needle holder (West)
Lead hand splint or similar, for immobilisation of hand during operation
6 cm (2½ in) straight round-bodied needles for transfixion of tendon during operation (optional)

Fig. 23.131 Method of uniting a large flat tendon. (Farquharson and Rintoul.)

Fig. 23.132 Method of repairing an extensor tendon severed over the proximal phalangeal joint. (Bailey.)

2 (3/0) Plain catgut or Dexon for ligatures
2 or 2·5 (3/0 or 2/0) Plain catgut or Dexon on a small half-circle cutting needle for subcutaneous sutures
33 SWG or 40 SWG stainless-steel wire or 1·5 (4/0) silk, polyester or polyethylene on a small curved non-traumatic needle for tendon sutures
Pearl button may be required for a 'pull through' suture
1·5 and 2 (4/0 and 3/0) Silk or nylon on small curved cutting needles for skin sutures
Malleable aluminium or plaster of Paris splint will be required.

OUTLINE OF PROCEDURE

For an end to end anastomosis, the cut tendon is exposed and fibrous tissue excised to effect mobility. The ends are approximated and straight round-bodied needles may be used to transfix the tendons and prevent the ends from retracting. The ends may or may not be trimmed with a knife, before suturing with stainless-steel wire or silk sutures, which are generally placed as modified mattress sutures.

Some surgeons use a 'pull through' wire technique in which a short strand of wire is included in the loop on one side of the anastomosis and is used to pull the wire suture out after the tendon has healed. This strand of wire is threaded on to a needle and passed through the skin at a point proximal to the anastomosis, and tied over a small pad of gauze. After the wire suture used for the anastomosis has been inserted in the distal part of the tendon, it is passed through the skin distal to this point (about 13 mm (½ in) to

Fig. 23.133 Successive stages in the operation of free flexor tendon grafting. (Rank.)

(A) The free graft placed in position and sutured to the terminal profundus tendon stump after resection of the damaged tendons and most of the tendon sheath. Note the two pulleys retained to prevent prolapse of the graft.
(B) The flap sutured back before proceeding to the proximal graft junction.

25 mm (1 in) away) and is tied over a pearl button. This 'pull through' technique of Bunnell may be used also to take the tension off a suture line. In this case the tendon is approximated in the usual manner with fine stainless-steel wire or silk sutures, and a 'pull through' wire inserted proximal to the point of anastomosis being tied over a button, with slight tension. This relieves the strain on the anastomosis until healing is complete. The technique is applied mainly to the repair of extensor tendons although it may be used equally well for flexor tendons, especially transposition procedures.

In the case of injuries to flexor tendons in the fingers, it is generally preferable to make the anastomosis in the palm. Although an end to end anastomosis may be possible, a length of tendon is usually transplanted from the forearm or foot to bridge the gap between the palm and the distal phalanx of the finger.

A mid-lateral incision is made in the affected finger, the flexor tendons identified and removed completely, or leaving a small tag where the profundus is inserted into the terminal phalanx. The tendon pulleys are preserved if possible. The palm is incised and the proximal portion of the tendon identified and drawn into the palm with tissue forceps.

A tendon graft of suitable length is removed from the flexor aspect of the forearm and wrist (palmaris longus), or a plantaris tendon or extensor tendon to the toe and is threaded through the tendon tunnel from the palm and under the finger pulleys to the terminal phalanx. At this point it is either sutured to the remaining tag of tendon or a hole is drilled through the terminal phalanx and the tendon approximated to its insertion with a suture which passes through the bone. This suture is tied over a pearl button for subsequent removal. The skin wounds of the finger and forearm or foot are closed in the usual manner.

The finger is placed in the correct degree of flexion and an anastomosis made with the proximal tendon and graft in the palm. This is achieved either by simple side to side suture, or by interweaving the tendons before suturing. The palm wound is closed and the finger, as for all tendon sutures, is immobilised with a malleable splint or plaster of Paris back slab, wool and bandages.

REFERENCES AND FURTHER READING

CRAWFORD ADAMS, J. (1976) *Standard Orthopaedic Operations*. Edinburgh: Churchill Livingstone.
FARQUHARSON, E. L. AND RINTOUL, R. F. (1972) *Textbook of Operative Surgery*. Edinburgh: Churchill Livingstone.
HALL, R. M. (1972) *Air Instrument Surgery Orthopaedics*. New York: Springer Verlag. (Courtesy Surgical Products 3M United Kingdom Limited.)
MACFARLANE, D. A. & THOMAS, L. P. (1972) *Textbook of Surgery*. Edinburgh: Churchill Livingstone.
RANK, Sir B. *et al.* (1973) *Surgery of Repair as applied to Hand Injuries*. Edinburgh: Churchill Livingstone.
ROBINSON, J. O. (1965) *Surgery*. London: Longman.
WILSON, J. N. (1976) *Watson Jones: Fractures and Joint Injuries*. Edinburgh: Churchill Livingstone.

24
PLASTIC OPERATIONS

Repair of cleft lip and cleft palate

DEFINITION

Closure of a harelip to establish continuity of muscle which is important for modelling the underlying bone and to produce a cosmetically acceptable lip; closure of a cleft palate and pushing back the soft palate so that it can approximate with the posterior pharyngeal wall.

POSITION

Harelip – supine. Cleft palate – supine, with sandbag between the shoulder blades and the neck in extension.

INSTRUMENTS

   Sponge-holding forceps (Rampley), 2
   Scalpel No. 9 with Nos. 11 and 15 blades (Bard Parker), 2
   Scalpel handles No. 5 with Nos. 11 and 15 blades (Bard Parker), 2
   Long fine dissecting forceps, toothed (Waugh), 2
   Long fine dissecting forceps, non-toothed (Waugh), 2
   Fine dissecting forceps, toothed (Gillies), 2
   Fine dissecting forceps, non-toothed (McIndoe), 2
   Artery forceps, curved on flat (Micron)
   Fine scissors, curved on flat, sharp points
   Fine scissors, straight, sharp points
   Fine tissue forceps (McIndoe), 2
   Skin hooks (Gillies)
   Angled tongue depressor
   Mouth gag with appropriate size of blade (Dott)
   Cleft palate raspatory, left and right patterns will be required, 2
   Cleft palate sharp hook; blunt hook may also be needed
   Raspatory (Howarth or Heath)
   Cleft palate sharp hook and raspatory
   Dissector (Macdonald)
   Harelip traction bow (Denis Browne)
   Cleft palate needle (Reverdin)
   Retractor, spring action (Kilner)
   Fine needle holder, fulcrum lever type with ratchet
   Fine needle holder (Gillies)
   Skin pen and sterile ink (e.g. Bonney's blue)
   Diathermy leads, electrodes and lead anchoring forceps
   Suction tubing, fine nozzles and tube anchoring forceps.

Fig. 24.1 Kilner Dott Insulated Mouth Gag with East Grinstead Blades.

Fig. 24.2 Denis Browne Hare Lip Traction Bow.

Fig. 24.3 Double End Cleft Palate Elevator (angled to side and on flat).

Fig. 24.4 Cleft Palate Sharp Hook and Raspatory.

Fig. 24.5 Cleft Palate Raspatories, Right and Left (Curved).

Fig. 24.6 Kilner Spring-Action Retractor

Fig. 24.7 Mitchell Trimmer.

Fig. 24.8 Gillies Skin Hook.

Figs. 24.1 to 24.8 Instruments for cleft lip and cleft palate. (Chas. F. Thackray Ltd.)

2 (3/0) Plain or chromic catgut or Dexon on cleft palate needles for cleft palate and harelip (mucosa)

1·5 or 1 (4/0 or 5/0) Silk or nylon on small curved non-traumatic cutting needles for harelip repair (skin).

OUTLINE PROCEDURE

Cleftlip. A Z-plasty type of incision is made, extending from the apex of the cleft to the mucosal edge of the lip. The tissues are undermined at each side of the cleft and if this extends up to the nose, the tissues of the cheek will be undermined towards the orbit in order to lessen tension when the wound is closed. The edges of the cleft are excised, drawn together and a fine silk suture inserted at the mucocutaneous junction in the centre. The muscles are approximated with catgut or Dexon sutures before completing the suture line with interrupted sutures of silk or nylon for the skin and fine plain or chromic catgut or Dexon for the mucosa. (Some surgeons apply a traction bow to relieve the tension on the suture line.)

Cleft Palate. A suitable mouth gag is inserted, an incision made on each side of the cleft soft palate and the edges of the cleft are freshened. Two flaps of mucosa and muscle with their bases posteriorly are raised on each side from the underlying hard palate.

These two flaps are transposed and sutured together in the midline, thereby leaving a defect. This defect is filled temporarily with a gauze pack and will eventually epithelialise.

N.B. *Cleftlip* cleft palate operations are rarely done as a combined procedure; the lip is repaired at about 12 weeks of age and the palate before the development of speech.

Fig. 24.10 Milton Gillies Needle Holder.

Fig. 24.9 Micron Artery Forceps.

Fig. 24.11 Reverdin Needles.

Figs. 24.9 to 24.11 Instruments for cleft lip and cleft palate (*cont'd.*). (Chas. F. Thackray Ltd.)

Fig. 24.12 The Mirault-Blair operation for cleft lip. The incisions are made between three points on each side of the cleft – A, B and C, and A′, B′ and C′. These points are determined by careful calculation, and are marked with tattooing before mobilisation. Points A and A′ are placed so that their approximation will correct the asymmetry of the nostrils. The distances A′C′ (curved as necessary) and B′C′ should equal respectively AC and BC; the approximation of C′ to C and of B′ to B should provide adequate depth to the lip. The vermilion border is constructed by imbrication, in order to prevent either notching or a redundant papilla. (Farquharson and Rintoul.)

Fig. 24.13 Operative repair of cleft palate (Wardill). This combines repair of the cleft with elongation of the soft palate. The margins of the cleft are pared, and the nasal mucosa is defined and separated upwards. Muco-periosteal flaps are raised by incisions placed in the manner shown, and are thoroughly mobilised. The posterior flaps are allowed to slide backwards, so that elongation of the soft palate is produced; to facilitate this, the hamulus is divided. The anterior flaps are brought together in the mid line. The cleft is then repaired in two layers – nasal mucosa first. (Farquharson and Rintoul.)

SKIN GRAFTS

Split-thickness Thiersch-type graft

DEFINITION

This is a graft which does not include all layers of the skin but only the epidermis and the tips of the papilla of the dermis. It is a useful type of graft which takes well and is therefore very widely used by surgeons. However, as healing takes place it contracts because it does not contain elastic fibres, does not have any sweat glands or hair, and may not, therefore, be cosmetically acceptable.

POSITION

This depends upon the location of the donor and recipient areas. In most cases where the graft is taken from the thigh for transference to an anterior area of the body, supine is suitable.

INSTRUMENTS

Sponge holding forceps (Rampley), 4
Scalpel handles No. 3 with Nos. 10 and 15 blades (Bard Parker), 2
Fine dissecting forceps, toothed (Gillies), 2
Fine dissecting forceps non-toothed (McIndoe), 2
Fine dissecting scissors, curved on flat, 10 cm (4 in) (Kilner)
Scissors, curved on flat 13 cm (5 in) (Mayo)
Long fine scissors, curved on flat 17 cm (7 in)
Fine artery forceps, straight or curved on flat (Mosquito), 10

Fig. 24.14 The varying thicknesses of the split-skin graft, showing the constituents of each. (McGregor.)

Fig. 24.15 Blair skin grafting razor with 178 mm fixed blade and protective guard.

Fig. 24.16 Braithewaite modified Humby skin graft knife, disposable blade.

Fig. 24.17 Net graft cutter.

Fig. 24.18 Eckhoff mapping pen.

Fig. 24.19 Gabarro graft board and measure.

Figs. 24.15 to 24.19 Skin grafting instruments. (Down's Surgical Ltd.)

Skin hooks (Gillies), 2
Skin graft boards (Metal Gabarro and teak), 2
Skin grafting razor (Blair) or
Skin grafting knife (Braithwaite modified Humby)
Net skin graft-cutter
Graft manipulators
Skin pen and sterile ink (e.g. Bonney's blue)
Towel clips (Backhaus or cross action), 6
Needle holders (Gillies), 2
Steel rule 15 cm (6 in)
Irrigation syringe and normal saline
Diathermy leads, electrodes and anchoring forceps
Thrombin, 5 ml syringe and hypodemic needles
1·5 (4/0) or finer, silk, braided nylon or Dexon on fine curved cutting needles sizes 12 to 16
Sterile gamgee tissue impregnated with proflavine emulsion, or polyurethane foam
Paraffin gauze dressing or similar
Cotton wool and crêpe bandages
Plaster of Paris may be required.

OUTLINE OF PROCEDURE

Unless it forms part of a fresh surgical defect, e.g., excision of tumour, debrided traumatic area, the recipient area is prepared by trimming excess granulation tissue to provide a smooth vascular bed for the graft. Haemostasis is secured by picking up blood-vessels and twisting them off or utilising diathermy.

The donor area is prepared by smearing lightly with sterile liquid paraffin or petroleum jelly and the graft is taken with a hand knife or dermatome.

A hand knife consists of a slender blade about 24 cm (9 in) long fitted to a handle. The knife may include also a guide, which is adjustable for various graft thicknesses. An example of the first type is the Blair knife, and of the second type, the Braithwaite knife (Fig. 24.15). When using a hand knife the skin is flattened by pressing a graft board at each end of the donor area.

There are two basic types of dermatome, the Paget's drum type and the mechanical oscillating blade type (Fig. 24.24A). The Paget's dermatome is prepared by adjusting the 'depth of graft' mechanism and coating the half cylinder with skin graft adhesive. Adhesive is applied also to the donor area, and the edge of the cylinder is placed at the point on the skin selected for the commencement of the graft. As the cylinder is rotated slightly, the skin adheres and is lifted so that the graft may be taken by oscillating the cutting blade. This manoeuvre is continued until the whole surface of the cylinder is covered with skin. The graft is then detached from the donor area and removed from the drum.

The mechanical type dermatome is adjusted for depth of graft and is operated with a 'planning action' over the selected donor area. A small amount of lubricant may be applied to the skin and under-surface of the dermatome before taking the graft. If a very thin graft is required, sterile adhesive tape or polyvinyl can be applied to the skin, which is cut with the tape still attached. This provides support to aid manipulation of the graft afterwards.

The graft is applied as a sheet, sutured at its periphery to the skin around the recipient area.

When insufficient skin is available or where fixation is difficult, as in the perineum or axilla, 'mesh grafting' may be employed. The graft is passed through an instrument which shreds it into a regular meshwork of skin (Fig. 24.22). Applying traction to the four corners of the mesh increases the areas, and although the final cosmetic result varies greatly, it allows skin to be applied to surfaces where other methods may fail.

Firm pressure is applied over the graft for a few minutes, and layer of petroleum jelly gauze is then placed over the whole area. A pad of polyurethane sponge or cotton-wool

Fig. 24.20 Cutting a graft with the Braithwaite knife. (McGregor.)

Fig. 24.21 The translucency of a thin split-skin graft (A), and a thick split-skin graft (B). (McGregor.)

Plastic Operations

Fig. 24.22 Meshing a skin graft. The split-skin graft, fed between the rollers, emerges meshed so that, stretched, it can be expanded to cover a much larger area. (McGregor.)

Fig. 24.23 The use of a mesh graft.
(A) Shows the mesh graft applied to a granulating area. (B) Shows the intermediate stage of healing by epidermal spread from the graft, seen by the increased blurring of the outline of the mesh. (C) The healed result, showing how the background of the original mesh is still visible. (McGregor.)

Fig. 24.24 Cutting a graft with the drum dermatome. (A) Painting drum with adhesive. (B) Skin lifted by drum. (C) Cutting the graft. (D) Stripping graft from drum. (McGregor.)

Fig. 24.25 Cutting a graft with the electric dermatome. (McGregor.)

impregnated with proflavine emulsion is very useful for exerting localised pressure on the graft and the dressing is completed with gauze and wool and crêpe bandages applied firmly.

Some surgeons inject a solution of thrombin under the skin graft before applying pressure. This serves to encourage adherence of the graft to the underlying tissues and helps to avoid accumulation of fluid which can prevent the graft taking. Finally, the

Fig. 24.26 The method of cutting a full thickness graft. (McGregor.)

operation is completed by dressing the donor area with petroleum jelly gauze, gauze, wool and bandages.

Unused portions of skin can be stored in a refrigerator at 1°C (34°F), spread on petroleum jelly gauze, and be placed in a sterile container with a few drops of normal saline. The grafts are then available for application as required in theatre or ward without administering an anaesthetic. Normal storage is up to three weeks.

Sometimes there is only limited skin available for auto-grafting, as for example in major burns involving 35–40 per cent of the body surface area. In such cases temporary skin cover may be provided with homografts from a skin bank, or by lyophilised homografts or zenografts.

Rejection of a skin homograft usually takes place in 8–10 days in a healthy individual, although this rejection may be delayed for 21 days in a burned patient. The development of tissue typing has enabled rejection to be postponed for up to 90 days for correctly matched skin (Roberts, 1976).

Application of homografts extends the period available to cover a burned area with autografts; a donor site on a patient can be used every 10–14 days. Ideally, eventually perfect matched skin from a skin bank will provide permanent cover, but present technology has not yet achieved this.

Skin bank. Skin for the bank is removed from cadavers under sterile conditions within 6–16 hours of death. Blood and spleen samples are also taken for tissue typing of the skin.

The homograft is spread and suspended in a film of 15 per cent glycerol with antibiotics, in a sealed nylon envelope. The envelope is mounted in a metal frame and the whole cooled with liquid nitrogen in a programmed freezing apparatus to $-100°C$, and then stored in liquid nitrogen at $-196°C$.

Whole skin graft   Split-skin graft

Fig. 24.27 The suturing and dressing of a whole skin graft and a split-skin graft showing the similarities and differences. Note the overlap of the split-skin graft being trimmed at the first dressing. (McGregor.)

To use the graft, the frame is immersed in sterile water at 37°C. Once thawed the viable graft cannot be re-frozen.

Lyophilised skin homograft. These are non-viable, freeze-dried homografts. They are collected from cadavers under clean conditions within 12–72 hours of death. After being freeze-dried they are packed in polythene envelopes, sterilised by ethylene oxide gas or gamma radiation and stored at room temperature.

The skin is re-constituted in sterile saline or Ringers solution for 15 minutes before use. The graft is applied to affected area, and although dead, provides a biological dressing and scaffolding for epithelialisation. With superficial burns, when the affected area heals, the lyophilised skin gradually peels off.

Used this way as a temporary dressing to cover burns or trauma defects after de-sloughing, the lyophilised homograft reduces evaporative fluid and capillary bleeding and helps to avoid infection. This contributes to preparing the bed for the final graft.

Lyophilised zenografts. These are grafts prepared from pigs skin and are available commercially as porcine skin graft (Corethum-Ethnor, Porcine Skin-Armour). They are used in a similar manner to lyophilised homografts.

Full-thickness Wolfe-type graft

DEFINITION

This is a free graft which includes all layers of the skin. Although it does not 'take' as easily as the Thiersch graft, it does not contract, contains sweat glands and hair and is therefore more cosmetically acceptable.

POSITION

This varies with the area to be grafted.

INSTRUMENTS

As for Thiersch graft
Sterile jaconet or polyvinyl sheet for patterns.

OUTLINE OF PROCEDURE

The recipient area is prepared as described previously by trimming granulation tissue. A pattern of the recipient area is made with a piece of sterile jaconet and this is used to outline the graft on the donor area with pen and ink.

An incision is made round this ink outline and deepened to the subcutaneous tissues. Starting at one end, the graft is undermined, held up with skin hooks and dissected free from the underlying fat. It is important that very little or no fat be included with the graft.

The graft is sutured at its periphery to the skin surrounding the recipient area. Fine silk or Dexon is used to obtain close approximation.

Pressure dressings are applied as for Thiersch graft.

Pedicle type flap

DEFINITION

This type of graft is a tube which includes skin and all subcutaneous tissue down to the muscle layer and is transferred to the recipient area with part of the tube still attached to the donor site. It is through this attachment to the donor site that the tube contains its blood supply and nourishment until it is established on the recipient area.

POSITION

This varies with the location of the donor and recipient areas.

INSTRUMENTS

As for Thiersch graft
Sterile jaconet or polyvinyl sheet for patterns.

OUTLINE OF PROCEDURE

The number of stages necessary for this procedure depends upon the distance of the donor site from the recipient area and also whether the two areas can be brought together into direct contact with each other, e.g., hand to abdomen.

Two-stage operation, e.g., hand to abdomen and cross leg flap

Abdominal Flap. A large defect in the skin of the hand may be replaced by raising an abdominal skin flap and attaching it to the hand which is immobilised on the abdominal wall until healing is complete.

A pattern of the defect is made on a piece of sterile jaconet and the outline transferred to the selected abdominal area, e.g., inguinal region, with pen and ink. The outlined flap and underlying fat are raised on three sides and a Thiersch graft applied to the raw area beneath.

Fig. 24.28 The basic types of flap transfer. (McGregor.)

The hand defect is prepared in the usual manner, is approximated to the donor site, and the flap sutured at its periphery to the skin surrounding the recipient area. Pressure dressings of petroleum jelly gauze, gauze, polyurethane sponge, proflavine wool, white wool and crêpe or adhesive bandages are applied.

Two or three weeks later, the fourth side of the flap is detached and sutured to the adjacent recipient skin edge. The donor site is trimmed at its periphery and if a defect remains where the flap has been detached, a further Thiersch graft is applied. Dressings are applied as before.

Cross Leg Flap. The recipient area, e.g., over the tibia, is prepared by excising excess granulation tissue and surrounding skin. A pattern of the defect, usually oblong in shape, is prepared on sterile jaconet. The outline of the pattern is transferred with pen and ink on to the calf of the other leg and an incision made round three sides of the outline. The base of the flap is always more anterior so that when the leg is crossed over the recipient site, the flap covers the defect without kinking.

The flap is sutured at its periphery to the skin surrounding the recipient area. The area underneath the raised flap on the donor leg is covered with a Thiersch graft from the thigh. Pressure dressings are applied in the usual way and the legs are immobilised with plaster of Paris bandages.

Three weeks later the flap is detached from its base and the fourth side sutured to the adjacent skin edge, followed by the application of dressings as before.

Multistage operation

If a pedicle graft needs to be transferred some distance, this is usually performed by raising a 'tubed flap' which can be moved in stages to the recipient area, e.g., abdomen to face.

A mobile area such as the inguinal region of the abdomen is selected and parallel incisions made for the entire length of tube required. The skin between these incisions is undermined and sewn together underneath to form a closed tube, the ends of which remain attached to the abdomen. The skin on each side of this raised tube is undermined and approximated with silk, nylon or Dexon sutures.

About 3 weeks later, one end of the tube is detached from the abdomen and sutured to a prepared area on the forearm. The wound caused by raising the tube on the abdomen is closed and the arm immobilised to the abdominal wall with pressure dressings of gauze, wool and bandages or adhesive strapping.

After a further 3 weeks, the tube is detached from the abdomen and sutured to the

Fig. 24.29 The classical cross-leg flap positions. (McGregor.)

Fig. 24.30 Raising a tube pedicle. (McGregor.)

prepared recipient area on the face. The arm is again immobilised whilst the facial attachment 'takes', and the wound caused when detaching the flap from the abdomen is closed with silk or Dexon sutures.

The final stage consists in severing the attachment of the tube from the hand and completing the suture of that end to the area on the face. The tube of skin is excised level with its attachment to the hand or forearm.

Rhinoplasty

DEFINITION

This term describes a wide variety of corrective procedures on the nose, any combination or all of the following may be carried out; excision of nasal hump, correction of sunken bridge, adjustment of length of the nose, narrowing of the nose, remodelling of the nasal tip, rotation or pedicle flap (with or without Z-plasty) to cover nasal defect. The operation is generally undertaken to restore to normal contour anatomy, deviations from the normal e.g., those arising from trauma, familial or racial deformity.

POSITION

Supine.

INSTRUMENTS

Scalpel handles No. 3 with Nos. 10 and 15 blades (Bard Parker), 2
Fine dissecting forceps, toothed (Gillies), 2
Fine dissecting forceps, non-toothed (McIndoe), 2
Fine artery forceps, straight, mosquito, 10
Fine artery forceps, curved or flat, mosquito, 10
Fine tissue forceps (McIndoe), 5
Skin hooks (Gillies), 4
Fine scissors, curved on flat, 10 cm (4 in) (Kilner)
Scissors, curved on flat, 13 cm (5 in) (Mayo)
Dissector (MacDonald or Durham)
Small retractors, double hook, 2
Small retractors, double end, 'rake' (Lane), 2
Fine needle holder (Gillies or Kilner)
Stent composition material or plaster of Paris moulded into a splint
2 and 1·5 (3/0 and 4/0) Plain catgut or Dexon for ligatures
2 (3/0) Plain catgut or Dexon on a half-circle cutting needle for subcutaneous sutures
1·5 or 1 (4/0 or 5/0) Silk, etc., on a small curved cutting needle (preferably non-traumatic) for skin sutures.

If a bone graft is contemplated
Cancellous bone from the bone bank (with bone-cutting forceps, etc.)
or instruments for taking a bone graft (Fig. 23.89A).

If nasal correction is contemplated
Nasal saw (Joseph)
Nasal rasp
Scissors, angled (Heyman)
Nasal septum forceps (Jansen Middleton)
Nasal raspatory (Hill or Howarth)
Nasal punch forceps, small and medium (Luc), 2
Nasal speculum, long (St Clair Thompson)
Dressing forceps, angled
Small gouges, 4 mm, 6 mm, 8 mm, 10 mm (Jenkins)
Small chisels, 4 mm, 6 mm, 8 mm, 10 mm
Ribbon gauze impregnated with 1 in 10,000 adrenaline.

If prosthesis is contemplated

Rhinoplasty implant e.g. SILASTIC® silicone elastomer implant designed for augmenting the sunken bridge of the nose (available in three sizes).

OUTLINE OF PROCEDURE

With the exception of external tissue defects (i.e. skin loss – excisions of tumours), the surgical approach is always from within the nasal cavity. The incisions are made on both sides between the upper and lower lateral cartilages, extending towards the top of the nasal septum. They are pushed through the membranous septum to separate the columella and septum. The skin of the nose is elevated with scissors up to the level of the nasal bones. The periosteum is then elevated from the nasal bones with a long raspatory.

Fig. 24.31 Removal of nasal hump with saw.

Fig. 24.32 SILASTIC® nasal implants and Safian technique for correction of sunken nasal bridge. (Dow Corning International.)

Fig. 24.33 Very extensive molluscum sebaceum (confirmed by biopsy) excised and repaired by simple glabellar flap. A modification is also shown which is useful when there is difficulty in closing the secondary defect of forehead. (McGregor.)

A nasal saw is used to remove a nasal bump, and the surfaces are smoothed with rasps. A sunken bridge can be corrected with a bone graft or SILASTIC® Rhinoplasty implant.

The nose may be narrowed by detaching the nasal bones from the septum in the midline and the maxilla laterally. These bones are then infractured and repositioned medially, thereby narrowing the nose. Shortening of the nose necessitates a triangular resection of the nasal septum.

Plastic remodelling of the nasal tip involves excision of height, width and length of the alar cartilage through a second incision at the junction of the skin and mucous membrane.

After evacuation of any blood clots from beneath the skin, subcutaneous sutures may be inserted followed by suture of the skin edges with Dexon or silk. A nasal pack is usually inserted in both nasal cavities; external splints of Stent or plaster of Paris may be applied.

Figure 24.33 illustrates the defect left following excision of an extensive molluscum sebaceum, repaired by a simple glabellar rotation flap. The area is dressed as for skin graft.

Operation for protruding ears

DEFINITION

The removal of segments of aural cartilage and reconstruction of antihelix.

POSITION

Supine, with the head turned to one side.

INSTRUMENTS

Scalpel handles No. 9 with Nos. 10 and 15 blades (Bard Parker), 2
Fine dissecting forceps, toothed (Gillies)
Fine dissecting forceps, non-toothed (McIndoe)
Fine artery forceps, curved on flat, mosquito, 5
Skin hooks (Gillies), 2
Fine tissue forceps (McIndoe), 2
Fine scissors, curved on flat, 10 cm (4 in) (Kilner)
Small retractors, double end, 'rake' (Lane), 2
Dissector (MacDonald)
Fine needle holder (Gillies or Kilner)
1·5 (4/0) Plain catgut or Dexon for ligatures
1·5 or 1 (4/0 or 5/0) Silk, etc., on a small curved cutting needle (preferably non-traumatic) for skin sutures.

OUTLINE OF PROCEDURE

The operation consists essentially of removing a portion of auricular cartilage so that when an appropriate amount of post-auricular skin is excised, approximation of the wound tends to draw the ears into a more normal position. Small vessels are ligated or twisted off and the wound closed with fine silk sutures.

Mammaplasty (Cronin technique)

DEFINITION

Prosthetic breast restoration as an augmentation procedure or following subcutaneous mastectomy, using a seamless, thin walled, contoured breast prosthesis (SILASTIC®).

POSITION

Sitting or supine possibly Trendelenberg.

INSTRUMENTS

General set (Figs. 14.1 to 14.28)
Local infiltration set (Fig. 10.35) plus 22 gauge spinal needle, with 0·5 per cent Lignocaine (Xylocaine) and 1 : 200,000 adrenaline, optional
Scissors, curved on flat, long, Metzenbaum

Fig. 24.34 SILASTIC® mammary prosthesis. (Dow Corning International.)

Retractors, Deaver, 25 mm (1 in), 2
Retractors, rake, medium, 2
Special template (not heat sterilisable)
Diathermy leads, electrodes and anchoring forceps
Irrigation syringe and saline or topical antibiotic solution
Long drainage tube and Redivac
2 (3/0) Dermalon sutures on medium curved cutting needles for skins.

OUTLINE OF PROCEDURE

The SILASTIC® Mammary Prosthesis features a seamless, thin walled silicone envelope designed to eliminate edge palpability of the prosthesis following augmentation procedures and subcutaneous mastectomy with prosthetic breast restoration. The uniquely contoured 'tear-drop' design closely simulates normal breast contour when implanted by providing desirable projection of the lower breast area with balanced upper area augmentation. In addition, thin, tightly woven Dacron net patches on the back of the prosthesis permit tissue ingrowth for positive fixation to the chest wall. Because body tissue or fluid will not invade the prosthesis itself, it retains initial softness when implanted while resisting absorption or degeneration.

The SILASTIC® Mammary Prosthesis is available in eight sizes to (1) meet the requirements of different operative procedures and patient conditions, (2) more adequately fulfil the demand for variations in tissue bulk, and (3) facilitate the achievement of symmetry. The extra-fill sizes are specifically designed for breast restoration following subcutaneous mastectomy.

The plastic template supplied with each prosthesis is designed to serve as a guide for both positioning of the implant and sharp or blunt dissection. A 13 mm (½ in) circumferential collar encircles each template.

In use, the template should be positioned over the breast to achieve the ultimately desired contour. A line is then marked on the skin around the edge of the template collar. This guide line provides the outer limits for the area requiring dissection.

With the patient in the sitting position, the inframammary fold is marked symmetrically beneath each breast. The small size can be inserted through a 6 cm (2½ in) incision, while shorter or longer incisions can be made for other sizes as appropriate. The line should be scratched in lightly with a needle prior to the skin prep. The template may be used as a guide to mark area of dissection.

Extending the patient's arms at right angles to her sides extends the pectoral muscles and facilitates dissection of the breast from the muscles. Bringing the arms to the sides of the body relaxes the skin and muscle and may ease the insertion of the implants. However, the complete operation can be done with the arms in either position.

Anaesthesia is usually general but the procedure is not infrequently performed under local anaesthesia. One half per cent lignocaine with 1:200,000 adrenalin is infiltrated, fan-shaped between the breast and the pectoralis major muscle using a 22 gauge spinal needle.

The incision is made through the skin and subcutaneous tissue down to the loose superficial fascia over the rib cage. The upper edge of the wound is lifted with a rake retractor and with sharp dissection, the anterior surface of the fascia over the pectoralis major muscle is exposed. From this point, blunt dissection with a tonsil sponge in a ring forceps or the gloved fingers may be efficacious. Not infrequently, however, the use of long handled scissors will be needed. Dever or Harrington retractors are helpful and sometimes the Trendelenburg position may help the illumination of the cavity. Some surgeons have used a headlight.

Of greatest importance is that the cavity be made of *generous* size, directing particular attention to dissection of the anterior axillary fold and superiorly and medially. Forcing the implant into a small cavity will result in undue firmness of the breast due to the pressure of the surrounding tissues. Hemostasis should be meticulous and is best accomplished by electrocoagulation. The space should be irrigated with saline, or, if preferred, with an antibiotic mixture such as neomycin – 0.5 gm, or Bacitracin – 10,000 units.

The breast is lifted up with a Dever retractor. To facilitate sliding the Dacron spots over the floor of the cavity, a wide ribbon retractor or a piece of plastic, such as Vi-drape, is inserted first. The implant is then gradually forced through the small incision with a ring forceps and the fingers, the thin flattened part inserted first. The retractors and/or plastic film are then removed and the exact positioning of the implant is completed by the manipulation and inspection of the two inferior Dacron spots to detect any undesirable rotation.

The wounds are closed in layers, the final skin closure being with a continuous 2 (3/0) Dermalon intradermal suture which can be left in for 2 weeks without leaving suture marks.

As with any large wound, serum accumulation may sometimes be troublesome, and is indicated by enlargement, firmness and discomfort of the breast. After sterilising the skin, an 18 to 20 gauge needle is inserted obliquely (to avoid damage to implant) through the skin and subcutaneous tissues inferiorly. Usually the fluid formation will subside after one to several aspirations. An alternative method is to insert a small polythene tube at the time of surgery and utilise Redivac.

Note: DOW CORNING® Medical-Grade Silicone Elastomers are among the most non-reactive implant materials available, however, dust, lint, talc, skin oils and other surface contaminants deposited on the prosthesis in handling can evoke foreign body reactions with subsequent fluid and fibrous tissue buildup. Extreme care with strict adherence to aseptic techniques must be employed to prevent contamination of the prosthesis and the possible resultant complications.

If the prosthesis becomes contaminated before sterilisation, scrub thoroughly with a clean, soft-bristled brush in a hot water-soap solution to remove possible surface contaminants. *Use a non-oily cleaner or mild soap. Do not use synthetic detergents or oil-based soap, as these soaps may be absorbed and may subsequently leach out to cause a tissue reaction.* Rinse copiously in hot water and follow with a thorough rinse in distilled water.

To sterilise: Autoclave by one of the following methods:

1. High speed instrument (flash) steriliser – Place on surgical towel in clean open tray. Sterilise 3 minutes at 130°C (270°F) at 28 p.s.i.
2. Standard gravity steriliser – Wrap in surgical towel and place in clean open tray. Sterilise 30 minutes at 120°C (250°F) at 15 p.s.i.

Do *not* use a prevacuum high temperature steriliser as this type of unit will cause the silicone gel to bubble and the prosthesis to swell.

Note: DOW CORNING® Medical-Grade Silicone Elastomers are not deteriorated by repeated autoclaving, thus this method of sterilisation is strongly recommended. Ethylene oxide sterilisation may also be used although it is not recommended unless sufficient data is available regarding the time required for complete gas emission from the product with the specific system employed. (SILASTIC® is the registered trade mark for Dow Corning's silicone elastomer products.)

Fasciectomy for Dupuytren's contracture

DEFINITION

Excision of hypertrophied palmar fascia which has contracted, thereby causing contracture of the fingers.

POSITION

Supine, with the hand extended on an arm table and the fingers separated by securing with a lead hand or similar splint.

INSTRUMENTS

Scalpel handle No. 3 with No. 10 blade (Bard Parker)
Scalpel handle No. 9 with No. 15 blade (Bard Parker)
Fine dissecting forceps, toothed (Gillies), 2
Fine dissecting forceps, non-toothed (McIndoe), 2
Fine scissors, curved (Kilner). Skin hooks (Gillies), 4
Small retractors, double end, 'rake' (Lane), 2
Fine artery forceps, curved on flat, mosquito, 10
Fine artery forceps, straight, mosquito, 10
Fine tissue forceps (McIndoe), 5
Dissector (MacDonald). Probe, malleable silver

640   Operating Theatre Technique

Fig. 24.35 A continuous multiple Z-plasty used in Dupuytren's contracture confined to the little finger ray.
The stages of the procedure are shown diagrammatically in Figure 24.36. (McGregor.)

Fig. 24.36 Planning and execution of the continuous multiple Z-plasty of the type used in the Dupuytren's contracture shown in Figure 24.35. The line of the long incision indicating the extent of the contracted fascia and the intended lines of the transverse limbs of the Z-plasty is shown (A). B shows the Z-plasty drawn to place the transverse limbs in the creases as planned. The good exposure obtained by the longitudinal incision is seen C. D shows the Z-plasty flaps incised, transposed for suture, E, and sutured (F). (McGregor.)

2 (3/0) Plain catgut or Dexon for ligatures
2 and 1·5 (3/0 and 4/0) Silk on small curved cutting needles for skin sutures.
(Instruments for skin graft (p. 621) may be required.)

OUTLINE OF PROCEDURE

A tourniquet is always used for this operation (Chapter 23).

An incision is made in line with the mid-palmar crease from one side of the hand to the other. The skin on each side of the incision is undermined and freed from the palmar fascia, care being taken to avoid 'button holding'.

Beginning proximally, the hypertrophied fascia is dissected from the underlying blood-vessels, nerves and tendons which supply the fingers. If the scar tissue extends to the fingers themselves, a mid-lateral or multiple Z-plasty incision is made and all the hypertrophied fascia excised.

Sometimes the fascia is so adherent to the skin that a segment must be excised, and in this case the defect may require skin grafting.

After fasciectomy is complete the tourniquet may be released and the divided bloodvessel ligated. Alternatively, the tourniquet remains inflated until a pressure dressing has been applied after wound closure.

The wounds are closed with fine silk sutures and petroleum jelly gauze applied followed by a pressure pad to the palm of sponge rubber, or wool impregnated with proflavine emulsion. The dressing is completed with wool and crêpe bandages applied firmly, so that the fingers are immobilised in the position of function.

Hypospadias operation (Denis Browne's procedure)

DEFINITION

The correction of a congenital abnormality where the urethral meatus lies at a point on the penis proximal to its normal position.

POSITION

Supine, with the legs separated.

INSTRUMENTS

Sponge-holding forceps (Rampley), 5
Hypospadias set (Fig 24.37) and lead anchoring forceps.

There is usually a contracted undersurface of the penis in addition to a displaced meatus. The first stage of the operation consists of freeing this contraction before making a new urethra.

A transverse incision is made in the skin just below the glans and extended into the prepuce on each side. The rudimentary corpus spongiosum is then peeled away from the main erectile tissue and reflected towards the penile base. The short fibrous bands which exist on each side of the chordee are divided and the transverse skin incision is closed longitudinally with fine plain catgut or Dexon to effect a lengthening of the penis.

The second stage of the operation follows at a much later date. A fine Malecot's catheter is inserted into the bladder with a fine introducer. A more rigid sound is then passed along this catheter and used to press its mid-shaft towards the perineum. A diathermy knife is then used to cut down on to the catheter which, when seen, is thrust out with the sound. This diverts urine from the operative area until healing has taken place, i.e., perineal urethrostomy.

A U-shaped insertion is made, commencing at one side of the glans, continuing along the undersurface of the penis, around and proximal to the displaced meatus and finishing at the other side of the glans. The skin edges are reflected widely on each side, leaving a central strip of skin extending from the glans to the displaced meatus. The skin edges are brought together to cover the strip of skin in a manner similar to closing a single-breasted coat.

Fig. 24.37 Hypospadias operation.

1. Scalpel handle No. 3 with No. 10 blade (Bard Parker).
2. Scalpel handle No. 9 with No. 15 blade (Bard Parker).
3. Fine dissecting forceps, toothed and non-toothed (Gillies and McIndoe).
4. Iris scissors, straight, sharp points.
5. Fine scissors, curved on flat, 10 cm (4 in) (Kilner).
6. Fine dissecting forceps, toothed, fixation.
7. Fine artery forceps, straight, mosquito, 6.
8. Fine artery forceps, curved on flat, mosquito, 6.
9. Towel forceps for penile holding.
10. Clamping forceps for aluminium collars (Denis Browne).
11. Catheter introducers, flexible and rigid (Denis Browne).
12. Catheter, self-retaining (Malecot), size 12 Charrière gauge.
13. Glass beads and aluminium collars (Denis Browne).
14. Size 5 (2) monofilament nylon and curved cutting needle.
15. 2 and 1·5 (3/0 and 4/0) chromic catgut or Dexon on 16 mm non-traumatic cutting needles.
16. Diathermy electrode and lead.
17. Towel clips, 4.
18. Fine needle holder (Kilner multiple joint).

Approximation is achieved by using monofilament nylon tension sutures held with a lead stop and glass bead at each side of the wound. The procedure is as follows; a glass bead is threaded on to stout monofilament nylon at the end of which has been placed a short piece of crushed lead or aluminium tubing. The nylon is threaded on to a needle and introduced through both skin flaps to emerge on the opposite side. Another bead is threaded on to the nylon followed by an aluminium stop, and both are pushed down the nylon until the correct tension is achieved. The aluminium stop is crushed and excess nylon cut off. The skin edges are then sutured together with very fine catgut or Dexon on a non-traumatic needle, and a longitudinal relaxing incision is made down the whole of the dorsum of the penis to prevent tension to the suture line and swelling.

If the operation area involves the scrotum, it is usual to make a small incision or incisions on each side of it, leading down to the central wound, so as to allow drainage and prevent accumulation of fluid in the scrotal tissues.

REFERENCES AND FURTHER READING

ROBERTS, M. (1976) The skin bank. *Nursing Mirror*, Sept. 2.
MCGREGOR, I. A. (1977) *Fundamental Techniques of Plastic Surgery*. Edinburgh: Churchill Livingstone.

25
UROLOGICAL OPERATIONS

Circumcision

DEFINITION

Partial excision of the penile foreskin.

POSITION

Supine.

INSTRUMENTS

Scalpel handle No. 3 with No. 10 blade (Bard Parker)
Fine dissecting forceps, toothed (Gillies)
Fine dissecting forceps, non-toothed (McIndoe)
Probe, malleable silver
Artery forceps, straight, 18 cm (7 in) (Spencer Wells) *or*
Bone cutters or sinus forceps
Scissors, straight, blunt points (Mayo 13 or 15 cm (5 or 6 in))

Fig. 25.1 Circumcision. (Swinney and Hammersley.)

Fine scissors, curved on flat, dissection points (Kilner)
Fine artery forceps, straight, mosquito, 5
2 (3/0) Chromic catgut or Dexon for ligatures
2 (3/0) Chromic catgut or Dexon on a small curved cutting needle, preferably non-traumatic, for prepuce sutures
Dressing of gauze impregnated with petroleum jelly, Tinct. Benz. Co., or Whiteheads varnish.

OUTLINE OF PROCEDURE

Two artery forceps are clipped to each side of the prepuce opening, and a probe inserted to separate the glans from the prepuce. More traction is applied to the foreskin and a pair of artery forceps or bone cutters is placed obliquely across the prepuce, but distal to the underlying glans. The excess foreskin is excised with a knife and the cut edge allowed to retract. The inner layer of the prepuce has to be slit up the dorsum of the penis to the glans and the redundant piece of skin excised. Any bleeding vessels are picked up and ligated before the cut edge of the skin is sutured to the inner layer of the prepuce.

Excision of hydrocele or encysted hydrocele of the cord

DEFINITION

Removal of a hydrocele sac (formed by the tunica vaginalis surrounding the testicle) or removal of an encysted hydrocele of the cord (formed by the prolongation of the tunica vaginalis from the testicle along the spermatic cord).

POSITION

Supine.

INSTRUMENTS

General set (Fig. 14.1 to 14.28)
Hydrocele trocar and cannula
Diathermy leads, electrodes and lead anchoring forceps
Corrugated drain
2 and 2·5 (3/0 and 2/0) Chromic catgut or Dexon for ligatures
2·5 and 3 (2/0 and 0) Chromic catgut or Dexon on a small half-circle round-bodied needle for deep sutures
2 (3/0) Silk or nylon on a small or medium curved cutting needle for skin sutures.

OUTLINE OF PROCEDURE

Hydrocele. The testicle is exposed through an incision made over the external inguinal ring, extending downwards and inwards towards the pubis. Unless the testicle is very large the incision stops just short of the scrotal skin. The spermatic cord is dissected free and traction applied until the hydrocele sac appears in the lower part of the wound. A trocar and cannula may then be inserted to drain the fluid, and the collapsed tunica vaginalis is cut away with scissors or a diathermy needle, and the innumerable vessels which have been divided during dissection are ligated or diathermised. When haemostasis is complete, a corrugated drain is inserted through a stab wound in the bottom of the scrotum, and the testicle is returned to its normal position.

The wound is closed in layers. Some surgeons remove a hydrocele through an upper scrotal incision, and instead of excising the sac it may be slit up the front, turned back and sutured behind the testicle.

An Encysted Hydrocele of the Cord. The incision, which generally is made over the swelling, usually lies over the inguinal canal, which is incised. The distended sac is freed from other structures of the cord, and ligated above and below before excision. The

Fig. 25.2 Three types of hydrocele. (A) Simple. (B) With Hernia. (C) Hydrocele of the Spermatic Cord. (Swinney and Hammersely.)

surgeon will search towards the internal ring in case there is an extension to the sac, which may form a hernia at a later date. Any sac so found is treated as a hernial sac (Chapter 15). The wound is closed in layers.

Orchidectomy

DEFINITION

Removal of the testicle.

POSITION

Supine.

INSTRUMENTS

General set (Figs. 14.1 to 14.28)
Corrugated drain
2·5 and 3 (2/0 and 0) Chromic catgut, Dexon or silk for ligatures
3 or 4 (0 or 1) Chromic catgut or Dexon on a small half-circle round-bodied needle for muscle (inguinal incision)
2·5 (2/0) Silk or nylon on a small or medium curved cutting needle for skin sutures.

OUTLINE OF PROCEDURE

The testicle is exposed through an inguinal (or scrotal) incision. The spermatic cord is dissected up and the vessels and vas deferens ligated individually, and the testicle is removed. A corrugated drain is inserted into the scrotum through a stab incision and the wound is closed. A pressure dressing is applied.

Urological Operations 647

Vasectomy

DEFINITION

Excision of part of the vas deferens.

POSITION

Supine.

INSTRUMENTS

Sponge-holding forceps (Rampley), 2
Towel clips, 4
Scalpel handle with No. 10 blade *or*
Diathermy scalpel with ball attachment
Fine dissecting forceps, toothed (Gillies), 2
Fine dissecting forceps, non-toothed (McIndoe), 2
Fine scissors, curved on flat (McIndoe or Lahey), 1
Scissors, curved on flat, 13 cm (5 in) (Mayo), 1
Fine artery forceps, curved on flat (Mosquito), 5
Artery forceps, curved on flat (Criles), 2
Tissue forceps, 15 cm (6 in) (Allis), 2
Special vasectomy mobilisation clamp (Tinkler), 1 (Optional)
Diathermy leads and electrodes
Local anaesthetic requisites (Fig. 10.34)
2·5 and 3 (2/0 and 0) Chromic catgut or Dexon for ligatures
2 or 2·5 (3/0 or 2/0) silk or nylon on straight or curved non-traumatic cutting needle for skin sutures.

Fig. 25.3 Vasectomy. (Swinney and Hammersley.)

OUTLINE OF PROCEDURE

The skin and underlying tissues are infiltrated with local anaesthetic. The vas is palpated and either mobilised between the fingers or with a special vasectomy clamp. The skin overlying the vas is incised longitudinally for a few centimetres and the vas is picked up out of the incision with tissue forceps. It is usual to infiltrate the covering sheath of the vas with a few millilitres of local anaesthetic before proceeding further.

The spermatic cord coverings are incised to display the vas deferens proper, a white avascular structure similar in appearance to a strand of spaghetti. The vas is gently lifted and the sheath teased away to free about 5 or 6 cm of vas. The vas is clamped at each end with an artery forceps and the segment between excised and sent for histological examination. The severed ends are ligated with catgut, Dexon (or silk) and a careful inspection made for haemostasis.

The skin is closed with mattress sutures of silk or nylon (some surgeons use catgut or Dexon to avoid having to remove the sutures) and the wound dressed with plastic spray solution such as Nobecutane.

Excision of varicocele

DEFINITION

The ligation and excision of varicose veins in the spermatic cord.

POSITION

Supine.

INSTRUMENTS

General set (Figs. 14.1 to 14.28)
2·5 and 3 (2/0 and 0) Chromic catgut or Dexon for ligatures
3 or 4 (0 or 1) Chromic catgut or Dexon on a small half-circle cutting needle for muscle tendon suture
2·5 (2/0) Silk or nylon on a small or medium curved or straight cutting needle for skin sutures.

OUTLINE OF PROCEDURE

An incision is made over the external inguinal ring and the spermatic cord dissected out. Some of the varicose veins are isolated from the rest of the spermatic vessels and are separated from the cord for about 8 cm (3 in) of their length. These vessels are ligated above and below the varicocele which is then excised. Some surgeons leave these ligatures long and tie them together, so pulling the testicle a little away from the scrotum. The wound is closed.

Orchidopexy

DEFINITION

Placing an undescended testicle into the scrotum (in a child).

POSITION

Supine.

Fig. 25.4 Orchidopexy. (A) Groin incision. (B) Mobilisation of testicle. (C) Excision of hernial sac. (D and E) Dissection of cord structures. (F) Testicle being brought down into scrotum. (G) Operation completed. (Swinney and Hammersley.)

INSTRUMENTS

General set (Figs. 14.1 to 14.28)
Fire artery forceps, curved on flat, mosquito, 10
Fine tissue forceps (McIndoe), 5
Fine-toothed dissecting forceps (Gillies), 2
Fine scissors, curved on flat, 10 cm (4 in) (Kilner or strabismus)
2 and 2·5 (3/0 and 2/0) Chromic catgut or Dexon for ligatures
2·5 (2/0) Chromic catgut or Dexon on a small half-circle or curved non-traumatic round-bodied needle for testicle fixation and hernial sac transfixion

Fig. 25.5   Clutton Bougie. Sizes available: 00/1, 0/2, ½/3, 1/4, 2/5, 3/6, 4/7, 5/8, 6/9, 7/10, 8/11, 9/12, 10/13, 11/14, 12/15, 13/16, 14/17, 15/18 Charrière gauge. Stainless steel.

Fig. 25.6   Lister Bougie. Sizes available: 6/10, 8/12, 10/14, 12/16, 14/18, 16/20, 18/22, 20/24, 26/30 and 28/32 Charrière gauge. Stainless steel.

Fig. 25.7   Clutton Bladder Sound. Sizes available: 9, 12, 15 and 18 Charrière gauge. Stainless steel.

Fig. 25.8   Nélaton Catheter. Sizes available: 8 to 30 Charrière gauge. Rubber or plastic.

Fig. 25.9   Tiemann Catheter. Sizes available: 10 to 26 Charrière gauge. Rubber or plastic.

Fig. 25.10   Olivary Tip Catheter. Sizes available: 5 to 30 Charrière gauge. Plastic.

Fig. 25.11   Coudé Catheter. Sizes available: 5 to 30 Charrière gauge. Plastic.

Fig. 25.12   'Whistle Tip' Catheter. Sizes available: 9 to 45 Charrière gauge. Rubber or plastic.

Urological Operations

Fig. 25.13 Bicoudé Catheter. Sizes available: 5 to 30 Charrière gauge. Plastic.

Fig. 25.14 Harris Catheter. Sizes available: 9 to 45 Charrière gauge. Rubber or plastic.

Fig. 25.15 Foley Self-Retaining Catheter. Sizes available: 5 to 15 ml balloon, 14 to 26 Charrière gauge. Latex or Plastic.

Fig. 25.16 Malecot Self-Retaining Catheter. Sizes available: 9 to 48 Charrière gauge. Rubber.

Fig. 25.17 Foley Self-Retaining Catheter, Haemostatic. Sizes available: 30 to 50 ml balloon, 14 to 26 Charrière gauge. Latex or Plastic.

Fig. 25.18 De Pezzer Self-Retaining Catheter. Sizes available: 12 to 39 Charrière gauge. Rubber.

Fig. 25.19 Alcock-Foley Irrigating Catheter. Sizes available: 14 to 26 Charrière gauge. Latex or Plastic.

Fig. 25.20 Catheter Introducer. (Chas. F. Thackray Ltd.)

Figs. 25.5 to 25.20 Examples of bougies, sound, and catheters. (Eschmann Bros. and Walsh Ltd.)

2·5 or 3 (2/0 or 0) Chromic catgut or Dexon on a small half-circle round-bodied needle for muscle sutures

2 (3/0) Silk or nylon on a small or medium curved cutting needle for skin sutures.

OUTLINE OF PROCEDURE

Through a groin incision, the testicle is mobilised and the hernial sac is excised and the neck transfixed. By dissecting the structures of the cord from the extraperitoneal tissues, the testicle is eventually brought down into the scrotum. It is retained there either by transposing the organ into the opposite side of the scrotum, or by sewing the testicle to the fascia lata in a tunnel constructed between the scrotum and thigh. A second operation is needed three months later, to separate the scrotum and thigh.

Bougies, catheters and sounds (Figs. 25.5 to 25.20)

These are available in a number of materials – rubber, plastic, metal (silver or stainless steel). Some catheters have one lumen, whereas others have several for the purpose of irrigation. They are obtainable with inflatable cuffs or balloons at their distal tip which prevent accidental withdrawal. Catheters at present are measured in the Charrière gauge, size being three times the nominal external diameter expressed in millimetres, usually stated to be a certain French size, e.g. 18FG, which equals 6 mm external diameter. Details of care and sterilisation of catheters are given in Chapter 6.

Cystourethroscopy

DEFINITION

Examination of the interior of the urethra or urinary bladder with an endoscope.

Fig. 25.21 Charrière catheter gauge.

Fig. 25.22 Cystourethroscope and accessories. (Stortz-Rimmer Bros.)

(A) Sheath with obturator.
(B) Catheter deflecting mechanism.
(C) Sheath with catheter deflecting mechanism and telescope in position.
(D) Biopsy or grasping forceps.
(E) Distal end of sheath with obturator.
(F) Telescope in 'position'.
(G) Catheter deflecting mechanism.
(H) Biopsy or grasping forceps.
(I) Ultra sonic suction tube.
(J) Diathermy electrode.

POSITION

Lithotomy or supine.

INSTRUMENTS

Cysto-urethroscope sheath with obturator (of appropriate diameter) (e.g., Stortz, Canny Ryall, Brown Beurger, Braäsch direct vision Geiringer, etc)
Sponge holding forceps (Rampley), 3

Fig. 25.23 Lowsley grasping forceps being used with a fibre optic for oblique telescope. (A.C.M.I.)

Telescopes (Forward oblique, lateral, straight forward retrospective)
Catheter deflecting mechanisms (may be integral with sheath)
Irrigating stopcocks and tubing
Biopsy or grasping forceps
Fibre light or electric cable, and light or low voltage source
Kidney dish
Penile clamp (if local analgesia being used).
Towel clips (Bachaus), 4.

A supply of sterile water, normal saline or 1·5 per cent w/v glycine solution (see Chapter 6, chemical disinfection) at a temperature of 34·5° to 35·5°C should be available to fill the bladder and provide irrigation. This fluid should be dispensed from closed inverted containers 1 or 2 litre, via a suitable connector, tubing and the cystoscope irrigation connection. If large quantities of fluid are required several containers can be interlinked with one another (Fig. 25.26). The flasks should be renewed for each operation.

OUTLINE OF PROCEDURE

Cystoscope optics. Since the first practical cystoscope was devised by Nitze and Leiter in 1879, and until recently, the basic design of cystoscopes has consisted of a small distal lamp and a telescope comprised of a series of small lenses. (Fig. 25.25a) (Wallace, 1975).

Fig. 25.24 Fibre optic illumination system. (Courtesy: Professor H. H. Hopkins, University of Reading.)

Fig. 25.25 Telescope optical systems. The symbols I_1, I_2, I_3 refer to the successive images that are formed. (Courtesy: Professor H. H. Hopkins, University of Reading.)

Two inventions in the last decade by Professor H. H. Hopkins of Reading University have resulted in considerable improvements in the optics of cystoscopes and other endoscopic instruments. These are the application of fibre optics and the development of the rod lens system.

The principals of fibre optics have already been described in Chapter 12. The reader will recall that two types of flexible glass fibres are utilised to convey light or images. When the fibres are arranged in any order in a bundle or in an annular fashion around the cystoscope tube they are said to be incoherent, and are used to transmit light to the distal end of the instrument (Fig. 25.24A).

When the glass fibres are arranged carefully so that the fibres at one end correspond with the fibres at the other, they are termed coherent and can transmit a visual image (Fig. 25.25B).

The second invention of Professor Hopkins was a redesign of the telescope to incorporate a rod lens system. A good deal of optic transmission is lost by the conventional lens system, because the light is dispersed on the sheath walls between the groups of lens. The

Fig. 25.26 Uromatic 'linked' 3 litre plastic irrigation containers. (1·5% w/v glycine solution) set up for cystoscopy. (Travenol Laboratories Ltd.)

Hopkins lens system, utilises a series of glass rods which reduces the light loss by the same principal of reflecting light from the surface of the rods. The ends of the rods are ground to reproduce the lens effect (Fig. 25.25C).

A number of significant advantages are claimed for the rod lens system, and these include wide viewing angle, bright and better light transmissions, natural colour reproduction, lens system occupies less space therefore smaller diameter instruments are possible, and more versatility in inter-changeability of telescopes between sheaths.

For anterior urethroscopy an instrument similar to the cystoscope shown in Figure 25.22A and having a concave tip is used. Alternatively an instrument incorporating a straight closed-end sheath, or a straight open-end sheath may be used e.g., the Canny Ryall or Geiringer respectively. For posterior urethroscopy, the end of the sheath is convex in shape, although the straight open-end instrument can be used for this also.

The lubricated instrument is inserted and if urethral constrictions are present, these are dilated first in the usual manner with sounds. The telescope is inserted, the light cable attached and the irrigation commenced.

Three types of telescopes are available, the fore-oblique, the right wide-angled field, and the direct vision. The fore-oblique telescope is similar to the one used for simple cystoscopy, when the surgeon generally wishes to examine a field of view which lies in front of, and a little to one side of the distal tip of the instrument. This type of instrument can be used for urethroscopy, but it is preferable to use a wide-angle lens telescope, which gives a field of view at right angles to the aperture in the tip of the instrument. The direct vision telescope can be used if the instrument has an open-end sheath.

The Braasch cystoscope does not incorporate a telescope and the surgeon views the interior of the urethra through a glass window in the proximal part of the instrument.

After the urethra has been examined, the instrument may be passed into the bladder, which is filled with solution and a general examination is carried out, unless this was performed at the beginning of the procedure.

A biopsy may be taken with biopsy forceps (Figs. 25.22D and 25.23). If bleeding is persistant after biopsy, the surgeon may complete the procedure by leaving an indwelling catheter.

During cystoscopy the dye excretion test may be carried out. In this instance intravenous 0·4 per cent indigo carmine is used.

Illumination of urological endoscopes is now generally accomplished by fibre optic systems and high intensity light sources. The reader is referred to Chapter 12 which describes the concept applied to gastroenterology and which is also applicable to urological instruments.

Ureteric catheterisation and retrograde pyelography

DEFINITION

The insertion of a ureteric catheter into the ureter and the kidney pelvis to obtain a specimen of urine from the kidney, or for the retrograde injection of a radio-opaque fluid for X-ray examination of the kidney.

POSITION

Lithotomy.

INSTRUMENTS

As for cystourethroscopy (p. 654) plus ureteric catheters and specimen tubes.

OUTLINE OF PROCEDURE

A lubricated catheterising cystoscope is inserted, the obturator removed and the telescope inserted to visualise the ureteric orifices. A ureteric catheter of appropriate size is passed into each orifice in turn by using the movable platform at the distal end of the instrument. The stilette is left in the catheters until it has been advanced a few centimetres into the ureter, and it is then removed before the catheter is advanced any further. The bladder is emptied, the light cable detached and the cystoscope carefully removed, leaving the catheters in position.

Fig. 25.27 Ureteric Catheter Cylindrical. Marked with blue or red bands to distinguish right and left. Sizes available: 3 to 12 Charrière gauge. Plastic.

Fig. 25.28 Ureteric Catheter Olivery. Marked with blue or red bands to distinguish right and left. Sizes available: 3 to 12 Charrière gauge. Plastic.

Fig. 25.29 Ureteric Catheter Flute End. Marked with blue or red bands to distinguish right and left. Sizes available: 3 to 12 Charrière gauge. Plastic.

The instrument nurse must ensure that the ureteric catheter marked with a red band at its proximal end is used for the right kidney. Similarly, the left ureter is catheterised with a catheter marked blue or green at its proximal end. Two test tubes marked Right and Left are strapped to each thigh (right and left respectively) to collect urine specimens from the kidneys. The catheters are each passed, either through the holes of a rubber teat which fits over the test tube, or through a cotton-wool plug in the neck of each tube. In the X-ray department, a radio-opaque medium such as 35 per cent Pyelosil or Hypaque will be injected into each catheter before making a radiographic examination of the kidneys.

Transurethral prostatectomy

DEFINITION

Transurethral removal of the prostate gland.

POSITION

Lithotomy.

INSTRUMENTS

Bladder sounds or bougies (Lister, Clutton, etc.), set
Supply of sterile water, etc., for irrigation (see cystoscopy)

Connecting tubing and nozzles for resectoscope
Electric resectoscope (Fig. 25.30A) or 'cold punch' instrument
Fibre light or electric cable and light or low voltage source. Electric cable and batteries
Diathermy leads, lead anchoring forceps and diathermy apparatus
Urethral catheter, self-retaining (Foley size 18, 20 or 22 Charrière gauge)
20 ml syringe and sterile water for inflating cuff of catheter.

OUTLINE OF PROCEDURE

The indifferent diathermy electrode is applied to the patient's thigh with the usual precautions. (Alternatively the resectoscope sheath incorporates the indifferent diathermy electrode.) Progressively larger sizes of sounds are passed into the urethra followed by the resectoscope. The obturator is removed and the telescope/resecting loops inserted. Irrigation and diathermy connections are made and the interior of the bladder examined together with the prostatic area.

The prostate is resected by advancing and withdrawing the diathermy loop with the current switched on. It may be necessary to change the diathermy loops several times during operation as they become charred.

A special electrode is used to coagulate bleeding vessels. A self-retaining catheter is inserted and the bladder irrigated until the water returns clear.

Alternatively, the 'cold punch' instrument is used for prostatic resection via the urethra. In this case the instrument is introduced in a similar manner to the electric resectoscope, but the hypertrophied prostate gland is excised with a punch mechanism at the distal end of the instrument.

Fulguration of bladder tumours

DEFINITION

Removal of bladder tumours or lesions by diathermy.

POSITION

Lithotomy.

INSTRUMENTS

As for cysto-urethroscopy (p. 654)
Operating cystoscope, preferably an irrigating instrument, having channels through which flexible diathermy electrodes can be introduced and manipulated: *or* an operating cystoscope which incorporates its own electrode at the distal end.
Diathermy electrodes, set of flexible variety leads and anchoring forceps
(Self-retaining urethral catheter occasionally required (e.g., Foley 18, 20 or 22 Charrière gauge).)

OUTLINE OF PROCEDURE

The indifferent diathermy electrode is applied to the patient's thigh with the usual precautions. The lubricated cystoscope is inserted, the obturator removed, the irrigation tubing and diathermy connections are made and the telescope inserted to visualise the lesion.

Fig. 25.30 Rapier resectoscope. (Chas. F. Thackray Ltd.)

(A) Resectoscope assembled in insulated sheath, 30 Charrière gauge. *Note.* Double-prong connector for light lead: small irrigating nozzle with tap.
(B) Obturator for above.
(C and D) Insulated sheaths, 28 and 26 Charrière gauge, with obturators.
(E) Cutting loops (active diathermy electrode slides inside sheath).
(F) Probe for cleaning.
(G) Large irrigation nozzle.
(H) Diathermy lead.
(I) Light lead.
(J) Resectoscope ready for use. *Note.* Irrigation tube attached to side nozzle; light lead coupled to double-prong connector.

Fig. 25.31 Lithotrite and Ellik evacuator. (Stortz-Rimmer Bros.)

The electrode is applied to the tumour and diathermy used until fulguration is complete. The bladder is emptied, the cystoscope removed and if necessary the catheter is inserted.

Lithotrity or litholapaxy

DEFINITION

Crushing and removal of bladder stones via the urethra.

POSITION

Lithotomy, with the head of the table slightly lowered.

INSTRUMENTS

As for cystoscopy
Lithotrite and sheath
Obturatur
Evacuator (Ellik or Bigelow)
Fibre light or electric cable and light or low voltage source

OUTLINE OF PROCEDURE

A cystoscopy is performed. When the stones have been visualised, the cystoscope is removed and progressively larger sizes of sounds are inserted followed by the lithotrite. The stone or stones are crushed, the lithotrite removed and an evacuation catheter inserted. The Ellik evacuator is used to irrigate the bladder and extract the fragments of stone by suction. It may be necessary to repeat this procedure several times before all the stone or stones have been completely crushed and removed.

Suprapubic cystostomy

DEFINITION

Temporary or permanent suprapublic drainage of the bladder.

POSITION

Supine, with some Trendelenburg.

INSTRUMENTS

General set (Figs. 14.1 to 14.28)
Suprapubic trocar
Catheter introducer
Catheter, self-retaining (De Pezzer, 30 to 34 Charrière gauge)
Spigot
Urethral catheter (Jaques or Nélation size 18 Charrière gauge). To distend bladder if required.
Catheter lubricant
Bladder syringe and warm irrigation solution
Corrugated drain and safety-pin
Suction tubing, nozzles and tube anchoring forceps
2·5 and 3 (2/0 and 0) Chromic catgut or Dexon for ligatures
3 or 4 (0 or 1) Chromic catgut or Dexon on a medium half-circle cutting needle for bladder and muscle sutures
2·5 (2/0) Silk or nylon on a medium or large curved or straight cutting needle for skin sutures.

OUTLINE OF PROCEDURE

If the bladder is not distended, it is first filled with irrigation solution. A 7–10 cm (3–4 in) midline incision is made just above the pubis. The incision is deepened and the rectus sheath opened in the midline, followed by a transverse opening in the transversalis fascia. The fascia and peritoneum are pushed upwards, and two stay sutures are inserted into the bladder wall and left long. Any veins in the vicinity of the proposed opening into the bladder are under-run and tied off. A stab incision is made, the bladder fluid suctioned away and a De Pezzer catheter inserted. The stay sutures are used to secure the catheter in position and these are reinforced if necessary with further interrupted sutures of chromic catgut or Dexon.

Some surgeons make a smaller incision in the abdomen and use a large trocar and cannula to insert the catheter. The wound is closed in layers with a corrugated drain in the lower part. The catheter is secured to the skin with a suture which is tied round the catheter near to the point where it emerges from the wound.

Transvesical prostatectomy

DEFINITION

Removal of the prostate gland via a suprapubic incision into the bladder.

POSITION.

Trendelenburg.

INSTRUMENTS

General set (Figs. 14.1 to 14.28)
Artery forceps, 20 cm (8 in) (Spencer Wells), 10

Fig. 25.32 Surgical approaches to the prostate. (A and B) Suprapubic transvesical approach. (C) Retropubic approach. (D) Transurethral approach. (Swinney and Hammersley.)

Fig. 25.33 Transvesical prostatectomy. (A) Incision in bladder. (B and C) The prostatic adenoma being freed from the false capsule with diathermy and blunt dissection. (D) Irrigation of the bladder. (Swinney and Hammersley.)

Long scissors, curved on flat (Nelson's)
Long dissecting forceps, toothed, 25 cm (10 in)
Long dissecting forceps, non-toothed
Deep retractors, narrow blade (Deaver or Paton), 2
Illuminated bladder retractor, self-retaining (Morson)
Vulsellum forceps (Teale), 2
Boomerang needles (Harris or Millin) for reconstruction of prostatic bed, 3 sizes
Ligature-carrying forceps (Harris or Millin), 2

Bladder syringe and irrigation solution at 43·3° to 46°C
Urethral catheter (Harris or Jaques size 18 Charrière gauge)
Large drainage tube or self-retaining catheter (De Pezzer size 36 Charrière gauge)
Catheter lubricant
Corrugated drain
Suction tubing, nozzles and tube anchoring forceps
Diathermy leads, electrodes and lead anchoring forceps
2·5 and 3 (2/0 and 0) Chromic catgut or Dexon for ligatures, and on ligature-carrying forceps for prostatic bed sutures
3 (0) Chromic catgut or Dexon on a small half-circle round-bodied needle for bladder sutures
3 or 4 (0 or 1) Chromic catgut or Dexon on a medium half-circle cutting needle for muscle
2·5 (2/0) Silk or nylon on a large curved or straight cutting needle for skin sutures
2·5 (2/0) Nylon on a large Colts needle for catheter suture.

OUTLINE OF PROCEDURE

There are several prostatectomy operations via this route and the following is a description of the Harris procedure:

If the bladder is not distended, it is first filled with sterile irrigation solution. A 13 cm (5 in) or longer midline incision is made just above the pubis. The incision is deepened and the rectus sheath opened in the midline, followed by a transverse opening in the transversalis fascia. The fascia and peritoneum are pushed upwards and two stay sutures are inserted into the bladder wall and left long. Any veins in the vicinity of the proposed opening into the bladder are under-run and tied off. A stab incision is made, the bladder fluid suctioned away, the incision extended and a self-retaining bladder retractor inserted.

The mucous membrane over the prostate is incised under direct vision with a pair of scissors. The retractor is removed and the gland shelled out with two fingers. The retractor is reinserted and any bleeding points picked up with forceps and diathermised. Using the boomerang needle, the torn mucous membrane is sutured well down into the prostatic cavity so that its posterior wall is covered.* A urethral catheter is inserted into the bladder and a figure-of-eight suture introduced in front of the catheter so that when it is tied, the side walls of the prostatic cavity are brought together. This manoeuvre largely obliterates the cavity and acts as a haemostatic suture also.

A long nylon suture is inserted through the abdominal wall at one side of the incision and passes into the bladder, through the tip of the catheter, and out again through the abdominal wall at the opposite side of the incision. When the incision has been closed, these ends are tied together over a gauze pad or are threaded through a short length of rubber tubing in the manner described for tension sutures (Chapter 15). This suture serves to suspend the catheter in the bladder until it is withdrawn about the tenth day post-operatively.

When all bleeding has stopped, the bladder drainage tube is inserted and the wound closed in layers around this tube. A corrugated drain extending down to the bladder is left at the lower end of the wound. The suprapubic drain and corrugated drain are usually removed on the fourth or fifth day post-operatively.

---

*The Harris or Millin boomerang needle (Fig. 25.34) consists of a spring-loaded holder to which the needle is attached. The needle has an open eye at its distal point and can be rotated through about 60 degrees by depressing the handle. In operation the surgeon approximates the needle to the tissues being sutured, and advances it through them by depressing the handle. The assistant positions a loop of suture material (usually catgut) in the open eye of the needle by means of ligature-carrying forceps and the surgeon releases the tension on the spring-loaded handle. The needle rotates back through track created by it, withdraws the catgut and thereby completes the suture. The boomerang needle may be used for single or continuous sutures.

Millin's retropubic prostatectomy

DEFINITION

Removal of the prostate gland through a suprapubic incision but without opening the bladder.

POSITION

Trendelenburg.

INSTRUMENTS

General set (Figs. 14.1 to 14.28)
Millin's prostatectomy set (Fig. 25.34)
Artery forceps, 20 cm (8 in) (Spencer Wells), 10
Long artery forceps, curved on flat (Gordon Craig), 5
Deep retractors, narrow blade (Paton or Deaver 25 mm (1 in))
Irrigation solution at 43·3° to 46°C

Fig. 25.34 Millin's retropubic prostatectomy.

1. Bladder syringe.
2. Long dissecting forceps, toothed (Millin).
3. Long scissors, curved, 23 cm (9 in) (Nelson).
4. Vulsellum forceps, 2.
5. Boomerang needles (Millin or Harris), 2.
6. Ligature-carrying forceps (Young).
7. Retractor self-retaining (Millin).
8. Malleable light with electric lead.
9. Bladder-neck spreader (Millin).

Fig. 25.35 Millin's Retropubic Prostatectomy. (A) Incision of prostatic capsule. (B and C) Prostatic adenoma being freed within false capsule. (D) Adenomatous mass is delivered through the capsular incision and dissected from overlying trigone. (E) Trigone seized with Vulsellum forceps; bladder neck and trigone excised. (F) Capsular incision sutured with boomerang needle. (Swinney and Hammersley.)

Urethral catheter (whistle tip or similar, Foley, size 20 Charrière gauge)
Catheter lubricant and Spigot
Suction tubing, nozzles and tube anchoring forceps
Diathermy leads, electrodes and lead anchoring forceps.

OUTLINE OF PROCEDURE

A transverse suprapubic incision is made and the prostate exposed behind the pubis. Blood-vessels running across the anterior aspect of the gland are ligated before opening the capsule in the front. The gland is enucleated, haemostasis secured with diathermy and sutures and a urethral catheter inserted into the bladder. The prostatic capsule is sutured and the wound closed in the usual manner with a corrugated drain down to the prostate capsule in the lower end of the wound.

With any form of prostatectomy the vas deferens may be ligated on both sides to prevent any possibility of infection reaching the testicles by this route.

Total cystectomy and ureterosigmoidostomy

DEFINITION

Removal of the urinary bladder, ureteric transplantation into the sigmoid colon.

POSITION

Trendelenburg.

INSTRUMENTS

General set (Figs. 14.1 to 14.28)
Laparotomy set (Figs. 15.1 to 15.7)
Fine tissue forceps (McIndoe), 5
Fine dissecting forceps, non-toothed (McIndoe), 2
Fine dissecting forceps, toothed (Gillies), 2
Scalpel handle No. 9 with No. 15 blade (Bard Parker)
Fine artery forceps, straight, mosquito, 10
Fine artery forceps, curved on flat, mosquito, 10
Intestinal occlusion clamps, curved (Doyen), 2
Suction tubing, nozzles and tube anchoring forceps
Diathermy leads, electrodes and lead anchoring forceps
Laparotomy ligatures and sutures
2 (3/0) Chromic catgut or Dexon on a small curved non-traumatic intestinal needle size 20 mm for ureteric anastomosis.

OUTLINE OF PROCEDURE

Sometimes the ureters are transplanted as a first procedure and the cystectomy follows at a later date.

Ureterosigmoidostomy. Through a lower midline incision, the sigmoid colon is mobilised. The posterior peritoneum is incised and the ureters are mobilised for a considerable length. A ligature is placed at the junction of each ureter with the bladder and they are divided proximal to this ligature.

Curved occlusion clamps are applied longitudinally to the colon at the point selected for the anastomosis. A small longitudinal incision is made in the bowel wall through the serosa, muscle and mucosa. The ureters are united to the colon mucosa by direct mucosa to mucosa sutures, using fine non-traumatic chromic catgut or Dexon sutures (Leadbetter's operation). The ureters may be immobilised further by suturing the serosa

Fig. 25.36 Ureterosigmoidostomy – Leadbetter's Technique. (Swinney and Hammersley.)

over them for a short distance from the anastomosis, and the sigmoid colon is immobilised to the wing of the pelvis. The wound is closed and a rectal tube inserted.

Cystectomy. If this is done as a second stage, the approach is as before. The peritoneum is stripped off the bladder, which is then dissected free from the surrounding tissue. The urethra is ligated and severed and the blood-vessels divided between forceps to complete mobilisation so that the bladder can be removed. The blood-vessels are diathermised or ligated, and when haemostasis is complete, the peritoneum is sutured to reconstruct the pelvic floor. The wound is closed in layers.

It may be mentioned here that the ureters can be transplanted into a loop of ileum (uretero-ileostomy) instead of the sigmoid colon. In this case 15 cm (6 in) or so of ileum is transected with the mesentery left intact, and the remaining proximal and distal bowel are anastomosed to re-establish intestinal continuity. The short section of ileum is closed at one end and the ureters transplanted in the manner previously described for ureterosigmoidostomy. The open end of the ileum is brought through the abdominal wall as for ileostomy (Chapter 15) and the urine drains into this, so forming an artificial bladder. It is usual to leave a small Paul's tube in the ileostomy, or apply an ileostomy bag immediately after operation.

Partial cystectomy

DEFINITION

Removal of part of the urinary bladder, and if necessary transplantation of one or both ureters to another part of the bladder.

POSITION

Trendelenburg.

INSTRUMENTS

As for cystectomy
Urethral catheter (Jaques or Nélation or Foley, size 18 Charrière gauge)
Bladder syringe and irrigation solution
3 or 4 (0 or 1) Chromic catgut or Dexon on a small half-circle round-bodied needle for bladder sutures.

Fig. 25.37 Removal of a Bladder Tumour by Partial Cystectomy. (Swinney and Hammersley.)

OUTLINE OF PROCEDURE

The bladder is distended with irrigation solution and an approach made through a lower midline incision.

Two stay sutures are inserted into the bladder wall and left long. Any vessels which are overlying the area for incision are under-run with chromic catgut or Dexon and tied. The bladder is opened and the fluid evacuated with the suction tube. The segment of bladder for removal is excised either by diathermy or by the clamp and cut method, whereby artery forceps are applied across the tissue before excision. If the ureter or ureters are involved in this area, they are divided and immobilised for sufficient of their length to enable transplantation into another part of the bladder by the direct mucosa to mucosa anastomosis. The bladder is closed with two layers of chromic catgut or Dexon sutures and a urethral catheter inserted. The wound is closed as before with drainage.

Adrenalectomy

DEFINITION

Removal of whole or part of one or both adrenal glands.

POSITION

Supine (the operation may also be performed through a posterolateral incision, and in this case the position is that for kidney operations).

INSTRUMENTS

Abdominal Approach
    General set (Figs. 14.1 to 14.28)
    Laparotomy set (Figs. 15.1 to 15.7)
    Long scissors, curved on flat, 23 cm (9 in) (Nelson)
    Long dissecting forceps, non-toothed, 25 cm (10 in)
    Long dissecting forceps, toothed, 25 cm (10 in)
    Silver ligature clips and insertion forceps (McKenzie)
    Suction tubing, nozzles and tube anchoring forceps
    Diathermy leads, electrodes and lead anchoring forceps
    Laparotomy ligatures and sutures.

Posterolateral Approach
    As nephrectomy, minus stone forceps, ureteric bougies and catheters.

OUTLINE OR PROCEDURE

Abdominal. A midline or paramedian approach is made and the upper pole of the kidney visualised by incising the posterior peritoneum and mobilising and retracting the overlying organs. The gland is palpated and grasped with tissue or sponge-holding forceps. It is carefully dissected free from the vena cava if it is on the right side. The adrenal vessels are clamped with long artery forceps or silver ligature clips and divided with the long scissors. The gland is removed and haemostasis secured either by ligatures, silver clips, chromic catgut or Dexon sutures or diathermy. The posterior peritoneum is reconstructed with chromic catgut or Dexon sutures and the wound closed in the usual manner.

Posterolateral. A posterolateral incision is made and the kidney exposed through the bed of the twelfth rib. Removal of the gland follows that described above except that the peritoneum is not opened. The wound is closed as for nephrectomy.

KIDNEY AND URETERIC OPERATIONS

Nephrectomy

DEFINITION

Removal of the kidney.

POSITION

Lateral, with kidney bridge elevated, Figure 4.10.

INSTRUMENTS

General set (Figs. 14.1 to 14.28)
Nephrectomy set (Fig. 25.38)
Artery forceps, 20 cm (8 in) (Spencer Wells), 10
Long artery forceps, curved on flat (Moynihan gall-bladder), 5
Long artery forceps, curved on flat (Gordon Craig), 5

Fig. 25.38 Nephrectomy and other kidney operations.

1. Rugine (Mitchell).
2. Rugine (Faraboeuf).
3. Rib raspatories (Doyen), left and right side.
4. Bone-holding forceps (Fergusson).
5. Bone-cutting forceps (Liston).
6. Bone-nibbling forceps, angled on side.
7. Bone-nibbling forceps, angled on flat.
8. Long-scissors, curved on flat, 23 cm (9 in) (Nelson).
9. Rib shears (Exner).
10. Kidney pedicle clamp.
11. Long artery forceps, curved on flat (Moynihan gall-bladder), 8.
12. Ureteric catheters.
13. Renal calculi forceps (Desjardin).
14. Renal calculi forceps (Thompson Walker).

Long dissecting forceps, non-toothed, 25 cm (10 in)
Long dissecting forceps, toothed, 25 cm (10 in)
Deep retractors, narrow blade (Deaver), set of 4
Deep retractors, broad blade (Winsbury-White and Worrall), 2
Long, medium-diameter drainage tube and safety-pin
2·5, 3, 4 and 5 (2/0, 0, 1 and 2) Chromic catgut or Dexon and silk or thread for ligatures
4 or 5 (1 or 2) Chromic catgut or Dexon on a large half-circle cutting needle for muscle sutures
2·5 (2/0) Silk or nylon on a large curved cutting needle for skin sutures.

Fig. 25.39   Incision along the Line of the Twelfth Rib. (Swinney and Hammersley.)

Fig. 25.40   Nephrectomy – clamping the ureter. (Swinney and Hammersley.)

Fig. 25.41 Nephrectomy – dividing the renal pedicle. (Swinney and Hammersley.)

OUTLINE OF PROCEDURE

An oblique incision is made commencing just below the mid-point of the last rib and continuing downwards and forwards towards the anterior superior iliac spine. The external oblique, transversus and internal oblique muscles are divided in line with the incision and the twelfth rib may or may not be excised.

The kidney is separated from its surrounding fat by blunt dissection and is delivered into the wound. The ureter and renal vessels are either clamped separately and divided distal to each forcep; or double ligatures are passed round each vessel and the ureter, which are divided between these ligatures. The kidney is removed and if artery forceps have been applied, the vessels and ureter are ligated. A drainage tube is inserted, the kidney bridge lowered and the wound closed in layers.

Nephrolitotomy, pyelolithotomy or partial nephrectomy

DEFINITION

Removal of a stone from the kidney, or pelvis of the ureter; excision of part of the kidney.

POSITION

Lateral, with kidney bridge elevated or break back position (Figs. 4.9 or 4.10).

INSTRUMENTS

As for nephrectomy
Arterial clamps, bulldog, 2
Self-retaining retractor (e.g., Ring)
Kidney cooling coils and temperature probe
Netalast sling
20 ml syringe, fine catheter and 1 litre plastic container with sterile irrigation solution (cooled in refrigerator).

OUTLINE OF PROCEDURE

Hypothermia. This technique is being used with increasing frequency for operations on the kidney; it enables the surgeon to occlude the blood supply to the kidney for an extended period whilst complicated intra pelvic procedures are undertaken. (Ward and Wickham, 1976). Normally, at body temperature of 37°C, ischaemia time of more than 30 minutes

Fig. 25.42 (A) Kidney exposed. (B) Kidney mobilised and suspended with slings. (Courtesy of Mr J. H. B. Yule, M.Ch., F.R.C.S., Consultant Surgeon and Mr J. R. Jenkins, Senior Medical Photographer, Victoria Hospital, Blackpool.)

can cause kidney injury, whereas if the kidney *in situ* is cooled to 15°–20°C the ischaemia time can be extended for up to two hours. This allows sufficient time in a 'non-bloody' operative field, for the removal of tumours or multiple calculi – particularly those of the staghorn type, which requires great care in searching through the kidney for all stones. There will also be a need to take X-rays of the kidney, during the operation, to locate the stones and check that all have been found.

Renal hypothermia is achieved by using cooling coils applied directly to the surface of the kidney. Utilising good exposure (Fig. 25.42A) the kidney is mobilized so that it is attached only by its pedicle of renal artery, vein and ureter. It is suspended by a Netalast sling (Fig. 25.42B) and the renal artery clamped with bulldog forceps. The sterile saucer-shaped coils are applied as illustrated in Fig. 25.43B).

Fig. 25.43 (A) Cooling coils positioned around kidney. (B) Kidney cooling coils. (C) Calculi removed from kidney. (Courtesy of Mr J. H. B. Yule, M.Ch., F.R.C.S., Consultant Surgeon and Mr J. R. Jenkins, Senior Medical Photographer, Victoria Hospital, Blackpool.)

Fig. 25.44 Hypothermia apparatus for kidney cooling coils. (Courtesy of Mr J. H. B. Yule, M.Ch., F.R.C.S., Consultant Surgeon and Mr J. R. Jenkins, Senior Medical Photographer, Victoria Hospital, Blackpool.)

Cooling is achieved by pumping cold water through the coils and this is done by connecting the coils to the renal hypothermia unit (Fig. 25.44). The temperature of the kidney is monitored by using a needle probe which is connected to a telethermometer fitted in the hypothermia unit.

Operative procedure. The kidney is exposed in the usual manner and freed from surrounding fat. For *nephrolithotomy*, the calculus is palpated by holding the kidney between the finger and thumb. The calculus is steadied carefully through the kidney substance and an incision made over it starting on the convex border of the organ. When the knife reaches the calculus it is removed and an examination made for others. Small fragments may be removed by irrigation. The incision is closed with two or three stout chromic catgut or Dexon sutures placed through the kidney substance, followed by several fine sutures to approximate the capsule. A drainage tube is inserted down to the kidney, the bridge is lowered and the wound closed in layers.

For *pyelolithotomy* exposure and mobilisation are the same as above, but care is taken to free the pelvis of the ureter by rotating the kidney forwards, as all the vessels pass in front of the ureter in their normal course. The calculus is palpated, steadied between the forefinger and thumb, and an incision made into the pelvis. The stone is extracted and the kidney probed for other stones, finally irrigating with sterile irrigation solution (e.g., saline). The incision is closed with fine non-traumatic sutures of chromic catgut or Dexon which may be reinforced with a piece of fat. A drainage tube is inserted down to the kidney, the operation table levelled and the wound closed in layers.

The operation of nephrolithotomy may be replaced by partial nephrectomy in suitable cases. In this procedure, the approach, dissection and closure follow that for nephrolithotomy. Hypothermia of the kidney may be carried out. The stone is located and the overlying capsule incised and carefully peeled off the area of excision. As bleeding is usually profuse, a vascular occlusion clamp is applied across the renal pedicle for a limited time.

Fig. 25.45(A to C) *Nephrolithotomy* (A) Vertical incision. (B) Exposure of calculus, after removal of main calculus fragments are washed out by irrigation. (C) Suture and drainage.

Fig. 25.45(D and E) *Pyelolithotomy* (D) Incision in posterior wall of pelvis. (E) Pyelotomy, using Randal's forceps.

Fig. 25.45(F to H) *Partial nephrectomy* (F) Incising renal cortex. (G) Suturing renal parenchyma. (H) Closing the renal capsule. (Fig. 25.45A to H, Swinney and Hammersley.)

A segment of kidney is removed together with the stone contained and the kidney pelvis may be irrigated. The stump of the calyx is closed with fine catgut and the substance of the kidney with several mattress sutures of strong chromic catgut which are so placed that when they are tied, the cut edges of the kidney tend to invaginate slightly. When haemostasis is complete, the capsule is sutured over the kidney with fine chromic catgut on a non-traumatic needle (Figs. 25.45F to 25.46A).

Ureterolithotomy

DEFINITION

Removal of a stone from the ureter.

POSITION

Supine, or lateral as for nephrectomy.

INSTRUMENTS

As for nephrectomy
20 ml syringe, fine catheter and irrigation solution
Fine rubber or plastic tubing, or nylon tape
2 (3/0) Chromic catgut or Dexon (or plain catgut at the surgeon's discretion) on a small curved rounded-bodied non-traumatic needle.

OUTLINE OF PROCEDURE

The ureter is approached either through an extension of the kidney incision, or through a paramedian incision. In the former case, the kidney incision is continued forwards to the centre of Poupart's ligament, deepened through the muscles to the peritoneum which is not opened but reflected inwards from the posterior abdominal wall.

The ureter lies on the psoas muscle and may be adherent to the peritoneum from which it is dissected free.

In the latter case, a lower midline incision is made and the peritoneum not opened but peeled inwards from the anterior and lateral abdominal wall. The ureter is then mobilised as before and the stone palpated.

A piece of tubing or nylon tape is passed around the ureter just above and below the stone, which is manoeuvred a little beyond the point of impaction. An incision is made into the ureter, the stone removed and the incision closed with fine non-traumatic catgut or Dexon sutures which pass through the muscular coats only. A drain is inserted down to the ureteric incision and the wound closed in layers. Some surgeons irrigate the ureter and probe with fine ureteric bougies to search for other stones.

Renal Transplantation

DEFINITION

Transplantation of a kidney from a living related donor, or a suitable cadaver.

POSITION

Supine.

INSTRUMENTS

    General set (Figs. 14.1 to 14.28)
    Laparotomy set (Figs. 15.1 to 15.7)
    Long scissors, curved on flat, 23 cm (9 in) (Nelson)
    Long dissecting forceps, fine, non-toothed, 25 cm (10 in), 2
    Long dissecting forceps, fine, toothed, 25 cm (10 in), 2
    Long dissecting forceps, fine toothed, 20 cm (8 in) (Waugh), 2
    Long dissecting forceps, fine, non-toothed, 20 cm (8 in) (Waugh), 2
    Vascular clamps (Potts, De Bakey or Satinsky), 2
    Large bulldog clamps (Potts), 4
    Small bulldog clamps (Potts), 4
    Long needle holders (Potts, Smith etc), 2
    Heparinised saline, and syringes with cannulae
    Suction tubing, nozzles and tube anchoring forceps
    Diathermy leads, electrodes and lead anchoring forceps
    Tantalum marker clips and insertion forceps
    Laparotomy ligatures and sutures
    1 and 0·75 (5/0 and 6/0) Silk or Ethiflex on small fine curved arterial needles for anastomosis.

OUTLINE OF PROCEDURE

Live donor transplant. A classical nephrectomy will usually be carried out through a lumbar or trans-abdominal incision. Instruments and procedure are similar to that described on page 671. Great care is taken when mobilising the renal pedicle, to avoid damage to the blood vessels and ureter. After removal of the kidney, excess perureteric tissue is dissected away and the kidney perfused with cold irrigating solution (Collins *et al.*, 1969; Sacks *et al.*, 1973; Fernando and Adams, 1976). The kidney is double-wrapped, and transferred to the recipient operating room for grafting.

Cadaveric donor nephrectomy. Kidneys from cadavers are used more frequently for transplants. They must be removed and perfused within one hour of cessation of renal blood flow.

Both kidneys are removed from a cadaver through a transverse or vertical transperitoneal incision. The aorta and inferior vena cava and ureters are carefully isolated, and mobilized from the diaphragm to the pelvic brim. The aorta and vena cava are clamped above and below the kidneys, which are then removed *en bloc* following careful perureteric dissection. The kidneys are then perfused with cold Collin's solution or Sack's solution through the aorta, or separately through the left and right renal artery. After separate dissection, and ligation of small blood vessel branches, each kidney is double-wrapped in sterile plastic bags and placed in ice for transplantation to the appropriate recipient hospital.

The kidneys can be perfused *in situ* with a special balloon catheter (Fernando and Adams, 1976). This permits an unhurried dissection of the kidneys following death (Fig. 25.46A). Gentle handling, meticulous aseptic techniques and observation of any anatomical abnormality are important at every stage of the procedure.

A collaborative scheme in Europe ensures that each available kidney is matched in terms of ABO and HLA compatibility, and the most suitable recipient is thereby chosen for transplantation.

Transplantation. The iliac fossa is used for transplantation, preferably the right side because of the sigmoid colon on the left.

Fig. 25.46 (A) *In situ* perfusion. (B) Anastomosis of renal vein to external iliac vein. (C) Anastomosis of renal artery to internal iliac artery. (D) Uretero-vesical anastomosis following revascularisation of kidney. (Courtesy of Mr O. N. Fernando and Miss. A. Adams, and *Nursing Times*.)

An oblique, muscle-cutting incision is made from above the iliac spine to the suprapubic region. The peritoneum is pushed medially and the iliac vessels are exposed carefully. The internal iliac artery is mobilised and its terminal branches ligated. If this artery is found to be unsuitable due to calcification or atheroma the external iliac artery is prepared.

The external iliac vein is mobilised and dissected in a similar fashion, and isolated between two vascular clamps. An incision is made anterolaterally between the clamps, the kidney removed from its storage bag and the renal vein is anastomosed to the window that has been created in the vein. An end to side anastomosis is carried out with fine silk or Ethiflex (Fig. 25.46B).

A distal ligature is applied to the internal iliac artery, which is then clamped at its origin from the common iliac artery. The vessel is divided obliquely, close to the ligature, and an end to end anastomosis made to the renal artery (Fig. 25.46C). Should the external iliac have been selected, an end to side anastomosis is carried out.

Before the anastomoses are completed, the vessels are flushed with heparinised saline to prevent embolisation of the kidney. The vascular clamps are released, and the kidney perfused to regain its normal colour and tension.

The procedure is completed by joining the ureter to the bladder, using an anastomosis similar to the anti-reflux technique of Leadbetter (Fig. 25.36A to D), except that a cystotomy is made in the bladder rather than colon.

Marker clips are placed at each pole of the kidney, to indicate the size and position, especially with a view to facilitating radiological control of X-ray therapy that may be given following transplantation. The kidney is placed in the iliac fossa and the wound closed with drainage. It is essential to make sure that there is no kinking of the anastomosis before wound closure.

FURTHER READING AND REFERENCES

COLLINS, G. M., BRAVO-SHUGARMAN, M. AND TERASAKI, P. I. (1969) *Lancet*, **ii,** 1219.
FERNANDO, O. N. AND ADAMS, A. (1976) *Nursing Times*, 1598.
LEADBETTER, G. W., JR., MONACO, A. P. AND RUSSEL, P. S. A. (1966) *Surg. Gynae. Obstet.* **123,** 839.
SACK, S. A., PETRITSCH, P. H. AND KAUFMAN, J. J. (1973) *Lancet*, **i,** 1024.
SWINNEY, J. AND HAMMERSLEY, D. P. (1963) *A Handbook of Operative Urological Surgery*. Edinburgh: Churchill Livingstone.
WALLACE, D. M. (1975) *Nursing Mirror*, July 17, 60.
WARD, J. P. AND WICKHAM, J. E. (1976) *Nursing Times*, 91.

26
OPERATIONS ON THE THYROID AND NECK

Radical cervical node dissection

DEFINITION

Removal of the submental, submaxillary and deep cervical glands, together with the sternomastoid muscle.

POSITION

Supine, with a sandbag under the shoulder blades, and the neck in extension (Fig. 4.13).

INSTRUMENTS

General set (Figs. 14.1 to 14.28)
Long scissors, curved on flat (McIndoe)
Large aneurysm needle
Artery forceps, curved on flat (Kelly Fraser), 10
Artery forceps, curved on flat (Dunhill), 25
Retractors, self-retaining (Travers and West), 2
Corrugated drainage tube and safety-pin or long plastic drainage tubing and Redivac suction bottle
Suction tubing, nozzles and tube anchoring forceps
Diathermy leads, electrodes and lead anchoring forceps
2, 2·5 and 3 (3/0, 2/0 and 0) Chromic catgut, Dexon or silk for ligatures
3 (0) Chromic catgut or Dexon on a medium half-circle round-bodied needle for muscle sutures
2·5 (2/0) Silk or nylon on a small or medium curved cutting needle for skin sutures
(Michel or Kifa clips may be used.)

OUTLINE OF PROCEDURE

An oblique incision is made from the mastoid process to the sternum. This incision is extended Y-fashion to the chin just beyond the midline. The skin flaps are reflected and the platysma incised at the lower end of the sternomastoid muscle which is then divided across. This muscle is dissected up and the lower part of the internal jugular vein clamped and ligated. Dissection is continued, turning up the sternomastoid muscle and jugular vein and removing all tissue which lies behind as far as the trapezius muscle. When the dissection reaches the bifurcation of the common carotid artery, the tissues below the chin, including the submaxillary gland, are then dealt with and reflected towards the carotid bifurcation also. The insertion of the sternomastoid muscle into the skull is severed and the mass of tissue removed, together with the lower pole of the parotid gland. During this dissection the facial artery and vein and the upper part of the jugular

Fig. 26.1 Drawing to show the position of the main vessels and nerves which are encountered in operations on the cervical lymph glands. (Farquharson and Rintoul.)

Fig. 26.2 Arterial supply and venous drainage of thyroid gland. (After Robinson.)

vein will be ligated, but the carotid vessels and the vagus and other essential nerves are carefully preserved. The wound is closed with drainage after haemostasis is complete.

Excision of parotid tumour

DEFINITION

Removal of a tumour in the parotid gland.

POSITION

As radical cervical dissection.

INSTRUMENTS

As radical cervical dissection, except
2 (3/0) Silk or nylon on a small curved cutting needle for skin sutures.

OUTLINE OF PROCEDURE

An incision is made commencing near the lobe of the ear and extending along the crease of the neck. The parotid gland is exposed and the tumour freed by dissection. Haemostasis is secured, a drain inserted and the wound is closed.

Excision of thyroglossal duct or cyst

DEFINITION

Removal of a congenital duct between the thyroid gland and the pharynx, which may be cystic, and have an external opening in the neck.

POSITION

As radical cervical dissection.

INSTRUMENTS

As radical cervical dissection
Small bone cutting forceps.

OUTLINE OF PROCEDURE

Sistrunk's operation consists of a transverse curved incision which is made over the site of the cyst, or an elliptical incision around the sinus opening. The cyst and sinus tract are grasped with tissue forceps and dissected down to the hyoid bone, the centre of which is removed, thereby dividing the bone. Dissection is continued down to the base of the tongue and the extent of this dissection confirmed by palpating through the mouth. The sinus and cyst are removed and the tissues of the tongue are closed with chromic catgut or Dexon sutures. The hyoid bone is approximated with chromic catgut or Dexon, a drain inserted and the wound closed.

Fig. 26.3 Partial thyroidectomy. A. Incision of deep fascia in the mid line. B. Mobilisation of the right lobe. C. Clamping of superior thyroid vessels. D. Exposure of the inferior thyroid artery. E. Division of the gland. F. Appearances after the subtotal removal. (Farquharson and Rintoul.)

D E F

Partial thyroidectomy or excision of adenoma of thyroid

DEFINITION

Removal of part of the thyroid gland or removal of thyroid adenoma.

POSITION

As radical cervical dissection.

INSTRUMENTS

General set (Figs. 14.16 to 14.28)
Thyroidectomy set (Fig. 26.4)
Long scissors, curved on flat (McIndoe)
Corrugated drainage tube and safety-pin
Suction tubing, nozzles and tube anchoring forceps
Diathermy leads, electrodes and lead anchoring forceps
Local infiltration requisites and adrenaline 1 in 400,000 in saline (Optional)

Fig. 26.4 Partial thyroidectomy, etc.

1. Thyroid dissector with eye at point (Kocher).
2. Thyroid dissector (Kocher).
3. Dissector (Durham).
4. Large aneurysm needle.
5. Thyroid-holding forceps (Laney), 2.
6. Artery forceps, curved on flat (Dunhill), 36.
7. Retractors, self-retaining, thyroid, 2 (Jackson Burrow, or alternatively one Joll type).
8. Small short blade retractors, thyroid (Kocher), 2.
9. Small, long blade retractors, thyroid (Kocher), 2.
10. Medium retractors (Czerny), 2.

2·5 and 3 (2/0 and 0) Chromic catgut or Dexon and silk for ligatures
2 and 3 (3/0 and 0) Chromic catgut or Dexon on small half-circle round-bodied needles for muscle and subcutaneous sutures
2 (3/0) Silk on a medium curved cutting needle for skin sutures *or* Michel or Kifa clips.

OUTLINE OF PROCEDURE

Some surgeons infiltrate the skin of the incision area and the platysma with a solution of 1 in 400,000 adrenaline in saline which acts as a vasoconstricting agent, lessens bleeding and provides a plane of cleavage between the platysma and the deeper structures.

A low transverse incision is made in the neck, in line with the skin creases. The skin flaps and platysma are reflected widely and a self-retaining retractor or retractors inserted. The deep cervical fascia is incised in the midline and the infra-hyoid muscles retracted laterally or divided. The gland is carefully freed one lobe at a time by first clamping and dividing the middle thyroid vein, and then elevating the upper pole with a gland enucleator and ligating the superior thyroid artery. The lower lobe of the gland is then dislocated forwards and the inferior thyroid artery is ligatured in continuity.

This process may then be repeated on the other lobe before any glandular tissue is excised. A small portion of the posterior part of one or both lobes which contains the parathyroid glands is left and the remainder excised, first clamping with forceps as the excision proceeds. These divided vessels and tissue are ligated to secure haemostasis, a drain is inserted through a stab incision in the deep fascia on each side, and the muscles and fascia are sutured. The skin is closed with sutures or skin clips.

For excision of adenoma, the gland is exposed in the usual manner, and artery forceps are placed along the line where the tumour has caused the gland tissue to thin out. An incision is made just in front of these into the adenoma capsule. The tumour is then shelled out and the resultant cavity sutured over. The wound is closed as above.

REFERENCE AND FURTHER READING

FARQUHARSON, E. L. AND RINTOUL, R. F. (1972) *Textbook of Operative Surgery*. Edinburgh: Churchill Livingstone.

27
THORACIC OPERATIONS

Bronchoscopy

DEFINITION

Examination of the trachea and main bronchi by means of an endoscope which is passed into their lumens.

POSITION

This will depend on whether a rigid or flexible instrument is used. It may be supine with flexion, or extension of the head as required, or sitting.

INSTRUMENTS

Bronchoscope (Flexible – Fig. 27.1 or rigid – Fig. 27.3)
Biopsy or grasping forceps (Flexible or rigid)
Cytology brush
Suction nozzles (long) (for rigid instruments only)
Suction tubing, tube anchoring forceps
Fibre light or electric cable
Light or electrical source
Pharyngeal spray and topical anaesthetic (lignocaine [xylocaine]) 2, and 4 per cent liquid, or 2 per cent gel.
Silicone liquid
Camera
Specimen tubes.

OUTLINE OF PROCEDURE

The introduction of the flexible fibreoptic bronchoscope has resulted in a safer procedure. The basic principles of this instrument have been described in Chapter 13, and the reader referred to page 308 for further information. In comparison with the rigid instrument the fibreoptic bronchoscope is about one third slimmer than the former (Fig. 27.1). This enables the instrument to be introduced through the nose under local analgesia. The bronchial tree can be examined to subsegmental level in all lobes; the upper lobes are not visible when using a rigid instrument.

The fibreoptic bronchoscope can be used in several ways. In addition to passing the instrument through the nose or mouth under premedication and local analgesia, it can be inserted through a rigid bronchoscope or endotracheal tube under general anaesthetic (Fig. 27.2).

If local analgesia is to be employed (in addition to premedication) the 4 per cent lignocaine (xylocaine) is sprayed into the nostril and also the throat. The fibrescope is lubricated with 2 per cent lignocaine (xylocaine) gel and the distal lens coated with a little silicone liquid to prevent misting (Clarke, 1975). The instrument is inserted through the nose and gently maneouvred round the turbinates, into the naso pharynx and thence behind the epiglottis to the larynx.

Fig. 27.1   Olympus bronchofibrescope. (Keymed.)

Fig. 27.2 (left)   The bronchofibrescope in use. The patient is under intravenous general anaesthetic and muscle relaxant. Oxygen venturi ventilation is in operation. The depth of insertion of the fibrescope is being controlled by the operator's right hand; the direction of the tip by his left. Any necessary suction is controlled by the left thumb here seen being applied to the black-grommetted control hole, punched in the side of the suction tube.

Fig. 27.3 (right)   Rigid bronchoscope in use. The larynx has been passed and the trachea entered.

Fig. 27.4 View during bronchoscopy.

(A and B) *Carina. Normal changes with quiet respiration.* The mucosa is moderately reddened, and there is a little frothy secretion present in the right main bronchus. The longitudinal mucosal corrugations on the posterior tracheal wall are well seen but not prominent. The carina is sharp on inspiration (A), but shortens and widens on expiration when the posterior wall of the lower trachea and main bronchi projects forward (B). This degree of movement on respiration is quite normal. The forward protrusion of the posterior wall during the expiratory phase, or during relaxation under general anaesthesia, may suggest a pathological cause posterior to the lower trachea, but raising the intra-bronchial pressure will rapidly abolish any doubt; rigid tissues, or posterior lymph-node enlargement, will prevent the normal backward displacement of the posterior wall expected with this manoeuvre.

(C) *Normal carina.* The carina edge in this case is extremely sharp. The submucosa is thin showing some senile atrophy, and the mucosa is drawing tightly over the carina and cartilages. The posterior longitudinal mucosa corrugations outlining the elastic bundles can be seen but are not prominent. The transverse ridges due to muscle bands in the membrane stand out more prominently than usual, particularly in the posterior wall of the left main bronchus. The mucosa is a little reddened and a slight increase in secretion can just be seen in the distal part of the right main bronchus.

(D) *Normal right main bronchus.* The cartilage outlines are well seen through the mucosa as far as the final division into middle and lower bronchi. The inferior lip of the upper branch orifice stands out well, making the surface itself easy to locate. The longitudinal mucosal corrugations on the posterior wall are not unduly prominent. The carina, in the left foreground is sharp and the orifice of a mucus duct is just visible beyond it on the medial wall. The normal secretion, seen on the posterior wall, has been swept into a transverse string by the bronchoscope.

Figure 27.4 is continued on page 694.

692   Operating Theatre Technique

Fig. 27.5   Negus Aspirating Bronchoscope – Fibre Lighting.

Fig. 27.6   Poppers Telescope.

Fig. 27.7   Jackson Bronchoscope – Fibre Lighting.

Fig. 27.8   Negus Laryngoscope fitted with fibre light carrier.

Figs. 27.5 to 27.8   Rigid bronchoscope, laryngoscope and grasping forceps (Down's Surgical Ltd.)

Thoracic Operations 693

Fig. 27.9 Chevalier Jackson Grasping Forceps with Negus Handle.

A. Forward grasping forceps.
B. 2/2 teeth claw forceps (Brünings).
C. Scoop cutting biopsy forceps (Brünings).
D. Side grasping forceps.
E. Rotation forceps.
F. Bronchial fenestrated biopsy forceps (Brünings).
G. Round foreign body forceps.

(E) *Chronic bronchitis. Main bifurcation.* The mucosa is generally reddened but swelling is not marked. Cartilages and carina are still well defined. A little increase in mucoid secretion is present, seen to the right of the carina. Longitudinal mucosal corrugations are only faintly visible, on the posterior tracheal wall. The carina does not lie in a true antero-posterior axis: this is a common variation and in this case the rotation is clockwise. The right upper orifice is somewhat more proximal than usual, being at carinal level.

(F) *Chondroma. Right main bronchus.* Partially occluding the right main bronchus is a large, irregular tumour arising from cartilage in the lateral bronchial wall, just beyond the upper bronchial orifice. Slight bleeding has been produced by suction. The tumour was of hard consistency with healthy smooth, overlying mucosa and was successfully removed by bronchotomy. Histology: simple chondroma. (Stradling.)

The larynx is then inspected and 2 ml of 4 per cent lignocaine (xylocaine) instilled directly on to the larynx. This usually causes the patient to cough and splutter a little for a few seconds, but after a pause of about 60 seconds, the bronchoscope can be carefully steered through the larynx and into the trachea. Further doses of 2 per cent lignocaine (xylocaine) are instilled into the trachea and main bronchi as the examination proceeds.

The trachea, carina and both right and left bronchial trees are examined. Biopsies are taken with forceps if any lesions are present, and under direct vision lung areas can be brushed or plugs of mucus aspirated for histology or microbiology.

The bronchofibrescope is removed, and the premedication usually wears off after a few hours.

Mediastinoscopy

DEFINITION

Examination of the mediastinal lymph glands or tumours, with an endoscope similar to a rigid bronchoscope.

POSITION

Supine.

INSTRUMENTS

Mediastinoscope (Carlins)
Biopsy forceps
Bronchus sponge holder
Sponge-holding forceps, 5
Towel clips, 5
Scalpel handle No. 3 with 15 blade (Bard Parker)
Dissecting forceps, toothed, small
Dissecting forceps, non-toothed, medium
Scissors, curved on flat 13 cm (5 in) (Mayo)

Fig. 27.10 Carlins mediastinoscope. (Genito Urinary Manufacturing Co. Ltd.)

Small needle holder (Kilner)
Diathermy leads, electrodes and lead anchoring forceps
Syringe, 20 ml with long fine needles
Suction tubing, long fine suction nozzles and tubes anchoring forceps
Local anaesthetic requisites (Fig. 10.34)
2 (3/0) Chromic catgut or Dexon on medium, half circle round bodied needle for subcutaneous sutures
2 (3/0) Silk or nylon on small curved cutting needle for skin.

OUTLINE OF PROCEDURE

A short transverse incision is made above the supra sternal notch, and the pre-tracheal fascia is exposed. A plane beneath the pre-tracheal fascia is developed by blunt dissection and the mediastinoscope introduced and advanced toward the mediastinum.

Manipulation of the scope enables visualisation of the trachea bifuration, bronchi, aortic arch and associated lymph nodes. Lymph nodal tissue for biopsy is aspirated to exclude vascular structure, and a piece of tissue excised for histology.

If bleeding occurs, pressure may be applied with a swab on a bronchus swab holder. If necessary diathermy may be used. The incision is closed first by suturing the subcutaneous tissue and then skin.

It is usual to combine this procedure with bronchoscopy (Cook, 1976).

Intercostal tube drainage (for empyema or haemothorax)

DEFINITION

The insertion of a tube for the drainage of a collection of pus or blood in the pleural cavity.

POSITION

Generally sitting with support.

INSTRUMENTS

Sponge-holding forceps (Rampley), 5
Towel clips, 5
Scalpel handle No. 3 with No. 11 blade (Bard Parker)
Trocar and cannula
Catheter, self-retaining (De Pezzer or similar, size 28 Charrière gauge)
Catheter introducer
Syringe and wide-bore needles
Underwater seal apparatus or pump
Local anaesthesia requisites (Fig. 10.34)
2 (3/0) Silk or nylon medium curved cutting needle *may* be required to secure the catheter.

OUTLINE OF PROCEDURE

Under local anaesthesia, a stab incision is made in the chest wall, and a trocar and cannula introduced between two ribs into the empyema cavity or haemothorax. The trocar is removed and the catheter introduced through the cannula, which is then removed. To prevent collapse of the lung and to allow drainage of pus or blood, the open end of the catheter is connected to an underwater seal apparatus and/or mechanical pump.

One or two skin sutures are inserted, left untied and rolled up in a small piece of gauze. These are tied immediately when the tube is removed, so that a pneumothorax, possibly of 'tension' type, does not occur.

An underwater seal apparatus consists of a sterile glass bottle, generally of 2 litres capacity, half-filled with sterile water and closed with a cap which incorporates two tube connections. One tube connection terminates below the water level in the bottle and the other terminates just inside the cap. The former connection is coupled to the chest tube and the latter remains open to the atmosphere but protected with a gauze filter.

The underwater seal apparatus reproduces the negative pressure which should be in the pleural cavity, and prevents air from entering from the atmosphere, but allows pus and air to escape from the expanding lung as the patient breathes out deeply. The pus collects in the bottle and the air bubbles out through the water. Any tendency for back suction will only result in the fluid being drawn slightly up the drainage tube connection.

Alternatively, a suction machine creating a small amount of air displacement may be used, and in this case the drainage tubing is connected to the collection bottle fitted to the apparatus.

Care must be taken that the drainage bottle is not elevated above the level of the patient. If this occurs, fluid may aspirate from the bottle and enter the patient's chest. During transportation of the patient, chest drains should be occluded with two clamps across each catheter.

Decortication of the lung (for empyema of haemothorax)

DEFINITION

Stripping or peeling off the fibrin layer from the lung following empyema or haemothorax, to allow full pulmonary expansion and obliteration of the empyema cavity.

POSITION. Lateral chest (Figs. 4.9 or 4.10).

INSTRUMENTS. As for thoracotomy.

OUTLINE OF PROCEDURE

The approach is as for thoracotomy. All free clot is removed from the pleural cavity, and the fibrin layer peeled off the lung to allow full re-expansion. Drainage tubes are introduced at the apex and base of the chest, and are connected to underwater seals or suction apparatus. These drainage tubes are to allow the escape of air and exudate.

Thoracotomy

DEFINITION

Opening the chest cavity as a preliminary to surgery of the thoracic organs.

POSITION

Lateral chest (Figs. 4.9 or 4.10).

Fig. 27.11 Thoracotomy.

(A) *The skin incision.*
(B) *Diathermy of bleeding points.*
(C) *Exposure of chest wall.* Entrance to muscle planes, incising through the fascial triangle and the underlying thomboid muscle until the chest wall is reached.
(D) *Incision of muscles.* The assistant's and the surgeon's index fingers are used to elevate the muscles, and they are then incised with diathermy parallel to the wound, picking up bleeding points meticulously as they meet. In this way, blood loss is kept to a minimum.

(E) *Incision and eversion of periosteum.* The periosteum is incised with diathermy in the mid-rib plane. The periosteum of the upper half of the rib is raised to avoid interference with the intercostal neurovascular bundle below the rib.

(F) *Entry into pleural cavity.* Entry into the pleural cavity is made by incising through the rib bed.

An intercostal incision is seldom employed, but some surgeons still prefer to resect the rib subperiosteally. Should subsequently the size of the thoracotomy appear to be restrictive, an increase in access can always be gained by prolonging the incision forwards, if necessary to the sternal border.

(G) *Introduction of retractor.* Adhesions in the neighbourhood of the incision between the chest wall and lung are first divided so that a large self-retaining retractor of the Tudor Edwards or Price Thomas type may be introduced, spreading the wound widely without tearing the lung. (Cleland.)

700 Operating Theatre Technique

Fig. 27.12 Nelson Rib Raspatory.

Fig. 27.13 Price Thomas Rib Raspatory

Fig. 27.14 Doyen Rib Raspatory.

Fig. 27.15 Price Thomas Rib Shears.

Fig. 27.16 Tudor Edwards Rib Shears for Anterior Ends.

Fig. 27.17 Lebesches Sternum Shears.

Figs. 27.12 to 27.22 Thoracic instruments. (Chas. F. Thackray Ltd.)

Thoracic Operations

Fig. 27.18 Morriston Davies Rib Approximator.

Fig. 27.19 Tudor Edwards Scapula Retractor.

Fig. 27.20 Allison Lung Retractor.

Fig. 27.21 Buckley's Modification of Finochietto's Rib Spreader.

Fig. 27.22 Tudor Edwards Double Rib Spreader With Key.

INSTRUMENTS

General set (Figs. 14.1 to 14.28)
Artery forceps, curved on flat (Kelly Fraser), 50
Artery forceps, straight, 20 cm (8 in) (Spencer Wells), 12
Long-toothed and non-toothed dissecting forceps, 25 cm (10 in)
Long scissors, curved (Nelson)
Small rugine (Faraboeuf)
Large rugine (Mitchell)
Rib raspatory (Doyen), left and right side
Bone-holding forceps (Fergusson) (Lion)
Gouge or bone-nibbling forceps, angled on side
Gouge or bone-nibbling forceps, angled on flat
Rib shears (Exner)
Rib shears (Price Thomas) (A variety of other rib shears may be required according to the site of thoracotomy.)
Rib approximator (Morriston)
Sponge-holding forceps (Rampley), 4
Lung artery forceps, right angled (O'Shaughnessy), 6
Lung artery forceps, curved on flat (Roberts or Tudor Edward), 20, lung artery forceps, curved on flat (Moynihan) (cholecystectomy) or (Gordon Craig), 6
Lung-holding forceps (Duval), 5
Large aneurysm needle, Nelson right and left, 3 of each
Lung retractors (Deaver or alternatively Allison 'fish slice' type), 2
Bronchus clamp (Thompson)
Lung tourniquet (Roberts-Nelson)
Long needle holder (Halstead)
Deep retractor (Winsbury – White)
Deep retractor (Worrall)
Double rib spreader (Tudor Edwards), complete with one set of blades
   Rib spreader keys
   Two sets of alternative sizes of blades
Suction tubing, nozzles and tube anchoring forceps
Diathermy leads, electrodes and lead anchoring forceps
2, 2·5 and 3 (3/0, 2/0 and 0) Silk on a small or medium half-circle round-bodied needle for transfixion sutures
4, 5 or 6 (1, 2 or 3) Chromic catgut, Dexon silk or thread for ligatures
5 or 6 (2 or 3) Chromic catgut, Dexon or stainless steel wire or large half-circle round-bodied needles for rib closure
3 (0) Nylon or silk on large curved or straight cutting needles for skin.

OUTLINE OF PROCEDURE

The site of the incision depends upon which part of the chest contents is to be approached. The incision may be posterolateral, lateral or anterolateral, and may be placed overlying the upper or lower part of the thorax.

The incision is deepened through fascia and muscle down to the intercostal muscles. Haemostasis is secured with diathermy or ligatures, and the chest is entered either between two ribs or through the bed of an excised rib. In the former case an incision is made through the intercostal muscles, and the pleura opened with scissors. In the latter case the periosteum is reflected off the rib anteriorly with a Faraboeuf's, Sembs or Price

Thomas rugine, and posteriorly by passing a Doyen's raspatory around and along the rib. The rib is excised, the pleura opened with scissors and a rib spreader inserted.

After the surgical procedure has been completed, an intercostal drain is inserted (see empyema), usually one apical and one basal. The drain is connected to the underwater seal and the wound is closed. Interrupted sutures of chromic catgut, Dexon or stainless-steel wire are inserted through the intercostal muscles above the upper rib of the wound into the chest cavity, and out again through the intercostal muscles below the lower rib. These sutures are left long until all have been inserted for the entire length of the wound.

Fig. 27.23 (left)   Price Thomas Bronchus Clamp. (A) Plain jaws. (B) 'Spiked' jaws.

Fig. 27.24 (right)   Bickford Bronchus Clamp. (L) Large jaws. (S) Small jaws.

A rib approximator is used to approximate the ribs and the interrupted sutures are tied. Further interrupted sutures may be inserted to reinforce this suture line. If a drainage tube has been used, this is connected to an underwater seal apparatus and the anaesthetist inflates the lung or lungs.

Interrupted or continuous sutures of chromic catgut, Dexon or stainless steel wire are used to close the intercostal muscles and other chest muscles. The skin is sutured with interrupted silk or nylon.

Lobectomy or pneumonectomy

DEFINITION

Excision of a lobe of the lung or total removal of the lung.

POSITION

Lateral chest (Fig. 4.6 or 4.7).

INSTRUMENTS

As thoracotomy (p. 702).

OUTLINE OF PROCEDURE

The chest is opened as for thoracotomy, with a posterolateral incision usually over the sixth interspace. The sixth rib, or alternatively the fifth or seventh rib, is excised and the chest entered through the bed of the excised rib.

704 Operating Theatre Technique

A

B

C

D

E

Fig. 27.25 Simple (left) pneumonectomy.

(A) Chest opened as described for thoracotomy, anterior adhesions of lung to chest wall being freed by blunt dissection. (B) Pulmonary artery dissection – the vagus nerve has been cut distal to its recurrent laryngeal nerve. (C) Artery ligated by passing a strong thread suture round it. (D) Lung retracted to expose the anterior aspect of the hilum – superior pulmonary vein dissected out and divided between ligatures. (E) Exposure of inferior pulmonary vein, pulmonary ligament divided – pericardium visible behind lung. (F) Bronchus clamped, bronchial artery ligated ready for division. (G) Bronchial incision started close to carina, retraction suture for lifting stump from mediastinum. Continuous suture of thread or wire to close bronchus. (H and I) Alternative method of closure of bronchus. (Cleland.)

706 Operating Theatre Technique

A

B

C

D

E

F

Fig. 27.26 Lobectomy and segmental resection of the lung.

Left lower lobectomy (A) Pulmonary artery and branches exposed. (B) Branches of pulmonary artery leading to lobe divided between ligatures, clamp applied across basal divisions of lower lobe bronchus.

Left upper lobectomy (C) Pulmonary artery and branches to upper lobe exposed. (D) Branches of pulmonary artery leading to upper lobe divided between ligatures. (E) Clamp or clamps are used to close and hold bronchi close to the line of section.

Right lower lobe lobectomy (F) Pulmonary artery and branches to lower lobe exposed. (G) The lower lobe artery has been divided, between ligatures, bronchus to apex of lower lobe divided – sutures on proximal stump shown. (H) The lobe has been removed – bronchial suture lines shown.

Segmental resection (I) After ligation of vessels and clamping of bronchi the segment is 'rolled off'. (Cleland.)

For lobectomy the affected lobe is held with lung forceps and any adhesions are freed with scissors or dissection swabs until the lobe is only attached by its main bronchus and vessels entering the hilum in the mediastium. The pulmonary artery and vein are isolated and clamped, divided and ligated. The bronchus is identified and clamped across with a special bronchus clamp. The rest of the chest is isolated with moist packs to prevent contamination as the lung is removed. Either the bronchus is divided by the cut and sew method, whereby sutures are inserted as the bronchus is divided; or a second clamp is applied and the bronchus divided between the two. With the latter method, the bronchus is oversewn before removing the clamp. In both cases a second and sometimes third layer of sutures (chromic catgut, Dexon, silk or stainless steel wire) are inserted to ensure a good closure. The stump of the bronchus is pleuralised, using interrupted silk, chromic catgut or Dexon.

For pneumonectomy the operative procedure is similar, but the dissection is more extensive, and the total lung is removed. The pericardium is incised and the dissection of the major vessels carried out through this opening in some cases.

If the pericardium has been opened, it is sutured with chromic catgut, Dexon or silk on a non-traumatic needle after haemostasis has been checked. The chest cavity *may* be irrigated with sterile saline, and chest drainage tubes inserted (usually one apical and one basal) and connected to the underwater seal. Low vacuum suction apparatus may be utilised for lobectomy, but not for pneumonectomy as this could cause mediastinal shift.

The chest is closed as for thoracotomy.

Thoraco-abdominal approach for oesophagogastrectomy

DEFINITION

Removal of part of the oesophagus and stomach for high gastric ulcer or tumour, oesophageal varices or oesophageal tumour. The operation is performed through a combined thoracic and abdominal incision. (Alternatively, laporatomy first to mobilise the stomach and perform a pyloroplasty followed by repositioning of the patient to make a thoracotomy incision to complete the resection.)

INSTRUMENTS

As for thoracotomy, page 702, plus:

- 5 (2) Chromic catgut, Dexon or silk or wire on a medium half-circle round-bodied needle for diaphragm
- 5 (2) Chromic catgut or Dexon on a large half-circle cutting needle for abdominal muscles.

OUTLINE OF PROCEDURE

A thoraco-abdominal incision is made, extending transversely across the epigastrium from the umbilicus, along the sixth or seventh intercostal space, to 5 cm (2 in) from the spine, i.e., behind the scapula. The sixth or seventh rib may be resected in the usual manner if insertion of a rib spreader indicates possible fracture of the ribs. The costal cartilage is cut across the diaphragm and peritoneum opened.

The tumour is palpated and resectibility determined. The oesophagus and upper end of the stomach are freed carefully, and vessels ligated with chromic catgut, Dexon or silk. Clamps are applied across the cardia of the stomach which is transected (if a tumour is present it would be distal to this point) and the lesser curvature narrowed by resection and closure with 2·5 or 3 (2/0 or 0) chromic catgut or Dexon on a non-traumatic needle.

Fig. 27.27 Closure of chest.

(A and B) If drainage is required an inter-costal drain is inserted, anterior to the mild axillary line below the incision. (C) Approximation of the ribs with instrument. (D) Periosteum sutured with interrupted thread, catgut or Dexon. (E) Muscle closed in layers with interrupted catgut, Dexon, nylon or wire, skin closed with interrupted sutures. (Cleland.)

Two occlusion clamps are applied across the oesophagus and the lesion is removed by dividing between the two clamps. The stomach is delivered into the chest and an end to end anastomosis made to the oesophagus with 'through and through' interrupted chromic catgut or Dexon non-traumatic sutures. The suture line is reinforced anteriorly and posteriorly with a serosa closure of interrupted silk sutures.

If the lesion is extensive, a total gastrectomy may be performed (Chapter 15) with oesophago-jejunostomy.

The diaphragm is closed with interrupted chromic catgut, Dexon or silk sutures, and the peritoneum with a continuous chromic catgut or Dexon suture. The chest cavity *may* be irrigated and an intercostal drainage tube is inserted through the eighth intercostal space. The chest muscles are sutured with interrupted chromic catgut, Dexon or wire, followed by interrupted silk or nylon for the skin.

The intercostal tube from the chest is connected to an underwater seal bottle.

Repair of diaphragmatic hernia (thoracic approach)

DEFINITION

The repair of an abnormal opening in the diaphragm (usually at the oesophageal hiatus), which allows a sliding hernia of stomach into the chest.

Fig. 27.28 The Belsey 'Mark IV' technique, viewed through left thoracotomy with patient lying on right side: (A) crural approximation sutures; (B) fastening stomach to oesophagus above the cardia; (C) placing second row of mattress sutures with the aid of cocktail spoon; (D) the completed repair. (Irvine.)

POSITION

Lateral chest (Fig. 4.9 or 4.10).

INSTRUMENTS

As for thoracotomy (p. 702)
Long tissue forceps (Littlewood or Vulsellum), 4
Ligatures and sutures as for thoracotomy
2·5 (2/0) Silk or stainless steel wire on a small half-circle round-bodied needle for diaphragm repair
Nylon tape or fine rubber tubing for oesophageal retraction.

OUTLINE OF PROCEDURE

A left posterolateral incision is made through the seventh intercostal space, and the chest opened as for thoracotomy. (A rib may, or may not be resected.) Rib spreaders are inserted, the mediastinal pleura opened, and the oesophagus mobilised and retracted with the nylon tape or rubber tubing.

The hernial orifice is identified, an incision made in the left dome of the diaphragm and the herniated organs returned to the abdomen. The edges of the orifice are grasped with tissue or Vulsellum forceps and the opening is repaired with interrupted silk or stainless steel wire sutures which are left long and are tied when all have been inserted. The incision in the left dome of the diaphragm is repaired in a similar manner.

The mediastinal pleura is approximated over the oesophagus and the chest closed in the manner usual for thoracotomy.

Sometimes the operation is performed through an abdominal or thoraco-abdominal incision, as described for oesophagectomy.

REFERENCES AND FURTHER READING

CLELAND, W. P. (1968) Surgery – Thorax. London: Butterworths.
COOK, F. (1976) *Nursing Times*, 1718.
CLARKE, S. W. (1975) *Nursing Mirror*, **47**, November 27.
IRVINE, W. T. (1971) *Modern Trends in Surgery* – 3. London: Butterworths.
STRADLING, P. (1976) *Diagnostic Bronchoscopy – An Introduction*. Edinburgh: Churchill Livingstone.

28
CARDIOVASCULAR OPERATIONS

This is a highly specialised and relatively new branch of surgery. The equipment and instruments used are extensive in range and often include many items which are of personal use only to a particular surgeon. In the following chapter it is possible only to cover those basic instruments for some cardiovascular procedures.

The reader is referred to Chapter 10 for a description of cardiac stimulant drugs, and Chapter 2 for the use of electric defibrillators and pacemakers which play an important part in heart operations.

A large proportion of heart and major blood vessels operations in the chest are performed under extracorporeal circulation (cardiopulmonary bypass, sometimes combined with hypothermia. With extracorporeal circulation, the blood is diverted from the heart and the circulation maintained by means of a mechanical pump or pumps and oxygenator (heart/lung machine, e.g., TMO oxygenator system). To achieve hypothermia, the patient's body temperature is first lowered to 30°C by physical cooling under anasthesia; after cardiopulmonary bypass has been established, the temperature can be lowered still further to 20°C. This is achieved by lowering the temperature in the oxygenator heat exchanger.

During operation the patient lies on, and is covered by special blankets which help to control the hypothermia. These blankets are made up of a series of rubber or plastic tubes through which fluid from a hypothermia machine circulates. The temperature of this fluid is adjusted to individual requirements and rewarming is started as soon as the patient is on the operating table.

Intracardiac procedures

Considerable developments have taken place, and intracardiac surgery is now an expanding specialty. There are many variations of technique for the same type of operation, each giving successful results in the hands of a particular team. Newer and more efficient prosthetic valve replacements are being designed, and in the not too distant future the use of auxiliary ventricles will become commonplace.

Cardiac surgery is complex and requires a specialised team of surgeons, anaesthetists, cardiologists, physiologists, technicians and nurses. Space will not permit more than a brief outline of surgical procedures for it would be easy to devote the entire book to describing these. In order to generalise, the descriptions depart from the format of the book hitherto. Exceptions are the description coarctation of the aorta and patent ductus arteriosus.

Intracardiac lesions vary considerably in severity, and in some cases the diseases overlap requiring several distinctly separate operative procedures during surgery. These lesions can be described as (a) and (b) congenital, they are listed together with the corrective surgery.

(A) ACQUIRED LESIONS

Mitral stenosis
  1. Closed valvulotomy
  2. Open valvulotomy (under direct vision)
  3. Valve replacement
Mitral insufficiency
  1. Valvuloplasty
  2. Valve replacement
Tricuspid stenosis, and/or insufficiency
aortic stenosis, and/or insufficiency
  1. Open valvulotomy
  2. Valvuloplasty
  3. Valve replacement
Coronary heart disease
  1. Revascularisation of the coronary arteries
Occlusive disease of the aorta
  1. Graft replacement
  2. Bypass
  3. Thromboendarterectomy
Thoracic aortic aneurysm
  1. Repair procedure
  2. Graft replacement
Chronic heart disease
  1. Transplantation

(B) CONGENITAL DEFECTS

Pulmonary stenosis
  1. Valvulotomy
Atrial septal defect
Ventricular septal defect
Tetralogy of Fallot
  1. Repair procedure
Patent ductus arteriosis
  1. Ligation and division
Coarctation of the aorta
  1. Resection and end to end anastomosis
  2. Resection and graft

Cannulation and cardiopulmonary bypass

Maintaining a patient's circulation by temporarily bypassing the blood from the heart enables protracted intracardiac procedures to be performed. Regardless of design the heart-lung machines, as they are known, consists basically of an oxygenator, arterial and venous pumps, heat exchanger, filter and arterial, venous and cardiotomy blood reservoirs.

The oxygenator takes the place of the patient's lungs, removing excess carbon dioxide from the venous blood and achieving oxygenation. It may consist of a screen, rotating discs, a bubbler, or a disposable membrane unit, but basically separates the blood into a thin film which is then exposed to an atmosphere of oxygen where the interchange of gases takes place.

Fig. 28.1 TMO membrane oxygenator modular system-cardiopulmonary bypass machine. (Travenol.)

Fig. 28.2 Cardiopulmonary bypass with TMO oxygenator. (Travenol.)

1 Venous line
2 Cardiotomy reservoir
3 Arterial line
4 Venous reservoir
5 Arterial reservoir
6 Filter
7 Oxygenator
8 Heat exchanger
9 Venous pump
10 Arterial pump

Cardiovascular Operations

A

B

C

D

The pumps, usually a set of rollers rhythmically massaging the outside of the arterial and venous tubes, maintain the flow of blood from the patient to the machine, and back after oxygenation. The output of the pump depends on the speed of rotation and therefore the perfusion rate can be varied but should approximate the resting cardiac output.

The heat exchanger is used to lower or raise the temperature of the blood after it has passed through the pump/oxygenator. In conjunction with suitable drugs, the heat exchanger provides a means of rapidly inducing hypothermia if required.

The filter is interposed between the cardiotomy reservoir and the venous reservoir. If a bubble oxygenator is used, it is necessary to interpose an arterial filter coated with a defoaming agent, between the oxygenator and the arterial line.

The arterial and venous reservoirs are joined by a recirculation tube to form the reservoir set. The venous reservoir is connected to the filter and cardiotomy reservoir, and has connections for venous drainage from the patient and delivering venous blood to the oxygenator. The arterial reservoir is connected to the exit part of the oxygenator and the arterial line back to the patient.

The cardiotomy reservoir collects blood suctioned from the heart or thoracic cavity. Its functions are to deform and remove debris from blood being returned from the operative site, to the extracorporeal circuit.

Cannulation is performed as a prelude to connecting the patient to the heart/lung machine. Venous blood is collected either from the superior and inferior venae cavae or the right atrium. If the venae cavae are cannulated Portex polyvinyl catheters 8 mm ($\frac{5}{16}$ in) are used; cannulation of the right atrium requires a larger size of catheter, 13 mm ($\frac{1}{2}$ in). A further plastic cannula is inserted into the left ventricle and connected to the venous blood reservoir on the heart/lung machine. This collects any blood pooling in the ventricular cavity, and is used to remove air from the heart immediately after bypass is stopped. A further suction line is also used to return aspirated blood into the venous blood reservoir.

Oxygenated arterial blood is returned either to a cannula inserted into the aorta or a cannulated femoral artery. The latter procedure is generally nowadays restricted to cardiopulmonary bypass for the repair of aortic aneurysms, or sometimes in re-operations where there may be danger of damaging the heart on re-opening.

During cannulation the polyvinyl catheters are inserted with their obturators in position, an exception being the finer femoral catheters. After insertion, these obturators are removed and the proximal end of the catheter clamped shut. The catheters are then connected to the heart/lung machine with polyvinyl tubing. This is done carefully under a constant flow of sterile saline to ensure air free connections. All tubing is secured to the drapes with sutures or towel clips, to prevent accidental withdrawal of the cannulae. If the myocardium is likely to be deprived of blood while the heart is ischaemic e.g., during aortic valve replacement coronary cannulae are inserted to perfuse the coronary system. Before going on bypass, intracardiac pressures are taken with a needle connected to a fluid filled manometer line incorporating a transducer, (this converts pressure to an electrical signal which is then amplified and displayed on a cardiac monitor). Normal values to be expected, are right atrium – 6 mm, right ventricle – 25/0 mm, left atrium – 11 mm, left ventricle – 12/0 mm and aorta – 120/0 mm (Linley, 1976). These values can of course vary considerably in the diseased heart. The measurements are checked again at the end of the procedure.

After total body heparinisation, removal of the clamps on the tubing puts the patients on partial bypass, that is some blood still passes into the heart. Complete bypass is accomplished by passing tourniquets around the venae cavae where they join the heart. These consist of 6 mm ($\frac{1}{4}$ in) wide nylon tape passed around the venae cavae with both ends threaded through a 10 cm (4 in) length of No. 5 rubber tubing. Tightening the rubber tubing down on to the tape constricts the venae cavae and prevents blood entering the heart, the patient is then on total bypass.

INSTRUMENTS REQUIRED

General basic
As for thoracotomy (p. 702)
Various vascular clamps, Satinsky, Brock, Potts Smith, Crafoord etc. (pp. 718–719)
Tissue forceps, Potts, 6
Long dissecting forceps, toothed, fine (Waugh)
Long dissecting forceps, non-toothed, fine (Waugh)
Long needle holders, (Potts Smith, Holmes Sellor, etc.) 2
Graduated jug for saline
Irrigation syringe and catheter
Coronary suction tip 2, and tubing
Assorted stop cocks, connectors and needles, etc.
Recording catheters and insertion needles

Cannulation and bypass
Polyvinyl cannulae pressure recording catheters/needles with connections to pressure tubing for cannulation
Connectors to attach catheters to heart/lung machine tubing
Nylon tape 6 mm ($\frac{1}{4}$ in) wide, 35 cm (14 in) long with 10 cm (4 in) lengths of No. 5 rubber tubing to act as tourniquets for major vessels

Closure
3 or 2·5 or 2 (0 or 2/0 or 3/0) Silk, polyester etc. on medium half-circle round-bodied needle for pericardium retraction and closure sutures
2·5 to 0·7 (2/0 to 6/0) Silk, polyester, polyethylene or Dacron etc., on small curved non-traumatic round-bodied or taper-cut needle for vascular sutures, valve replacements and closure of the atrium. The size varies according to the vessel and surgeon's preference. A size 3(0) may be used for closing ventricular incisions, combined with a Teflon felt reinforcing buttress. This may also be used as a purse-string suture for the cannulation sites, and appendage in closed mitralvalvulotomy.
Routine thoracotomy sutures

Special Instruments
Valvulotomy
Dilators, valvulotomes (Brock, etc.), various sizes
Scissors, angled (Potts), set of 3
Leaflet retractors

Figs. 28.3 to 28.6   (opposite page). (Travenol.)

(A) Exploded viewing Travenol TMO oxygenator; a closed system which eliminates oxygenator produced micro bubbles, providing independent control of O_2 and CO_2 gas transfers, reducing the damage to the blood, preserving better platelet function and reducing particulate matter micro-embolised. *Key* – 1. Shim, 2. Case, 3. Shimtube, 4. Spacer, 5. Manifolds, 6. Blood filmer, 7. Membrane.
(B) Oxygenator mounting bracket assembly.
(C) TMO adaptor kit with bracket mounting arm and reservoirs fitted.
(D) TMO oxygenator disposable equipment. *Key* – 1. Cardiotomy reservoir, 2. Miniprime heat exchanger, 3 and 4. Arterial and venous reservoirs.

Fig. 28.7   Aorta Clamp, Potts-Smith.

Fig. 28.8   Bulldog Clamp, Glover, straight, 6·5 cm (2½ in) long.

Fig. 28.9   Bulldog Clamp, Glover, right angle, 6 cm (2¼ in) long, 27 mm jaw length.

Fig. 28.10   Bulldog Clamp, Glover, Satinsky shape jaws, 6·5 cm (2½ in) long.

Fig. 28.11   Bulldog Clamp, Potts', half curved, 4 cm blades.

Fig. 28.12   Bulldog Clamp, DeBakey, with ring handles, right angle jaws, 10·5 cm (4⅛ in) long.

Fig. 28.13   Bulldog Clamp, DeBakey, with ring handles, 45° angle jaws, 12·5 cm (5 in) long.

Fig. 28.14   Bulldog Clamp, DeBakey, with ring handles, curved on flat, 12·5 cm (5 in) long.

Fig. 28.15   Vessel Clamp, Waterston's, delicate model, 16 cm (6½ in) long with 1·5 cm and 2 cm straight portion of jaws.

Figs. 28.7 to 28.15   Cardiovascular instruments. (Genito Urinary Manufacturing Co. Ltd.)

Fig. 28.16 Ductus Arteriosus Clamp, Potts' angled and straight, 20 cm (8 in) long.

Fig. 28.17 Dissecting Clamp, Crafoord's, full curve.

Fig. 28.18 Auricular Clamps, Brock's, set of three varying curves.

Fig. 28.19 Multi-purpose Clamp, DeBakey, obtuse angle 60°, 24 cm (9½ in) long with 4 cm jaws.

Fig. 28.20 Vascular Clamp, Satinsky's, with 4 cm and 5 cm straight portion of jaws.

Fig. 28.21 Aorta Clamp, Brock's, with Potts' teeth, 4 cm straight portion of jaws.

Fig. 28.16 to 28.21 Cardiovascular instruments (*cont'd.*) (Genito-Urinary Manufacturing Co. Ltd.)

Fig. 28.22 Cardiac Punch, Brock's, for infundibular stenosis, 7·5 mm, 10 mm and 12 mm blade.

Fig. 28.23 Dilator, Brock's, for pulmonary stenosis, opening to 24 mm.

Fig. 28.24 Dissecting Scissors, Hedgeman's, delicate, angled on edge 25°, 19 cm (7½ in) long.

Fig. 28.25 Aortic Dilator, Brock's, three blade.

Fig. 28.26 Cardiac Retractors, Brainbridge's, 23 cm (9 in) long.

Fig. 28.27 Cardioplegia Coronary, Cannula, Brainbridge's, 50° and 90° angle, 3·0 mm dia. distal end, with 5 mm olive for ¼ in tubing, stainless steel.

Fig. 28.28 Needle Holder, Abrams, modified Sellors', for fine non-traumatic needles, 20 cm (8 in) long.

Fig. 28.29 Needle Holder, DeBakey, with extended ring on one side, 19 cm (7¾ in) long.

Figs. 28.22 to 28.29 Cardiovascular instruments. (Genito Urinary Manufacturing Co. Ltd.)

Valve replacement
  Prosthetic heart valve, e.g., Starr Edwards, heterograft
  Valve holder
  Scissors, angled (Potts), set of 3
  Suture to secure valve, usually 2·5 (2/0) polyester etc. on double ended 25 mm taper cut non-traumatic needle.

Septal defects
  Teflon or similar prosthetic repair material for patch
  Suitable sutures as detailed above.

Types of valve replacement. Often by the time the patient presents himself for the treatment of an acquired heart valve malfunction, the valves are so affected by calcification or disorganisation, that valve replacement, not repair is the preferred procedure (Paneth, 1975).

Replacement valves can be considered under two headings:
1. *Mechanical valves* – (a) ball and socket, e.g., Starr-Edwards, De Bakey, Magovera-Cromie., (b) Floating discs, e.g., Bjork-Shiley.
2. *Biological valves* – (a) homograft fresh free or mounted, and preserved – free or mounted; (b) heterograft preserved – mounted.

The mechanical valves in group 1, although having superior mechanical durability compared with the biological graft, exhibit thrombogenic tendency to a greater or lesser degree. This requires anti-coagulant therapy for an indefinite period.

Conversely although biological valves have a greater mechanical failure rate, they are for all practical purposes free from the danger of formulation of thrombus. Patients do not require anticoagulant therapy to avoid thrombus interfering with valve function or causing systemic embolism.

Preparation of homograft is difficult and time consuming. They must be removed within 12 hours of death and after antibiotic sterilisation, are stored at 4°C for a limited period; usually not more than 14 days.

There has been an increasing use of heterograft valves, in the form of porcine valves, prepared in gluteraldehyde and mounted on a frame (Lockie, 1975; Pagliero, 1975). These pig valves are preserved by a special tanning technique to render the valve leaflets more durable. They are not visible when implanted but this is not disadvantageous compared with initially viable homograft. Examination of implanted valves after predetermined

Fig. 28.30 Heart valve replacements. (Courtesy E. Lockie and *Nursing Times*.)

Fig. 28.31 Mitral valve replacement (A) left atrial incision. (B and C) Excision of mitral valve – stay sutures placed in mitral leaflets to facilitate exposure, excision started along attached margin of aortic leaflet, division of posterior papillary complex, followed by division of anterior papillary complex and incision of remaining attached portions of the aortic and mural leaflets. (D) Doubled armed sutures in position through mural leaflet portion of the mitral annulus, sutures being placed through the remainder of annulus, method of attachment to cloth portion of valve prosthesis. (E and F) All sutures in position, prosthesis is passed down into its bed. (Cleland.)

Fig. 28.32 Aortic valve replacement. (A and B) Aortic cross-clamped, opened transversely; aortic valve being palpated. (C) Excision of aortic valve. (D) Measurement of aortic root and annulus to determine type of prosthesis. (E and F) Double armed sutures are used to secure cloth edge of valve prosthesis, these are tied after the valve (G) has been passed down in place. (Cleland.)

periods have shown that the viable valves quickly lost all living cells. In addition, homografts in many instances became distorted and damaged, probably due to inflammatory rejection, whereas this was avoided by non-viable valve transplant (Lockie, 1976).

Careful consideration is necessary before deciding whether a hetero valve graft or a mechanical valve should be the method of choice. For example, a young woman of child bearing age may be more suitable for a heterograft to avoid continuous anti coligulant therapy. Similarly, a manual labourer may be subjected to frequent minor injuries, especially to his limbs (Gilbert, 1972). In cases of re-operation due to failure of a valve graft, the patient may demand the superior durability of a mechanical valve. In all instances meticulous care, in preparation of grafts, sterilisation and surgical technique are paramount in rate of success.

PROCEDURES

Mitral valvulotomy. The chest is opened through a right posterior lateral incision or mediastinal split. The pleura is opened with scissors and a rib spreader inserted. With the posterior lateral approach it may be necessary to resect a rib; the lung is retracted.

For closed valvulotomy. The pericardium is incised and retracted with interrupted silk sutures. The left appendage is identified and an appendage clamp applied. A purse-string suture may be placed in position beneath the clamp. An opening is made in the appendage tip and the clamp loosened to admit the surgeon's finger. (The purse-string suture may be tightened if there is a leak of blood.) If dilatation of the stenosed valve is impossible with the surgeon's finger, he withdraws it and inserts a dilator. After adequate dilatation has been accomplished, the dilator is removed and the appendage clamp applied. The opening in the appendage tip is closed with two rows of 2 (3/0) silk on non-traumatic needles.

Alternatively, a dilator may be passed from the ventricle. In this case the instrument is introduced through the ventricle wall, and after dilatation the opening in the myocardium is closed with 2 (3/0) silk on non-traumatic needles.

The pericardium is irrigated with warm saline and sutured with interrupted 2 (3/0) silk on round-bodied needle. The chest is closed in the usual manner for thoracotomy.

For open valvulotomy the chest is entered through a right posterior lateral incision or mediastinal split, the pericardium is opened and secured to the chest wall with 2 or 2·5 (3/0 or 2/0) silk or polyester etc.

After the establishment of total bypass, an incision is made into the left atrium. The mitral valve is opened under direct vision and the atrium then closed with 3 (0) silk or polyester etc. The patient is put onto partial bypass by releasing the venae cavae tourniquets, clamps are then placed on the tubing leading to the heart/lung machine and the bypass is discontinued. Filling of the heart chambers is started before the final sutures are tied, in order to evacuate the air. After removing the cannulae, the incisions in the atrium are closed with 3 (0) silk or polyester, and the chest is closed in the routine manner.

Mitral valve replacement. Similar to the above except the valve is excised and a valve prosthesis inserted and secured with 2·5 (2/0) silk or polyester etc.

Mitral valvuloplasty. Similar to valvulotomy except the incompetent valve is plicated with sutures of 2 or 2·5 (3/0 or 2/0) silk or polyester etc.

Tricuspid valvulotomy, valvuloplasty, or valve replacement. Essentially the same as the mitral procedures described except the right atrium is opened to visualise the valve.

Aortic valvuloplasty or valve replacement. During this procedure, which is performed under bypass, the normal coronary circulation will be compromised. It is essential to incorporate coronary perfusion in the bypass and this can be accomplished in several ways. A tube from the main arterial supply is split into two with a Y connection. The two

Fig. 28.33 Mitral valvulotomy. (A) Non crushing clamp applied to base of appendage, tip of appendage amputated to provide a lumen sufficient to admit index finger to second interphalangeal joint. (B) Momentarily release of clamp to washout any loose thrombi. (C) Palpation of valve; it may be possible to dilate the valve with the index finger or dilator from this approach. (D) Transventricular dilatation. (E and F) Suture of appendage. Inset in (F) Suture of the pericardium.

Fig. 28.34 Ventricular septal defect. (A) Seen through incision in right ventricle. (B) Inspection of defect before repair. (C and D) Mattress sutures are first placed in the margins of the defect and through the Teflon patch. (E and F) When all sutures are passed, the patch is lowered down and the sutures tied. Additional reinforcing sutures may be required after testing for completeness of closure.

tubes are then used to perfuse both coronary arteries one method being via hand-held metal suction ends.

The venous blood is collected from the right atrium via a 13 mm ($\frac{1}{2}$ in) Portex polyvinyl atrium catheter. Total bypass is accomplished by clamping the main pulmonary artery. Frequently the bypass is combined with hypothermia to minimise the hazards associated with interrupting the normal coronary blood supply.

After establishing complete bypass the aorta is clamped, incised and coronary perfusion started. Aortic valvulotomy, reconstructive valvuloplasty or valve replacement is then performed using 2·5 (2/0) polyester etc. on a 17 taper cut needle. After this has been completed the aorta is closed rapidly, for in order to do so the coronary perfusion has to be stopped. Saline 'slush' is often put into the chest cavity to produce some local hypothermia thereby protecting the myocardium until normal coronary circulation is started. Partial bypass is started by unclamping the pulmonary artery, and when the patient's condition is satisfactory, this is discontinued and the chest closed in the normal manner. The sternum is generally approximated with stainless steel wire size No. 25 SWG.

Pulmonary valvulotomy. This can be performed under hypothermia without cardiopulmonary bypass. The approach is through a sternal splitting incision with the patient supine. Tape tourniquets are placed in position round the major vessels (aorta, venae cavae and pulmonary vessels).

A Potts clamp (which constricts only one third of the vessel lumen) is placed on the pulmonary artery a few centimetres from the valve, and a longitudinal incision of about 2 cm is made in the segment held by the clamp. The heart is emptied of blood by tightening the tourniquets on the venae cavae, and when the chambers are empty the pulmonary artery and aorta are occluded. A careful note is made of the time that the tourniquets are applied. Pulmonary valvulotomy is then performed under direct vision after removing the Potts clamp. This is then reapplied to the pulmonary artery and the circulation started again, usually within 3 minutes or so of its cessation, by releasing the tourniquets. (First the venae cavae constrictions are released, then the pulmonary artery side clamp is applied, and finally the pulmonary artery and aorta tourniquets released.) The opening in the pulmonary artery is closed with 1 (5/0) silk or polyester etc. on a non-traumatic needle. If ventricular fibrillation is present, this is dealt with by electrical stimulation.

It should be noted that various arterial clamps may be used to occlude the major vessels as an alternative to tourniquets.

With the indirect Bourie procedure, a Bisch dilator (or Bisch knife) is passed into the right ventricle through the myocardium, pushed through the valve, opened 15 or 20 mm,

Fig. 28.35 Normal heart and vessels as compared with characteristics of Tetralogy of Fallot. (Courtesy Evans and *Nursing Times*.)

thereby dilating the valve or cutting in two planes. The opening in the myocardium is closed with 2 (3/0) silk or polyester etc. on a non-traumatic needle.

Intraventricular pressures are reassessed, and the pericardium is irrigated and closed as described before.

The chest is closed as for thoracotomy.

Atrial septal defect. One of the most common of the congenital cardiac defects, it causes shunting of blood from the left to the right side of the heart. The gradual pressure build up and volume in the right heart and increased pulmonary resistance eventually causes a reverse of this shunt from right to left with consequent right heart failure. Surgical treatment of this condition consists of repairing the defect under direct vision, with complete bypass.

The approach is via a sternal splitting incision and the procedure approximates that for open mitral valvulotomy. The right atrium is opened and the intraseptal defect either sutured, or repaired with a Teflon patch. The atrioventricular valves may also require some reconstructive surgery. The atrium is closed with 3 (0) silk or polyester etc. bypass discontinued and the chest closed in the usual manner.

Ventricular septal defect. This again produced a left to right shunt of blood within the heart which may eventually 'balance' due to an increase in the right ventricular and pulmonary pressures. The reconstructive procedure is similar to repair of atrial septal defect except that the right ventricle is incised, and is closed with 3 (0) silk or polyester etc. combined with Teflon patches.

Fig. 28.36 Operative photograph of a double vein graft. One vein graft has been attached to the aorta, whereas the other has been attached to the previously inserted vein graft as an end-to-side anastomosis. It courses transversely across the field to connect to the anterior descending coronary artery. The initial graft was anastomosed distally to the termination of the right coronary artery. (Irvine.)

Fig. 28.37 Operative photograph of double vein grafts implanted in the aorta. The vein graft in the centre of the field was anastomosed distally to the anterior descending coronary artery, while the graft in the upper right portion of the field was attached to the circumflex coronary artery. (Irvine.)

Tetralogy of Fallot. This is a simultaneous occurrence of pulmonary stenosis; intraventricular septal defect; dextraposition of the aorta; and hypertrophy of the right ventricle. This results in increased pressure within the right ventricle due to pulmonary stenosis and a right to left shunt of blood via the ventricular septal defect with decreased oxygenation of the systemic blood.

The corrective procedure is similar to aortic valvulotomy under direct vision, and repair of the ventricular septal defect. The patient is placed on complete bypass.

During all open heart surgery it is generally necessary to arrest the heart beat by using a fibrillator which administers a constant D.C. shock. The effect is reversed with a defibrillator.

Revascularisation of the coronary arteries. There are several operations carried out in the surgical treatment of coronary heart disease. Varied success has been reported on performing myocardial mammary artery implantation, coronary endarterectomy, and saphenous vein graft between the aorta and coronary artery beyond the blocked segment (Rowe, 1978). Of these, the latter procedure has gained a degree of popularity in the United Kingdom (Waugh, 1975). An appropriate length of long saphenous vein is removed from either leg, and the cut side branches are ligated; it is then placed in heparinised saline solution. Alternatively, if the patient has had an operation for varicose veins, the vein graft may be removed from the arm.

The heart is approached through a sternum – splitting incision; the pericardium is opened and cardio pulmonary bypass established. A 1 cm incision is made longitudinally in the coronary artery beyond the stenosed segment. The end of the vein graft is cut obliquely and anastomosed end-to-side to the slit in the coronary artery, using 0·75 (6/0) Dacron or other non-absorbant material. It is essential to ensure that the vein is anastomosed the correct way round i.e., valves opening towards the coronary anastomosis.

The vein graft is then cut to the required length, and anastomosed end-to-side to the aorta after removing a 7 mm disc of aortic wall. If necessary, further bypass grafts are inserted and the heart is then allowed to take over the circulation, cardio pulmonary bypass being discontinued.

Fig. 28.38 (A) Divided pulmonary artery and implantation of coronary arteries. (B) The completed 'transposition' operation. Aorta connected to left ventricle, pulmonary artery connected to right ventricle. (Foster.)

Great care is taken to secure haemostasis. Heparinisation of the patient is reversed and drainage tubes inserted in the pericardial cavity and chest cavity just behind the sternum. The chest is closed in the usual way.

Transposition of the great arteries. (TGA) One of the commonest forms of cyanotic congenital cardiac defects, TGA generally consists of the aorta arising from the right ventricle and the pulmonary artery from the left ventricle. The result of this, is two completely separate circulations, and for a baby to survive at birth a ventricular septal defect, (VSD) atral septal defect (ASD) or patient ductus arteriosus must be present (Foster and Hibbert, 1977).

For many years the only operative surgery possible consisted of a physiological type of correction, where the pulmonary venous blood was redirected to the right ventricle and systemic venous return redirected into the left ventricle (Mustard operation). Now in certain cases, it is possible to transpose the great arteries to their anatomically correct ventricles.

The pulmonary artery is divided transversely above the pulmonary valve. The right ventricle is incised and the ASD or VSD repaired with a Dacron patch. The right and left coronary arteries are excised with a disc of aorta, and anastomosed to the sides of the pulmonary artery root. The holes left in the aorta are repaired either with a patch of Dacron or Dura mater. The aorta is then divided and anastomosed to the pulmonary artery root.

To achieve continuity between the aortic root and the pulmonary artery, it is usual to interpose a connecting Dacron tube. The cardiopulmonary bypass is discontinued and the chest closed in the usual manner.

Thoracic aortic aneurysm. This is performed through a left posteriolateral thoracotomy.

With the repair procedure, the distal portion of the aneurysm is clamped across both proximally and distally. The aorta is divided and sutured circumferentially back on itself to close the false channel. The aorta is then re-anastomosed.

Replacement with a graft or woven Dacron or aortic homograft is accomplished after excising the aneurysm between two aortic clamps. The graft is sutured with 2·5 (2/0) polyester etc.

Fig. 28.39 Thoracic aortic aneurysm. (A) The aorta is divided through the intimal tear, and catheters inserted into one or both coronary artery orifices for perfusion with cooled blood from the oxygenator. The separated intima and adventibia are sutured circumferentially. (B) It may be necessary to insert a valve prosthesis if the aortic valve has been deformed. (C) Anastomosis of the aorta. (D) Insertion of a Teflon aortic graft. (Cleland.)

Correction of patent ductus arteriosus

DEFINITION

The ligation or division of a patent ductus which is a remnant of foetal circulation and allows blood to pass from the aorta into the pulmonary artery.

POSITION

Right lateral chest (Fig. 4.10).

INSTRUMENTS

As for thoracotomy (p. 702)
Ductus clamps (Potts), 3
Aortic clamp (Potts)
Large bulldog clamps (Potts), 3
Scissors, angled (Potts Smith), set of 3
Long needle holders (Potts Smith or Holmes Sellor, etc.), 2
Irrigation syringe, rubber catheter and sterile warm saline
Nylon tape or fine rubber tubing prepared for tourniquets
Routine thoracotomy ligatures and sutures
Sterile liquid paraffin
3 (0) Silk or polyester etc. for ligation of ductus
2 (3/0) Silk or polyester etc. on a small half-circle round-bodied needle for mediastinal pleura
1 (5/0) Silk or polyester etc. on a small curved non-traumatic needle for ductus suture.

OUTLINE OF PROCEDURE

A left posterolateral incision is made and the chest entered through the fourth interspace or the bed of a resected fifth rib. A rib spreader is inserted and the lung retracted to expose the region of the ductus and the mediastinal pleura which is incised.

The aortic arch and pulmonary artery are dissected free on both sides of the ductus, using blunt and sharp dissection. In order to allow adequate mobilisation, some small vessels in the ductus region may require ligation. The vagus nerve is identified and retracted with tape or rubber tubing.

Fig. 28.40 Patent ductus arteriosus. The ductus is seen communicating with the pulmonary artery and the aorta. (Farquharson and Rintoul.)

The ductus may be ligated with 3 (0) silk or polyester etc. ligatures which are placed at the aortic and pulmonary end of the ductus. Alternatively, the ductus may be divided after placing ductus clamps near to the pulmonary artery and aortic junction. With the latter method, the ductus is then divided and the ends closed with a continuous 1 (5/0) silk or polyester etc. on a non-traumatic needle, followed by an outer layer of interrupted sutures.

The clamps are then removed, haemostasis is secured and the mediastinal pleura sutured over the operation area with 2 (3/0) silk or polyester etc. The chest cavity is irrigated with saline and the thorax closed in the usual manner, with underwater drainage.

Correction of coarctation of the aorta

DEFINITION

Resection of a congenital narrowing of the arch or descending part of the aorta, and re-establishment of aortic continuity by end to end anastomosis.

POSITION

Right lateral chest (Fig. 4.10).

INSTRUMENTS

As for thoracotomy (p. 702)
Coarctation clamps, straight and curved (Crafoord, Potts, etc.), 2 of each
Clamps (Blalock), 2
Large bulldog clamps (Potts), 6
Various other arterial clamps (Blalock, etc.)
Long dissecting forceps, toothed, fine (Waugh)
Long dissecting forceps, non-toothed, fine (Waugh)
Long fine scissors (tonsil or McIndoe)
Long needle holders (Potts Smith or Holmes Sellor, etc.), 2
Irrigation syringe, rubber catheter and sterile warm saline
Nylon tape or fine rubber tubing prepared for tourniquets
Routine thoracotomy ligatures and sutures
Sterile liquid paraffin
2 (3/0) Silk or polyester etc. on a small half-circle round-bodied needle for mediastinal pleura
1 (5/0) Silk or polyester etc. on a small curved non-traumatic needle for anastomosis
Prepared homograft or fabric prosthesis may be required (Chapter 27).

OUTLINE OF PROCEDURE

A left posterolateral incision is made and haemostasis of the many collateral vessels is secured. The chest is entered through the fourth interspace or bed of a resected fifth rib. A rib spreader is inserted, the lung retracted, and the mediastinal pleura incised to expose the aortic arch. The aorta is freed by sharp and blunt dissection and tapes or rubber tubing passed above and below the stenosed area. Alternatively, arterial clamps may be employed.

Vessels which leave the aorta at the point of resection are ligated, and this may include the left subclavian artery which commonly rises at the stenosis.

734

A

B

C

D

E

F

The vagus nerve is identified and retracted before applying coarctation clamps or Blalock clamps above and below the stenosed segment, which is then excised. The gap is closed either by end to end anastomosis with 1 (5/0) silk or polyester etc., or the interposition of a homograft or fabric (Teflon) tube prosthesis. The homograft or fabric prosthesis is anastomosed to each end of the cut aorta in the usual manner.

Haemostasis secured, the mediastinal pleura is sutured over the operation area, and the chest cavity irrigated before closing in the usual manner, with underwater drainage.

Heart transplantation

Note: Human cardiac transplantation is now a clinical reality, although in the United Kingdom few operations have been carried out (Laguea et al., 1979), it is a well established procedure in the United States (Ballinger et al., 1972; Jamieson et al., 1979). The ethical aspects of donor selection and immune reaction will remain for some time to come.

POSITION AND INSTRUMENTS

As for major intra cardiac surgery (p. 717), but equipment for two individual cardiopulmonary bypasses will be required.

OUTLINE OF PROCEDURE

Donor operation. Until 1979, it was necessary to undertake a transplant immediately following removal of the donor heart in an adjacent operating theatre. However, following the development of a technique at Stanford University Medical Centre, California (Jamieson et al., 1979), it is possible to remove donor hearts in distant centres and transport them within three hours to the recipient. This is provided the myocardial temperature is reduced sufficiently to preserve the donor heart.

In this instance, a cardiac team travels to the hospital concerned to remove the heart. A thorough examination of the donor is undertaken to exclude congenital cardiac defects or cardiac trauma. If the donor is suitable, he is taken to the operating theatre where the heart is exposed and thoroughly examined. After pronouncement of death, heparine is administered, the heart arrested, followed by infusion of cold cardioplegic solution through the coronary arteries. After mobilisation, the venae cavae and pulmonary veins are divided at the atrium. Transection of the pulmonary artery is carried out following division of the atrial septum. The aorta is divided beyond the coronary ostia, the heart filled with cold cardioplegic solution, and placed in cold saline at 4°C. Transferring to several further bowls of cold saline ensures maximum cooling. The heart is finally placed in a sterile plastic bag of cold saline, covered with several more sterile plastic bags and stored in an ice container for rapid transport to the recipient.

Throughout this procedure, communication is maintained with the recipient hospital so that removal of the donor heart can be coordinated with the start of the recipient operation.

Recipient operation. On arrival, the donor heart is removed from the protective bags, and still kept in cold saline, is dissected and tailored to fit the recipient vessels. This

◄ Fig. 28.41 Coarctation of the aorta. (A) Mobilization of the aorta. (B) Control of the right intercostal arteries. (C) Occlusion of the aorta and excision of coarctation. (D) Anastomosis. (E) Removal of clamps – additional sutures may be required to control oozing. (F) Teflon graft replacement for long coarctations.

usually consists of trimming fat off the aorta and pulmonary artery, followed by an incision from the inferior vena cava towards the superior vena cava, curving upwards to the right atrial appendage and avoiding the sinuatrial node (Jamieson et al., 1979). This opens up the right atrium. The left atrium is then opened up by incisions connecting the pulmonary veins on the posterior surface of the heart.

After exposure of the heart, the recipient is placed on cardiopulmonary bypass. As there must be complete absence of tubes in the region of the heart, peripheral cannulation of the venae cavae is carried out through the right internal jugular and left saphenous veins.

Occlusion of the intra pericardial venae cavae is achieved with rubber tourniquets. The pulmonary trunk and aorta are mobilised just above their semi lunar valves, and the atria are excised, leaving intact portions of the right and left atrial walls and atrial septum. The redundant heart tissue is then removed.

The donor heart is placed in position, and sutures at each end of the atrial cavity (of the recipient) are united to the extent of the donor heart left atrium. Simple over and over sutures are then used to unite first the left atria, and then the right atria. Preservation of the myocardium is continued by continuous pericardial irrigation with cold saline. On completion of the atrial anastomosis, irrigation of cold saline is continued through a tube inserted through the left atrial appendage. This maintains cooling and helps to expel air from the left atrium and ventricle.

The aortic anastomosis is carried out and just before the suture line is complete, any air remaining in the chambers of the heart is expelled by manipulation of the heart and inflation of the lungs. The aortic clamp is removed to allow perfusion of the coronary vessels by blood returning from the cardiopulmonary bypass machine.

The heart is generally in ventricular fibrillation at this time and the pulmonary artery anastomosis is carried out. The donor pulmonary artery is occluded, the venae cavae tourniquets released and a needle inserted in the apex of the ascending aorta to allow any residual air to be expelled. The heart usually defibrillates spontaneously; if not a small electric shock restores sinus rhythm.

Temporary cardiac pacing wires are positioned on the donor right atrium. These are for direct ECG recording and pacing if necessary. After a 20 minute period of partial bypass, the cardiopulmonary bypass is discontinued, and the chest closed in the usual manner, meticulous care being taken with haemostasis, apposition of tissues and insertion of the two chest drains. It is usual to leave an indwelling catheter inserted suprapubically to minimise the risk of transurethral infection.

REFERENCES AND FURTHER READING

BALLINGER, W. F., TREYBAL, J. C. AND VOSS, A. B. (1972) *Alexander's Care of the Patient in Surgery.* C. V. Mosby Co.
CLELAND, W. P. (1968) *Surgery – Thorax.* London: Butterworths.
EVANS, J. (1978) *Nursing Times,* 918.
FARQUHARSON, E. L. AND RINTOUL, R. F. (1972) *Textbook of Operative Surgery.* Edinburgh: Churchill Livingstone.
FOSTER, G. A. (1977) *Nursing Times,* 1193.
GILBART, R. (1972) *Nursing Times,* 1439.
ILLINGWORTH, C. (1973) *A short Textbook of Surgery.* Edinburgh: Churchill Livingstone.
IRVINE, W. T. (1971) *Modern Trends in Surgery.* London: Butterworths.
JAMIESON, S., STINSON, E. AND SHUMWAY, N. (1979) *Nursing Mirror,* **24,** June 21st.
LAGUEA, J., CROWIE, D., WALKER, C. AND WILLIAMS, J. (1976) *Nursing Mirror,* **19,** November 29th.
LINLEY, G. (1976) *Nursing Mirror,* **52,** June 24th.
LOCKIE, E. (1976) *Nursing Times,* 1190.
PAGLIERO, K. M. (1975) *Nursing Times,* 925.
PANETH, M. (1975) *Nursing Mirror,* **58,** August 7th.
ROSS, et al. (1976) *British Medical Journal,* **1,** 1109.
ROWE, G. C. (1978) *Lancet,* **i,** 264.
WRIGHT, J. E. C. (1975) *Nursing Mirror,* **53,** August 7th.

29
ABDOMINAL VASCULAR OPERATIONS

Excision and graft for aneurysm of the aorta

DEFINITION

Excision of a dilated portion of the abdominal aorta and insertion of a synthetic fabric prosthesis, e.g., Teflon, Dacron.

POSITION

Supine.

INSTRUMENTS

General set (Figs. 14.1 to 14.28)
Laparotomy set (Figs. 15.1 to 15.7)
Long fine dissecting forceps, toothed, 20 cm (8 in) (Waugh), 2
Lone fine dissecting forceps, non-toothed, 20 cm (8 in) (Waugh), 2
Dissecting forceps, toothed, 25 cm (10 in)
Dissecting forceps, non-toothed, 25 cm (10 in)
Long scissors, curved on flat, 23 cm (9 in) (Nelson)
Scissors, curved on flat, 18 cm (7 in) (Mayo)
Scissors, angled (Potts Smith), set of 3
Vena cava occlusion clamps, 2
Aortic clamps (Potts), 2
Large bulldog clamps, 6
Small bulldog clamps, 6
Long needle holders (Potts Smith or Holmes Sellor, etc.), 2
Polythene tubing or nylon tape
20 ml syringe, needles and blunt cannula
Heparin 10,000 units in 2 ml and protamine sulphate 100 mgm (*Note.* 1 mg of heparin is equivalent to 100 units, and for neutralisation the equivalent of 1 mg of protamine sulphate is given for each 100 units of heparin.) or polybrene
Laparotomy ligatures and sutures
2 and 1 (3/0 and 5/0) Silk, etc., on small curved arterial needles for anastomosis
Occlusion cuffs (tourniquets) for both thighs.

OUTLINE OF PROCEDURE

A midline or left paramedian incision is made from the xyphisternum to the symphysis pubis. The bowel is retracted with moist packs and the posterior peritoneum opened over the aorta. The ureters are identified and retracted, and the inferior mesenteric artery is divided between ligatures.

The aorta is mobilised above the aneurysm and the aorta or the iliac vessels below, and polythene tubing or nylon tape passed round them. Adjoining vessels are retracted in a similar manner, and after systemic heparinisation, the aorta above the aneurysm (but below the renal arteries) is occluded with an occlusion clamp. The common iliac arteries are occluded with bulldog clamps, the aneurysm is mobilised and the anterior wall excised.

Fig. 29.1 (left)   A small abdominal aortic aneurysm exposed at operation, tapes around normal vessels in vicinity of aneurysm. These will be clamped and ligated before the anterior wall of the aneurysm is excised.

Fig. 29.2 (right)   Bifurcated Dacron graft replacing the aneurysm seen in Fig. 29.1. (Courtesy Mr A. P. Wyatt, F.R.C.S. and *Nursing Mirror*.)

The aortic defect is bridged with a bifurcated fabric prosthesis (e.g., Teflon, Dacron, Fig. 29.2), and the anastomosis carried out with continuous non-absorbable sutures. Synthetic fabric prostheses of Teflon or Dacron are either of the knitted or woven type. The knitted type have a wider mesh and required 'pre-clotting'. This is done by immersing the graft for at least 20 min in 30 ml of patient's blood taken before heparinisation. After the anastomoses are completed, the clamps are carefully released one after another to test the integrity of the suture line. If necessary, the anastomoses may be reinforced with further interrupted sutures of non-absorbable material. Thigh occlusion cuffs may be applied and inflated before release of the iliac occlusion clamps, and gradually released subsequently to avoid possible fall of blood-pressure. The action of the heparin is neutralised by the appropriate amounts of protamine sulphate.

Should occlusion of the aorta above the renal arteries be required hypothermia, a temporary bypass graft, or an extracorporeal circulation may be required.

The posterior peritoneum is closed with absorbable sutures and the abdominal aspirated free of blood before closure of the wound. Tension sutures are usual as paralytic ileus is frequent.

Splenorenal shunt

DEFINITION

Anastomosis between the splenic and renal veins to relieve hypertension in the portal venous system.

POSITION

Supine or right lateral chest for a left side approach.

INSTRUMENTS

Abdominal approach. As for laparotomy (p. 327)
Thoraco-abdominal approach. As for thoracotomy (p. 702)
Both routes
   Long fine dissecting forceps, toothed, 20 cm (8 in) (Waugh), 2
   Long fine dissecting forceps, non-toothed, 20 cm (8 in) (Waugh), 2
   Dissecting forceps, toothed, 25 cm (10 in)
   Dissecting forceps, non-toothed, 25 cm (10 in)
   Long scissors, curved on flat, 23 cm (9 in) (Nelson)
   Aorta clamps (Potts and Blalock), 2 of each, optional
   Large bulldog clamps (Potts), 6
   Small bulldog clamps, 6
   Long needle holders (Potts Smith or Holmes Sellor, etc.), 2
   Manometer, three-way tap, rubber or plastic tubing and exploration needle
   Polythene tubing or nylon tape
   20 ml syringe, needles and blunt cannula
   Heparin 10,000 units in 2 ml and protamine sulphate 100 mgm or polybrene
   Laparotomy or thoracotomy ligatures and sutures
   1 and 0·75 (5/0 and 6/0) Silk or other non-absorbable material, etc., on small curved non-traumatic arterial needles for anastomosis.

OUTLINE OF PROCEDURE

For abdominal approach, a long, left paramedian incision with 'T' or 'L' extension as required is made and the peritoneum opened in the usual manner.

For thoraco-abdominal approach, the incision is made through the bed of the ninth rib which is resected, and extends across the epigastrium transversely. The left diaphragm is divided and a rib spreader inserted to obtain exposure.

The pressure in the splenic vein may be measured with a needle and manometer before mobilising the spleen, either directly from the vein or by splenic puncture. The spleen is freed and removed as described for splenectomy in Chapter 13, but leaving a maximum length of the vein by mobilising from the tail of the pancreas. The splenic vein is divided distal to the occlusion clamp applied close to the hilum of the spleen.

The left kidney is exposed and mobilised, and the renal vein is identified and marked with polythene tubing or nylon tape. Occlusion clamps or tubing tourniquets with rubber stops are applied to the renal vein to isolate a suitable segment for the anastomosis.

Fig. 29.3 Splenorenal shunt. (A and B) Site of incision. (C) Spleen mobilised, splenic vein dissected free and held with tape. (D) Kidney exposed, spleen removed, splenic vein transected, renal vein occluded with tape-tourniquet, before longitudinal incision made at site of anastomosis. (E) Splenorenal anastomosis completed. (Ross.)

It is wise to have temporary control of the renal artery with occlusion clamps at this stage also. The end of the splenic vein is trimmed before making an end to side anastomosis with 1 or 0·75 (5/0 or 6/0) non-absorbable sutures. Alternatively, a nephrectomy may be carried out to permit end to end anastomosis to the renal vein, but this method is avoided if at all possible. Heparin may be injected systematicaly before the clamps are applied and the anastomosis made, followed by an injection of the appropriate amounts of protamine sulphate after release of the clamps.

The wound is closed in the usual manner for laparotomy or thoracotomy.

Portacaval shunt

DEFINITION

Anastomosis between the portal vein and the inferior vena cava.

POSITION

Supine or left lateral chest for a right side approach.

INSTRUMENTS

As for splenorenal shunt except that the operation is on the other side.

OUTLINE OF PROCEDURE

The exposure is identical to that for splenorenal shunt but on the right side.

The portal vein and inferior vena cava are mobilised in the usual manner and either an end to side anastomosis or side to side anastomosis made. A laterally placed partial occlusion clamp on the inferior vena cava avoids obstruction to the venous drainage of the kidneys and lower part of the body during the formation of the shunt.

REFERENCES AND FURTHER READING

ROBB, C. (1976) *Vascular Surgery*. London: Butterworths.
WYATT, A. R. (1976) *Nursing Mirror*, **52**, August 11–19.

30
PERIPHERAL VASCULAR OPERATIONS

Development of the binocular microscope during the last decade has enabled considerable advances to be made in the field of microsurgery (see Chapter 12). This is particularly so in peripheral vascular operations. Previously, the surgeon was restricted to operations on vessels which were large enough to visualise either by normal eyesight, or by limited magnification afforded by using spectacles or binocular lenses. Using an operating microscope and the ultra-fine suture needles and suture material now available, it is possible

Fig. 30.1 Microvascular repair of a 1 mm vessel. (See also Fig. 12.14.)

(A) Three sutures have been inserted on the anterior wall. The clear circle of one of the sutures is evident.
(B) The clamps have been turned over and the gaping posterior vessel edges are obvious. The posterior repair is completed in a similar fashion after inserting a central suture first. (O'Brien.)

Fig. 30.2 Repair of 1 mm vein.

(A to C) Sometimes, in a confined space, it may be necessary to repair the posterior vessel edges first from an anterior approach after placing guide sutures.
(D) The posterior repair of the vein is almost complete. The micro needle holder grasps the metalized needle of the nylon microsuture.
(E) A final suture is being placed in the posterior wall of the 1 mm vein repair, tying the suture with the needle holder in the right hand and number 5 jeweller's forceps in the left hand.
(F) Completed posterior wall repair.
(G) Final microvascular repair, the scale is measured in millimetres. (O'Brien.)

A

B

C

D

E

F

G

to repair blood vessels and nerves with a diameter of only 1 mm or less. This technique has revolutionised the surgery of trauma, enabling reimplantation of digits which previously would have been amputated.

Microvascular surgery requires meticulous, painstaking technique. The principles of vascular anastomosis is described in some of the operations included in this chapter. For more detail, the reader is advised to consult a specialised text book on the subject. However, the basic technique can be appreciated in the following illustrations and Figures 30.4 to 30.10 give an indication of the delicate instrumentation required.

Fig. 30.3   End to side anastomosis of an 0·9 mm artery using 0·2 (10/0) nylon.

(A) Second guide suture being inserted.
(B) Posterior wall repair completed – central anterior suture being inserted.
(C) Anterior wall repair completed.
(D) Patent anastomosis on release of clamps. (O'Brien.)

Operations for varicose veins (Trendelenburg's operation and vein stripping)

DEFINITION

Ligation and division of the long saphenous vein at the point where it joins the femoral vein and of the terminal long saphenous vein tributaries. In the stripping operation, a flexible stripper is used to remove a length of the diseased vein from the leg.

POSITION

Supine, with the legs slightly abducted.

INSTRUMENTS

General set (Figs. 14.1 to 14.28)
Vein stripper, if stripping operation is to be performed
2·5 and 3 (2/0 and 0) Chromic catgut, Dexon or silk for ligatures
3 (0) Chromic catgut or Dexon on a small half-circle round-bodied needle for deep sutures
2·5 (2/0) Silk or nylon on a medium curved or straight cutting needle for skin sutures.

OUTLINE OF PROCEDURE

For Trendelenburg's Operation an incision is made in the upper thigh, parallel to the crease in the groin over the saphenous opening. Dissection is made through the fat down to the point where the saphenous vein joins the femoral vein. (Small tributaries are ligated as the dissection proceeds.) The saphenous vein is isolated, divided, and both ends ligated at the femoral junction. The wound is closed in layers. The operation may require to be supplemented by ligation of the deep perforating veins, or stripping.

For the Stripping Operation, before the groin wound is closed, an incision is made at the ankle and a stripper threaded up the saphenous vein to the groin. The lower part of the divided saphenous vein in the ankle is secured to the bulbous end of the stripper by a ligature, and the whole withdrawn through the groin incision, thereby pulling the saphenous vein out of the leg. The short saphenous vein is treated by division and

Fig. 30.4 Microscissors. (Genito Urinary Manufacturing Co. Ltd.)

746 Operating Theatre Technique

Fig. 30.5 Micron Artery Forceps.

Fig. 30.6 Yasargil Micro Vessel Clips.

Fig. 30.7 Razor Blade Fragment Holder.

Fig. 30.8 Hoskin Forceps.

Fig. 30.9 Micro Groove Forceps Curved.

Fig. 30.10 Micro Groove Forceps Straight.

Figs. 30.5 to 30.10 Micro instruments. (Chas. F. Thackray Ltd.)

Fig. 30.11 Stripping operation for varicose veins.

(A) Trendelenburg operation. Long saphenous vein ligatured and divided at junction with femoral. Tributaries divided between ligatures. (The stripper will not be seen emerging from the cut saphenous vein until a later stage of the operation.)
(B) Lower end of long saphenous vein exposed in front of medial malleolus. Stripper inserted, and ligature around vein ready to be tied.
(C) Ligature tied to anchor vein against acorn-head of stripper, and vein divided.
(D) The complete vein after avulsion, telescoped against the head of the stripper.

(Farquharson and Rintoul.)

ligation at the sapheno-popliteal junction and stripped between there and an incision on the outer side of the tendino Achilles. A crêpe bandage is applied after the wounds have been closed. The patient has the foot of his bed elevated on blocks after operation, but is mobilised as soon as possible.

Arterial and venous embolectomy

DEFINITION

Removal of a blood clot which has become impacted in an artery or vein and is interfering with the circulation below that point. The most common sites for an arterial embolism to occur are at the arterial bifurcations, such as that of the abdominal aorta, the femoral and popliteal arteries. Similarly, venous emboli are also common at venous bifurcations such as the junction of the vena cava with the common iliac vessels. This is an emergency operation.

POSITION

Depends upon the site of the embolus.

INSTRUMENTS

General set (Figs. 14.1 to 14.28)
Scalpel handle No. 9 with No. 15 blade (Bard Parker)
Fine dissecting forceps, toothed (Gillies), 2
Fine dissecting forceps, non-toothed (McIndoe), 2
Fine dissecting forceps, micro (various sizes and shapes)
Fine scissors, curved on flat, 10 cm (4 in) (Kilner or iris)
Fine needle holders, 2
Fine needle holders, micro, 2
Vascular occlusion clamps (Yasargil, Carrel) 6 or more will be needed
Suction tubing, fine nozzles, rubber catheter with connection
Irrigation syringe, rubber catheter and non-pyrogenic saline
20 ml syringe, needles and blunt cannula
Fogarty embolectomy catheters 3FG to 7FG (Balloon inflation according to catheter size, i.e., 0·5 ml to 2·5 ml)
Fogarty irrigating catheters 4FG to 6FG (Balloon inflation according to catheter size, i.e., 0·5 ml to 2·5 ml)
Heparin 10,000 units in 2 ml and protamine sulphate 100 mgm or polybrene
Local anaesthetic requisites may be required (Fig. 10.34)
2·5 and 3 (2/0 and 0) Chromic catgut, Dexon or silk for ligatures
1·5, 1 or 0·7 (4/0, 5/0 or 6/0) Silk or polyester etc. on a small curved non-traumatic arterial needle for vascular suture
Appropriate sutures for that area of the body.

OUTLINE OF PROCEDURE

Method 1. An incision is made over the point at which the embolus has lodged. Dissection is made down to the vessel and an adequate exposure obtained. Polythene tubing or nylon tape is passed round the vessel and any immediate branches above and below the clot. This tubing or tapes can be threaded through short pieces of rubber or plastic tubing, as shown in Fig. 30.12, which can be slid down to occlude the vessel. Alternatively, bulldog or other vascular occlusion clamps (e.g., Carrel's) are applied to occlude the vessels. Heparin solution may be injected systemically before the application of clamps. An incision is made in the vessel wall and the clot milked or suctioned out. After as much of the clot as can be seen and palpated has been removed, the patency of the vessels below the thrombosed section is checked by momentarily releasing the constrictions and allowing the blood to flow. When the surgeon is satisfied that all the thrombus has been removed, the vessel incision is closed with 1 (5/0) silk or polyester and if the heparin has been injected, it is neutralised with protamine sulphate (or polybrene), following which the blood circulation is recommenced.

The wound is closed in layers.

Fig. 30.12 Embolectomy (A to E) methods of temporary control of the artery.
(F to H) Clot may be removed by extraction, 'milking' or a 'corkscrew' wire.
(I to J) Testing for patency of the artery.
(I) Backflow indicates clearance to at least one sizable branch but this is not necessarily sufficient.
(J) Full flow from above – this must be an obvious full bore flow to be accepted as evidence of complete clearance above the arteriotomy. A conical and arterial cannula attached to a syringe filled with saline can also be used to test for patency.
(K) Resuture of the arteriotomy. (Martin.)

Method 2. Using the Fogarty embolectomy balloon catheter for saddle emboli, iliac artery and peripheral artery emboli.

Bilateral incisions are made over the common femoral arteries and the superficial and deep femoral arteries are isolated. After applying suitable arterial clamps, incisions are made at the junction of the superficial and deep femoral arteries. Appropriate sizes of embolectomy catheters are threaded distally as far as they will go, inflated with fluid and withdrawn to remove the distal thrombus. After removal, 20 mg of heparin in 50 ml of saline is injected into the distal arterial tree via irrigation catheters. This procedure is repeated by passing a catheter through the common femoral artery and into the aorta, inflating the balloon with fluid and withdrawing to extract the thrombus.

The incisions in the vessels are then closed with 1 or 0·7 (5/0 or 6/0) silk or polyester etc. and the groin incision is closed in the usual manner.

Method 3. Vein emboli. Using the Fogarty embolectomy balloon catheter for ileo-femoral emboli. An incision is made over the sapheno-femoral junction on the unaffected side. The largest major tributary is isolated, ligatured distally and its stump utilised to introduce an embolectomy catheter. The catheter is passed up the iliac vein to the vena cava where it is left uninflated.

An incision is then made in the femoral triangle on the affected side and the common, superficial and deep femoral vessels identified. If dissection is difficult the balloon catheter already inserted is inflated with fluid to prevent movement of emboli up the vena cava.

Through a venotomy at the junction of the superficial and deep femoral veins on the affected side, a further balloon is introduced until it is obstructed by the previously inflated catheter. It is then inflated and withdrawn until it lies within the proximal iliac vein segment – the first catheter is then deflated.

A second catheter is then inserted proximally into the affected side and when it reaches the inflated balloon, is itself inflated with fluid. Withdrawal of this catheter extracts the

Fig. 30.13 Fogarty embolectomy catheter. (Genito-Urinary Mfg. Co. Ltd.)

Fig. 30.14 Fogarty embolectomy catheter in use. (Genito-Urinary Mfg. Co. Ltd.)

thrombus. Further catheters may be inserted distally into the limb to extract distal thrombus after which 20 mg of heparin in 50 ml of saline is injected.

Femoral popliteal bypass graft

DEFINITION

The creation of a channel for arterial blood to bypass an occluded segment of the femoral artery. The patient's long saphenous vein is generally used as a graft but if unsuitable, thrombo endartectomy may be performed as an alternative procedure.

POSITION

Supine, with the leg slightly abducted and flexed.

INSTRUMENTS

As arterial embolectomy, minus embolectomy catheters
Graft introducing tube and obturator
Long crocodile forceps
Solution for inflating vein graft which is made up at commencement of operation as follows:
    Normal saline 500 ml
    Heparin 5,000 units in 1 ml
    Procaine hydrochloride 2 per cent, 10 ml.

OUTLINE OF PROCEDURE

Longitudinal incisions, separated by small skin bridges, are made over the course of the long saphenous vein from the groin crease to behind the knee. (This relieves tension

Fig. 30.15 Technique of femoro-popliteal by-pass operation. (A) Removal of vein. (B) Suture of localized varix. (C) Preparation of end of vein. (D) Injection of heparin solution into distal segment of artery. (E) Mattress sutures in place. (F) Completion of suturing. (G) Distension of segment of vein. (H) Mattress suture taking the adventitia of the thickened artery. (I) Progressively deeper bites of artery. (J) Constriction of vein graft if initial bite is too deep. (Martin.)

from the suture line and preserves skin vitality.) The long saphenous vein is exposed and inspected. If found suitable it is removed at a later stage in the operation.

Systemic heparinisation with 10,000 units in 2 ml is now carried out. The common femoral artery and its branches in the femoral triangle are exposed and isolated with tapes of polythene tubing. The popliteal artery is also exposed and mobilised so that it may be brought up into the superficial part of the wound. In order to select a patent length of healthy artery suitable for receiving the distal end of the graft, it may be necessary to divide both the tendon of adductor magnus and the medial head of the gastrocnemius muscle. Small arterial branches are controlled either with small bulldog clamps or double-looped slings of strong silk or polyester.

Fig. 30.16 Disobliteration of 'rebore': (A) is the cross-section of the diseased artery. The dotted line shows the plane of cleavage within the wall of the artery around the atheromatous inner layer and the solid centre of old thrombosis. In (B) the core has been lifted out and in (C) the core has been divided and an artery stripping loop threaded over it, preparatory to being thrust up the affected length of artery. (Figures 30.16 and 30.17 by kind permission of Prof. A. Harding Rains and the *Nursing Times*, published May 1964.)

After ligating its tributaries, the vein is removed and cleaned of adventitia. To test for leaks and size, the proximal end of the vessel is clamped and a suitable arterial cannula tied into the distal end. Using a 20 ml syringe the vein is 'blown up' with a solution of saline/heparin/procaine. Sections of the vein which appear narrow may be due to spasm or constricting adventitia; removal of the latter will allow it to dilate.

The graft introducing tube is inserted, with gentle pressure, from the popliteal fossa, through the adductor canal to emerge in the groin incision. The vein graft is reversed and pulled through the tube with long forceps. The tube is then removed and the proximal end of the vein anastomosed (only three-quarters of the anastomosis being completed at this stage) end-to-side to the popliteal artery using 1 or 0·7 (5/0 or 6/0) silk or polyester as a continuous running suture. The proximal anastomosis of the narrow (distal) end of the vein to the common femoral artery, also end-to-side is completed. Distal, then proximal clamps are released to test for distal reverse flow and to wash out any clots from the graft. The clamps are then re-applied, the distal anastomosis completed and the clamps removed for a second time.

Surgicel may be applied locally to control small leaks, but larger ones will require insertion of further sutures. Heparinisation is reversed with appropriate amounts of protamine sulphate.

Wounds are closed with interrupted skin sutures only with closed Redivac suction drainage.

Disobliteration (Re-bore thrombo endarterectomy)

DEFINITION

Removal of a central atheromatous obstructive core of an artery leaving an outer layer which is free from disease, usually performed on the aorta, iliac, femoral, or popliteal arteries, also the vertebral, subclavian and carotid arteries.

POSITION AND INSTRUMENTS

As femoral popliteal bypass graft
Cannon's endarterectomy ring strippers or similar.

Fig. 30.17 The atheromatous core after it has been stripped out of the femoral artery (the mark indicates 1 cm).

Fig. 30.18 Cannon endarterectomy ring strippers.

OUTLINE OF PROCEDURE

A long thrombo endarterectomy may be performed if the long saphenous vein is not suitable as a graft (see previous operation). This may occur if the vein is too narrow, or has been thrombosed, or is varicose, or absent.

The thrombo endarterectomy is carried out from patent artery above to patent artery below, through multiple arteriotomies. These are repaired using patches of vein graft or Dacron to prevent narrowing.

Through the arteriotomies, the atheromatous core is divided and the loop of the instrument is threaded over one end of the core. Holding this core with artery forceps, the loop is pushed along the plane of cleavage between the core and the vessel wall thereby affecting separation.

At the most distal arteriotomy, the intima is tacked down to the subjacent media by 3 or 4 0·7 (6/0) silk or polyester sutures tied on the outside. This prevents flap formation or 'dissection' which results in occlusion.

There are a number of ring strippers and dissectors in use including Cannon's ring strippers and MacDonald's dissector. A method has been developed using high pressure CO_2 gas which acts in a similar manner.

Short occlusions are treated by localised thrombo endarterectomy and the arteriotomy is repaired by vein or Dacron patches.

REFERENCES AND FURTHER READING

FARQUHARSON, E. L. AND RINTOUL, R. F. (1972) *Textbook of Operative Surgery*. Edinburgh: Churchill Livingstone.
MARTIN, P. (1968) *Indications and Techniques in Arterial Surgery*. Edinburgh: Churchill Livingstone.
O'BRIEN, B. McC. (1977) *Microvascular Reconstructive Surgery*. Edinburgh: Churchill Livingstone.

31
PLASTER OF PARIS TECHNIQUE

For further details of plaster techniques, the reader is referred to *Gypsona Technique* by Smith & Nephew, and to English, M. (1957). *Plaster of Paris Technique*. Edinburgh: Livingstone.

Although metal and wooden splints are still used for the immobilisation of some fractures, plaster of Paris has almost entirely superseded these, and offers many advantages. The basic constituent of plaster of Paris is gypsum or calcium sulphate which is quarried in rock form. The gypsum is ground into a fine powder and heated to evaporate most of the water content to form plaster of Paris. The powder is mixed with chemical solvents and cellulose. Combined with a heating process, the liquid is impregnated on to an open woven, interlocked fabric which holds the plaster uniformly. The impregnated fabric can then be fashioned into bandages and slabs of various sizes. The addition of resin to the basic process of manufacture helps to minimise plaster loss after moistening the bandage, thereby reducing the number of bandages needed for each cast.

Gypsona, manufactured by Smith & Nephew Ltd., is a brand of plaster of Paris which is used extensively in orthopaedics today. The booklet *Gypsona Technique* provides an excellent treatise on all aspects of the 'art and craft' of plastering. This chapter provides a basic outline of plaster procedure related to the operating theatre and readers are referred to *Gypsona Technique* for a more extensive exposition.

Requirements for plaster of Paris application

A deep pail or bowl for soaking the plaster bandages. (This should be three parts filled with tepid water 25 to 35°C.)
Plaster bandages of various widths
Prepared slabs in Gypsona dispenser
Cotton bandages 5 cm and 7·5 cm (2 in and 3 in)
Crepe bandages of various widths
Macintoshes, or disposable paper towels
Plaster wool and orthopaedic felt for padding
Tubular stockinet of various widths
Plaster scissors (usually of the Böhler type)
Heavy angled dressing scissors
Plaster shears
Plaster benders
Plaster knife
Tape measure and marking pencil
A suitable table top or glass sheet for the preparation of slabs
Dusting powder or olive oil may be needed for application to the patient's skin before plastering is commenced, especially if a tight plaster cast is being applied
An electric plaster saw may be required for the removal of a dry cast.

Application of plaster of Paris

Some surgeons prefer to apply their own plaster casts but this may be left to experienced plaster staff who specialise in the art.

The person applying plaster usually wears rubber boots and apron. Rubber gloves may be worn although this is a matter for individual preference.

Plaster slabs

Some operations such as tendon suture of the hand and certain fresh fractures require only the application of a plaster slab for immobilisation, followed by a gauze or crêpe bandage. This provides a well-fitting splint which is quick to prepare and easy to remove for dressings, etc.

There are four methods of preparing plaster slabs:
(a) By unrolling dry plaster bandages,
(b) By unrolling wet plaster bandages,

Fig. 31.1 Dry method of preparing plaster slabs.

(c) By using 5 or 6 thickness plies material from a dry plaster dispenser,
(d) The pattern technique.

(a) The slab is prepared from either dry or wet Gypsona plaster bandages folded out on a smooth surface. The most usual way is to use dry plaster bandages, for the operator may measure and cut the slab at his own speed without fear of the plaster setting before this has been completed.

The dry bandage is placed alongside the limb and the length required marked with a pencil or cut. Alternatively, a tape measure may be used and the length required marked on a bandage which has been unrolled sufficiently on the table-top. The necessary thickness, usually four to six layers, is obtained by unwinding the bandage 'to and fro'. Care must be taken to ensure that all layers extend for the same distance and short ends are discarded. Ten per cent additional length is allowed for shrinkage.

To apply, the slab is lightly folded from each end to the centre, immersed in water and immediately removed. After submergence, surplus water may then be removed by compression, which must be moderately light, for strong squeezing will cause quick setting and vice versa.

After extending the squeezed slab, it is placed on the table-top and carefully smoothed out to remove air bubbles. Failure to do this may cause the finished slab to crack or crumble after application.

Widths of slabs vary according to the individual surgeon's requirements, but the nurse will find generally that a 10 to 15 cm (4 to 6 in) wide slab is suitable for the forearm or a child's leg, but a 15 to 20 cm (6 to 8 in) wide slab will be needed for the lower limb. A larger cast such as a spica may incorporate wider slabs described in the pattern technique.

(b) With this method the bandage is unrolled for about 5 cm (2 in), *held* (not gripped) in the hand and lowered into the water until all bubbling has ceased, usually 5 to 10 seconds. Gripping of the bandage should be avoided because it tends to force plaster out

Fig. 31.2 Method of wetting a plaster slab. (From *Gypsona Technique*.)

of the fabric. The bandage is then lifted out of the water, and the two edges squeezed towards the centre and each other with the thumb and forefinger of each hand. This will allow excess moisture to run out of the bandage, but will retain the greater part of the plaster.

The slab is made by pressing the end of the bandage on to the table-top and holding it there with the left hand. The bandage is then unrolled with the right hand, 'to and fro', to form the correct length and thickness of slab. The air bubbles are smoothed out and the slab applied immediately. The nurse will find it useful to place a stout rod through the centre core of the bandage before unrolling during the preparation of a slab.

(c) The required length of 6 thickness plies (5 thickness low plaster loss) is withdrawn from a dry plaster dispenser. This is quicker and more reliable than the unrolling method. The slab is applied as described under (a).

(d) Another method is the pattern technique by which standard dry plaster slabs are prepared before they are required, using wide Gypsona material.

The patterns described in this chapter are for hip, shoulder and spinal jacket.

The patterns allow for shrinkage after the slabs have been moistened. If the slabs are cut to individual measurements and not the patterns, 10 per cent should be added to these measurements to compensate for this shrinkage.

The slabs are moistened by submerging flat in a sink filled to a depth of 8 to 10 cm (3 to 4 in). The surplus water is removed by drawing the slab over the edge of the sink as it is lifted out. Air bubbles are expressed by smoothing the slab on the table-top, after which it is applied immediately, moulded to the part, and held in place by open wove or Gypsona bandages.

Any slab may be reinforced to withstand additional stress by ridging or girdering. Ridging consists of raising the centre of the slab for 10 mm ($\frac{3}{8}$ in) along its length, after which it is applied carefully to the cast. Girdering is accomplished by superimposing a ridged slab which is about 10 cm shorter than the underlying one.

If the cast has dried, the surface should be roughened and moistened before the application of further slabs.

Application of plaster bandages

Plaster bandages may be used either to make a cast or to complete one after slabs have been applied.

Fig. 31.3 Method of wetting a plaster bandage.

Bony prominences are padded with plaster wool or felt after applying tubular stockinet if required. The stockinet should be longer than the completed plaster to allow turning back for 2·5 cm (1 in) or so just before the final bandages are applied.

The bandages are submerged in tepid water in the manner described for the preparation of wet slabs. They are applied, using even circular turns with no reversing and with a rolling action, not as an ordinary bandage. Any threads which work free from the bandage as it is applied should be cut away, otherwise tightening may occur afterwards. Each turn of the bandage should cover approximately two-thirds of the previous turn. Smooth pleats can be made in the upper or lower edges of the bandage, to allow it to 'sit' evenly when following the contour of a limb. A pause is made after each bandage has been applied, to mould the plaster to the part and allow the layers to set. As the finished plaster cast should be an homogenous mass rather than a series of layers, the moulding is very necessary, together with the exclusion of air between each plaster bandage.

The nurse holding the limb should support it with extended palms to avoid indentations from her finger tips which can cause pressure sores at the point of indentation. She should be very careful to maintain the correct position during the whole period of application.

After application, the plaster cast should be supported on macintosh covered pillows until it has dried. Drying may be hastened in the ward with a heat cradle, but care must be taken to protect exposed areas of the patient's skin from burns, especially if he is unconscious.

An unpadded plaster is very rarely applied to fresh fractures due to the subsequent swelling which always occurs. Even with padding, it may be necessary to bi-valve or cut the plaster along its entire length to allow for this swelling. As the swelling subsides and the plaster becomes loose, it may need to be reapplied (with little padding) to ensure immobilisation.

If it is known that a plaster cast may require splitting, a greased rubber or plastic tube should be placed anteriorly along the length of the limb before plastering is commenced. This tube may be pulled out of the completed plaster easily, leaving a channel inside which simplifies cutting afterwards.

Control of setting time

Normally tepid water (25 to 35°C) should be used for moistening plaster bandages; cold water may cause involuntary muscular contractions if the patient is conscious, and hot water will cause the plaster to set too quickly.

Gypsona bandages set in four to six minutes using tepid water. It is possible to retard this setting time by adding borax to the water.

The setting may be retarded for 1 minute by adding two heaped teaspoonfuls of borax to 1 gal (0·5 per cent); for 7 minutes by adding four level dessertspoonfuls of borax to 1 gal (0·75 per cent); and for 15 minutes by adding one heaped tablespoonful of borax to 1 gal.

TYPES OF PLASTER CASTS

Arm

Colles' fracture

After reduction, the hand is maintained in a position of full pronation and ulnar deviation. A simple fracture is then immobilised with an incomplete forearm plaster, and a severe fracture is immobilised with a mid-arm pronation plaster.

For an incomplete plaster, the elbow is flexed to 90 degrees and the arm is covered with stockinet or a thin layer of plaster wool bandage. A dorsal slab is made from 15 cm (6 in) wide 5 or 6 ply plaster bandage, the length of the slab being 15 cm (6 in) more than the measurement from the elbow to the metacarpal heads. The slab is applied and extends 2·5 cm (1 in) from the olecranon process (where it is folded obliquely to avoid pressing

Fig. 31.4 Colles fracture. Slab bound with wet gauze bandage.

Fig. 31.5 Colles fracture plaster completed.

into the antecubital fossa when the elbow is flexed) to 13 mm ($\frac{1}{2}$ in) proximal to the metacarpal heads. The slab must be well moulded and extend round the ventral surface of the radius and base of the first metacarpal to prevent radial deviation. The slab is fixed to forearm with a *wet* gauze bandage or a crêpe bandage which is applied from the elbow to the wrist where it is carried across the palm.

For a complete plaster, stockinet is applied and the elbow flexed to 90 degrees with full pronation of the hand. Plaster wool bandage is used at the elbow and at mid-arm. A short Colles' plaster is applied as previously described, followed by a U-slab made from 10 cm (4 in) wide 5 or 6 ply plaster bandage which is applied to the upper arm. This slab is secured with a wet gauze bandage or crêpe bandage, followed by a 10 cm (4 in) wide by 2·74 m (3 yd) plaster bandage, which extends below for one turn only.

Both these plasters may be completed after swelling has subsided by applying plaster bandages circular fashion round the forearm and upper arm.

Alternatively, a completed plaster cast may be applied over plaster wool bandage and is changed for a skin-tight plaster when swelling has subsided.

Scaphoid fracture

The wrist is maintained in a position of radial deviation and dorsiflexion. A modified short arm Colles' plaster which incorporates the thumb up to the distal joint is applied.

Fig. 31.6 Scaphoid fracture. Dorsal slab applied.

Fig. 31.7 Scaphoid fracture. Plaster completed.

The slab is prepared by cutting a notch to accommodate the thumb, and it is then bound to the dorsum of the arm and hand with a *wet* gauze bandage in the usual manner.

When the swelling has subsided, the plaster is completed with circular turns of two 10 cm (4 in) wide by 2·74 m (3 yd) plaster bandages. Alternatively, a completed padded cast may be applied at first and renewed when it becomes loose.

Fractures of the radius and ulna

There are two types of plasters – full flexed elbow and straight arm. The flexed elbow plaster is most generally used unless contraindicated by the position of the fracture, as straight arm plasters tend to cause a stiff elbow joint, especially in adults.

For a flexed arm plaster, the forearm is generally in a position of mid-pronation, although some fractures may require full pronation or supination. The fracture is reduced with counter-traction applied by means of a sling round the upper arm. Stockinet is applied, followed by plaster wool bandage round the wrist, elbow and upper arm. A U-slab is prepared from 10 cm (4 in) 5 or 6 ply wide 2·74 m (3 yd) plaster bandage and is

Fig. 31.8 Forearm fractures, flexed elbow plaster. U-slab applied to forearm and secured with a few turns of a circular plaster bandage.

Fig. 31.9 Full arm plaster cast completed. (From *Gypsona Technique*.)

Fig. 31.10 Forearm fractures. Straight arm plaster cast completed.

applied along the dorsal aspect of the forearm, extending from 13 mm (½ in) behind the knuckles, round the elbow and along the palmar aspect to finish at the wrist crease. This slab is retained with a few turns of a circular plaster bandage and after it has set the counter-traction sling is removed.

A second U-slab is prepared from 10 cm (4 in) 5 or 6 ply wide by 2·74 m (3 yd) plaster bandage sufficiently long to extend from the axilla round the elbow and up the outer aspect of the arm to just below the shoulder. This slab is retained with a few turns of a circular plaster bandage in the usual manner, and the elbow section is strengthened with one 10 cm (4 in) wide by 2·74 m (3 yd) plaster bandage applied obliquely from upper to lower arm round the elbow.

If swelling increases, the gauze bandage is cut and a fresh one applied. As swelling decreases, fresh or additional gauze bandages are applied to take up the 'slack'. When swelling has completely subsided, the cast is completed with circular turns of one or two plaster bandages.

Alternatively, a complete padded plaster may be applied at first, and changed when it becomes loose.

For a straight arm plaster, the elbow is extended and stockinet applied, followed by plaster wool bandages to the wrist, elbow and upper arm. The wrist is placed in a position of pronation and a dorsal slab made from 10 cm (4 in) 5 or 6 ply plaster bandage is applied. This should extend from the axilla to the wrist for olecranon fractures, and from just below the axilla to 13 mm (½ in) proximal to the metacarpal heads for all forearm fractures. The slab is held in position by a wet gauze bandage, and when swelling has subsided the cast is completed with plaster bandages in the usual way.

Fractures of the humerus

Middle and Upper Third. The patient stands or sits with his trunk inclined towards the injured side and his upper arm hanging vertically. The forearm is supported with the elbow flexed to 90 degrees and adhesive felt is applied to pad the outer end of the clavicle and acromium process. A thin layer of plaster wool bandage may be applied from the elbow to the axilla and any tendency to outward angulation of a high shaft fracture is countered with a pad of wool placed to keep the elbow away from the body.

Fig. 31.11 Upper and middle third fractures of the humerus. Slab applied and secured with wet gauze bandage or crêpe bandage and arm supported with collar and cuff sling. (From *Gypsona Technique*.)

A slab is made from 15 cm (6 in) 5 or 6 ply plaster bandage, and is applied from the axilla, along the inner aspect of the arm, round the elbow, up the outer aspect of the arm and over the shoulder where 15 cm (6 in) excess (allowed in the slab length) is turned back and secured with strapping. The slab is bound to the arm with a *wet* gauze bandage or a crêpe bandage, and the forearm is supported with a collar and cuff sling.

Lower Third. A U-slab is applied in the manner just described, and a strip of wet lint is placed over the forearm and lower part of the U-slab. A short slab about 40 cm (16 in) long is prepared and applied to the dorsal aspect of the forearm. This slab extends from the wrist to just above the elbow, and is secured with a *wet* gauze bandage or crêpe bandage. The wet lint prevents adherence of the two slabs so that the lower slab can be removed after an interval of two weeks or so.

Alternatively, a padded complete plaster may be applied at first and renewed if necessary.

Shoulder

Shoulder abduction spica

This is used for some upper humeral or shoulder fractures and post-operative immobilisation for shoulder arthrodesis.

The cast is applied with the patient seated on a backless stool or supported sitting up on the operation table. The arm is abducted about 60 degrees from the side, being carried well forward in front of the coronal plane and with some 15 degrees lateral rotation. The correct position for ankylosis should enable the hand to reach the mouth by flexion of the elbow alone. An assistant supports the elbow and forearm.

A stockinet lining is applied followed by adhesive felt pads over the iliac crests, either side of the spinous process, across the clavicle on the affected side and under the elbow with a small hole to accommodate the medial epicondyle. Plaster wool bandages are then applied to cover the area to be enclosed.

A light layer of plaster bandage is applied over the plaster wool. Plaster slabs, 15 cm (6 in) wide, are applied from the iliac crests under the axilla to the elbow; from the axilla on the soundside across the affected shoulder and upper arm, anteriorly and posteriorly (Fig. 31.12). In addition 15 cm (6 in) wide slabs can be applied from the suprasternal notch to the symphysis pubis and posteriorly from the seventh cervical vertebra to the sacrum. The cast is completed with circular plaster bandages.

Using the pattern technique, identical posterior and anterior body sections are prepared from six layers of 90 cm (24 in) wide plaster material. A combined shoulder, arm and forearm slab is made in a similar manner, using the pattern technique as illustrated. The length A-B equals the distance (plus 10 per cent) between the base of the neck and upper aspect of the flexed elbow joint (point E), plus half the circumference of the forearm. The length C-D is the distance from the same point E to the knuckles, plus half the circumference of the arm. The distances M-L and B-N are the circumference of the arm and of the forearm respectively. The distance A-S usually equals that between the base of the neck and the point of the shoulder. The shaded portions are cut away and reserved for reinforcement of the cast.

Stockinet and felt padding is applied as previously described followed by the anterior and posterior body sections which are moulded carefully and secured with one or two 10 cm (4 in) wide by 2·74 m (3 yds) plaster bandages. The arm section is then applied, moulded and secured with plaster bandages in a similar manner, and the axilla is strengthened with the surplus plaster material remaining from the wide pieces.

Fig. 31.12 Method of applying slabs for shoulder abduction spica and completed spica cast. (From *Gypsona Technique*.)

Fig. 31.13 Shoulder abduction spica. Pattern for shoulder and arm section.

Fig. 31.14 Shoulder abduction spica. Pattern for anterior and posterior body sections.

If a strut is desired, this may be made from the cores of the bandages, cut to length, covered with plaster material and fixed between the body and arm with a few turns of plaster bandage.

The cast is trimmed as indicated in Figure 31.12 and the edges made neat by turning back and securing the edges of the stockinet lining.

Leg

Fractures of the tarsus, metatarsus, internal and external malleoli, and stable Potts fractures

These fractures are immobilised with below-knee casts. The fracture is reduced (if necessary) and the knee flexed as shown in the illustration, with the foot dorsiflexed. Alternatively, a padded knee rest may be used and the leg supported by an assistant. Stockinet and plaster wool bandage are then applied from just below the knee to the toes.

A plaster stirrup may then be prepared from 10 cm (4 in) plaster bandages and applied commencing just below the knee, continuing down the leg, round the heel, to finish just below the knee on the outer side where any excess is turned back. This stirrup is bound loosely in place with a plaster bandage.

Fig. 31.15 Below-knee plaster cast. Leg supported with foot dorsiflexed.

A back slab is prepared from 15 cm (6 in), 5 or 6 ply plaster bandage (10 or 12 ply if the plaster stirrup has not been used) and is applied extending from just below the knee, round the heel (where a cut is made to accommodate the ankle) and along the sole of the foot where excess slab is temporarily dropped over the toes, or in front of the surgeon's knees if the plaster is being applied with the leg flexed over the end of the table. The slab

Fig. 31.16 Below-knee plaster cast. Stirrup applied and secured with plaster bandage.

is secured with two 15 cm (6 in) wide by 2·74 m (3 yd) plaster bandages from just below the knee to include the ankle. The excess slab is turned back to make a double thickness of plaster which extends just beyond the toes (toe platform). This foot portion of the slab is secured with one or two 10 cm (4 in) wide by 2·74 m (3 yd) plaster bandages and another similar bandage is applied round the ankle to provide reinforcement. The toe platform portion of the slab must not be bent upwards, as contracture of the extensor tendons may occur.

Fig. 31.17 Below-knee plaster cast. Back slab applied and excess turned over toes temporarily.

Fig. 31.18 Below-knee plaster cast. Showing how toe platform is made by turning back slab.

Severe Potts fractures; fractures of the lower third of the tibia; and fractures of the upper tibia when the patient is immobilised in bed.

These fractures are immobilised with mid-thigh casts. If the fracture is comparatively stable, the below-knee portion of the cast is applied first as described previously, but with the stockinet extended to mid-thigh. Plaster wool bandage is then applied round the knee joint and thigh.

Anterior and posterior slabs 76 cm (30 in) long are each prepared from two 15 cm (6 in) wide by 2·74 m (3 yd) plaster bandages. These are applied from a point 20 cm (8 in) below the knee joint to mid-thigh, where any excess bandage is turned back. The slabs are secured to the limb in the usual manner with two 15 cm (6 in) wide by 2·74 m (3 yd) plaster bandages.

If the fracture is unstable, it is usually easier to apply the upper and lower portions of the cast in one operation. A thin layer of plaster wool is applied to the limb and the fracture is reduced. The limb is supported by two padded wedges, as illustrated, one under

Fig. 31.19 Below-knee plaster cast, alternative method. Back slab applied and excess turned back in front of surgeon's knees temporarily.

Fig. 31.20 Below-knee plaster cast, alternative method. Plaster bandages applied spirally to secure back slab. Note how toe platform is made.

Fig. 31.21 Below-knee plaster cast completed.

the knee joint and one under the fracture, or alternatively, this second wedge is dispensed with and the fracture area supported by an assistant.

Two anterior slabs are prepared from six layers of wide plaster material, or alternatively, from 15 cm (6 in) wide by 2·74 m (3 yd) plaster bandages. These slabs are applied on each side, from mid-thigh along the anterolateral aspect of the limb, and round the sole of the foot. They are moulded carefully and secured with two 15 cm (6 in) wide by 2·74 m (3 yd) plaster bandages, leaving two small gaps where the limb is supported by the wedges or assistant.

When the anterior slabs have set, the lower wedge or support is withdrawn and a back slab made from two 15 cm (6 in) wide by 2·74 m (3 yd) plaster bandages is applied from behind the knee to the toes, where it forms the toe platform. The slab is secured with two 15 cm (6 in) wide by 2·74 m (3 yd) plaster bandages applied spirally.

The knee wedge is removed and another back slab prepared from two 15 cm (6 in) wide by 2·74 m (3 yd) plaster bandages. This slab is applied to the back of the thigh, extending down beyond the knee, and is secured with two 15 cm (6 in) wide by 2·74 m (3 yd) plaster bandages.

Fig. 31.22 Mid-thigh plaster cast for unstable fractures of the lower leg. Supporting wedges in position.

Fig. 31.23 Mid-thigh plaster cast for unstable fractures of the lower leg. Anterior lateral slabs applied.

When the swelling has subsided and the plaster becomes loose, it will be changed to a full length tuber bearing plaster, which is in effect a mid-thigh cast extending to the tuber ischii where it is padded similarly to a walking caliper.

Hip

Hip spica

This is used for immobilisation of infective conditions of the knee, femur and hip; fractures of the femur and hip; osteotomy of the femur; pelvic injuries and arthrodesis of the hip. The double hip spica is the cast most frequently applied in theatre and this will be described.

The patient is placed on extension apparatus as illustrated, and all bony prominences are padded with adhesive felt, i.e., the anterior superior iliac spines, the sacrum, head of the fibula, both malleoli and the tendo achillis. Stockinet is applied to the trunk and legs. Other padding depends upon the type of patient. A thin patient will require a good deal of padding in the form of plaster wool, whereas a stout patient will require very little.

The cast consists of a series of circular bandages and reinforcing slabs, 15 cm (6 in) wide applied as illustrated in Fig. 31.24. The hip section is reinforced by slabs positioned anteriorly and posteriorly from the lower ribs on each side around the hip to the groin and also from the lower ribs down to the lateral side of the knee. The cast is completed by circular bandages; 20 cm (8 in) used in a figure of eight manner around the pelvis and the hip, and 15 cm (6 in) bandages from the hip joint to the knee joint. Using the pattern technique the main part of the spica consists of slabs which are made from wide plaster material. For a double hip spica five slabs are required: a posterior section of seven or eight layers, two anterior sections of four layers, a complete long leg section of eight layers, and a thigh and pelvic section of eight layers. One heaped tablespoonful of borax may be added to a sink filled with tepid water to a depth of about 8 cm (3 in), and this retards setting of the plaster and allows time for adequate moulding.

The posterior body section is soaked, drained, smoothed and applied. The slab is moulded carefully and secured with a few turns of a 20 cm (8 in) wide by 2·74 m (3 yd) plaster bandage.

Fig. 31.24 Hip spica. Method of applying reinforcing slabs to right hip. This manoeuvre is repeated for the left side in a double hip spica. (From *Gypsona Technique*.)

The first anterior body section is then soaked, drained, smoothed and applied, followed by the second anterior section which is reversed so that each thigh section can be moulded carefully round the upper part of the leg.

The long leg section is then soaked, drained, smoothed and applied to the lateral aspect of the body, thigh and lower leg, so that the pelvic section stretches roughly from the opposite anterior superior iliac spine to the tuber ischii on the slab side, and the leg section extends down to the foot stirrup. The thigh and leg sections are carefully moulded and the back of the hip is reinforced with the surplus material remaining from the cut slabs.

The short thigh section is soaked, drained, smoothed and applied to the opposite pelvis and thigh. This section is finished just proximal to the knee joint so that full flexion is possible afterwards. The ankle section is completed with 10 cm (4 in) wide by 2·74 m (3 yd) plaster bandages and this may be extended to include the foot if required.

The whole spica is secured firmly with several 15 and 20 cm (6 and 8 in) wide plaster bandages and the stockinet is turned back at the upper and lower limits of the plaster in the usual manner. If the spica is required to incorporate the upper ribs, the depth of body sections must be increased accordingly.

770 Operating Theatre Technique

Fig. 31.25 Hip spica, pattern technique. Posterior body section applied.

Fig. 31.26 Hip spica, pattern technique. Anterior body section applied.

Fig. 31.27 Hip spica completed.

Fig. 31.28 Hip spica. Pattern for posterior body section.

Fig. 31.29 Hip spica. Pattern for anterior body section.

Fig. 31.30 Hip spica. Pattern for leg sections.

Spine

Spinal jacket

This is used for immobilisation of a fractured spine. The patient is placed in a position of hyperextension between two tables as illustrated or standing erect. Cervical traction may be used if standing, to give extension to the spine and to overcome spasm of the erector spinae muscles. Stockinet is applied to the trunk and leg and adhesive felt pads are applied to the manubrium sternum, the symphysis pubis and over the fracture area.

Stockinet is applied followed by felt padding over the iliac crests and down either side of the spinous processes. The whole area is covered with plaster wool compressed with a light covering of plaster bandages. Plaster slabs 15 cm wide (6 in) are applied (as illustrated in Fig. 31.32) followed by 15 or 20 cm (6 or 8 in) plaster bandages to complete the cast (Fig. 31.34). Using the pattern technique, two slabs are made from six layers of wide plaster material and are soaked, drained, smoothed separately and applied to overlap as illustrated. The overlap anteriorly should be 15 cm (6 in) and the slab extends from the manubrium sternum to the symphysis pubis. Posteriorly the shorter edges overlap in the lumbar region. The slabs are secured with several 15 cm (6 in) wide plaster bandages and the edges turned over where necessary to avoid trimming. The stockinet is turned back at the periphery of the jacket in the usual manner.

Fig. 31.31 Plaster spinal jacket. Position of patient.

Fig. 31.32 Plaster spinal jacket. Application of plaster reinforcing slabs. (From *Gypsona Technique*.)

Fig. 31.33 Plaster spinal jacket. Pattern technique.

Fig. 31.34 Plaster spinal jacket. Completed cast. (From *Gypsona Technique*.)

Plaster of Paris is likely to remain the dominant material used in fracture splinting for many years to come, although alternatives are being developed. This is particularly appropriate in the field of orthopaedics where lightness, high strength to weight ratio and durability of casts are important for young and elderly patients.

A decade ago an attempt was made to achieve these requirements with the development of Glassona, a fibre glass-based splinting material. This material, in the form of fibre glass impregnated bandages was activated by immersion in an acetone solvent. Apart from the dangers inherent in the flammable nature of acetone there were instances of skin reactions to the solvent. A glass-based material is now available called Crystona which offers strength and lightness similar to Glassona, but with the advantage of being water activated.

Crystona bandages comprise two major components, an alumino silicate glass and acrylic acid polymer, on a cloth base. The glass controls the rate at which the bandage sets and reinforces the cement. In the presence of water, the polymer reacts with the glass to form a rigid water-insoluble matrix. The unique reactive glass compound has been formulated specially for Smith and Nephew by Chance Pilkington Ltd.

It is possible to produce a cast with Crystona bandages which is only two-thirds of the weight of a conventional plaster of Paris cast. The initial setting time is 9–12 minutes, and casts are load-bearing within an hour, which enables earlier patient mobility.

Crystona casts have a high durability and resistance to moisture; complete immersion in water results in less than 10 per cent reduction in strength, and full strength is restored on drying out. The material has a high moisture vapour permeability, minimising the risk of skin masceration. The lower bulk of casts and increased translucency facilitates check X-ray procedures.

Crystona can be used for any of the casts described in the previous pages. It is particularly useful for cast bracing, body casts and 'frog' plasters although generally not recommended for the splinting of fresh fractures.

The main difference in application compared with plaster of Paris is that after immersion the bandages are shaken – not squeezed which would accelerate the setting process. Within two minutes of application, the bandages 'gel' to form a rubbery cast which sets rigid after about ten minutes.

Because Crystona is water resistant, it could adhere to the hands when set. It is recommended therefore, that disposable gloves are worn during application. As the material dries, it has a small shrinkage, giving a well-fitting cast. It should be applied over a layer of orthopaedic padding, and checked for comfort of fit after 30 minutes.

The following procedure is recommended by the manufacturer:

1. *Water temperature*
   Cool water (20°C).
2. *Soaking the bandage*
   a. Immerse one bandage at a time at an angle of 45° until large bubbles cease to escape (3·5 seconds).
   b. Shake excess water from the bandage but do not squeeze. Squeezing may make unrolling difficult, and will shorten working time.
3. *Drying the cast*
   a. Immediately after setting, the cast will exude surface water droplets. This process (Syneresis) lasts for about 10 minutes; clothing and/or bedding should be protected.
   b. Do not cover the cast, but allow a free circulation of air around it.
4. *Loud bearing*
   a. The cast will enable loud bearing in one hour, and achieves full strength within 24 hours.
5. *Cast removed*
   Crystona casts may be removed in the same way as plaster of Paris as with most dusts, including plaster of Paris, steps should be taken to minimise inhalation.

32
RADIOACTIVE MATERIALS IN THE THEATRE

Radium is an element emitting powerful rays which are used for the destruction of malignant or other abnormal tissue.

These rays are energy liberated as a result of constant disintegration of the element, and consist of three forms: alpha, beta and gamma radiation. It is gamma rays which are utilised for therapeutic purposes, the alpha and beta rays generally being excluded by using metal screens made of platinum 0·5 to 1·0 mm thick, although beta rays are sometimes used therapeutically.

Radium is generally used in the form of radium sulphate and is virtually indestructible, for its 'half-life' is about 1,700 years.

Over-exposure to the radiation from radium or radioactive products is dangerous, and care must be taken to ensure that this does not occur, either to the patient or staff.

Radium needles and tubes

Practically all the radium used medically today is prepared as needles or tubes. The needles, made from platinum, are hollowed to contain the radium salt and have a trocar point and an eye to which thread may be attached. Radium for use in gynaecology is in tubes, having no trocar and sometimes an eye. There are varying sizes of needles and tubes containing from 0·5 to 50 mg of radium salt.

If needles are used individually, they are threaded with strong silk, tying the thread near but not on the eye, and leaving it about 15 cm (6 in) long. The silk threads may be of different colours, according to the strength of radium packed in the needle and help in the sorting and handling of various types, although the needles are engraved accordingly and vary in length. The knot should not be tied actually on the eye for it may break during or after insertion into the tissues.

Larger amounts of radium may be prepared by packing various sizes of needles or tubes into a silver or plastic box or tubes, making applicators which are covered with plastic or rubber before disinfection and insertion.

The needles and applicators are disinfected by pasteurisation in a suitable container, care being taken to avoid tangling of the threads. These should be clipped individually with artery forceps or arranged in slots incorporated in the container.

Other radioactive products for therapeutic use

Radium is being superseded by isotopes prepared by treating elements in the atomic reactor.

Radioactive cobalt, Co 60, 'half-life' of 5·3 years, and *radioactive caesium 137*, 'half-life' 30 years, has replaced radium to some degree. The cobalt/caesium element is placed in the atomic reactor and after radio-activation is prepared as needles and tubes in a similar manner to radium. Large amounts of radioactive cobalt Co 60 or caesium 137 are also incorporated in the beam unit for teletherapy.

Radioactive tantalum wire and radioactive gold-198 seeds 'half-life' 2·7 days are often used therapeutically, the radioactive gold seeds having superseded radon. As the emanation is for a limited time, these seeds may be left buried in the tissues, but are sometimes removed owing to the value of the containers.

All these radioactive isotopes require very careful handling as the radiation may be equally lethal to that of a similar amount of radium or radon.

Methods of radium application

1. *Surface application* is made by embedding the needles or applications in a mould made from plaster of Paris, Stent composition, Acrylic, or sorbo rubber, etc. These moulds are placed in position over the area being treated for the requisite period.

2. *Teletherapy* is a form of treatment with a large amount of radioactive cobalt Co 60 or caesium 137 which is enclosed in a thick lead-walled chamber having an aperture through which the rays may be directed on to the area being treated. This is often called the radium or cobalt beam unit, but alternately deep X-rays are used, generated by machines using several million volts of electricity.

3. *Interstitial irradiation* is applied by inserting radium needles, radioactive tantalum wire or radioactive gold seeds into the tissues.

4. *Cavitary irradiation* is applied by inserting applicators into the natural cavities of the body, e.g., the vagina or cervical canal.

Of the four methods of radium or radioactive isotopes application, only the last two are generally performed in the theatre. Surface application and teletherapy are performed on patients in the radiotherapy department either as inpatients or outpatients.

A technique called 'after loading' may be used with cobalt-60 or caesium 137, whereby the empty containers are positioned in the patient before the radioactive tubes are inserted within them (Mould, 1978). This reduces the radiation dose to those personnel involved in the operation.

Precautions during the handling of radioactive products

1. All radioactive needles, applicators, wires, seeds are manipulated with long-handled forceps, the jaws of which are covered with rubber or plastic. *On no account should they be picked up by hand.*

2. All radioactive products must be carried in a special lead-lined container during transport between radium safe and the theatre. This container should be carried by the long handle or strap provided.

3. Any preparation of needles, wires or applicators must be performed behind special lead screens, using the long manipulation forceps.

4. Proximity to radioactive products should be minimal. All persons coming into regular contact with these are issued with personal monitoring films from which the physicist can determine the radiation dose received by the person concerned. Blood tests may be made regularly to ensure that the white cell-count remains within normal limits, especially if a suspected high dose has been recorded on the monitoring film.

5. The theatre sister or nurse is responsible for checking the radium, etc., when it arrives at the theatre and after disinfection.

Used needles and applicators are entered on the record sheet, and unused ones checked and placed in the transport container for immediate return to the radium custodian. If it is necessary to keep radioactive materials in the theatre for any length of time, a special lead-lined safe must be provided and the key retained by the person accepting responsibility for the materials.

Fig. 32.1 Radium insertion instruments.

1. A, B, C, Radium needle probes.
2., 3., 4. Radium needle insertion forceps (Finzi).
5., 6. Radon seed introducers (Christie Cancer Hospital).
7. Radium needle-holding forceps (Chester Williams).

6. The success of the treatment is dependent upon a carefully calculated dosage. The time at which the radium treatment is due to start and terminate must be carefully noted and strictly adhered to, for the time of contact with the tissues is one factor which affects dosage.

It is usual to use special record charts for the guidance of ward staff and others responsible during the course of treatment. In theatre on this card or chart is entered all relevant details, including the number, strength and position of needles, applicators, wires or seeds. The time inserted and time due for removal is also entered on this record chart. This record is sent to the ward when the patient returns. There may also be a duplication which is returned to the radium custodian after the radioactive products have been inserted.

Radium, cobalt and other products are very valuable as well as very dangerous. Careful checking at each stage of handling is important to avoid accidental loss. Radium containers left lying about the wards or departments, or radium needles, etc., which may have slipped out of their proper place and are lying in contact with healthy tissues are in the first case a danger to the staff, and in the second case a danger to the patient.

Misplacement or loss of any radioactive element must be reported immediately either to the radiotherapist or to the physicist. Strict observance of the instructions regarding handling of the radioactive materials makes this work completely safe nowadays.

REFERENCE

MOULD, R. F. (1978) *Nursing Mirror*, **15,** August 31, September 23.

Appendix I

TABLE I
SHOWING THE PRESSURE/TEMPERATURE RELATIONSHIP OF PHASE BOUNDARY STEAM AND THE ACTUAL TEMPERATURES ACHIEVED IN AN AUTOCLAVE CHAMBER WITH PARTIAL AIR DISCHARGE

lb p.s.i.	Pure steam and complete air discharge Degrees C	Degrees F	Two-thirds air discharge 20 in vacuum Degrees C	Degrees F	One-half air discharge 15 in vacuum Degrees C	Degrees F	One-third air discharge 10 in vacuum Degrees C	Degrees F
15	121	250	115	240	112	234	109	228
20	126	259	121	250	118	245	115	240
25	130	267	126	259	124	254	121	250
30	135	275	130	267	128	263	126	259

This chart indicates the importance of temperature, as pressure which is a mixture of air and steam has a much lower temperature than that of pure steam. Partial air discharge means a much longer sterilisation period than if complete air discharge had been achieved from the chamber.

TABLE II
MEDICAL GAS CYLINDER CAPACITIES AND PRESSURES

Gas	Pressure of a full cylinder (lb p.s.i.)	Capacities of cylinders in common use — Boyle's machine	Transportable circle circuit machines
Oxygen, O_2	1,500/2,000	24 cubic feet	36 or 72 gallons
Nitrous oxide, N_2O	600/700	200 gallons	100 or 200 gallons
Carbon dioxide, CO_2	1,000	2 pounds weight	2 pounds weight
Cyclopropane, C_3H_6	90	40 or 80 gallons	40 or 80 gallons

TABLE III
CALIBRATIONS OF ROTAMETERS ON ANAESTHETIC MACHINES

Gas	Calibration	Maximum measurable flow per minute
Oxygen, O_2	In 100 ml divisions	2,000 ml or 2 litres
Carbon dioxide, CO_2	...	...
Nitrous oxide, N_2O	In 1,000 ml or 1 litre divisions	10 litres
Cyclopropane, C_3H_6	In 50 ml divisions	750 ml

NOTE: A bypass is usually incorporated adjacent to the flowmeter bank whereby an increased flow of oxygen (and sometimes nitrous oxide also) can be obtained. This increased flow is not measurable without additional instruments, but in the case of oxygen is probably in the region of about 6 to-8 litres per minute.

TABLE IV
RECOMMENDED SIZES OF TWIST DRILLS TO BE USED FOR VARIOUS SCREWS OR BOLTS

SCREW OR BOLT, OUTSIDE DIAMETER	DRILLS, OUTSIDE DIAMETER
Finger screws, 1·6 mm ($\frac{1}{16}$ in)	No. 55, 1·2 mm ($\frac{3}{64}$ in)
Wood screws, 2·8 mm ($\frac{7}{64}$ in)	2·3 mm ($\frac{3}{32}$ in)
Wood screws, 3·6 mm ($\frac{9}{64}$ in)	2·8 mm ($\frac{7}{64}$ in)
Sherman, Phillips, or cruciform screws – 3·6 mm $\frac{9}{64}$ in	No. 31 (3·0 mm)
4·0 mm ($\frac{5}{32}$ in)	3·6 mm ($\frac{9}{64}$ in), or 3·2 mm ($\frac{1}{8}$ in)
Transfixion screws, 4·4 mm ($\frac{11}{64}$ in)	3·6 mm ($\frac{9}{64}$ in), cancellous bone; 4·0 mm ($\frac{5}{32}$ in), cortical bone
Wilson bolts, 3·6 mm ($\frac{9}{64}$ in)	3·6 mm ($\frac{9}{64}$ in)
Barr bolts, 4·3 mm ($\frac{11}{64}$ in)	4·0 mm ($\frac{5}{32}$ in)
Johannson lag screws, 4·0 mm ($\frac{5}{32}$ in) (shaft diameter)	4·8 mm ($\frac{3}{16}$ in) for 3·2 mm ($\frac{1}{8}$ in) depth, followed by 4·0 mm ($\frac{5}{32}$ in) for total depth of screw
Venable hip screws, 6·4 mm ($\frac{1}{4}$ in)	No. 4 (5·3 mm)
Venable hip screws, 5·5 mm ($\frac{7}{32}$ in)	4·8 mm ($\frac{3}{16}$ in)

METHOD OF REPROOFING VENTILE OR SCOTCHGUARD IN THE LAUNDRY[*]
(Based on a 250-lb load)

After washing and rinsing the material three times, the machine is filled with cold water to a 30 cm (12 in) dip.

Add 3¼ pints of 50 per cent acetic acid previously diluted with an equal amount of cold water and rotate the machine for 3 minutes.

Add 25 lb of Mystolene M.K.7[†] previously diluted with its own weight of cold water and raise the temperature slowly to 49°C to 54·5°C, when the milky liquor should have cleared. Turn off the heat and continue running the machine for a further 2 to 3 minutes.

Run the liquor to waste and add cold water until the materials are cool enough to handle when they can be removed, hydro-extracted and finished in the usual way.

This method produces a reproofed dense fabric which possesses more advantages than most disposable products yet available. It is a method which can easily be absorbed into the normal hospital laundry service and has the advantage that larger pieces than one square yard can be used. (The average size of a disposable drape.) The latter are useful as water-repellent layers in theatre packs or perhaps as drapes for lotion bowl stands.

There is no reason why the material should not be used as ordinary drapes, and it is particularly suited to making up abdominal 'slit' sheets. Used over the incision area in conjunction with Vi-Drape or similar plastic, the water-repellent sheet is ideal, particularly where excessive soiling is likely to occur, as in Caesarean section.

VENTILATORS – A METHOD OF DECONTAMINATION – THE CAPE VENTILATOR IN PARTICULAR
(Based on an article by Mr D. I. Ankrett, Dudley Road Hospital, Birmingham, reproduced by kind permission of NATNews)

Freshly prepared 20 volume hydrogen peroxide should be used each time. This should be made by diluting a solution of 100 volume hydrogen peroxide 1 in 5 with distilled water or freshly drawn tap water in areas supplied by high quality soft mains water.

A flow rate of 15 litres per minute is required to drive a suitable nebuliser (e.g. Ohio). A direct oxygen supply can be used if the pressure is sufficient; the valve on the top of the nebuliser set at 60 per cent to prevent build-up of pressure and possible release of peroxide through the safety valve. (Alternatively a De Vilbiss or LKB NB 100 nebuliser may be used as described on page 264, Chapter 10.)

The ventilator should be running with the respiratory volume set at 1000 mls per respiration; the respiration rate is adjusted to 25 per minute and expiratory assistance set exactly in the midway position between minimum and maximum. Failure to do this will cause a section of the expiratory circuit to remain unexposed to the aerosol. The oxygen inlet must be closed with a plug or cap during the process.

(Cape ventilator: the three drainage taps should be opened and left open with the machine running for 2–3 minutes, then closed and the drain tap cover door closed. This is to remove any moisture which may have accumulated and could neutralise nebulised hydrogen peroxide.)

[*] Published in the *Nursing Times*, 11th December 1964.
[†] Mystolene M.K.7 is obtainable from Catomance Ltd., 94 Bridge Road, Welwyn Garden City, Herts.

Nebulised hydrogen peroxide is introduced at the air intake and allowed to escape directly into the atmosphere at the inspiratory port. This is continued for a period of 60 minutes and its effectiveness monitored by a potassium iodide indicator paper placed by the inspiratory port. The indicator paper should turn deep brown within 5 minutes of the process commencing.

The same procedure is then carried out by introducing nebulised hydrogen peroxide for 60 minutes into the expiratory port, the aerosol emerging at the air outlet. This should be similarly monitored with the potassium iodide indicator placed at the air outlet. To save time two nebulisers can be used simultaneously.

This method will not decontaminate the length of tubing from the valve block to the spirometer outlet. If a spirometer has been used, decontamination can be achieved by an additional 10 minutes nebulisation on the expiratory side with the spirometer control held in the 'in' position.

The ventilator should be adequately aired after this process. After removing the nebuliser, drainage taps are opened and the ventilator allowed to run for 10 minutes. The drainage tubes are then closed and the ventilator allowed to run until peroxide can no longer be detached in the air passing through inspiratory port, air outlet or respirometer outlet; a period of 2–4 hours will be required in some instances. At the end of the airing process, drainage taps should again be opened for 10 minutes. If the respirometer has been decontaminated, at least 30 minutes venting will be required with the spirometer control held in the 'in' position.

Detection of residual peroxide vapour: if potassium iodide indicator strips held at the outlets described do not show detectable brown discoloration, the ventilator may be considered free of peroxide vapour. These indicator strips are prepared by the immersion of filter papers in a saturated solution of potassium iodide in distilled water followed by drying in a peroxide-free atmosphere.

VOLT/AMP METER MAY BE SUBSTITUTED FOR LAMP

Voltage Diagram

Appendix II

The Lewin Report* included guides to job descriptions for nurses and operating department assistants. Although it was accepted that these may need modification in accordance with local policy, it was thought useful to include them in the Report to facilitate the understanding of the type of organisation in the operating department envisaged by the Committee.

The job descriptions are outlined here, although readers are advised to consult the Lewin Report in full in order not to read them out of context.

Guide to Job Description: Nursing Officer: Operating Department Superintendent

Role. Programming and implementing policies formulated by Senior Nursing Officers. Formulating and programming, as a member of the Operating Department Committee, departmental policies within the overall framework of the Health Authority, Management policies. Ensuring that operational policies aimed at a high standard of patient care, staff welfare and training are implemented. As a registered nurse the operating department superintendent has responsibilities involving the storage, checking and administration of drugs.

Experience. Charge Nurse/Operating Department Sister.

Minimum Qualifications. State Registered Nurse
　　　　　　　　　　　　Middle Management Course
　　　　　　　　　　　　Successful assessment following operating department training

Functions

Management of the Operating Department

1. Controlling and co-ordinating the work of non-medical staff within the operating department, allocating staffing according to need, applying maximum delegation compatible with safety, and ensuring that high standards of service and good order are provided and maintained.

2. Reporting to the Senior Nursing Officer and the hospital administrator (in the case of ancillary staff) on current staffing situations and future requirements, staffing difficulties and problems; co-ordinating annual leave arrangement.

3. Reviewing the organisation and management of the department and reporting to the appropriate personnel, the efficiency of existing operational policies particularly in relation to:
　　　A. the allocation of theatres
　　　B. provision for emergency surgery
　　　C. length of operating sessions.

4. Initiating and developing new ideas and controlling the introduction of new methods in consultation with senior nursing officers, the operating department committee and departmental staff, within the limits of Health Authority, Management policies.

5. Maintaining and updating procedure manuals in consultation with teaching staff.

6. Maintaining responsibility for the custody and registration of all scheduled drugs used in the operating department. Supervising custody and stock levels of drugs, lotions, and anaesthetic agents held in the department in co-operation with the hospital pharmacist.

7. Exercising responsibility for the control of stock levels within the department and ordering new equipment in consultation with medical and administrative staff.

8. Receiving and recording details concerning mishaps, complaints and defects in supplies and equipment; investigating the circumstances in collaboration with appropriate staff and reporting findings to a senior nursing officer and other staff in accordance with hospital policy.

---

* The Organisation and Staffing of Operating Departments (1970). A report of a Joint Subcommittee of the Standing Medical Advisory and Standing Nursing Advisory Committee. London: HMSO.

9. Ensuring that policy relating to operating department record-keeping is followed.

10. Co-operating with medical and other staff in research procedures, including clinical trials and evaluation of equipment and supplies.

11. Arranging and participating in programmes for professional visitors to the operating department.

Communication and Liaison

12. Controlling alterations to operating lists, informing all relevant personnel in the operating department, other hospital departments and ward units of proposed list changes.

13. Ensuring that ward and recovery room staff receive the necessary information on which to base nursing care and in emergency situations reporting details of the patient's condition to appropriate hospital staff.

14. Conferring with ward staff and representatives of other departments, e.g. Theatre Sterile Supply Units/Hospital Sterilising and Disinfecting Units/Central Sterile Supply Departments, education, supplies, pharmacy, pathology, X-ray, medical photography, hospital administration and housekeeping services.

15. Conferring with, and co-ordinating the work of medical and paramedical staff concerned with procedures in the operating department from time to time (e.g. radiological Protection Officer, Control of Infection Officer, Microbiologist).

16. Attending operating department and procedure committee meetings, hospital and area (hospital) nursing meetings, to report on the work of the department.

17. Conferring with representatives of surgical firms to obtain information on new products and to report on products currently in use.

18. Collaborating with senior nursing officers to provide operating department planning guidance for building project team.

Safety

19. Ensuring that agreed safety procedures are known and followed by theatre staff especially measures concerning swab, instrument and needle counts; the storage and administration of blood and drugs; ionising radiation; static electricity/explosion hazards; fire; departmental cleaning.

20. Checking, receiving and relaying to the appropriate staff information concerning environmental conditions; interior fabric maintenance; planned maintenance and the integrity of piped gas supplies.

Education

21. Organising and participating (in consultation with the teaching division and other appropriate staff) in training programmes for post qualification, student and pupil nurses and operating department assistants.

22. Organising in-service training (in consultation with appropriate staff) for nursing and ancillary staff. Participating in collaboration with the medical staff as appropriate in instruction for medical students within the department.

23. Participating in general hospital staff training programmes in the Hospital Education Centre by lecturing on subjects such as theatre techniques and procedures.

24. Arranging visits by departmental staff to operating departments in other hospitals.

Personnel

25. Participating with appropriate staff in the recruitment and selection of operating department staff.

26. Organising and participating in the orientation of new staff in consultation with appropriate nursing and administrative staff.

27. Counselling staff on professional and personal problems.

28. Preparing reports and discussing the progress of operating department staff in training with appropriate officers; compiling reports on operating department staff in accordance with hospital policy.

29. Encouraging staff to pursue further studies and discussing with senior nursing officers or the hospital administrator where appropriate the suitability of staff for further courses of study.

30. Ensuring that procedures to safeguard staff health and welfare during working hours are implemented.

31. Participating as an assessor in the selection of operating department staff in other hospitals.

32. Attending professional conferences, careers conventions and making contacts with professional colleagues in other hospitals.

Guide to Job Description: Charge Nurse: Operating Department Sister

Role. Management of an operating suite or a small operating department according to local policy. Implementing policy formulated by Nursing Officer in consultation with the Operating Department Committee, directed towards high standards of patient care, staff welfare, and staff training in the operating department. As a registered nurse the Operating Department Sister/Charge Nurse has responsibilities involving the storage, checking and administration of drugs, and may also at times act as a scrubbed assistant in surgical procedures. The Sister/Charge Nurse may carry out the duties of the Nursing Officer in her absence.

Experience. Operating department staff nurse.

Minimum Qualifications. State Registered Nurse.
Successful assessment following operating department training, including first-line management course.

Functions

General

1. Supervising the work of all staff in the area under her control. Checking that work is carried out in accordance with agreed policy and ensuring that high standards of service and good order are provided and maintained.

2. Reporting to Nursing Officer on the current state of staffing, seeking or offering support as available. Advising Nursing Officer of likely future alterations in staffing requirements or special off-duty or 'time off in lieu' requests. Submitting annual leave requests to Nursing Officer for approval and reporting problems associated with the health of operating department staff (e.g. infected lesions).

3. Reviewing the efficiency of departmental operational policies and reporting on matters affecting policy to Nursing Officer. Communicating policy changes to relevant staff.

4. Developing and discussing with Nursing Officer new ideas and methods of procedure.

5. Participating in the maintenance and review of procedure manuals in consultation with teaching staff.

6. Maintaining the custody and register of controlled and scheduled drugs used in the area under her control. Checking and witnessing the administration of drugs in accordance with hospital policy.

7. Maintaining or delegating responsibility for levels of supplies in accordance with departmental policy.

8. Reporting to Nursing Officer incidence of accidents, complaints, and defects in drugs, supplies or equipment.

9. Supervising maintenance of the operations register in co-operation with appropriate staff.

10. Co-operating with medical and other staff in research procedures, including clinical trials and evaluation of equipment and supplies.

11. Advising Nursing Officer of proposed changes in the operating list order.

12. Participating in discussions with Nursing Officer concerning the repair or renewal of major equipment.

13. Establishing personal contacts with patients through ward and/or anaesthetic room visits in accordance with hospital policy.

14. Participating as a scrubbed assistant in surgical procedures.

15. Arranging for the care of patient's property in emergency situations.

16. Carrying out duties of Nursing Officer (operating department superintendent) in an 'acting up capacity', in the absence of the former.

17. Reporting on the work of the operating suite to Nursing Officer.

18. Participating in programmes for professional visitors to the operating department.

Liaison and Communication

19. Relaying to ward and recovery room staff details of the patient's physical condition and other information affecting nursing care of the patient.

20. Co-operating with medical, receptionist and ward staff in calling patients to the operating department when required, in accordance with hospital policy.

21. Co-operating with medical and paramedical staff from other departments in procedures carried out in the operating department from time to time, e.g. radiological protection officer, control of infection officer, microbiologist.

22. Participating in regular meetings of operating department staff and hospital nursing staff meetings at the appropriate level.

23. Co-ordinating the arrival and departure of patients, and staff from departments such as X-ray of laboratory, in co-operation with medical and receptionist staff.

Safety

24. Ensuring the implementation of safety measures concerning swabs, instrument and needle counts, the storage and administration of blood and drugs, ionising radiation, static electricity/explosion hazards, fire, and departmental cleaning.

25. Checking, receiving and relaying to Nursing Officer reports concerning the state of the following within the department:
- Heating
- Lighting
- Ventilation
- Fabric maintenance
- Routine maintenance
- The integrity of piped gas supplies.

Education

26. Implementing and participating in training programmes (including in-service training) for all grades of staff.
27. Instructing staff in new procedures as these are introduced.

Personnel

28. Introducing new members of staff to their duties.
29. Counselling operating department staff on personal and professional matters.
30. Discussing reports, on operating department staff and nursing progress reports on staff in training with Nursing Officer in accordance with hospital policy.
31. Taking all possible steps to safeguard the welfare and safety of staff in the operating theatre during working hours.
32. Encouraging staff to pursue further studies.
33. Attending professional conferences, careers conventions, and making contact with professional colleagues in other hospitals.

Guide to Job Description: Operating Department Staff Nurse

Role. To provide nursing care in the operating department and as a skilled member of the theatre team, to act as the scrubbed or circulating assistant during surgical procedures. As a registered nurse the Staff Nurse has responsibilities involving the storage, checking and administration of drugs. The Staff Nurse may carry out duties of Charge Nurse in her absence.

Experience. Post-registration training course and operating department experience.

Minimum Qualifications. State Registered Nurse.
Successful assessment following operating department training.

Functions

General

1. Providing nursing care for patients within the operating department.
2. Performing operating department work in accordance with agreed policy, e.g.
    A. Participating as a scrubbed member of the theatre team and carrying out safety checks of swabs, instruments and needles, in conjunction with a second person, and reporting on the same to the surgeon.
    B. Acting as a circulating member of the theatre team.
    C. Assisting with other members of the team in the preparation and clearing of theatres.
    D. Assisting in compiling the operations register.
    E. Checking and labelling and despatch of laboratory specimens.
    F. Providing assistance to the anaesthetist and surgeon as required.
    G. Checking, witnessing and administering controlled and scheduled drugs.
    H. Co-operating with appropriate departmental and ward staff in sending for patients to the operating department.
    I. Advising Charge Nurse of proposed changes in the order of operating lists.
3. Participating in the supervision of junior staff and staff in training.
4. Discussing departmental policies and developing and discussing new procedures with Charge Nurse. Communicating policy changes to relevant staff.
5. Assisting in the compilation of procedure manuals.
6. Ensuring that appropriate stock levels are maintained in the operating suite if required to do so.
7. Reporting to Charge Nurse incidents of accidents, complaints, defects in drugs, supplies or equipment.
8. Participating in clinical trials of new equipment and supplies and the evaluation and serviceability of existing equipment.
9. Co-operating with medical or other staff in research procedures.
10. Assisting when required in bacteriological investigations in the operating department.
11. Assisting medical and paramedical staff from other departments with procedures carried out in the operating department as required.
12. Participating in programmes for professional visitors to the department.
13. Carrying out the duties of Charge Nurse in her absence.

Liaison and Communication

14. Ensuring the maintenance of good relationships, communications and teamwork with all disciplines within the department and other departments of the hospital concerned with operating department work.
15. Participating in regular meetings of operating department staff.

16. Implementing safety measures in relation to:
    Swabs, instruments and needle count
    Storage and administration of blood and drugs
    Ionising radiations
    Static electricity/explosion hazards
    Fire.

Education
17. Participating in teaching programmes for staff in training.

Personnel
18. Assisting with the orientation of new staff.
19. Assisting Charge Nurse in the assessment of nurses in training and a compilation of staff progress reports.

Guide to Job Description: Operating Department State Enrolled Nurse

Role. To provide nursing care for the patient in the operating department and to act as a scrubbed or circulating member of the theatre team. The responsibility accorded to her and the degree of supervision under which she carries out her work is a matter for local professional assessment.

Experience. Two months' appraisal if no pupil nurse training in operating department.
        Post-enrolment training course and operating department experience.

Minimum Qualifications. State Enrolled Nurse.
        Successful completion of operating department state enrolled nurse training.

Functions

General
1. Providing nursing care for patients within the operating department.
2. Performing operating department work in accordance with agreed local policy including:
   A. Participating as a scrubbed member of the theatre team and carrying out safety checks of swabs, instruments and needles in conjunction with a second person and reporting on the same to the surgeon if in accordance with agreed local policy.
   B. Acting as a circulating member of the theatre team.
   C. Assisting with other members of the team in the preparation and clearing of theatres.
   D. Assisting in compiling the operation register.
   E. Assisting in the labelling and despatch of specimens for laboratory examination.
   F. Providing assistance to the anaesthetist and surgeon as required.
   G. Checking, witnessing and administering controlled and scheduled drugs in agreed circumstances.
3. Discussing departmental policies and new procedures with staff nurse or Charge Nurse in appropriate circumstances.
4. Assisting in the compilation of procedure manuals.
5. Ensuring where appropriate that stock levels are maintained if required to do so.
6. Reporting to the staff nurse or Charge Nurse incidents of accidents, complaints, defects in drugs, supplies or equipment.
7. Participating in clinical trials of new equipment and supplies and the evaluation and serviceability of existing equipment.
8. Co-operating with medical or other staff in research procedures.
9. Advising staff nurse or Charge Nurse of proposed changes in the order of operating lists.
10. Assisting medical and paramedical staff from other departments with procedures carried out in the operating department as required.
11. Participating in programmes for professional visitors to the department.

Liaison and Communication
12. Ensuring the maintenance of good relationships, communications, and teamwork with all disciplines within the department and other departments of the hospital concerned with operating department work.
13. Participating in regular meetings of operating department staff.

Safety
14. Implementing safety measures, in accordance with agreed local policies in relation to:
    Swabs, instruments and needle counts
    Storage and administration of blood and drugs
    Ionising radiations
    Static electricity/explosion hazards
    Fire.

Education
    15. Participating in in-service training programmes.

Personnel
    16. Assisting with the orientation of new staff.

Guide to Job Description: Operating Department Assistant

Role. To provide skilled assistance in the operating department and act as a member of the theatre team. To care for specified equipment relevant to his skills.
Experience. Two years' operating department training.
Minimum Qualifications. Successful assessment following operating department training.

Functions

General
1. Performing operating department work in accordance with agreed operational policies.
2. Participating as a scrubbed member of the theatre team in surgical procedures and carrying out safety checks on swabs, instruments, and needles in conjunction with a second person and reporting on the same to the surgeon.
3. Providing assistance as a circulating member of the theatre team including:
    A. Positioning and any preparation of a patient on the operating table as required by the surgeon and anaesthetist.
    B. Assisting the anaesthetist and surgeons as required, including assistance with blood transfusions and intravascular procedures.
    C. Assisting, with other members of the team, in the preparation and clearing of operating theatres, e.g. moving apparatus and lights and cleaning up during and after an operation.
    D. Preparing splints and plasters in the operating department.
4. Assisting in movement of patients in the operating department.
5. Acting as a member of the resuscitation team.
6. Cleaning, preparation and minor maintenance of instruments where appropriate.
7. Maintaining in an effective condition anaesthetic, inhalation and resuscitation equipment in accordance with local policies.
8. Cleaning, care and day-to-day maintenance of all equipment in general use in the operating department.
9. Operating autoclaves within the operating department where appropriate.
10. Assisting in the care, labelling and despatch of specimens for laboratory examination.
11. Assisting in compiling the operations register in co-operation with other staff.
12. Maintaining appropriate stock levels if delegated this task within the suite or department.
13. Reporting to Charge Nurse or Senior Operating Department Assistant, as appropriate, accidents, complaints, defects in drugs, supplies or equipment.
14. Participating in clinical trials of new equipment and supplies and the evaluation of existing equipment in collaboration with medical and nursing staff.
15. Assisting as required in research procedures.
16. Reporting to Charge Nurse and/or Senior Operating Department Assistant on the state of fabric maintenance and any deviation from accepted standards of operating department cleaning.
17. Proposing new ideas and procedures for discussion with Senior Operating Department Assistant or Charge Nurse.
18. Such other duties as may be determined by the Operating Department Superintendent and the Operating Department Committee.

Liaison and Communication
19. Attending departmental staff meetings.
20. Ensuring the maintenance of good relationships, communications, and teamwork with all disciplines within the department and other departments in the hospital concerned with operating department work.

Education
21. Participating in in-service training programmes.

Personnel
22. Assisting with the orientation of new staff.

Safety
23. Ensuring that safety procedures agreed by the Operating Department Committee are carried out in relation to swabs, instruments and needle counts and in relation to hazards from ionising radiation, static electricity/ explosion, and fire.

Guide to Job Description: Senior Operating Department Assistant

Role. To perform all the duties of an operating department assistant and in addition duties requiring special skill and ability in at least one particular branch of work including in appropriate circumstances the supervision of an operating suite. To implement agreed policies directed towards high standards of patient care, staff welfare and staff training.

Experience. Two years' experience in qualified grade (or possibly less according to educational qualifications).

Minimum Qualifications. Successful assessment following one year's training for the senior grade.

Functions

General

1. Co-ordinating the work of operating department assistants where this is appropriate.
2. Participating as a scrubbed assistant in general and specialised surgical procedures including responsibility for carrying out safety checks in conjunction with a second person.
3. Providing specialised assistance to the anaesthetist and acting as a member of the resuscitation team.
4. Exercising responsibility for effectiveness of anaesthetic and resuscitation equipment in the department, and dispersed throughout the hospital, if in accordance with local policy.
5. Exercising responsibility for the care, cleanliness and day-to-day maintenance of specialised equipment and assisting with their use in the theatre, e.g., pressure transducers, blood gas analysers within the department and hospital, if in accordance with local policy.
6. Advising Charge Nurse or Nursing Officer of proposed changes in the order of operation lists.
7. Ensuring the correct care, labelling and despatch of laboratory specimens.
8. Supervising the work of operating department assistants in training.
9. Ensuring if appropriate, or if required to do so, that stock levels (except drugs) are maintained in the operating suite or department.
10. Reporting to Nursing Officer or Charge Nurse as appropriate, accidents, complaints, defects in drugs, supplies or equipment.
11. Co-operating with medical or other staff, in consultation with Nursing Officer, in research procedures, including clinical trials and the evaluation of equipment and supplies.
12. Assisting when required in routine bacteriological investigations in the operating department under the direction of a microbiologist.
13. Discussing with Nursing Officer or reporting to Nursing Officer the current state of operating department assistant staffing and possible future staffing requirements and consulting with nursing officer in charge in respect of annual leave or time off 'in lieu' requests for operating department assistants.
14. Discussing departmental policies with Charge Nurse or Nursing Officer. Communicating policy changes to relevant staff.
15. Developing and discussing with Nursing Officer or Charge Nurse new ideas and methods of procedures.
16. Assisting in the compilation of procedure manuals, in consultation with teaching staff.
17. Encouraging the development of managerial skills in operating department assistants by the delegation of tasks.
18. Participating in programmes for professional visitors to the operating department.

Liaison and Communication

19. Co-operating with medical, receptionist and ward staff in appropriate circumstances in calling patients to the operating department when required according to local policy.
20. Assisting medical and paramedical staff from other departments with procedures carried out in the operating department from time to time, e.g. radiological protection officer, control of infection officer, microbiologist.
21. Reporting on the work of the suite (if appropriate) to Nursing Officer.
22. Ensuring the maintenance of good relationships and teamwork between other disciplines and staff under his supervision.
23. Participating in regular meetings of operating department staff.
24. Organising meetings of operating department assistants.
25. Co-ordinating, in appropriate circumstances, the arrival and departure of patients, and staff from other departments such as X-ray or laboratory.

Safety

26. Ensuring, in appropriate circumstances, the implementation of safety measures in relation to swabs, instruments and needle counts; the storage and administration of blood and drugs, ionising radiation, static electricity/explosion hazards, fire and departmental cleaning.
27. Checking, receiving and relaying to Nursing Officer reports concerning the state of the following within the department:

Heating
Lighting
Ventilation
Fabric maintenance
Routine maintenance
The integrity of piped gas supplies.

28. Participating in discussions with Nursing Officer or Charge Nurse concerning the repair or renewal of major equipment.

29. Reporting to Nursing Officer or Charge Nurse as appropriate (*a*) the need for fabric or plant maintenance and (*b*) the satisfactory implementation of the planned maintenance programme.

Education

30. Assisting Nursing Officer in the compilation of training and teaching programmes for operating department assistants.

31. Participating in training and teaching programmes for all operating department staff.

32. Instructing staff in accordance with agreed policies, in new procedures and the use of new equipment.

Personnel

33. Encouraging operating department assistants and other ancillary staff to pursue further studies.

34. Counselling operating department assistant staff.

35. Discussing progress reports on trainee operating department assistants with Nursing Officer and with the staff concerned.

Guide to Duties: Operating Department Receptionist/Clerk Typist

To receive patients and direct their escorts on arrival in the operating department; to co-ordinate communications within the operating department and with wards and other departments. Staff in these grades should have clerical and typing experience and receive in-service training. Whether the duties of receptionist and clerk typist are separated will depend upon the size of the department. Normally the following duties will be involved:

Communications
1. Receiving and relaying messages.
2. Maintaining communication and liaison with other hospital departments and with outside callers.
3. Providing information regarding location of departmental staff.

Reception
1. Receiving and directing patients and escorts on arrival at the operating department.
2. Receiving and directing visitors to the operating department.

Clerical
1. Maintaining appropriate departmental records in accordance with local policy.
2. Dealing with departmental correspondence in association with Nursing Officer in charge.
3. Typing departmental information including:
    Off-duty and emergency rosters
    Departmental procedures
    Notices
    Operating lists where appropriate
    Study programmes
    Visitors' programmes.
4. Preparing requisitions for equipment, supplies, stationery in consultation with relevant staff.
5. Such other duties as may be determined by operating department superintendent.

Guide to Duties: Domestic Assistant

1. Clearing and cleaning scrub-up and changing rooms as required during working hours.
2. Checking and clearing or cleaning as required wash hand basins, W.C.'s and showers.
3. Receiving and sorting clean non-sterile linen and topping up to pre-determined levels.
4. Topping up changing room linen.
5. Checking and topping-up supplies of cleaning materials, disposal bags, hand towels.
6. Serving refreshments.
7. Clearing and washing up crockery.

8. Clearing pantry.
9. Assisting in the preparation of patients' trolleys.
10. Removing waste materials, i.e. changing room linen bags and pantry waste to the appropriate disposal area within the operating department.
11. Such other duties as may be determined by the Nursing Officer and Domestic Superintendent not demanding a higher level of responsibility than those listed above.

Guide to Duties: Operating Department Orderly

Role. To carry out portering and general duties in the operating department.

Duties
1. Lifting patients and moving them between beds, trolleys and special tables.
2. Preparing patients' trolleys.
3. Receiving and sorting stores.
4. Moving and storing equipment.
5. Assisting in the maintenance of stock levels.
6. Clearing theatre and assisting with cleaning within the department.
7. Caring in general way for theatre equipment, e.g. operating table, lights, etc.
8. Changing of medical gas cylinders.
9. Operating autoclaves within the operating department, where appropriate.
10. Providing messenger service within the operating department.
11. Cleaning theatre footwear.
12. Such other duties as may be determined by the operating department Superintendent and the Operating Department Committee.

INDEX

A

Abdominal incisions, 327
    Battle incision, 330
    closure of, 328
    Kocher's incision, 329
    Mayo Robinson, 330
    McBurney incision, 332
    midline incision, 327
    paramedian incision, 329
    Pfannenstiel's elliptical incision, 329
Abdominal operations, 327
    draping of, 198
    vascular, 737
Abdominal packs, 98
    method of packing for sterilising, 101
Abdominoperineal resection of the rectum, 354
    draping of, 212
Ablative surgery of brain whitematter, 468
Abortion, curettage for, 434
Abscess, brain, 459
    breast, 374
    incision for quinsy, 415
    intrapelvic, 334
Acoustic neuroma, 401
Acrylic bone cement, 587
Active antipollution scavenging system, 253
Active electrode, diathermy, 56
Adams regulators, 234
Adaptors, electric, 34
Adenoidectomy, 287, 416
Adenoma, of breast, 374
    of thyroid, 686
Adrenalectomy, 287, 670
Adrenaline, (epinephrine), 266, 270, 283, 284
Advancement, or strabismus operation, 287, 496
After loading of radioactive materials, 775
Air, bacteriological sampling, 20
Air changes, number of, 19
Air conditioning, 19
    filters, 17
    heating by, 26
    humidity, 17, 26, 69
    laminar/linear air flow, 20
    pressures, 17
Air elimination from steriliser chamber, 128, 134
Air encephalography, 289, 454
Air flows, smoke test, 20
Air turbine, 549
Airway, anaesthetic, 207, 244

Airway (*continued*)
    disinfection of, 159
    in unconscious patient, 277
Alarm, ventilator, 258
Albee technique for congenital dislocation of the hip, 287
Aleudrin (isoprenaline), 266, 280, 283
Alloferin (Toxiferone), 232, 266
Althesin, 232
Aluminium foil for diathermy electrode, 59
Amethocaine (Decicaine), 232
Aminophylline, 266, 284
Amputation, of arm,
    through humerus, 609
    of breast, 374
    of cervix, 431
    of forearm, 608
    of leg, below the knee, 609
        mid-thigh, or above the knee, 610
    of tongue, 426
    through upper arm, 609
Anaesthesia, 228
    airway, 277
    endotracheal intubation, 267
    epidural or spinal, 273, 289
    general, 232, 264, 277
    hypothermia, heating of the theatre, 26
    induction of, nurses' duties, 277
    inhalation, 232, 264
    intravenous, 232, 266, 277
    local or regional, 232, 269
    preparation for, 233
    relaxants, 266
    stages of, 278
    types of, 231
Anaesthetic apparatus, disinfection of, 159
    maintenance of, 228
Anaesthetic assistant, 276
Anaesthetic breathing attachments, B.S.I. layout, 242
Anaesthetic circuit, 236, 244
    semi-closed, 236
Anaesthetic equipment, 233,
    checking of, 229
    explosions, 66
    storage of, 229
Anaesthetic gas cylinders, 233, 777
    carbon dioxide, 232, 777
    cyclopropane, 232
    oxygen, 232
Anaesthetic gases, extraction of, 20, 252
    danger of accumulation, 20, 66

Anaesthetic machines, 234
   Blease/Northwick Park, 250
   Boyle's absorber unit, 245
   Boyle International, 247
   breathing attachments, 242
   closed circle circuit layout, 244
   corrugated tubes, 160, 242
   Ether vaporiser, 236
   expiratory and inspiratory valves, 243
   face masks, 243
   Fluothane (halothane) vaporiser, 236
   gas cylinders, 233, 777
   harness, 243
   inspection of, 87
   maintenance of, 228
   nitrous oxide, 232, 234, 777
   oxygen, 232, 234, 777
   pin index cylinders, 233, 234
   pin safety system of filling vaporisers, 239, 241
   regulators for reducing gas pressures, 234
   reservoir bag, 241
   rotameters, 235, 777
   rubber harness, 243
   semi-closed circuit, 236
   soda lime canister, 244, 246
   thermocompensated vaporiser, 236
   Trilene vaporiser, 235, 243
   types of, 234
Anaesthetic nurse, assistant or technician, 228, 276
Anaesthetic room, 1, 27, 228, 276
   ventilation of, 19
Anaesthetic screens for operation table, 202
Anaesthetic technician, 228
Anaesthetic swabs or mops, 98
Anal fissure, 371
Analgesia, spinal and epidural, 273
Anastomosis, 287
Ancillary rooms, theatre, 6, 27
   staff, 1
Aneurysm of the aorta, 713, 731, 737
Angiography, 287, 452
Ankle, arthrodesis of, 570
Ansolysen (Pentolinium), 232
Anterior resection of rectum, 359
Antibacterial agent for skin preparation, 194
   swabs for skin preparation, 194
Antipollution systems for expired anaesthetic gases, 252
Antipollution valve, 249
Antistatic floor, 69
Antistatic rubber, 67
Antrostomy, 287
   intranasal, 410
   radical (Caldwell Luc operation), 410
Antrum instruments, 409
Aorta, aneurysm of, 713
   occlusive disease, 713
Aortic grafts, 713
Aortic valve replacements, 721, 724
Aortic valvuloplasty, 724
Aramine (Metaraminol), 266, 280
Arbralene, 178

Arfonad (Trimetaphan), 232
Appendectomy, 287, 330
Arm, amputation through humerus, 609
   amputation through forearm, 608
   holding for intravenous injection, 276
   plaster of Paris application, 759
Arm support, Carter Braine, 78
Arm table, for transfusion, 77, 202
Arterial operations, 713, 737, 741
   bypass graft, 751
   embolectomy, 747
   graft, aorta, 713
   microsurgery, 742
Arteriotomy, 287
Artery forceps, 324
Arbralene, 177
Arbralon, 176
Areas of skin preparation, 195
Arteriectomy, 287
Arthrectomy, 287
Arthrodesis, 287
   of ankle (fibula graft), 570
   of hip, Brittain extra-articular fusion, 576
      Charnley central dislocation, 576
   of knee, Charnley compression, 573
   of shoulder, 575
   of spine, 600
   of toes, 569
   of wrist, Brittain fusion, 577
   stabilisation of foot, 571
Arthrography, 287
Arthroplasty, 287
   of fingers, Nicholle, 604
   of hip, Austin Moore or Thompson operation, 579
      Charnley, 529
      Howse, 579, 589
      McKee Farrar, 579, 585
   of metatarsophalangeal joint for hallux rigidus, 604
Arthroscopy, 287, 564
Arthrotomy, 287
   of knee, 565
Aspiration of a joint, 562
Assisting the surgeon, 194, 218, 225
Atrial septal defect, 713, 728
Atropine, 266
Austenitic stainless steel, 520, 534
Austin Moore, arthroplasty of hip, 579
   prostheses, 581
   pins for femoral neck, 543
Australia antigen patients, 225
Autoclave, gravity displacement type, 128, 129
   double ended, 129
   high-vacuum, high-pressure type, 128
   indicator tape, 110
   jacket, 129
   load simulator, 134
   portable, 150
   steam condensate line, 130
   temperatures, 128, 131, 144, 777
   vacuum leak test, 140
Autoclaving, 127
Autogenous bone grafts, 556

Autogenous bone grafts (*continued*)
   iliac strips and chips, 560
   inlay, 560
   tibia, 440
Axilla operation position, 79

B

Bacillus stearothermophilus, spore test, for steam sterilisation, 133, 154
   for ethylene oxide sterilisation, 151
Bacillus subtilis (globigii), spore test, 148
Bacteria, destruction of, 126
   dissemination of skin particles, 86
   effect of chemicals, 127
Bacterial contamination, of dilute antiseptic solutions, 159
   infected operation, 225
   of operating suite, 86
Bacterial structure, 126
Balanced flaps for ventilation system, 20
Bags for sterilisation, heat seal, 110
   Kraft plain top, 110
Bandages, packing for sterilisation, 100
   plaster of Paris, 756
Bankart operation for recurrent dislocation of shoulder, 288, 596
Barbiturates for intravenous anaesthesia, 232, 266
Barium strand in swabs for location, 95
Barnet ventilator, 261
Bartholinian cyst, excision of, 429
Bassini herniorrhaphy, 367
Batchelors zygoma hooks, 515
Batteries, care of, 43
Battle incision for appendectomy, 330
Beam splitter, for microscopes, 299
Bell table, 535
Benique gauge for catheters, 344
Benzalkonium chloride, 157
Betadine, 28, 88, 158
Bicarbonate of soda, intravenous, 280, 283
Billroth I gastrectomy, 288, 344, 345
Biopsy, of brain, 459
   of cervix, 435
Bird respirator, 261
   disinfection of, 261
Bistouries, 189
Blackburn skull calipers, 515
Bladder instruments, 665
Bladder operations, 661, 667
   partial cystectomy, 669
   suprapubic cystotomy, 661
Bladder tumours, fulguration of, 659
   partial cystectomy for, 669
Blalocks operation, 288
Blankets in theatres, 67
Blease/Northwick Park anaesthetic machine, 250
Blepharotosis, sutures for, 172
Blin lighting system, 37

Blinds for theatre windows, 17
Block dissection of cervical glands, 681
Blood transfusion pump, Martin, 231
Blood vessel operations, 742, 745
   ligation of, 168, 745
Boiling, of instruments, 149
Bolts, Webb, 601
Bone bank, 556
Bone cement, 587
Bone cutting forceps, 517
Bone fracture instruments, 516
Bone grafts, autogenous, inlay, 560
   onlay, 556
   fibula for ankle arthrodesis, 570
   for cranioplasty, 468
   from iliac crest, 560
   to spine, 'H', 600
Bone plates, 520, 530
Bone saw, 537, 549, 559
Bone tumours, 608
Bonney Reverdin suture needles, 188
Boomerang needles, Harris or Millen, 664
Boots, antistatic, 67
Bougies, catheters and sounds, 650
Bourie pulmonary valvulotomy, 727
Bowel opening of, soiling drapes, 222
Bowel resection, 350
Bowie-Dick autoclave test, 138
Boyle's absorber unit, 245
Boyle's anaesthetic machine, 234, 247
Boyle's vaporisers, 235
Boxes for sterilisation, 112
Braasch cytoscope, 657
Bracheal plexus block, 269
Braided nylon, 176
Braided silk, 173
Brain abscess and cysts, 459
Brain, biopsy of, 459
Brain instruments, 457
Brain operations, 452
Breast abscess, 374
Breast adenoma, 374
Breast operations, 374
Breast position for surgery, 79
Brietal (Methohexitone), 232, 266
Brigden, Kuntscher nail extractor, 544
Bripac boxes for sterilisation, 112
British Standard for anaesthetic circuit, 242
Brittain arthrodesis, of hip, 576
   of wrist, 577
Bronchofibrescope, 688
Bronchoscopes, sterilisation of, 160
Bronchoscopy, 288, 687
Browne, Denis, operation for hypospadias, 641
Browne's formaldehyde test, 148
Browne's tubes for sterilisation tests, 132, 161
Brushes, for scrubbing up, 88
Bunnell 'pull through' tendon sutures, 615
Bupivacaine (Marcaine), 232, 270, 273
Burns diathermy, prevention of, 202
Burr hole in skull, 459
Butyrophenone tranquillisers, 232

C

Cadavaric kidney donor, 678
Caecostomy, 288
Caesarean section, 288, 449
Calcium chloride for cardiac arrest, 283
Caldwell Luc operation on the antrum, 410
Calnan arthroplasty of metacarpophalyngeal joints, 604
Calona soda lime, 247
Cancellous iliac bone grafts, 560
Cape-2000 ventilator, 254
   disinfection of, 779
Caps for nurses and surgeons, 86
Capsulectomy, 288
Capsulorrhaphy for recurrent dislocation of the shoulder, 288, 596
Capsulotomy, 288
Carbolic acid, 155
Carbon dioxide, absorption circle closed circuit, 244
Carbon dioxide cylinder contents/pressures, 777
Carbon dioxide/ethylene oxide sterilising mixture, 150
Carbon steel, 521
   instruments, sterilisation of, 126, 142
Cardiac arrest, treatment of, 279, 280
Cardiac defibrillator, 48, 54, 280
Cardiac massage, 279
Cardiac monitor, 48, 50
Cardiac pacing, 53
Cardio-circulatory arrest, 279
   trolley, 282
Cardio-pulmonary bypass, 713
Cardioscope, 49
Cardiotomy reservoir, for cardiopulmonary bypass machine, 715
Cardiovascular instruments, 718
Cardiovascular operations, 712
Carlin's endobronchial tube, 269
Carlin's mediastinoscope, 695
Carter Braines arm support, 78
Cartilage, excision of, 565
Cartilage knives, 189
Case notes, patient, 91
Castors, antistatic, 68
Cataract extraction, 502
Cataract knives, care of, 126, 142
Catgut, manufacture of, 164
   method of handling, 170
   sizes of, 168
   sterilisation of, 126
   storage of, 162
Catheterisation, ureteric, 657
Catheters, 190, 650
   care of, 121
   gum elastic, 125
   sizes of, comparison gauge, 652
   sterilisation of, 154
   ureteric, 658
Caudal block, 288
Cauterization of cervix, 435
Cautery, 61
Cavitary irradiation, 775
Central sterile supply, 2, 6, 29, 102, 111

Cerebellar craniotomy, position, 81
Cerebral vascular tree, serial x-ray examination of, 452
Cervical dislocation, 515
Cervical node dissection, 681
Cervical laminectomy, position for, 81
Cervicectomy, 288
Cervix, amputation of, 431
   biopsy of, 435
   cauterisation of, 435
   dilatation of, 434
Cetavlon, CTAB, 157
Cetrimide, 157
Chalazion, excision of, 489
Chamber and jacket pressure gauges, autoclave, 129
Changing to theatre clothing, 86
Changeover or transfer section, 6
Charnley arthrodesis of hip, 576
Charnley arthroplasty of hip, 579, 590
Charnley body exhaust ventilation system, 24
   compression arthrodesis of knee, 573
Charnley Howarth operating enclosure, 21, 24
Charrière gauge for catheters, 652
Chart, of autoclave temperatures, 144, 777
   of catheter sizes, 652
   of disinfection by chemicals, 152
   of drill and bone screw sizes, 777
   of gas cylinder capacities, 777
   of rotameter calibrations, 777
   of pre-operative skin preparation, 195
   of sterilisation by dry heat, 145
Cheatle transfer forceps, 88
Check labels for swabs, 94
Checking swabs or sponges, 94, 218
Chemical disinfection, 154
   benzalkonium chloride (Roccal, Zephrian), 157
   carbolic acid, 155
   cetrimide (Cetavlon), 157
   chlorhexidine (Hibitane), 157
   chloroxylenol (Dettol), 156
   formaldehyde, 159
   glutaraldehyde, 159
   hexachlorophane, 157
   hycolin, 155
   iodine, 158
   lysol (cresol), 155
   Povidone-iodine, 158
   Printol, 155
   Savlon, 157
   sodium hypochlorate, 158
   Sudol, 155
   tests for sterility, 133
Chemical indicator test, ethylene oxide sterilisation, 110
Chest electrodes, 52
Chest instruments, 700
Chest operations, 688
   positions, 75
Chisels, 549
Chlorhexidine (Hibitane), 156
Chlorine disinfectants, 158
Chloros, 158
Chlorpromazine (Largactil), 232

Index

Chloroxylenol (Dettol), 156
Cholecystectomy, 288, 337
Cholecystenterostomy, 288, 339
Cholecystogastrostomy, 339
Cholecystostomy, 335
Choledochoduodenostomy, 340
Choledochotomy, 288, 339
Chromic catgut, 165
Cidex, 120, 159, 160
Chordotomy, 288
Cinchocaine (Nupercaine), 232, 273
Circulating nurses (or runners), 90
   swab check, 94, 218
Circulation, clean and dirty traffic, 6
Circumcision, 288, 644
Citanest (Prilocaine), 232
Clamps, bone holding, 519
   Charnley compression for knee, 573
   vascular, 718,
Clausen harness, 243
Cleaner, ultrasonic, 114
Clean zone in operating departments, 6
Clearsol, 156
Cleft palate and hare lip repair, 617
Clips, ligature, 179
   suture, 179, 183, 190
   sterilisation of, 163
Closed circuit for anaesthesia, 244
Closed gloving technique, 93–95
Clothing, theatre, 86
Clutton sounds, 650
Coagulation by diathermy, 56
   of bacteria, 126
Coarctation of the aorta, correction of, 713, 733
Cobalt, radioactive, 293, 774
Coccygectomy, 288
Cold disinfection, 154
Cold punch, transurethral prostatectomy, 659
Colectomy, 288, 351, 354
Collagen tape, 172
Colles fracture, plaster case, 759
Colonofibrescope, 318
Colonoscopy, 318
Colostomy, 288, 361
   closure of, 362
Colpoperineorrhaphy, 431
Colporrhaphy, 288
Colpotomy, 288
Commissurotomy, 288
Common bile duct operations, 339
Compressed air cylinders, 777
Condensate steam valve, 130
Condensation, process of during sterilisation, 128
Conductive floors, 69
Congenital dislocation of the hip, 594
   gill operation, 594
   shelf operation, 594
Connell head harness, 243
Conn pneumatic tourniquet, 512
Conray contrast medium, 452
   for angiography, 452
Construction of theatre, 11, 14

Contaminated wounds, 194
Controlled drugs, 228
Coramine (nikethamide), 266
Corneal transplants, 497
Corneoplasty, 288
Corneoscleral trephining, 488
Coronary heart disease operation, 713, 729
Corrosion of orthopaedic implants, 522
Corrugated tubes, anaesthetic machine, 242
   disinfection of, 160
Cottonoid (or lintine), 100
Cotton blankets, 67
Cotton thread, 175
Coventry infant lag screw, 550, 554
Cranial operations, 452
   draping of, 207
   prone position, 81
   sitting position, 82
   supine position, 80
   supine and prone position, draping of, 207
Craniectomy, 288, 459
Cranioplasty, 288, 467
Craniotomy, 288, 459, 463
Cronin mammaplasty, 636
Cross-leg skin graft flap, 630
Cryoprobe for stereotactic surgery, 470
Cryosurgery, 289
   ophthalmic, 507
CSSD, 2, 6, 29, 102, 111
Culdoscopy, 289
Curare (Tubarine), 232, 266
Curettage, 289
   of uterus, 434
Cushing stitch for closing bowel stump, 223
Cushing's (or McKenzie's) ligature clips, 179
Cyclotomy, 289
Cyclopropane gas cylinders, 232, 234, 777
Cylinder contents gauge, 234
Cystectomy, 289, 667
   partial, 668
   total, and ureterosigmoidostomy, 667
Cysternal puncture, 455
Cystocele, repair of, 431
Cystodiathermy, 289
Cystoscope optics, 655
Cystoscopes, care of, 120
   sterilisation of, 154
Cystoscopy, 289
   draping of, 212
Cystostomy, 289
   suprapubic, 661
Cystourethroscopy, 652
Cysts, sebaceous of face, 428
Cysts, brain, drainage of, 234

D

D & C, 434
Dacrocystectomy, 289
Dacrocystorhinostomy, 289, 492
Dacron, 176

Index

Dandy's operation, 482
Daptazol, 266
Daystar shadowless light fitting, 38
Debridement, 289
Decicaine (Amethocaine), 232
Decortication of the lung, 289, 697
Defibrillation, 55,
Defibrillator, cardiac, 48, 54, 280
De Martel clamp, 355
Denis Browne's operation for hypospadias, 641
Dental operations, 379
Depressed fracture of the skull, 463
De Pezzer catheters, 651, 662
Dermal ulcer of the face, excision of, 428
Dermalene, 177
Dermatomes for skin grafting, 623, 626
Design, of anaesthetic room, 1, 27
　of theatre, 6
Detergent disinfectants, 157
Dettol, 156
De Wecker's eye scissors, 190
Dexon ligatures and sutures, 172
Diak controls for sterility tests, 133
Diaphragmatic hernia, thoracic approach, 710
Diastol glove powder, 123
Diathermy, 56, 289
　active electrode, 56
　electro-coagulation, 56
　electro-section, 56
　endoscopic accessories, 317
　for ophthalmic operations, 507
　for urology (genito-urinary) operations, 59
　indifferent electrode, 56
　machine, 48, 60, 87
　precautions for use, 202
　sterilisation of electrodes, 160
　strength of current, 60
Dichrotic coating on light reflectors, 38
Digoxin, 284
Dilatation of cervix (D and C), 434
Disinfection, by chemicals, 126
　by heat, subatmospheric steam, 146
　chart, 152
　of anaesthetic apparatus, 159
　of endoscopes, 160
　of ventilators, 261, 779
Disintegration or decay of radioactive materials, 293
Disfex, 88, 157
Disobliteration (thrombo endarterectomy), 289, 754
Dispenser, nailbrush, 28, 162
　anaesthetic equipment, 230
　syringe, 229
Disposable face masks, 87
Disposal room, 29
Disposal zone, 6
Dissection, operation, tonsillectomy, 419
　swabs, preparation of, 99
Diuretic, cardiac arrest, 280
Domestic assistant in operating department, 787
Dorsal recumbent position, 75
Double vacuum technique for sterilisation, 128
Drainage, suction, breast 377

Drainage tubing, care of, 121
　sterilisation of, 190
Draping of operations, abdominal, 198
　cranial, 207
　ENT, 208
　eye, 211
　limb, 202
　lithotomy, 212
　neck, 209
　neuro, 207
　spinal, 210
　thoracic, 202
Draping the Mayotable, 214
Draping the operation area, 194
　to prevent soiling of drapes, intestinal operations, 222
Dressings, preparation of, 97
　sterilisation of, 132
Drills, for bone, 520, 522, 778
Droperidol (Proleptan), 232
Dropleptan (droperidol), 232
Drugs, checking of, 254
　controlled, 228
　register, 229
　storage of, 273
Dry heat sterilisation, 126, 142
　indicator tape, 110
　of instruments, 127
　period of exposure, 145
Dry heat steriliser, gravity convection type, 143
　mechanical convection, 143
　tests, 110, 132
Drying cycle of steam sterilisation, 134, 148
Ductus arteriosus, correction of, 713, 732
Duodenofibrescope, 313
Duodenum, examination of, 317
Dupuytren's contracture, fasciectomy, 639
Durasorb, soda lime, 247

E

Ear operations, 385
　draping of, 208, 210
　position for, 75
　surgical approach to, 386
Ears, protruding, 636
Earth-free patient circuits, electromedical apparatus, 44
Earthed patient circuits, electromedical apparatus, 45
Earthing of electrical apparatus, 43
E.c.g., 48, 50
Ectopic gestation, 289
　examination through laparoscope, 439
Ectropion correction, 406
Edinburgh pre-set tray system, 103
Egger bone plates, 528
Electric adaptors, danger of, 34
Electrical apparatus, care of, 42
　defibrillator, 48, 54, 280
　disinfection of, 160
　earthing of, 43, 44

Electrical apparatus (*continued*)
  low voltage circuits, 41
  pacemaker, 53
  plugs, 34
  sterilisation of, 160
  suction machine, 61
  switchgear, spark-free, 33, 60
  wiring, colour code, 34
Electricity, in the theatre, 33
  static, 66
Electrocardiograph, 49
Electro-coagulation, diathermy, 56
Electrode jelly, 53
Electrodes, chest, 51
  diathermy, 56
  defibrillator, 55
  limb, 52
  monitoring, 49, 51, 52
  pacemaking, 53
Electrohydraulic operation table, 72
Electromedical equipment, 33, 43
  safety precautions, 47
Electro-section, diathermy, 56
Electrostatic ignition, 67
Ellick evacuator, 660
Embolectomy, 289, 747
Emergency light fittings, mobile, 34
Emergency lighting, 33, 41
Empyema operations, 696
Encephalography, 289, 454
Encysted hydrocele of the cord, 646
Endarterectomy, 289
Endaural surgical approach to ear, 386
Endobronchial tubes, 269
Endocardial pacemaker, 53
Endoscopes, care of, 120
  disinfection of, 160
  sterilisation of, 154, 160
Endoscopic accessories,
  for diathermy, 317
Endoscopy, 289
Endoscopy, fibreoptics, 308
  position for, 85
Endotracheal intubation, 267
Endotracheal tubes, 243, 268, 282
English gauge for catheters, 652
ENT operations, 385
  draping of, 208, 210
Enterostomy, 289
Entropian, correction of eyelid deformity, 491
Enucleation, 289
  of the eye, 509
Ependymoma, 481
Epididymectomy, 289
Epidural anaesthesia, 273, 289
Epiphyseal arrest with staples, 551
Episiotomy, 289
Epontal (propanidol), 232, 266
Equipment, anaesthetic storage of, 273
Equipment for theatre, 26
E.R.C.P. catheterisation, 313
Esmarch's tourniquet, 511

Ether, 232, 236
  open mask, 264
  vaporiser, 235
Ethibond polyester thread, 176
Ethicot, cotton thread, 175
Ethmoidectomy, fronto, 414
  intranasal, 412
Ethmoidosphenoidal exenteration, 476
Ethylene oxide sterilisation, 150
  indicator tape, 110
  packing of items for sterilisation, 151
Exflow clean zone ventilation unit, 25
Exhaust filter for suction machines, 64
Exostosectomy, 607
Expiratory valves, anaesthetic machine, 243
Explosions, anaesthetic, 33, 66
External cardiac massage, 279
External defibrillation, 55
Extracapsular cataract extraction, 504
Extracorporeal blood circulation, 713
Extradural haematoma, 464
  neoplasm, 481
Eye anatomical cross section, 488
Eye operations, 488
  draping of, 211
  position for, 75
Eyelid deformities, 489, 491

F

Fabrics, sterilisation of, 129
Face mask, anaesthetic, 243
  disinfection of, 159
  for personnel, 87
Face operations, 428
Face, superficial ulcer of, 428
Fallopian insufflation and salpingography, 435
Fallot, tetralogy of, correction, 713, 728
Fascia sutures, 172
Fasciectomy for Dupuytren's contracture, 639
Fasciotomy, 290
Femoral artery, bypass graft, 751
Femoral epiphysis, slipped, 543
  position for operation, 84
Femoral herniorrhaphy, 367
Femoral neck fractures, nailing of, 541, 543
  position for, 84
Femoral shaft fractures, Kuntscher nail, 544
Femur, upper end fractures, types of, 538
Fenestration, 290
Fentanyl (sublimaze), 232
Fibre bronchoscope, 688
Fibre light bundle, 308
  source, 308
Fibre optic endoscopes, care of, 311
Fibre optic endoscopy, 308
Fibre optic system, 655
Fibrescopes, 311
Filter, heat absorbing for shadowless light fittings, 38
Filters, for air conditioning, 17
  high efficiency particulate (HEPA), 21, 24

Filters (*continued*)
   for cardiopulmonary bypass machine, 715
   for suction machine exhaust, 63
   for ventilators, 257, 258
Fistula in ano, 372
Flammable gases accumulation, 20, 33
Flasks for sterile hand lotion, 31
Flaxedil (gallamine triethiodide), 232, 266
Floor, antistatic, 69
   construction, 14
Flow generators, ventilators, 255
Fluothane, 232, 236
Fluothane vaporiser for an anaesthetic machine (Fluotec), 235, 236
Focus of shadowless light fittings, 35
Fogerty embolectomy catheters, 750
Folded-top sterilisation bags, 118
Foley catheters, 651
Foot, stabilisation of, 571
Footwear for theatre, 86
Forearm, amputation of, 608
   fracture of, 760
Formaldehyde, 159, 777
   for disinfecting ventilators, 263
Formaldehyde/low temperature steam sterilisation, 120, 146, 160
Fortral (pentazocine), 232, 266
Fothergills operation, 290, 431
Fractures, of the femur, intertrochanteric, 538
     neck, 535
     shaft, 544, 768
   of the hip, 768
   of the humerus, 762
   of the leg, 765
   of the mandible, 382
   of the nose, 402
   of the olecranon, 525
   of the radius and ulna, 760
   of the scaphoid, 760
   of the shoulder, 763
   of the tibia, shaft, 547
   open reduction, 516
   plating and screwing of, 533
   wiring of, 533
Frangenheim laparoscope, 438
Freeman-Watts prefrontal leucotomy, 468
Frontal sinus operations, 414
Fronto ethmoidectomy, 414
Fronto-thalmic association fibres, severance of, 468
Frusimide (lasix), 280, 284
Fulguration of bladder tumours, 290, 659
Furniture in theatre, antistatic testing, 68

G

Gain on cardiac monitor, adjustment of, 50
Gallomine triethiodide (Flaxedil), 232, 266
Gall-bladder operations, 335
   instruments, 336
   position for, 76
Gallie herniorrhaphy, 172, 290, 367

Gallie fascia needles, 188, 192
Gamma irradiation, 126
Ganglionectomy, 290
Gas cylinders, anaesthetic, 233, 777
Gases, anaesthetic, accumulation of, 20, 66, 252
Gastrectomy, 290, 343, 350
Gastroenterostomy, 290, 342
Gastrointestinal endoscopy, 316, 318
Gastrointestinal fibrescopes, 315
Gastrojejunostomy, 290, 342
Gastroscopy, 290, 316
Gastrostomy, 290
Gauges, steriliser, 129
Gauze rolls, 98
Gauze swabs, 97
General anaesthesia, 232, 264, 277
General instruments, 322
Generator, electricity, emergency, 33
Genito-urinary (urology) operations, 644
Gerrard Reading anaesthetic equipment dispenser, 230
Gibbon catheters, 650
Gigli wire saw, 458
Gill technique for congenital dislocation of the hip, 594
Gilliam's operation, 290, 449
Girdlestones operation, 290
Glabellar skin flap, 635
Glassware, sterilisation of, 127, 161
Glossectomy, 290
Glove powders, 123
Gloves, rubber, care of, 101
   disposable, 92
   method of putting on,
     closed, 93–95
     open, 92
   opening packets, 113
   packing for sterilisation, 122
   sterilisation of, 132
   testing of, 122
Glutaraldehyde, 159
GNC, syllabus, 2
Gold radioactive, 775
Gouges, 549
Gowns, folding of, 100
   method of putting on, 91
   shelf in scrub room, 28
   sterilisation of, 161
   Ventile/scotchguard fabric, 21, 86, 88
Grafts, aortic, 713, 731, 737
   bone, 556
   femoral artery bypass, 751
   skin, 621
   tendons, 615
Gravity convection, dry heat steriliser, 143
Gravity displacement, autoclave, 128
   of air in autoclave, 128
Grid iron incision (McBurney), 332
Guedel airway, 207, 244
Guedel stages of anaesthesia, 278
Guillotine operation for tonsillectomy, 420
Guiot stereotactic frame, 469
Gum elastic catheters, 125
Gynaecological operations, 429

H

Haemathorax, 696
Haemorrhoidectomy, 290, 370
  position for surgery, 79
Hagedorn suture needles, 188
Half-life of radioactive materials, 293
Hallux rigidus, arthroplasty procedure, 604
Hallux valgus, Keller's operation, 603
Halogenation of bacteria, 127
Halogens and halogen compounds, 158
Haloperiodol, 232
Halothane, 232, 236
  vaporisers, 235
Halstead mattress sutures, 222
Hammer toes, 569
Hanalux light fittings, 38
Hand drills, 532
Hand lotion, sterilisation of, 161
  rinse after scrubbing up, 158
Hands, drying of after scrubbing up, 90
  rinsing of after scrubbing up, 158
Harelip and cleft palate repair, 617
Harris catheters, 651
Harris modified Müller osteotomy plate, 553
Harris prostatectomy, 290, 664
Haslinger or Negus head support, 85
Heart lesions, acquired, 713
Heart/lung machine, 713
Heat sterilisation by, table of, 144, 145
Heart valve replacement, 721
Heat disinfection, 146
Heat-labile instruments, sterilisation of, 154
Heat-seal paper bags, 118
Heating, by ventilation system, 26
Heidbrink expiratory valve, disinfection of, 243
Heirsch airway, 244
Hemicolectomy, 290, 351
H.E.P.A. filters, 21
Heparine, storage of, 273
Hepatectomy, 290
Hepatitis patients, 225
Hernia, diaphragmatic, thoracic approach, 710
Hernia, femoral, 367
  inguinal or scrotal, 364, 367
  strangulated, 370
  umbilical, 368
  ventral, 368
Herniorrhaphy, 175, 290, 367
Hexachlorophane, 157
  solution, 88
Hibitane, 120, 156, 160
  hand rinse after scrubbing up, 88
  for disinfection, 156
  skin preparation, 114
Hicks bone plates, 528, 530
High-vacuum autoclave, high-pressure, 128,
High vacuum suction apparatus, 62
Hip, arthroplasty, Austin Moore or Thompson
  operation, 579
  Brittain arthrodesis, 576
  Charnley arthrodesis, 576

Hip (continued)
  congenital dislocation, 594
  lateral position, 77
  plaster of Paris spica, 768
  prostheses, 581–583
  supine position, 75
Holding time for steam sterilisation, 132, 138
Homogenous bone grafts, 556
Homografts, skin, 627
Hopkins rod lens system, 655
Hospital Sterilising and Disinfecting Unit, 2, 6, 29, 102, 111
Hot air sterilisation, 142, 161
Howarth Surgicair enclosure, 24
Howse hip arthroplasty, 579, 589
Hudson endotracheal head harness, 268
  skull brace, 457
Humby skingraft knife, 622
Humerus, amputation through, 609
  plaster of Paris cast, 762
Humidifier for ventilators, 258
Humidification during ethylene oxide sterilisation, 153
Humidity of the theatre, 17, 26, 69
Hycolin, 155
Hydrocele, 646
Hydrocortisone, 284
Hygrometer for measuring humidity, 26
Hydrogen peroxide disinfection of ventilators, 261, 779
Hydrolosis of bacteria, 127
Hymenectomy, 290
Hypáque contrast medium, 452
Hypophysectomy, transphenoidal, 290, 473
Hypospadias, Denis Browne's operation, 641
Hypothermia, induced, 232
  renal, 674
  temperature in theatre, 26
Hysterectomy, 290
  abdominal, 440
  vaginal, 443
  Wertheim's 443
Hysteropexy, 290, 448
Hysterotomy, 291

I

Identification of patients, 5, 276
Ileocolostomy, 291
Ileocystoplasty, 291
Ileoureterostomy, 291
Ileostomy, 291, 362
Iliac bone graft, 560
Impacted wisdom tooth, 380
Incise drapes, 219
Incisions, Kochers, 329
  mid-line, 327
  paramedian, 329
  Pfannensteil, 329
Indicator tape autoclave, 110
  dry heat and ethylene oxide, 110
Indicator tubes for sterility tests, 132, 161

Indifferent electrode, diathermy, 56, 58, 59
Indox ethylene oxide indicator tape, 110
Induction and training programmes, 2
Induction of anaesthesia, nurses' duties, 277
Infected case, precautions for, 225
Inguinal colostomy, 361
Inguinal herniorrhaphy, 364
Instrument nurse, 88, 198, 213
   non-touch technique at operation, 191, 216
   position at operation, 207
Instrument check, 218
Instrument defects, 115
Instrument lube, 115
Instrument sets, packing of, 27, 103
Instrument trays, 103
Instrument trolleys, preparation of, 88, 213
Instruments, boiling of, 149
   care of, 114
   chemical disinfection of, 154
   cleaning after operation, 114
   general set, 322
   handling of during operation, 214
   in polypropylene tubes, 108, 111
   sharps, 116
   soiled during operation, 115
   sterilisation of, 127, 161
   washing machine, 124
Insufflation of the Fallopian tubes, 435
Insuprel (isoprenaline), 266, 283
Intercostal tube drainage, 696
Interdental eyelet wiring, 382
Interstitial irradiation, 775
Intervertebral disc prolapse, operation for, 272
Intestinal instruments, 344
Intracapsular cataract extractions, 504
Intracerebra tissue, biopsy of, 459
Intramedullary fixation, of femoral neck fracture,
   Smith Petersen nail, 535
   femoral shaft fracture, Kuntscher nail, 544
   of femoral trochanteric fracture, McKee nail, 538
Intrapelvic abscess, 334
Intraval, 232
Intravenous anaesthesia, 232, 277
Intravenous needles, 272
Intussusception, 350
Iodine, 158
   skin preparation, 194
Iodophors, 88, 158
Irradiation for sterilisation, 149
Iridectomy, 291, 499
Isoprenaline (Aleudrin, Isuprel), 266, 280, 283

J

Jack knife position, 83
Jackson bronchoscope, 690
Jaques catheters, 650
Jaw, fracture of, 382
   partial excision of, 427
Jejunostomy, 291
Jewett femoral nail, 540, 543

Job description, charge nurse, 781
   domestic assistant, 782
   nursing officer, 780
   operating department assistant, 785
   orderly, 788
   receptionist, 787
   staff nurse, 783
   state enrolled nurse, 784
   senior operating department assistant, 786
Joint, aspiration of, 562
Jones, tenotomy knives, 189

K

Kehr's T-tube, 336, 339
Keller's operation for hallux valgus, 291, 604
Keratectasis, keratoconus, 291
Ketalar (ketamine hydrochloride), 232, 266
Kidde tourniquet, 513
Kidney operations, 670
   draping of, 202
   position for, 77
Kidney cooling coils, 674
Kifa and Michel suture clips, 179, 183, 190
Kifa operation table, 74
Kirschner wires, 515, 521, 570
Knee, arthrotomy, 565
Knee/elbow (rabbit) position for surgery, 83
Knee, Charnleys arthrodesis, 573
Knee, plaster of Paris, 765
Knives, 189, 622
   care of, 116
   sterilisation of, 127
Knowle pins, 543
Kocher's abdominal incision, 329
Kraft bags for sterilisation, heatseal, 118
   folded top, 118
Kuntscher, femoral nails, 544
   extractor, 544
Kymograph, 435

L

Labels, patient identity, 5
Labrynthectomy, 401
Lacrimal sac, opening into, 492
Lag screws, 524
Laminar/linear airflow, 22
Laminectomy, 291, 477
   draping of, 210
   for prolapsed intervertebral disc, 477
   for spinal cord tumour, 481
   position for surgery, 81, 82, 83
Lamp, changing of, in shadowless light fitting, 39
   circuits, parallel, 41
   in shadowless light fittings, burning position, 41
   testing apparatus, 43
   type for metal reflector shadowless light fittings, 37
Langton Hewer mattress for Trendelenberg position, 76

Lanz incision, 330
Laparatomy, 291
   set of instruments, 327
Laparoscopy (peritoneoscopy), 437
Largactil (chlorpromezine), 232
Laryngectomy, 291, 424
Laryngofissure, 291, 424
Laryngoscope, 267
Laryngoscopes, care of, 120
Laryngoscopy, 291, 415
Laryngotomy, 291
Lasix (frusemide), 280, 284
Latent heat in sterilisation, 128
Lateral position of extension for surgery, 77
Leadership, qualities of, 3
Leakage, current in electrical apparatus, 44
Leg, amputation of, below the knee, 609
      mid-thigh, 610
   draping of, for surgery, 202
   fracture, 765
   plaster of Paris, 765
Leksell frame for stereotactic surgery, 469
Lembert inverting sutures, 223
Lemperts surgical approach to the ear, 394
Lethidrone (nalorphine), 266, 284
Leucotomy, prefrontal, 291, 468
Levallorphan (Lorfan), 266, 284
Levophed (noradrenaline), 266
Lewin Report, 2, 4, 5
   job descriptions, 780
Ligation of blood vessels, assistants' duties, 218
Ligature clips, Cushing's and McKenzie's, 179
Ligature materials, storage of, 164, 182, 191
Ligature trolley, 182
Ligatures, absorbable, 164, 172
   Catgut, 168
   Dexon, 172
   handling of, 182, 191, 216
   non-absorbable, 173
     cotton thread, 175
     linen thread, 174
     nylon, 175
       thread, 176
     silkworm gut, 173
     Terylene (polyester), 176
     wire, 177
   serum proofing, 174
   sterilisation and storage, 163
Light field, task area, 34, 37
Lighting, artificial, 14, 33, 34
   Blin system, 37
   daylight, 14
   emergency, 17, 41
   in theatre, 15, 34
   shadowless, types of, 34, 37, 38, 87
   terminology, 34
Light source, fibre optic, 308
Lignocaine, 232, 270, 283
Limb electrodes for monitoring, 52
Limb operations, draping of, 202
Linear accelerator used for sterilisation, 149
Linear/laminar flow ventilation, 20

Linear polyethylene, 177
Linen, infected, disinfection of, 155
Linen for operation, 101
   folding of, 102
   sterilisation of, 161
Linen thread, 174
   sizes and tensile strength, 174
   sterilisation of, 163
Lintine, or Cottonoid, 100
Lists, operation, preparation of, 5
Lithotomy position for surgery, 79
   draping of, 212
Lithotrity or litholapaxy, 291, 660
Live donor, kidney transplant, 678
   heart transplant,
Live electrode, diathermy, 56, 58
Living sutures, 172
Load simulator for sterilising, 134
Lobectomy, thoracic, 291, 703
Local anaesthesia, 232
   for gastrointestinal endoscopy, 316
   ophthalmic, 488
Loose bodies of knee, 565
Lorfan (levallorphan), 266, 284
Lotions, for cystoscopy, 656
   sterilisation of, 161
Low voltage apparatus, 41
   checking of, 42
   circuit, 42
   rheostat, 42
   testing apparatus circuit, 42
Lowsley grasping forceps, 654
Lube, instrument, 115
Lumbar sympathectomy, 482
Lung, decortication of, 697
   removal of, 293, 703
Lymph adenectomy, 291

M

Macbic lotion flasks, 161
Macintoshes, sterilisation of, 162
   disinfection of, 162
Mackintosh, arthroplasty of knee, 591
Magill, anaesthetic expiratory valve, 243
   catheter connection, 243
Malleoli fractures, plaster of Paris casts, 765
Manchester repair, 291, 431
Malecot catheters, 651
Mammaplasty (Cronin operation), 636
Management, 3
Mandible, excision of, 427
Mandible fractures, 382
Mannitol, 284
Manley Servovent anaesthetic ventilator, 247
Marcaine (bupivacaine), 232, 270, 273
Martensitic stainless steel, 521
Martin transfusion pump, 231
Masks, anaesthetic, 243
Masks, face, for personnel, 87
Massage, cardiac, 279

Mastectomy, 291
  radical, 375
  simple, 374
Mastoidectomy, 292, 388, 392, 394
  draping of for surgery, 208
Matburn operation table, 73
Mattress, ribbed, 76
Mattress sutures, 222
Mayo Robinson abdominal incision, 330
Mayo scissors, 189
Mayo suture needles, 187
Mayo trolley, 213, 214
McBurney abdominal incision, 332
McKee intertrochanteric plate, 539
McKee trifin nail, 539
McKee-Farrar hip prosthesis, 579, 585
McKenzie's or Cushing's ligature clips, 179
McLaughlin intertrochanteric pins and plates, 539
McMurray's displacement osteotomy of the femur, 548
Meatal atresia and microtia of the external auditory canal, 394
Mechanical convection dry heat steriliser, 143
Mechanical heart valves, 721
Mediastinoscopy, 695
Medical gas cylinders, capacities and pressures, 777
Megger D.C. electrical tester, 68
Megimide, 266
Ménièrés disease, 401
Meningocoele, 477
Meniscectomy, 292, 565
Metacarpophalangeal joint replacement, 604
Metaraminol (Aramine), 266, 280
Metal corrosion of orthopaedic implants, 522
Metatarsus fractures, plaster of Paris casts, 765
Methedrine, 266
Methohexitone (Brietal), 232, 266
Methoxamine (Vasoxyl, Vasoxine), 266
Methoxyflurane, (Penthrane), 232
Methylamphetamine, 284
Metrizamide, 454
Meurig Williams spinal plates, 601
Michel and Kifa suture clips, 179, 183, 190
Micro-organisms, destruction of, 126
Micropore adhesive skin closures, 180
Microscope operating, 296, 389
  care and maintenance, 303
  draping of, 211
Microtia and atresia of external auditory canal, 394
Midline incision, 327
Mid-thigh amputation, 610
Millen's retropubic prostatectomy, 665
Mirault Blair operation for cleft lip, 620
Mitral insufficiency, 713
Mitral stenosis, 713
Mitral valvulotomy, valve replacement, 295, 713, 724
Mobilisation of stapes, 396
Modular operating theatre, 13, 18
Moist heat sterilisation, 132
Mölnlycke swab system, 97
Monitoring, diathermy circuit, 56
  equipment, 48, 50

Monofilament, nylon, 175
  silkworm gut, 173
Mop, See Swabs
Mouth operations, 379
Moynihan suture needle, 183
Müller compression apparatus, 529
Müller staples, 551
Myelography, 454
Myodil contrast medium, 454
Myomectomy, 292, 443
Myringoplasty, 397
Myringotomy, 292, 388

N

Nail brushes, dispenser, 28, 162
  for wound cleansing, 194
  sterilisation of, 162
Nalorphine (lethidrone), 266
Nasal endotracheal tubes, 269
Nasal fracture, reduction of, 402
Nasal packing, pre-operative, 401
Nasal polypectomy, 405
Nasal punch forceps, 404
Nasal speculum, 404
  Septum, submucous resection, 407
Neck anatomy, 682
Neck operations, 681
  draping of, 209
  position for surgery, 80
Needle holders, 193
Needles, hypodermic, 118, 190
  intravenous, 272
  suture, 182, 184
    care of, 117
    handling of, 216
    sterilisation of, 143
Negus or Haslinger head support, 85
Negus bronchoscope, 688
Nelaton catheters, 650
Nephrectomy, 292, 670
  partial, 673
Nephrolithotomy, 673
Nephropexy, 292
Nephrostomy, 292
Nerve repair by anastomosis, 292
Neurectomy, 292
Neurofibroma, 481
Neuroleptanalgesia, 232
Neuroma, acoustic, 401
Neuroma, excision of, 486
Neuroplasty, 292
Neurorrhaphy, 292
Neurosurgical operations, 452
  draping of, 207
  instruments, 457
  microsurgery, 298
  patties, 100
Nicholle arthroplasty, 604
Nikethamide (Coramine), 266, 284
Nitrous oxide, 232, 234, 77

Non-absorbable ligatures and sutures, 164, 172
Non-touch technique, 216
Non-traumatic sutures, 171
Non woven fabric theatre suits, 21
Noradrenaline (Levophed), 266
Northwick Park anaesthetic trolley, 250
Nose operations, 401
Novocaine (procaine), 232, 270
Nupercaine (cinchocaine), 232, 273
Nurses' caps, 86
Nurses' suits, 86
Nursing officer, job description, 780
Nursing process, 274
Nylon, braided, 176
    monofilament, 176
    sterilisation of, 163
Nylon, static electricity, 67
Nylon darn for hernia repair, 367
Nylon suture materials, sizes and tensile strength, 175
Nylon tubing, sterilisation of, 154

O

Ouabain (strophanthin), 284
Observer tubes for microscope, 299
Oesophagectomy, 292
Oesophagogastrectomy, 708
Oesophagoscope, 315
    sterilisation of, 160
Oesophagoscopy, 292, 316
Olecranon fracture, 525
Oophorectomy, 292, 446
Open ether, 264
Operating department, 1
    assistants, 2
        job description, 785
    committee, 4
    construction, 6
    design, 11, 14
    sessions, length of, 5
    suite, 1
    theatre, 1
    theatre, modular, 14
    ventilation, 11, 17
    walls, 14
    zones, 6
Operating microscopes, 296
    care and maintenance, 303
Operation area, draping of, 194, 198
    abdominal, 198
    cranial, 207
    ENT, 208
    kidney, 202
    limb, 202
    neck, 209
    ophthalmic, 211
    perineal, 212
    spinal, 210
    thoracic, 202
    preparation of, 194

Operation linen, 101
    folding of, 102
Operation lists, preparation of, 5
Operation, preparation for, 112, 114
Operation records register, 5
Operation table, 71
    position of patient, axilla and breast, 79
    cranial, prone, 81
    cranial, sitting, 82
    cranial, supine, 81
    endoscopy, 85
    gall bladder, 76
    jack knife, 83
    laminectomy, 82
    lateral, 77
    lithotomy, 79
    neck, 80
    supine, 75
    supine hip, 84
    trendelenberg, 76
Operidine (phenoperidine), 232, 266
Ophthalmic instruments, 490
    sterilisation of, 154
Ophthalmic operations, 488
    draping for, 215
    suture needles, 184
Op Site, PVC sheet, 198
Orchidectomy, 292, 645
Orchidopexy, 649
Orthopaedic implants, 109
Orthopaedic instruments, 516
Orthopaedic operations, 511
Orthopaedic scalpels, 116, 189
Osteoma of external auditory canal, 395
Osteoplastic flap, craniotomy, 465
Osteoplasty, 292
Osteotomes, 549
    care of, 116, 549
    sterilisation of, 161
Osteotomy, 292, 548
    of femur, McMurray's, 548
    of tibia, 550
    plates, 550
Osteotomy, Wainwright, 550
Oxidation of bacteria, 127
Oxygen, 232, 234, 777
Oxygenator, cardiopulmonary bypass, 713

P

Pacemaker, cardiac, 53
Pacing, 53
Packet system of sterilisation, 88, 101, 103, 107, 114, 119, 120
    Edinburgh pre-set tray, 103
Packs, abdominal, preparation of, 98
Padgett skin graft dermatome, 623
Pallidotomy, 292
Pancreas, radical excision of head, 340
Pancreatectomy, 292
Pancreatico jejunostomy, 340

Pancuronium bromide (Pavulon), 232, 266
Papaveretum, 232
Paramedian abdominal incision, 329
Parietal operations, position for, 80
Parathyroidectomy, 292
Parotid tumour, excision of, 683
Partial cystectomy, 668
Partial gastrectomy, 343
Partial nephrectomy, 673
Pasteurisation, in water, 126, 148
    of endoscopes, 146, 148
    in subatmospheric steam, 146
Patellectomy, 292, 568
Patent ductus arteriosus, 713, 732
Patient in theatre, 274, 276, 284
    indentification, 276
    monitoring, 48, 50
Patties for neurosurgery, preparation of, 100
Paul-Mikulicz operation, 292
Pavulon (pancuronium bromide), 232, 266
Pedicle skin grafts, 629
    'tubed' flap, 481
Pedicles, ligation of, 168
Pelvic operations, position for, 76
Penis, circumcision of, 288, 644
Pentazocine (Fortral), 232, 266
Pentec, thermocompensated anaesthetic vaporiser, 241
Penthrane, 232
Penthrane vaporiser, 241
Pentolinium (Ansolysen), 232
Pentothal (thiopentone sodium), 232, 266
Pericardectomy, 292
Perineal operations, draping of, 212
Perineorrhaphy, 292, 430
Perineum, rupture of, 430
Peripheral nerve repair, 483
Peripheral pulsometer, 52
Peripheral vascular operations, 742
Peritoneoscopy (laparoscopy), 437
Peritoneum, suture of, 169
Peritonsillar abscess, 415
Permapak boxes, 112
Permeatal surgical approach to the ear, 386
Personnel, theatre, 2, 86
Pethidine, 232, 266
Pfannenstiel's elliptical abdominal incision, 329
Pharyngo laryngectomy, 292
Pharyngotomy, 292
Phase boundary stream, 128, 132, 777
Phemister bone grafts, 562
Phenol derivatives, 155
Phenoperidine (operidine), 232, 266
Phillips airways, 244
Phillips, screws, 522
PHisoHex, 28, 88, 157
Phlebotomy, 292
Photoadaptor for microscopes, 299
Phrenic avulsion, 292
Piles, excision of, 290, 370
Pilonoidal sinus, draping of for surgery, 210
Pin index, anaesthetic gas cylinders, 234
Pin safety system for vaporisers, 238

Pipeline suction apparatus, 61
Pituitary tumours, excision of, 473
Plans, theatre, 8, 10, 12, 15, 16
Plaster of Paris, 756
    control of setting time, 759
Plaster of Paris casts, below knee, 767
    Colles fracture, 759
    fracture of humerus, 762
    fracture of radius and ulna, 760
    fracture of scaphoid, 760
    hip spica, 768
    shoulder abduction spica, 763
    slabs, 756
    spinal jacket, 771
    technique, 754, 759
Plastic isolator for surgery, 25
Plastic and hand surgery, 300, 617
    instruments, 618
Plastics, sterilisation of, 162
Plates for bone, 520, 530
Plating and screwing of bone, 533
Plating for skull defects, 467
Plenum air-conditioning system, 17
Plethysmograph, 52
Plugs, electric, 34
Pneumonectomy, 293
Pneumothorax, artificial, 293
Pollution by anaesthetic gases, 20, 252
Polyamides (nylon), ligatures and sutures, 175
Polya resection of stomach, 345
Polyolefins, ligatures and sutures, 177
Polyester (Terylene) ligatures and sutures, 176
Polyethylene sutures, 177
Polyglycolic acid sutures, 172
Polypectomy, cervical, 435
    colonic, 318
    nasal, 405
    uterine, 436
Polypropylene tubes for instruments, 108, 111
Polypropylene sutures, 177
Polytetramethylene adipate (polybutylate) coating for
    sutures, 176
Polyvinyl chloride, sheet for skin drapes, 198
Polyvinyl chloride, sterilisation of, 162
Portacaval shunt operation, 738
Positioning of patient for operation, 93
Positions for surgery, breast, 79
    cranial, prone, 81
        sitting, 82
        supine, 75
    endoscopy, 85
    gall-bladder, 76
    hip, lateral, 77
        supine, 84
    jack-knife, 83
    laminectomy, 82
    lateral extension, 77
    lithotomy, 79
    neck, 80
    supine, 75
Post aural surgical approach to the ear, 386
Posterior fossa exploration, 467

Posterior tympanotomy, 388
Post-operative care, 275
Potassium chloride, for cardio pulmonary arrest, 284
Potts fracture, plaster of Paris cast, 765
Povidone-iodine, 88, 158
Powders, for rubber gloves, 123
    sterilisation of, 162
Prefrontal leucotomy, 468
Premedication, 92
Pre-operative visits, 275
Preparation/lay-up room, 1, 29, 192
Preparation of operation area, 194
Preparation for operation, 86
Pre-set tray system, 27, 103, 129
Pressure generator, ventilators, 255
Presurgical wash, 88
Prevacuum steam pulsation, 134
    in subatmospheric sterilisation, 147
Prilocaine (citanest), 232
Printol, 155
Procaine amide, (Pronestyl), 280
Procaine (Novocaine), 232, 270
Proctoscopy, 293, 321
Prolapsed intravertebral disc, removal of, 477
Prolene sutures, 177
Pronestyl (procaine amide), 280
Propanidid (Epontal), 232, 266
Prostatectomy, 293
    Millin's retropubic, 665
    transurethral, 658
    transvesical, 662
Prostheses, for arterial surgery, 713
    for orthopaedic surgery, 581–583
Prostigmine, 266
Protective clothing, theatre, 86
Protective zone, 6
Prone cranial position for surgery, 81
Protruding ears, correction of, 636
Ptosis, sutures for, 172
Pugh hip nail, 540
Pulmonary stenosis, 713
Pulmonary valvulotomy, 727
Pulsometers peripheral, 52
Pulvertaft tendon sutures, 183
Pudenz valve, 473
Purse string sutures, 223
Putti-Platt operation for recurrent dislocation of the shoulder, 596
P.V.C., sterilisation of, 162
Pyelography, 293
    retrograde catheterisation of the ureters, 657
Pyelolithotomy, 293, 673
Pyloric stenosis, 341
Pylormyotomy, 296
Pyloroplasty, 293

Q

Quaternary ammonium compounds, 157
Quinsy, incision of abscess, 415

R

Radiators in the theatre, 27
Radiation, 293
    for sterilisation, 149
Radical cervical node dissection, 681
Radical excision, head of pancreas, 340
Radical mastectomy, 375
Radioactive materials, 774
    precautions in handling, 775
Radio-opaque filament in swabs, 96
Radiotherapy, 293, 774
Radium, 293, 774
Radius and ulna fractures, plaster of Paris casts, 760
Ramstedt's operation, 293, 341
Rayon, static electricity formation, 66
Rayon swabs, 97
Raytec swabs, 95, 97
Razor skin grafting, 622
Rebore thromboendarterectomy, 754
Rebreathing bags, disinfection of, 159
Receptionist, job description, 787
Reciprocating pump suction machines, 62
Recorder chart of sterilisation, 144
Records of operation, 5
Recovery area, postanaesthetic, 93, 275, 284
Rectocele, repair of, 431
Rectosigmoidectomy, 293
Recurrent dislocation of shoulder, 596
Reducing regulators, anaesthetic gases, 234
Rectal operations (lithotomy), draping of, 213
Rectum, abdominal perineal resection, 354
    anterior resection, 359
Redivac suction device, 376
Regional or local anaesthesia, 269
Register of drugs, 229
Register, operation, 4, 96
    swab check, 94, 218
Regulators for anaesthetic gases, 234
Relaxants for anaesthesia, 232, 266
Renal, hypothermia, 674
    operations,
    transplantation, 677
Reproofing Ventile or Scotchguard, 778
Resection, of a rib, 697
    of small bowel, 350
    operations for squint, 496
Resectoscope, Rapier, 660
Reservoir bag, anaesthetic, 241
Retinal detachment, 506
Retractors, 577
    use during operation, 219
Retrograde pyelography, 293, 657
Retropubic prostatectomy, 665
Retroversion of the uterus, 448
Revascularisation of coronary arteries, 713, 729
Rheostat, low-voltage, 43
Rhinoplasty, 293, 633
Rib instruments, 700
Rib, resection of, 697
Ribbed mattress, for operating table, 76
Ringleb cytoscope, 289

Roccal, 157
Rockwell hardness scale, 521
Rotameters, 235, 777
Rotary compressor suction machine, 63
Rowbothan endotracheal connectors,
Rubber, antistatic, 67
Rubber floors, 9
Rubber glove powders, 123
Rubber gloves, care of, 101
    disposable, 92
    method of putting on, closed technique, 93–95
        open technique, 92
    packing for sterilisation, 122
    reusable, testing of, 122
    sterilisation of, 162
Runners or circulating nurses, 90

S

Safety, electrical apparatus, 43
Saline, for hand lotion, 29
    sterilisation of, 161
Salpingectomy, 293, 446
Salpingography, 435
Salpingo-oophorectomy, 293
Salt solution for diathermy, 56
Saw, power, 537, 549, 559
Savlon, 157
Scalpels, Bard Parker, 182, 188
    cartilage, 189
    solid variety, 189
Scaphoid fracture, plaster of Paris cast, 760
Scavenging system for expired anaesthetic gases, 20, 252
Scheduled drugs, 228
Schimmelbusch anaesthetic mask, 265
Schlemn, canal of excision, 501
Schnitker scalp retractor, 457
Schoemaker gastrectomy, 343
Scissors, 190
    care of, 116
    sterilisation of, 116, 161
Scialytic light fitting, 35
Scleral encircling, 508
    identation, 508
Scotchguard/Ventile, 86, 88, 108
Scoline (suxamethonium), 232, 266
Scotchguard, 86, 88, 108
    method of reproofing, 778
Screen, anaesthetic, 202
Screwdrivers, 526
Screwing and plating, 533
Screws for bone, 520, 522
    sizes of, 520, 522, 778
Scrotal herniorrhaphy, 364, 367
Scrub nurse, 2, 88, 90, 213
    handling ligatures, 182, 191, 216
    opening sterile packets, 118, 121, 123
    position at operation, 216
    preparation of trolleys, 88, 118
    swab check, 94, 218

Scrub up solutions, 28
Scrubbing up, 88
Scrubbing up areas, 1, 19, 28
Scrub suit, 86
Sellick manoeuvre, 278
Semi-closed anaesthetic circuit, 236
Senior operating department assistant, job description, 786
Sensible heat (sterilisation), 128
Serum proofing of ligature and suture materials, 174
Shadowless light fittings, changing the lamp, 39
    cleansing of, 35
    Daystar, 38
    focussing of, 35
    Hanulux,
    multiple reflector type, 37
    multiple reflector wall lights, 38
Shadowless light fittings, scialytic, 35
    types of, 35
Shaving operation site, 194
Sharp instruments, care of, 121
Shea teflon piston prosthesis, 396
Shelf operation for congenital dislocation of the hip, 293, 594
Shephards grommet drain, 389
Sherman bone plates, 527, 530
Sherman screws, 523
Shoes, anti-static, 68
Shoulder, arthrodesis of, Smith Petersen nail, 451
    anterior exposure of, 597
    recurrent dislocation of, 596
Shoulder spica, 763
Showers, pre-operative, 86
Shropshire horse, 535
Shut off towel, 204
Sigmoidoscopy, 293, 321
Silastic implant for rhinoplasty, 634
    mammary, 637
Silk sutures, 173
    sizes of, 173
    sterilisation of, 163
    tensile strength, 173
Silkworm gut, 173
    sizes of, 173
Simulator for autoclaves, 134
Sistrunk's operation for thyroglossal cyst, 683
Skeletal traction, 294
    of limbs, 513
    of skull, 515
Skin antiseptic, 194
Skin bank, 628
Skin closure tape, 180
Skin grafts, for tympanoplasty, 397
    full-thickness, Wolfe type, 628
    homo, 627
    pedicle type flap, 629
    split skin, Thiersch, 621
    zeno, 627
Skin or tetra towels, application of, 210
Skin preparation, contaminated wounds, 194
    elective procedures, 158, 194
    plastic cubes for antiseptic, 99

Skin preparation (*continued*)
  table of areas of preparation, 195
Skin sutures, 175, 224
Skull, depressed fracture of, 463
Skull instruments, 457
Skull operations, 452
Skull traction, 515
Sliming, manufacture of catgut, 175
Slipped upper femoral epiphysis, 543
Small bowel resection, 350
Smillie cartilage knives, 189
Smillie epiphyseal staples, 551
Smith Petersen nail, for fracture of the femoral neck, 535
  for arthrodesis of the shoulder, 575
SMo stainless steel for implants, 520
Smoke test, for ventilation system, 20
S.M.R. operation, 407
Soda lime, 247,
Sodium bicarbonate, intravenous, 280, 283
Sodium hypochlorate, 158
Solar heat gain related to design, 14
Sounds, bladder, 650
Spark-free apparatus, 33, 60
Spark-gap diathermy machine, 57
Sparkless electrical sockets/switches, 33
Spark-static, 66
Sphenoidectomy, intranasal operation, 473
Spica, hip, 768
  shoulder, 763
Spike arthrodesis of toe, 569
Spina bifida, repair of, 477
Spinal anaesthesia, 273, 289
Spinal canal, x-ray examination of, 454
Spinal cord tumour, excision of, 479
Spinal decompression, draping of, 210
Spinal fracture, plaster of Paris jacket, 771
Spinal fusion, 600
Spinal operations, draping of, 210
Spinal plates, 601
Spitz-Holter valve, 473
Splenectomy, 294, 364
Splenorenal shunt operation, 739
Sponge checking, 97, 221
Spores, bacterial, destruction of, 126
Spotlights, shadowless, 231
Squint, 287, 494
Stabilisation of foot, 572
Staffing of operating departments, 1
Staff nurse, job description, 783
Stainless steel, austenitic, 520
  martensitic, 521
Stainless steel wire, sizes of, 177
Stallards ophthalmic suture needles, 186
Stanmore knee prosthesis, 592
Stapedectomy, 294, 396
Stapes, mobilisation of, 396
Staples, for epiphyseal arrest, 551
State enrolled nurse, job description, 784
Statens seruminstitut *B. subtilis*, spore test, 151
Static electricity, 66
  anti-static rubber, 66, 68

Static electricity (*continued*)
  dangers of, 66
  dissipation of charges, 67
  generation of, 66
  tendency of certain materials to form, 67
  theatre floor, 66
Steamclox indicators for sterilisation tests, 133
Steam, penetration during sterilisation, 128
  phase boundary, 128, 132, 777
  under subatmospheric pressure, 120
Steam pulsation technique, 128
Steam sterilisation,
  of fabrics, 128
  of instruments, 127, 161
  of rubber, 162
Steinmann pins, 514, 521, 543, 573
Stereomicroscopes, 296
Stereotactic surgery, 294, 469
Stericol disinfectant, 158
Steridrape, 194, 195, 198
Sterile lotion, for cystoscopy, 656
  for hands, 161
Sterile packets, 88, 101, 103, 107, 114, 119, 120
Sterile zone, 6
Sterilisation, 127
  application of methods, 159
  bags, Kraft, heatseal top, 118
    folded top, 118
  by dry heat, 142
    exposure period, 145
  by ethylene oxide, 150
  by heat, table, 144
  by irradiation, 149
  by moist heat, 132
  by steam, 134
    drying cycle, 134, 148
    fabrics, 129
    holding times, 134
    instruments, 127
    pre-vacuum, 127
  by subatmospheric steam/formaldehyde, 146, 160
  indicator tape, 110
  of airways, (disinfection), 159
  of bandages, 100
  of braided suture materials, 162
  of brushes, 162
  of carbon steel instruments, 127
  of catgut, 126, 168
  of catheters, 126, 154
  of compressed-air drills, 127
  of cryoprobes, 154
  of cystoscopes, 154, 160
  of diathermy electrodes, 160
  of drainage tubing, 190
  of drapes, 161
  of dressings, 126, 132
  of electrical apparatus, 160
  of endoscopes, 154, 160
  of endotracheal tubes, 162
  of fabrics, 129
  of glassware, 127, 161
  of glove powder, 162

Sterilisation (*continued*)
  of gloves, rubber, 132
  of gowns, 161
  of instruments, dry heat, 127
    moist heat, 161
  of knives, 127
  of ligature materials, 183
  of linen, 161
  of linen thread, 163
  of lotions, 161
  of macintoshes, 162
  of metal wire and mesh, 163
  of nail brushes, 162
  of nylon sutures, 163
  of plastics, 162
  of powders, 162
  of rubber gloves, 132
  of rubber goods, 162
  of saline and water, 161
  of scissors, 116, 161
  of suture clips, 163
  of suture materials, 162, 163, 183
  of suture needles, 143
  of syringes, 143
  of tubing, 154
  of ventilator components, 261
  packet system, 88
  penetration of steam, 128
  pre-set trays, 28, 103, 107, 116, 136
  spacing of load, 129
Steriliser chamber and pressure gauges, 129
Steriliser function tests, 138
Steriliser, high vacuum/high pressure, 133
Steriliser holding times, 132
Sterilising facilities, 29
Sterility tests, 132
  Bacillus stearothermophilus, 133, 154
  Bowie-Dick, 138
  Browne's tubes, 132, 161
  for ethylene oxide, 110, 151
  thermocouples, 133
  vacuum leak, 140
Steristrip skin closures, 220
Stimulants, 266, 284
Stockinette cuffs for theatre suits, 86
Stomach, examination of, 317
  suture of, 169
Storage of drugs, 273
Storage of sterile packets, 112
Strabismus operations, 287, 494
Strangulated hernia, 370
Stripping of varicose veins, 745
Stryker screwdriver, 526
Student nurses, 2
Subatmospheric steam/formaldehyde pasteurisation, 120, 146, 160
Subcapital fracture, neck of femur, 538
Subcutaneous tissue, suture of, 170
Subcuticular suture, 223
Subdural haematoma, 464
Sublimaze (Fentanyl), 232
Submucous resection of the nasal septum, 407

Subtemporal decompression, 464
Subtotal hysterectomy, 296, 440
Subtrochanteric fracture of femur, 538
Sucrose, intravenous, 280, 284
Suction drainage, breast, 376
Suction machines, 61, 87, 229
  adjustment of vacuum, 63
  anaesthetic room, 229
  filter for exhaust, 63
  pipeline, 63
  portable, 61
  precautions for use, 64
  rotary compressor, 63
Suction nozzles, 183, 457
Suction tubing, cleansing of, 122
Sudol, 155
Suits for nurses, 21, 86
Supine position for surgery, 75
  cranial, 80
  hip, 84
Supplementary sterile items,
  preparation of, 109, 122, 123
  opening of, 122
Suprapubic cystotomy, 661
Surgeon's assistant, 194, 213, 218, 225
  caps, 86
Surgery, positions for, 71
  axilla and breast, 79
  cranial, prone, 81
    sitting, 82
    supine, 75
  endoscopy, 85
  gall-bladder, 76
  hip, lateral, 77,
    supine, 84
  laminectomy, 82
  lateral extension, 77
  lithotomy, 79
  neck, 80
  supine, 75
  Trendelenburg's, 76
Surgical cautery, 61
  checking for faults, 62
Surgical diathermy, 56, 289
Surgical plastic isolator, 26
Surgical toilet of wounds, 194
Suture clips, Kifa and Michel, 179, 183, 190
  sterilisation of, 163
Suture needles, 182, 184
  care of, 117
  ophthalmic, 186
  sterilisation of, 143
Sutures, absorbable, 164
  assistant's duties, 182, 191, 216
  catgut, 168
  collagen tape, 172
  Dexon, 172
  frontal muscle sling, 172
  handling of, 182, 192, 216
  linear polyethylene, 177
  living, fascia and tendons, 172
  non-absorbable, 173

Index

Sutures (continued)
    serum proofing, 174
    sterilisation and storage, 163
  non-traumatic, 171
  nylon, 175
  polyester, 176
  polyethylene, 177
  Pulvertaft, 183
  silk, 173
  silkworm gut, 173
  skin, 175
  sterilisation of, 162
  tension, 192
  types of, 219, 222
  wire, 177
Suxamethonium (Scoline), 232, 266
Swab register, 94, 218, 221
Swabs, anaesthetic (coloured), 98
  dissection, 99
  location (checking) of, 94, 218
  preparation of, 97
Switchgear in theatre, 33
Symond's fish-hook needles, for suture, 188
Sympathectomy, lumbar, 294, 482
  draping of, 210
Synovectomy of knee, 294, 568
Synthetic suture materials, 175
Syringes, care of, 118, 190
  dispenser, 229
  sterilisation, by dry heat, 119, 143

T

Table, of autoclave temperatures, 144, 777
  of disinfection by chemicals, 152
  of drill and bone screw sizes, 777
  of gas cylinder capacities, 777
  of pre-operative skin preparation, 195
  of rotameter calibrations, 777
  of sterilisation by dry heat, 145
  operation, 71
Talc granulomata, danger of, 123
Tantalum wire, 775
Tape, collagen, 172
Tarsorrhaphy, 294
Tarsus fractures, plaster of Paris cast, 765
Technical terms, 286
Teeth, extraction of, 379
  impacted wisdom, 380
Teflon, arterial prostheses, 713
  piston, 396
Telescopes, types for cystoscopy, 657
Teletherapy, 775
Temperature of the theatre, 26
Tendon advancement, strabismus, 287, 494
Tendon graft and suture, 615
  suture material, 612, 614
Tenoplasty, 294, 615
Tenorrhaphy, 294, 615
Tenotomy, 294
  knives, 189

Tension sutures, 192
Tensile strength, of catgut, 166
  of cotton, 175
  of Dexon, 172
  of linen thread, 174
  of nylon, 175
  of silk thread, 174
Terrazo floors, 9
Terylene for ligatures and sutures, 176
Test circuit, low voltage, 42, 77
  for steriliser function, 138
Testicle, excision of, 292, 645
  undescended, operation for, 649
Tests for sterility, 132
Tetra or skin towels, application of, 210
Tetrology of Fallot, 713, 728
Thackray operation table, 71
Theatre, air pressures, 17
  ancillary rooms, 6, 27
  clothing, 86
  committee, 4
  construction and materials used, 11, 14
  design of, 6
  equipment, 26
  floor, anti-static properties, 11, 69
    colour and materials, 11, 69
    conductive properties, 69
  footwear, 86
  humidity, 17, 26, 69
  lighting, 14, 33, 34
  modular, 13, 18
  preparation of, 112, 114
  protective clothing, 86
  sterile supply unit or service, 2, 6, 29, 102, 111
  switchgear, 33
  temperature of, 26
  walls, colour of and materials used, 14
  zones, 6
Thermal death time, dry heat, 126
  moist heat, 126
Thermo compensated vaporiser, 236
Thermocouples for steriliser tests, 133
Thermostatic valve for autoclave, 130
Thermotop bags, 110
Thiersch skin grafts, 621
Thiopentone (Pentothal), 222, 266
Thompson arthroplasty, 579
Thoracic instruments, 700
Thoracic operations, 688
  draping of, 202
Thoracoplasty, 294
Thoracoscopy, 294
Thoracotomy, 294, 697
  instruments, 700
Thread, cotton, 175
  linen, 174
  silk, 173
  Terylene, 176
Throat operations, 415
Thrombo-endarterectomy, 294, 754
Thymectomy, 294

Thyroglossal cyst or duct, excision of, 683
Thyroid adenoma, excision of, 686
Thyroid and neck operations, 681
Thyroidectomy, 294, 686
    position for operation, 80
Tibia, bone graft from, 556
    fracture of, Kuntscher nail, 547
    osteotomy of, 550
    plaster of Paris casts, 766
Tiemann catheters, 653
Time cycling ventilators, 255
Tissue forceps, 326
Tissue reaction to implanted metals, 522
Titanium, 520, 521
Toes, arthrodesis of, 569
Tongue, partial amputation of, 426
Tonsillectomy, 294, 416, 419, 420
    instruments for, 417
Torkildsen operation for hydrocephalus (ventriculo cysternostomy), 471
Tourniquets for limb surgery, 511–513
Towels, abdominal, 100
    folding of for operation, 101
    sterilisation of, 161
Toxiferine (Alloferin), 232, 266
Trabeculectomy, 501
Trachelorrhaphy, 294
Tracheostomy, 294, 420
Tracheostomy position, 80
Tracheostomy tubes, 420
Traffic in theatre, 6
Transfer trolley for patient, 276
Transfer area, 6
Transfixion screws, 523
Transformer for surgical cautery, 42
Transfusion arm table, 202
Transfusion cannulae and needles, 272
Transfusion pump, 231
Transphenoidal hypophysectomy, 473
Transposition of the ulnar nerve, 487
    of great arteries, 730
Transplantation of heart, 713, 735
    of kidney, 677
Tranquillisers, 232
Transurethral prostatectomy, 658
Transvesical prostatectomy, 662
Trays for instruments, 88, 101, 103, 107, 114, 119
Trendelenburg's operation for varicose veins, 294, 745
Trendelenburg's position for surgery, 76
Trephine, 294
    corneoscleral, 488
Tricuspid stenosis, 713
Trigeminal neuralgia, division of posterior root of nerve, 482
Trilene, 232
    vaporiser, 235, 236, 243
Trimetaphan (Arfonad), 232
Trolley, drapes, 108
    loading for steriliser, 42
    patient, side transfer, 274
T.S.S.U., 2, 11, 29

Tubal patency, laparascopy, 439
Tubarine (curare), 232, 266
Tubes, instrument, 108, 111
Tubing, cleansing of, 122
    sterilisation of, 154
Tumours of bone, 608
    of spinal cord,
Turbinectomy, 407
Turbinotomy, 409
Twist drills, 520, 522, 778
Tympanic membrane, incision of, 388
    repair of, 397
Tympanoplasty, 397

U

Ulnar nerve, transposition of, 487
Ultraclean environments, 21
Ultrasonic cleaner for instruments, 114
Ultrasonic nebuliser for disinfecting ventilators, 264
Ultraviolet light radiation for sterilisation, 154
Umbilical herniorrhaphy, 368
Unconscious patient, care of after operation, 93, 275
    maintenance of airway, 276
    observations during anaesthesia, 276
    supporting the jaw, 276
Underwater seal for chest drainage, 697
Undescended testicle, 649
Unidirectional valves in anaesthetic machines, 244
Ureteric catheterisation and retrograde pyelography, 657
Ureteric catheters, 658
Ureteric operations, 667
Ureteric transplantation, 667
Ureterileostomy, 294, 667
Ureterocolostomy, 294
Ureterolithotomy, 294, 677
Ureterosigmoidostomy, 667
Urethral operations, 652
Urethrocystoscope, 653
Urethroscopy, 652
Urethrotomy, 295
Urevert, 280, 284
Urology operations, 644
Uterus, biopsy of, 435
    curettage of, 434
    excision of, 296, 440
    polypectomy, 436

V

Vacuum, during sterilisation, 128, 134
    residual, in suction machines, 65
Vacuum leak test, 140
Vaginal operations, draping of, 212
    hysterectomy, 443
Vagotomy, 295, 348
Valve diathermy machine, 57

Index

Valvuloplasty, 713
    aortic, mitral, tricuspid, 724
Vapourphase inhibitor paper, for steam sterilisation, 188
Vaporisers, Boyle, 235
    Ether, 236
    out of circuit (VOC), 236
    thermocompensated, 236
    trilene, 235, 243
Valve generator, diathermy, 57
Valve replacement, 713, 721
    mitral, 724
Valvulotomy, mitral, 295, 713, 724
    pulmonary, 727
Varicocele, excision of, 648
Varicose veins, ligation of, 745
Vascular instruments, 718, 744
Vascular operations, abdominal, 737
    cardiac, 712
    peripheral, 742
Vasectomy, 295, 647
Vasoxine (methoxamine), 266, 284
Vasoxyl (methoxamine), 266, 284
Vein stripping, 745
Venable plates, 530
Venous embolectomy, 742, 747
Ventilation, air flow, 11, 17
    balanced flaps, 20
    Charnley enclosure, 23
    Charnley body exhaust system, 24
    heating, 26
    humidity, 17, 26, 69
    laminar/linear flow, 20
    outward flow pattern, 19
    smoke test, 20
Ventilators, 255
    Barnet, 261
    Bird, 261
    disinfection of, 261, 779
    failure alarm, 258
    flow generators, 255
    on anaesthetic machine, 247
    pressure generators, 255
Ventile, 86, 88, 108
    for gowns, 21
    for suits, 21
    reproofing, 778
Ventricles, drainage to cysterna magna, 471
Ventral herniorrhaphy, 368
Ventricular asystole, 280
Ventricular cannula, 458
Ventricular fibrillation, 44, 280
Ventricular septal defect, 713, 728
Ventriculo-atrial peritoneal shunt, 295, 471, 473
Ventriculo-cysternostomy, 295, 471
Ventriculography, 295, 454
Ventrosuspension of the uterus, 295
Verres needle for laparoscopy, 439
Vertebral column, defects of, 477
Vi-drape, 198
Vitallium, or Vinertia, 520, 521
Volume cycling ventilators, 255
Vulva, excision of, 295, 439
Vulvectomy, 295, 439

W

Wainwright osteotomy plate, 550, 552
Walls, surface of, 14
Ward staff in theatre, 91
Washing machine for instruments, 124
Wardill operation for cleft palate, 617
Water, sterile, for hand lotion, 29
    sterilisation of, 161
Water-repellent materials, 95, 114
Waters to-and-fro carbon dioxide absorber, 247
Wertheim's hysterectomy, 295, 443
Wessex caskets for instruments, 109
Whistle tip catheters, 650
Williams screwdriver, 526
Wilson spinal plates, 601
Wire, sizes of, 177
    sterilisation and storage of, 163
Wiring, of fracture, 533
    of mandible fracture, 382
    sterilisation of, 163
Wisdom tooth, impacted, excision of, 381
Wolfe skin grafts, 629
Wood screws, 524
Wool balls, 99
    rolls, method of packing for sterilisation, 100
Wounds, cleansing of, 156–158
Wrap-over surgeons gowns, 91, 100
Wrapping materials, for packet sterilisation, 101
Wrist, Brittain arthrodesis, 577

X

X-ray, detectable swabs, 94, 95
Xylocaine (lignocaine), 232, 270, 283

Z

Zephiran, 157
Zones, theatre, 6
Zygoma hooks, 515